Pediatric Complaints and Diagnostic Dilemmas
A Case-based Approach

Pediatric Complaints and Diagnostic Dilemmas
A Case-based Approach

Editors

Samir S. Shah, M.D.
Fellow, Divisions of General Pediatrics and Infectious Diseases
The Children's Hospital of Philadelphia
Instructor, Department of Pediatrics
University of Pennsylvania School of Medicine
Philadelphia, Pennsylvania

Stephen Ludwig, M.D.
Associate Physician-in-Chief for Education
Department of Pediatrics
The Children's Hospital of Philadelphia
Professor, Department of Pediatrics
University of Pennsylvania School of Medicine
Philadelphia, Pennsylvania

Radiology Consultant:
Richard I. Markowitz, M.D.
Senior Radiologist
The Children's Hospital of Philadelphia
Professor of Radiology
University of Pennsylvania School of Medicine
Philadelphia, Pennsylvania

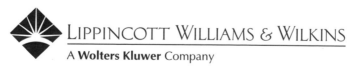

LIPPINCOTT WILLIAMS & WILKINS
A **Wolters Kluwer** Company
Philadelphia · Baltimore · New York · London
Buenos Aires · Hong Kong · Sydney · Tokyo

Acquisitions Editor: Timothy Y. Hiscock
Developmental Editor: Erin McMullan
Production Editor: Melanie Bennitt
Manufacturing Manager: Benjamin Rivera
Cover Designer: Brian H. Crede
Compositor: Lippincott Williams & Wilkins Desktop Division
Printer: Maple Press

© 2004 by LIPPINCOTT WILLIAMS & WILKINS
530 Walnut Street
Philadelphia, PA 19106 USA
LWW.com

Printed in the USA

Library of Congress Cataloging-in-Publication Data

Pediatric complaints and diagnostic dilemmas : a case-based approach / editors, Samir S. Shah, Stephen Ludwig ; radiology consultant, Richard I. Markowitz
    p. ; cm.
  Includes bibliographical references and index.
  ISBN 0-7817-4188-2
    1. Children—Diseases—Diagnosis—Case studies. 2. Teenagers—Diseases—Diagnosis—Case studies. 3. Pediatrics—Case studies. 4. Adolescent medicine—Case studies. I. Shah, Samir S. II. Ludwig, Stephen, 1945–
  [DNLM: 1. Pediatrics—Case Report. 2. Adolescent Medicine—Cse Report. 3. Diagnostic Techniques and Procedures—Child—Case Report. 5. Diagnostic Techniques and Procedures—Infant—Case Report. 6. Signs and Symptoms—Adolescent—Case Report. 7. Signs and Symptoms—Child—Case Report. 8. Signs and Symptoms—Infant—Case Report.
  WS 200 P37046 2004]
  RJ50.P425 2004
  618.92′0075-dc22

                                        2003060157

---

10 9 8 7 6 5 4 3 2 1

This book is dedicated to our parents, siblings, and extended families for providing a nurturing environment and a zest for our work on behalf of other families.

To Suresh and Meena Shah, Mala, Grishma, Hans, and the rest of my family.

To Abraham (a constant memory) and Rose Ludwig, Stelle, and the rest of my family.

Contents

Contents by Diagnosis

Contributing Authors

Debra Boyer, M.D. *Instructor, Department of Pediatrics, Harvard Medical School; Assistant in Medicine, Department of Medicine, Children's Hospital-Boston, Boston, Massachusetts*

Marina Catallozzi, M.D. *Instructor, Department of Pediatrics, University of Pennsylvania; Fellow, Craig-Dalsimer Division of Adolescent Medicine, The Children's Hospital of Philadelphia, Philadelphia, Pennsylvania*

James P. Cavanagh, M.D. *Clinical Assistant Professor, New York University School of Medicine, New York, New York*

Heather C. Forkey, M.D. *Clinical Associate, Department of Pediatrics, University of Pennsylvania School of Medicine; Attending Physician, Department of Pediatrics, The Children's Hospital of Philadelphia, Philadelphia, Pennsylvania*

Eric J. Frehm, M.D. *Fellow, Division of Neonatology, The Children's Hospital of Philadelphia, Philadelphia, Pennsylvania*

Stephen Ludwig, M.D. *Associate Physician-in-Chief for Education, Department of Pediatrics, The Children's Hospital of Philadelphia; Professor, Department of Pediatrics, University of Pennsylvania School of Medicine, Philadelphia, Pennsylvania*

Christina L. Master, M.D. *Clinical Assistant Professor, Department of Pediatrics, University of Pennsylvania School of Medicine; Assistant Director, Pediatric Residency Program, Department of Pediatrics, The Children's Hospital of Philadelphia, Philadelphia, Pennsylvania*

David Munson, M.D. *Fellow, Division of Neonatology, The Children's Hospital of Philadelphia, Philadelphia, Pennsylvania*

Robert A. Nordgren, M.D., M.P.H. *Adjunct Assistant Professor, Department of Pediatrics, Dartmouth Medical School, Lebanon, New Hampshire; Executive Director, Child Health Services, Manchester, New Hampshire*

Jacqueline Owusu-Antwi, M.D. *Instructor, Department of Pediatrics, University of Pennsylvania School of Medicine; Fellow, Division of General Pediatrics, The Children's Hospital of Philadelphia, Philadelphia, Pennsylvania*

Jeanine Ronan, M.D. *Primary Care Pediatrician, Society Hill Pediatrics, Philadelphia, Pennsylvania*

Samir S. Shah, M.D. *Fellow, Divisions of General Pediatrics and Infectious Diseases, The Children's Hospital of Philadelphia; Instructor, Department of Pediatrics, University of Pennsylvania School of Medicine, Philadelphia, Pennsylvania*

Phillip Spandorfer, M.D. *Assistant Professor, Department of Medicine, University of Pennsylvania School of Medicine; Attending Physician, Division of Emergency Medicine, The Children's Hospital of Philadelphia, Philadelphia, Pennsylvania*

Nathan L. Timm, M.D. *Assistant Professor, Department of Clinical Pediatrics, University of Cincinnati College of Medicine; Attending Physician, Division of Emergency Medicine, Cincinnati Children's Hospital Medical Center, Cincinnati, Ohio*

Lisa B. Zaoutis, M.D. *Clinical Assistant Professor, Department of Pediatrics, University of Pennsylvania School of Medicine; Director of Inpatient Services, Division of General Pediatrics, The Children's Hospital of Philadelphia, Philadelphia, Pennsylvania*

Preface

The conceptual framework for this book is based on a traditional model of medical education—case-based learning. Despite advances in medical science, the emergence of evidence-based medicine and the vast changes in medical technology, many physicians still learn from a case-based model. In the understanding of what happens in individual cases, one is able to generalize to similar situations and incorporate basic principles of practice. Early in the course of medical education, one seeks to teach and learn pattern recognition. We are taught the classic signs and symptoms of common diseases and disorders. From repetitive review of these patterns we learn the elements of common conditions. As the stages of medical education advance, one becomes more oriented to the exceptions in the routine patterns. It is the minor exception from the usual that leads to more advanced diagnostic skills. The astute physician will see the variance from the typical pattern, make the more unusual or exceptional diagnosis, and pick up on the rare complication of a common condition.

In the education of pediatric house officers at the Children's Hospital of Philadelphia, there is a tradition of special rounds for the senior residents. The senior rounds are organized and conducted by the chief residents and supported by the faculty. It is within the context of these educational seminars that our residents are able to move and mature from pattern recognition to pattern deviation. We hope that in this effort they will move from good pediatricians to exceptional pediatricians. Many house officers accomplish the goal set out for them. This book is a collection of those cases presented at the Children's Hospital of Philadelphia Senior Rounds. Most cases start with common complaints on the part of the child or the parent. The cases presented in this text have common complaints, but despite the protean presenting signs and symptoms, the cases evolve to challenging diagnostic dilemmas. Many of the final diagnoses are rare and we expect that the reader will be challenged. The format of the book involves chapters that begin with the complaint and the exploration of the sign or symptom that brings the patient to the physician. Following an exploration of the complaint and some of the pertinent questions associated with the complaint, a series of cases detail twists and turns that lead to the final diagnosis. Following each case presentation there is a final diagnosis and an exploration of core material about that diagnosis. For the book to be enjoyed most, we suggest that the reader review the case and try to arrive at their known differential diagnosis and plan of evaluation. Then read on and find out how the "mystery" was solved.

We thank the many Chief Residents, Dr. Christina Master, Dr. Heather Forkey, Dr. James Cavanagh, Dr. Colette Desrochers, Dr. Philip Spandorfer, Dr. Deborah Boyer, Dr. Robert Nordgren, and Dr. Marina Catallozzi, who prepared some of these cases and the many house officers and faculty members who discussed them and agonized over the actual care of the children and their families. Many former chiefs have served as chapter authors.

My thanks also to my co-editor Samir Shah, M.D., who was recently the beneficiary of this kind of training and now is quickly becoming a master teacher in his own right. Nothing can give a teacher more satisfaction than to watch a former student surpass the teacher. Such is the case with Dr. Shah. I am certain that you will be seeing his name on many publications in the future. I am honored to have had a role in his first major publication and I value the relationship that has transformed from teacher-student to respected colleague.

We also thank Mona Mahboubi for her tireless work in helping us to locate figures, photos, and other material. Richard Markowitz, M.D., was our radiologic editor and we thank him for all of his advice and contributions. Carolyn Trojan was, as usual, invaluable in her skills and assistance. Our appreciation to Marybeth Helfrich for providing the blood smears and hematology figures. Our Department Chair, Alan Cohen, M.D., and our Division Chiefs, Louis Bell, M.D., and Paul Offit, M.D., also have our appreciation and respect.

We thank our editors, Timothy Hiscock and Erin McMullan, and the staff at Lippincott Williams & Wilkins for their guidance and patience.

Finally we thank our families for their encouragement and support. Our families have been the best "case examples" for how to lead our lives both personally and professionally.

Stephen Ludwig, M.D.
Philadelphia, Pennsylvania

1

Wheezing

Samir S. Shah

APPROACH TO THE PATIENT WITH WHEEZING

I. Definition of the Complaint

Noisy breathing, as opposed to the usual silent breathing patterns of infants, is a common presenting complaint. The first step in formulating a differential diagnosis is to characterize the type of sound heard. Stertor, a rattling inspiratory noise, is frequently heard in infants with nasal congestion. Stridor, a harsh, high-pitched respiratory sound typically heard on inspiration, often indicates laryngeal obstruction. Wheezing, a musical sound heard on expiration, is caused by partial obstruction of the lower airway. In young children, sometimes expiratory noises cannot be easily distinguished from inspiratory ones, and at times both may be present. Among these causes of noisy breathing, wheezing is the most common. In lower airway

II. Complaint by Cause and Frequency

The causes of wheezing in childhood vary by age (Table 1-1) and may also be grouped in categories based on the following mechanisms: (a) anatomic (extrinsic or intrinsic to the airway), (b) inflammatory/infectious, (c) genetic/metabolic, or (d) miscellaneous causes (Table 1-2).

III. Clarifying Questions

Thorough history taking is essential to arriving at an accurate diagnosis in a child who presents with wheezing. Consideration of age at onset, course and pattern of illness, and associated clinical features provides a useful framework for creating a differential diagnosis. The following questions may help provide clues to the diagnosis.

TABLE 1-1. *Causes of Wheezing in Childhood by Age*

Disease prevalence	Neonate/infant	School age child or adolescent
Common	Bronchiolitis Asthma	Asthma

Less common	Pulmonary aspiration
	  Gastroesophageal reflux
	  Swallowing dysfunction
	Foreign body aspiration
	Bronchopulmonary dysplasia
	Cystic fibrosis
		Foreign body aspiration
		Anaphylaxis
		Atypical pneumonia

Uncommon	Congenital heart disease
	Defective host defenses
	  Immune deficiency
	  Immotile cilia syndrome
	Congenital structural anomalies
	  Tracheobronchomalacia
	  Vascular ring
	  Lobar emphysema
	  Cystic abnormalities
	  Tracheoesophageal fistula
		Defective host defenses
		Mediastinal tumors
		Enlarged mediastinal lymph nodes
		Parasitic infection
		Pulmonary hemosiderosis
		α_1-Antityrpsin deficiency

TABLE 1-2. *Causes of Wheezing in Childhood by Mechanism*

Diagnostic category	Cause
Anatomic	‒ Extrinsic to airway
	Lymphadenopathy
	Tumor
	Diaphragmatic hernia
	Vascular ring/Aberrant vessel
	‒ Intrinsic to airway
	Tracheobronchomalacia
	Foreign body aspiration
	Endobronchial tuberculosis
	Vocal cord dysfunction
	Bronchopulmonary dysplasia
	Congestive heart failure/pulmonary edema
	Pulmonary cysts
	Congenital lobar emphysema
	Pulmonary sequestration
Inflammatory/infectious	Asthma/Reactive airways disease
	Bronchiolitis
	Respiratory syncytial virus
	Influenza viruses A and B
	Parainfluenza viruses
	Adenovirus
	Bronchitis
	Pneumonia
	Mycoplasma pneumoniae
	Chlamydia pneumoniae
	Aspiration pneumonia
	Bronchiectasis
	Bronchial papillomas
	Hypersensitivity pneumonitis
	α_1-Antrypsin deficiency
	Pulmonary hemosiderosis
Genetic/Metabolic	Cystic fibrosis
	Immotile cilia syndrome
	Kartagener syndrome
	Metabolic disturbances
	Hypocalcemia
	Hypokalemia
Miscellaneous	Psychosomatic illness
	Emotional laryngeal wheezing

- What was the age at onset of wheezing?

  — Onset at birth or during early infancy suggests congenital structural abnormalities. Congenital diaphragmatic hernias (CDHs) are usually detected on prenatal ultrasound. Vascular rings and aberrant vessels can cause wheezing or other respiratory symptoms early in life. Infants younger than 2 years of age are more susceptible to lower respiratory tract infection (e.g., bronchiolitis), whereas adolescents are more likely to have asthma or *Mycoplasma pneumoniae* infection.

- Is the wheezing of new onset or recurrent?

  — The initial episode of wheezing in a previously healthy infant in conjunction with symptoms of upper respiratory tract infection usually indicates bronchiolitis. The sudden onset of wheezing is also characteristic of anaphylaxis; particularly in the presence of urticaria, stridor, or environmental exposure. Recurrent episodes of *timing/precipitating factors.*

wheezing may suggest gastroesophageal reflux (GER). However, if precipitated by upper respiratory infections, recurrent wheezing may suggest reactive airways disease. Recurrent wheezing or "difficult-to-control asthma" should lead to consideration of cystic fibrosis, immotile cilia syndrome, recurrent aspiration, immune deficiency, or anatomic abnormalities.

- Is the wheezing episodic or persistent?

  — Persistent wheezing suggests mechanical obstruction from a variety of causes, such as airway foreign body, congenital airway narrowing, or external compression by a mediastinal mass or vascular anomaly.

- Was the episode of wheezing preceded by choking or gagging? *preceding factors*

  — Aspiration of a foreign body is sometimes associated with the sudden onset of symptoms after gagging or choking. Foreign body aspiration is most common in children between the ages of 1 and 4 years. Symptoms depend on the size and location of the foreign body. The wheezing may be unilateral, and secondary bacterial infection may occur.

- Was the wheezing preceded by upper respiratory tract infection? *preceding factors*

  — Antecedent upper respiratory tract infection is suggestive of an underlying inflammatory or infectious etiology.

- What is the child's weight and height? */growth*

  — Features suggestive of cystic fibrosis include failure to thrive, steatorrhea, and recurrent infections.

- Is there a history of recurrent bacterial infection?

  — Children with cystic fibrosis often have recurrent respiratory tract infections. Ciliary dyskinesis is associated with frequent cough, sinusitis, and otitis media.

- Is there a history of preterm birth, or did the child require mechanical ventilation or prolonged supplemental oxygen after birth?

  — Bronchopulmonary dysplasia should be considered.

- Does the patient have allergic shiners, Dennie lines, nasal crease, or atopic dermatitis?

  — The presence of atopy increases the likelihood of asthma.   *Atopy*

- Are symptoms exacerbated by feeding?

  — GER and tracheoesophageal fistula (TEF) should be considered.

- Was the mother tested for sexually transmitted diseases during pregnancy?

  — *Chlamydia trachomatis* pneumonia may present during the 2nd month of life, with nonpurulent conjunctivitis, wheezing, and pneumonia without fever.

The following cases represent less common causes of wheezing in childhood.

Case 1-1: 8-Month-Old Girl

I. History of Present Illness

An 8-month-old girl presented to the emergency department for the third consecutive day with parental complaints of wheezing and cough. Two days before admission she was seen in the emergency department, diagnosed with bronchiolitis and otitis media, and discharged on amoxicillin, nebulized albuterol, and prednisolone. One day before admission, she was again evaluated in the emergency department for continued wheezing and cough, which improved with nebulized albuterol. A chest roentgenogram demonstrated hyperinflation and peribronchiolar thickening. There was no cardiomegaly or pleural effusion. On the day of admission, her cough was accompanied by two episodes of perioral cyanosis. She had decreased oral intake and urine output and was febrile to 39.7°C at home.

II. Past Medical History

Her past history was remarkable for frequent episodes of wheezing since 5 months of age. She had received nebulized albuterol intermittently, including every 4 hours for the past month, without significant improvement in her wheezing. Her cough was worse at night but did not seem to be worse with feeding or supine positioning. Her birth history was unremarkable, and the prenatal ultrasound was reportedly normal.

III. Physical Examination

Temperature (T), 38.3°C; respiration rate (RR), 60/min; heart rate (HR), 110 bpm; blood pressure (BP), 110/55 mm Hg; and pulse oximetry (SpO_2), 100% in room air

Height, 25th percentile; weight, 25th percentile; head circumference, 25th percentile

Initial examination revealed a well-nourished, acyanotic infant in moderate respiratory distress. Physical examination was remarkable for purulent rhinorrhea and buccal mucosal thrush. Moderate intercostal and subcostal retractions were present. There was fair lung aeration with diffuse expiratory wheezing. No murmurs or gallops were heard on cardiac examination, and femoral pulses were palpable. No hepatomegaly or splenomegaly was present.

IV. Diagnostic Studies

Laboratory analysis revealed 14,600 white blood cells (WBCs)/mm³, with 38% segmented neutrophils, 53% lymphocytes, and no band forms. The hemoglobin was 11.0 g/dL, and there were 580,000 platelets/mm³. Electrolytes, blood urea nitrogen, and creatinine were normal. Polymerase chain reaction performed on nasopharyngeal aspirate was negative for *Bordetella pertussis*. Antigens of adenovirus; influenza A and B viruses; parainfluenza virus types 1, 2, and 3; and respiratory syncytial virus (RSV) were not detected by immunofluorescence of nasopharyngeal washings. However, RSV subsequently grew in viral culture of the nasopharyngeal aspirate. Blood and urine cultures were negative.

V. Course of Illness

The patient was diagnosed with bronchiolitis. Her tachypnea and wheezing improved with nebulized albuterol and oral prednisolone. She was discharged after 3 days of hospitalization, receiving albuterol every 4 hours. A radionuclide milk scan was scheduled on an outpatient basis to assess for the presence of GER and pulmonary aspiration.

Ten days later, the patient returned to the emergency room with increased wheezing and recurrence of her fever. She had poor oral intake, which had not improved significantly since the last admission and was now accompanied by frequent emesis. She was admitted for treatment and further evaluation. Her radionuclide milk scan, which had been performed between admissions, revealed GER without pulmonary aspiration. During her current admission, careful examination of the chest radiograph suggested the diagnosis (Fig. 1-1A,B). Magnetic resonance imaging (MRI) of the chest confirmed this diagnosis (Fig. 1-1C).

DISCUSSION: CASE 1-1

I. Differential Diagnosis

The causes of recurrent or persistent wheezing in the infant are diverse. Common causes of recurrent wheezing in infancy include bronchiolitis, reactive airways disease, and GER with microaspiration. Less commonly, recurrent wheezing is caused by congenital abnormalities of the lung or respiratory tract (cystic adenomatous malformations, TEF), diaphragmatic abnormalities (paralysis of the diaphragm, diaphragmatic hernia), cystic fibrosis, or immunologic defects (congenital absence of thymus, DiGeorge syndrome, chronic granulomatous disease, gammaglobulin deficiencies). Rarely, anomalies of the major arterial branches of the aorta or pulmonary blood vessels compress the trachea and bronchi of the infant, causing acute or progressive respiratory distress. The features of this case that prompted additional evaluation included recurrent episodes of wheezing, incomplete resolution of wheezing despite prolonged β-agonist therapy, and episodes of cyanosis.

II. Diagnosis

The chest radiographs revealed a midline trachea with bilateral indentations in the anteroposterior projection (Fig. 1-1A) and anterior bowing of the trachea on the lateral projection (Fig. 1-1B). These findings suggested the diagnosis of double aortic arch. MRI of the chest showed the bifurcation of this double arch as the "horseshoe"-appearing structure surrounding the trachea in the center of the image (Fig. 1-1C). There were no associated structural defects of the heart. **The diagnosis is double aortic arch.**

III. Incidence and Anatomy of Vascular Rings and Slings

Vascular anomalies, commonly referred to "vascular rings and slings," can cause tracheal or esophageal compression leading to respiratory symptoms or feeding difficulty. The term *vascular ring* refers to any aortic arch anomaly in which the trachea and esophagus are completely surrounded by vascular structures. The vascular structures need not be patent. For example, a ligamentum arteriosum may complete a ring. A vascular or pulmonary sling is an anomaly in which vascular structures only partially surround the lower trachea but cause tracheal compression. Vascular rings are seen in fewer than 1% of congenital cardiac anomalies.

The most commonly occurring rings and slings are described in the following paragraphs (Fig. 1-2).

Double aortic arch. This is the most common clinically recognized form of vascular ring; as the name implies, both right and left aortic arches are present. "Left" and "right" refer to which bronchus is crossed by the arch, not which side of the midline the aortic root ascends. The ascending aorta divides anterior to the trachea into left and right arches, which then pass on either side of the trachea. The right arch is usually higher and larger and gives rise to the right common carotid and right subclavian arteries. The right arch travels posteriorly and indents the right side of the trachea and the right and posterior portions of the esophagus, as it passes behind the esophagus to join the left arch at the junction of the left-sided descending aorta. The left arch gives rise to the left common carotid and left subclavian arteries. The left arch is located anteriorly and indents the left side of

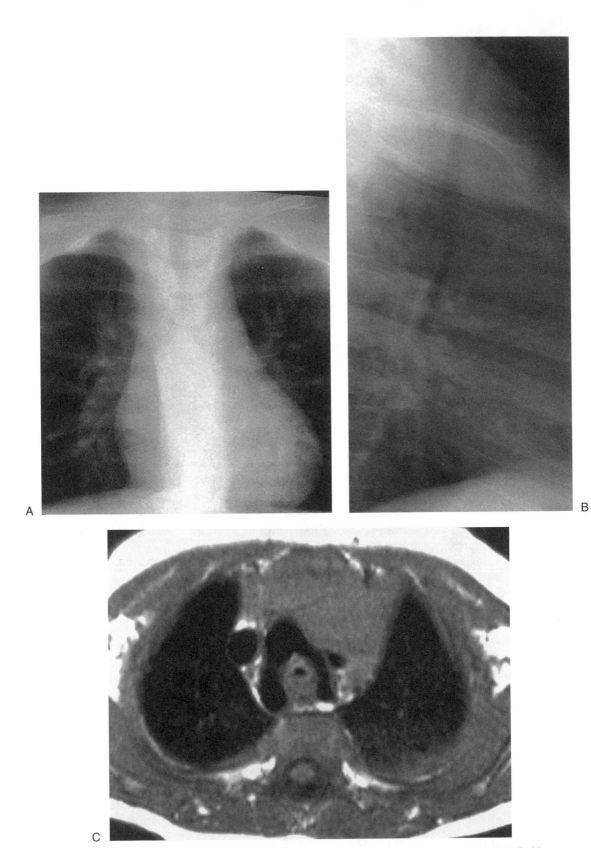

FIG. 1-1. Case 1-1. **A,** Anteroposterior chest radiograph. **B,** Lateral chest radiograph. **C,** Magnetic resonance image of the chest.

Anatomy

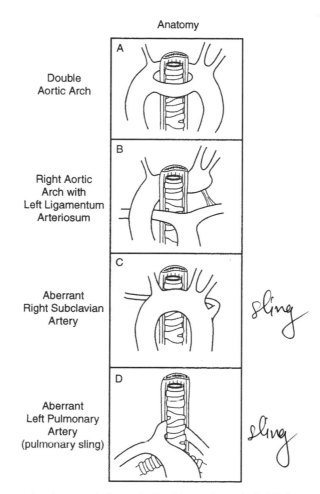

Double
Aortic Arch

Right Aortic
Arch with
Left Ligamentum
Arteriosum

Aberrant
Right Subclavian
Artery

sling

Aberrant
Left Pulmonary
Artery
(pulmonary sling)

sling

FIG. 1-2. Anatomy of vascular rings and slings. **A**, Double aortic arch. **B**, Right aortic arch with anomalous left subclavian artery and left ligamentum arteriosum. **C**, Aberrant right subclavian artery. **D**, Aberrant left pulmonary artery.

the trachea and esophagus as it joins the descending aorta. Double aortic arch is rarely associated with congenital heart disease. If congenital disease is present, tetralogy of Fallot is the most common condition, and transposition of the great arteries is occasionally seen. Surgical division of one of the arches, usually the smaller one, is curative. Respiratory symptoms may persist for months postoperatively due to prolonged deformity of the tracheobronchial tree.

Aberrant right subclavian artery. This condition is also known as left aortic arch with retroesophageal right subclavian artery. It is the most common aortic arch malformation noted on postmortem examination. The incidence of this abnormality in the general population is approximately 0.5%. Aberrant right subclavian artery was found in 0.9% of 3,427 consecutive patients undergoing cardiac catheterization at The Children's Hospital of Philadelphia; it represented 20% of aortic arch anomalies found at catheterization. It is also seen in approximately one third of patients with Down syndrome and congenital heart disease. The left aortic arch has a normal course to the left and anterior to the trachea. However, the right subclavian artery arises as the last branch of the arch and runs posteriorly from the descending thoracic aorta to reach the right arm, passing obliquely up to and right behind the esophagus, indenting it posteriorly. Although most patients with this anomaly are asymptomatic, an older patient may complain of dysphagia. Symptomatic anterior tracheal compression results if there is a common origin of both carotid arteries in conjunction with a retroesophageal aberrant right subclavian artery. Rarely, an anomalous right subclavian artery in association with a left aortic arch, retroesophageal descending aorta, and right ligamentum arteriosum produces a symptomatic vascular ring.

Right aortic arch with anomalous left subclavian artery and left ductus arteriosus or ligamentum arteriosum. The aortic arch passes to the right of the trachea, becomes retroesophageal, and descends on left. The first branch is the left carotid artery; the second, the right carotid artery; the third, the right subclavian artery; and the fourth, the left subclavian artery, which arises from the descending aorta. The ductus arteriosus originates from a retroesophageal diverticulum of the descending aorta, courses to the left, and connects to the pulmonary artery. Patients are usually asymptomatic. However, some patients present with wheezing or stridor due to tracheal compression and require surgical division of the ligamentum arteriosum. Older children with dysphagia may require relief of esophageal compression by actual division of the aortic arch. The retroesophageal portion is mobilized, and reanastomosis of ascending and descending portions of the aorta is completed with the use of a graft.

Aberrant left pulmonary artery (pulmonary sling). A normal pulmonary artery is absent, and the left lung is supplied by an anomalous left pulmonary artery that arises from the distal right pulmonary artery. The vessel courses to the right of the trachea and then passes between the trachea and the esophagus, causing compression of the right main stem bronchus, trachea, and esophagus. The resulting compression of the right main stem bronchus and trachea leads to airway obstruction, primarily affecting the right lung. Two thirds of affected infants present in the first month of life with wheezing, stridor, or apnea. Dysphagia is rare. There may be associated collapse or hyperinflation of the right lung. Aberrant left pulmonary artery is frequently associated with complete cartilaginous rings in the distal trachea, resulting in tracheal stenosis. It usually appears as an isolated abnormality but can be associated with other congenital cardiac defects, particularly tetralogy of Fallot. Surgical repair involves division of the left pulmonary artery from the right and their reanastomosis in front of the trachea. Bronchoscopy is performed at the time of surgical repair because of the frequent association of complete cartilaginous rings causing tracheal stenosis.

IV. Clinical Presentation of Vascular Rings and Slings

Most infants present with symptoms in early infancy. Superimposed viral infection with edema of the trachea or bronchi may account for or contribute to the respiratory symptoms. Asymptomatic infants, particularly those with aberrant right subclavian artery, are sometimes diagnosed incidentally on the basis of a chest roentgenogram taken during a viral respiratory illness.

The symptoms of a vascular ring or sling are caused by tracheal compression and, to a lesser degree, esophageal compression. Symptoms of tracheal compression include wheezing, stridor, and apnea. Some infants hyperextend their necks to reduce tracheal compression. Symptoms related to esophageal compression include emesis, choking, and nonspecific feeding difficulties in infants and dysphagia in older children. Less severe obstructions may cause recurrent respiratory infections as a result of aspiration or inadequate clearing of respiratory secretions.

V. Diagnostic Approach

Clinicians should have a high index of suspicion for a vascular anomaly in the evaluation of an infant with recurrent wheezing. Chest roentgenography and barium esophagography should be considered in the initial evaluation.

Chest roentgenogram. The diagnosis of a vascular ring may be suspected before a barium esophagogram is performed. The chest roentgenogram should be examined to assess laterality of the aortic arch and for evidence of tracheal or bronchial compression. The following features on chest roentgenogram are suggestive of a vascular anomaly and require additional evaluation. (a) A midline trachea in which there is no rotation of the patient or a sharp indentation on the right side of the trachea above the carina suggest a right aortic arch; the normal infant's trachea is slightly displaced to the right by the normal left arch. (b) Lateral displacement of the right mediastinal pleural line indicates a right descending aorta. (c) Anterior bowing of the trachea rather than a normal posterior convexity on the lateral view indicates compression. Generalized or focal areas of hyperinflation due to tracheal or bronchial compression can be mistakenly diagnosed as a foreign body aspiration.

Barium esophagogram. Posterior (vascular ring) or anterior (pulmonary sling) indentation of the esophagus is frequently seen and suggests the diagnosis.

Magnetic resonance imaging. MRI has been shown to give excellent anatomic detail and is helpful in planning reconstructive procedures.

Angiogram and transthoracic echocardiogram. In the absence of any other cardiac defect, angiography is probably unnecessary for diagnosis. It may be helpful in delineating the anatomic detail necessary for surgical correction. Transthoracic echocardiography is important to detect associated congenital cardiac defects but is less reliable at delineating vascular and tracheal anatomy.

Bronchoscopy. This allows direct visualization of compression on the trachea and is indicated for suspected tracheal stenosis present.

VI. Treatment

Surgical management is necessary to relieve symptomatic obstruction of trachea and esophagus. Surgery should also be considered if the infant has frequent respiratory infections or is failing to thrive. The infant with severe preoperative respiratory symptoms is likely to have postoperative tracheomalacia from prolonged compression by the vascular ring. However, feeding difficulties resolve rapidly.

VII. References

1. Berdon WE, Baker DH. Vascular anomalies and the infant lung: rings, slings, and other things. *Semin Roentgenol* 1972;7:39–63.
2. Edwards JE. Malformations of the aortic arch system manifested as "vascular rings." *Lab Invest* 1953;2:56–75.
3. Goldstein WB. Aberrant right subclavian artery in mongolism. *Am J Roentgenol* 1965; 95:131–134.
4. Hawker RE, Celermajer JM, Cartmill TB, et al. Double aortic arch and complex cardiac malformations. *Br Heart J* 1972;34:1311–1313.
5. Moes CAF, Freedom RM. Rare types of aortic arch anomalies. *Pediatr Cardiol* 1993;14:93–101.
6. Weinberg PM. Aortic arch anomalies. In: Emmanouilides GC, Riemenschneider TA, Allen HD, et al., eds. *Moss and Adams' heart disease in infants, children, and adolescents, including the fetus and young adult,* 5th ed. Baltimore: Williams & Wilkins, 1995:810–837.

Case 1-2: 3-Year-Old Boy

I.   History of Present Illness

A 3-year-old boy was referred to the emergency department for evaluation of wheezing, cough, and increased work of breathing. He had been well until 3 days before admission, when he developed rhinorrhea and cough without fever. Nebulized albuterol was prescribed for wheezing and retractions, with little improvement. On the day of admission, the child's respiratory distress had continued and his cough had worsened and was accompanied by mild sternal discomfort exacerbated by coughing. He had received nebulized albuterol every 4 hours during the day of admission without significant relief. There was no vomiting or diarrhea. The onset of wheezing was not accompanied by an episode of choking or gagging. There was no history of trauma.

II.   Past Medical History

His past medical history was unremarkable. There were no prior episodes of wheezing. He was born at 39 weeks gestational age without perinatal complications. There was no family history of atopic dermatitis or asthma.

III.   Physical Examination

T, 37.7°C; RR, 52/min; HR, 130 bpm; BP, 108/70 mm Hg; SpO$_2$, 95% in room air
Weight, 50th percentile
Physical examination revealed a fair-haired Caucasian boy in mild respiratory distress. On examination, there was no conjunctival injection or chemosis. Clear rhinorrhea was present. He had mild intercostal and subcostal retractions. Lung examination revealed dullness to percussion, diminished breath sounds, and prominent wheezing at the left base. There was good aeration without wheezing, rales, or rhonchi in the remainder of the left lung and throughout the right side. A I/VI vibratory systolic ejection murmur was present at the left sternal border. His abdomen was thin and soft, with active bowel sounds and no organomegaly or palpable mass. The remainder of the physical examination was normal.

IV.   Diagnostic Studies

Laboratory analysis revealed 15,100 WBCs/mm^3, with 0% band forms, 52% segmented neutrophils, 33% lymphocytes, and 5% eosinophils. The hemoglobin, platelet count, electrolytes, blood urea nitrogen, and creatinine values were normal.

V.   Course of Illness

The lung examination results did not change after administration of nebulized albuterol. A chest roentgenogram revealed the diagnosis (Fig. 1-3).

DISCUSSION: CASE 1-2

I.   Differential Diagnosis

The most likely cause of a first episode of wheezing in a 3-year-old boy, particularly in the context of an upper respiratory tract infection, is asthma. Foreign body aspiration should also be strongly suspected in this age group, especially if there are asymmetries on lung examination. Less common causes in this age group include anaphylaxis, which is typically associated with urticaria or other features of a systemic allergic response, and airway compression caused by mediastinal tumors, lymph nodes, or other structures. In the immunocompromised host, *Pneumocystis carinii* pneumonia (PCP) often results in a presentation with tachypnea, wheezing, and respiratory distress in the absence of fever. Children with cystic fibrosis usually have poor weight gain, pancreatic insufficiency, and

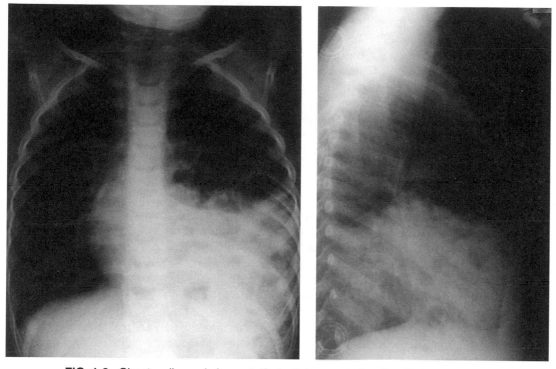

A

B

FIG. 1-3. Chest radiograph (case 1-2). **A,** Anteroposterior view. **B,** Lateral view.

recurrent respiratory symptoms. The features of this case that prompted additional evaluation included hypoxia, progressive respiratory distress that was unresponsive to β-agonist therapy, and the presence of focal wheezing on lung examination.

II.   Diagnosis

The chest roentgenogram (Fig. 1-3) revealed a heterogeneous opacity overlying the lower half of the left lung, consistent with the appearance of small or large bowel in the thorax. The mediastinal structures were displaced rightward. **The diagnosis is posterolateral congenital diaphragmatic (Bochdalek) hernia with delayed presentation.**

III.   Incidence and Epidemiology

CDH is a simple anatomic defect in which a hole in the diaphragm allows abdominal viscera to herniate into the thorax. CDH defects are usually left-sided (80%). The incidence of CDH is estimated to be 1 in every 2,000 to 5,000 births. Although most cases of CDH are diagnosed prenatally or during the neonatal period, approximately 10% to 20% have delayed presentation (age greater than 1 month). They are thought to occur most often as a sporadic developmental anomaly, although familial cases have been reported. The recurrence risk in a first-degree relative is approximately 2%. Population-based studies of CDH among liveborn, stillborn, and spontaneously aborted fetuses suggest that approximately 30% of fetuses who have CDH die before birth, usually from chromosomal or lethal nonpulmonary malformations. Approximately 40% of liveborn patients with CDH have one or more associated anomalies, including cardiac (60%) genitourinary (23%), gastrointestinal (17%), central nervous system (14%), and chromosomal (10%) abnormalities.

CDHs vary in size and occur in various portions of the diaphragm. Types of CDH include posterolateral or Bochdalek (59.5%), anteromedial or Morgagni (2.6%), hiatal (23.3%), and eventration (14.6%). Posterolateral diaphragmatic hernias result from an absence or defective fusion of the septum transversum dorsally and the pleuroperitoneal membrane posterolaterally. There appear to be two groups of patients with delayed presentation of posterolateral CDH. In the first group, the defect is long-standing, but the viscera are confined by a hernia sac or obturated by a solid organ. Presentation occurs when the sac ruptures or the intraabdominal pressure is raised, causing the viscera to herniate. A previously normal chest radiograph is supportive. Members of the second group also have a congenital defect, but they present only if a complication of the herniated contents, such as volvulus, strangulation, or acute or recurrent respiratory distress, develops.

IV. Clinical Presentation

Many patients with CDH are diagnosed antenatally by ultrasound. In such instances, other congenital anomalies, particularly those affecting the cardiovascular and central nervous systems, should be sought. The presentation of CDH in the neonatal period is determined primarily by the severity of the pulmonary hypoplasia and pulmonary hypertension. The most severely affected infants show obvious respiratory signs within the first 24 hours of life. Classically, these infants are born with a scaphoid abdomen and develop progressive respiratory distress as swallowed air causes intestinal distention followed by worsening lung compression and mediastinal shift. These infants may have cyanosis, increased work of breathing, and respiratory failure.

In contrast, the presentation of diaphragmatic hernia outside the neonatal period is extremely varied and may be associated with misleading clinical and radiologic assessments. Children who have CDH with delayed presentation may have recurrent respiratory distress, chronic pulmonary infection, or acute gastrointestinal symptoms caused by gastric volvulus or intestinal obstruction.

V. Diagnostic Approach

Prenatal ultrasound. CDH may be diagnosed by ultrasound during routine obstetric screening or during investigation of polyhydramnios, which complicates up to 80% of pregnancies in which CDH occurs. The accuracy of prenatal diagnosis varies, depending on the site of the lesion and the presence of corroborating criteria such as mediastinal shift and abnormal fetal abdominal anatomy. The diagnosis is suggested strongly by the presence of a fluid-filled stomach or intestine at the level of the four-chamber view of the heart.

Associated studies. Once the diagnosis of CDH in a neonate has been confirmed, a careful search for associated anomalies should be performed. Additional studies to consider include renal and cranial ultrasonography, echocardiography, and karyotyping.

Chest roentgenogram. The diagnosis is confirmed by a chest radiograph that demonstrates loops of intestine within the chest. The location of the gastric bubble should also be noted, and its position can be confirmed by placement of a nasogastric tube. Occasionally, a large multicystic lung lesion, such as a congenital cystic adenomatoid malformation, has the appearance of a CDH on plain radiography. In these instances, ultrasonographic visualization of an intact diaphragm or a computed tomographic (CT) scan of the chest may be necessary. In an older child, the radiographic appearance of CDH may be misinterpreted as a pneumothorax, pneumatocele, or lobar consolidation.

Upper gastrointestinal barium series. Confirmative barium studies represent an unnecessary delay in appropriate therapy for the neonate, but in the older child they serve to confirm the diagnosis. Additionally, up to 30% of children with delayed presentation of CDH have associated abnormalities of bowel fixation or rotation that require repair.

VI. Treatment

Prenatal care. Antenatal diagnosis of CDH has allowed optimal immediate care of affected infants. Birth at a tertiary care center that has pediatric surgery and neonatology services as well as advanced strategies for managing respiratory failure, including extracorporeal membrane oxygenation (ECMO), usually is most appropriate. A spontaneous vaginal delivery should be anticipated unless obstetric issues dictate otherwise.

Fetal therapy. The role of *in utero* surgery for CDH remains controversial. Fetal intervention is currently focused on temporary occlusion of the fetal trachea for those fetuses who have CDH and liver herniation above the diaphragm, in an attempt to correct the severe pulmonary hypoplasia that is often associated with CDH. Normally, fetal lungs produce a continuous flow of fluid that exits the trachea into the amniotic space. In the presence of tracheal obstruction, the lungs grow, and there is gradual reduction of herniated viscera back into the abdomen. After a period of intrauterine tracheal occlusion sufficient to cause a reversal of pulmonary hypoplasia, the fetus is delivered and maintained on placental support until the tracheal obstruction is relieved and an adequate neonatal airway is established. Other forms of antenatal therapy include pharmacologic strategies that target pulmonary growth and development.

Delivery room and intensive care. Immediate resuscitation includes prompt endotracheal intubation, avoidance of bag-mask ventilation, placement of a nasogastric tube to provide intestinal decompression, and ongoing care in an intensive care nursery by individuals experienced in the management of newborns with CDH.

Surgical repair in the neonate. Historically, neonates who had CDH were rushed to the operating room under the mistaken belief that decompression of the lungs by reduction of the abdominal viscera offered the greatest chance of survival. This disorder is no longer thought to require immediate surgery, because the primary problem after birth is not herniation of abdominal viscera into the chest but severe pulmonary hypoplasia and associated pulmonary hypertension. Average time to surgery now ranges from 3 to 15 days after birth. New treatments, including ECMO and permissive hypercapnia with gentle ventilation to minimize barotrauma, have led to incremental increases in survival rates, which now range from 78% to 94%. Other treatments, such as partial liquid ventilation, inhaled nitric oxide, surfactant-replacement therapy, and maternal corticosteroid therapy before birth, require additional study in patients with CDH.

Surgical repair in the child with delayed presentation. Repair of CDH in patients who present beyond the neonatal period typically occurs within days after presentation, or earlier if symptoms are acute. The prognosis in late-presenting CDH is good. It does not depend on lung hypoplasia, as in neonatal CDH, but relates to accurate diagnosis of the condition and immediate operative correction in symptomatic cases. Complications of delayed repair in the symptomatic patient include incarceration or strangulation of herniated bowel and cardiorespiratory arrest due to mediastinal compression by the herniated viscera.

VII. References

1. Berman L, Stringer D, Ein SH, et al. The late-presenting pediatric Bochdalek hernia: a 20-year review. *J Pediatr Surg* 1988;23:735–739.
2. Fotter R, Schimpl G, Sorantin E, et al. Delayed presentation of congenital diaphragmatic hernia. *Pediatr Radiol* 1992;22:187–191.
3. Skarsgard ED, Harrison MR. Congenital diaphragmatic hernia: the surgeon's perspective. *Pediatr Rev* 1999;20:e71–e78.
4. Stolar CJH, Dillon PW. Congenital diaphragmatic hernia and eventration. In: O'Neill JA Jr, Rowe MI, Grosfeld JL, et al., eds. *Pediatric surgery,* 5th ed. St. Louis: Mosby, 1998:819–837.
5. Thibeault DW, Sigalet DL. Congenital diaphragmatic hernia from the womb to childhood. *Curr Probl Pediatr* 1998;28:5–25.
6. Van Meurs K, Short BL. Congenital diaphragmatic hernia: the neonatologist's perspective. *Pediatr Rev* 1999;20:e79–e87.

Case 1-3: 5-Week-Old Boy

I.   History of Present Illness

A 5-week-old boy presented to the emergency department with a 1-day history of fever and "wheezing." His visit to the hospital was prompted by a rectal temperature of 38.6°C. His respiratory difficulty seemed worse with feeding. There had been no emesis, diarrhea, rhinorrhea, cough, or cyanosis. He had been drinking approximately 4 ounces of a cow's milk-based formula every 3 hours. His only ill contact was his mother, who had had cough and rhinorrhea for 1 week.

II.   Past Medical History

He was born by spontaneous vaginal delivery at 39 weeks gestation. His birth weight was 3,900 g. The pregnancy, labor, and delivery were uncomplicated. Prenatal ultrasound revealed polyhydramnios but was otherwise normal. The mother's prenatal laboratory studies included a negative group B *Streptococcus* screen. Testing for antibodies to human immunodeficiency virus (HIV) had not been performed. The infant had not previously been hospitalized.

III.   Physical Examination

T, 38.5°C; HR, 180 bpm; RR, 70/min.; BP, 62/40 mm Hg; SpO$_2$, 96% in room air

Length, 25th percentile; weight, 50th percentile

The infant was ill-appearing and in moderate respiratory distress. His anterior fontanelle was open and flat. There was no conjunctival injection or discharge. There was intermittent grunting and nasal flaring. Moderate intercostal and subcostal retractions were present. Breath sounds were diminished throughout the left chest. The right lung was clear to auscultation. There was no wheezing. The heart sounds were normal. The

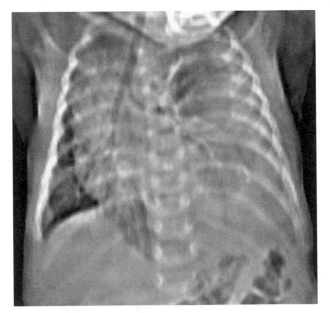

FIG. 1-4. Chest radiograph (case 1-3).

14

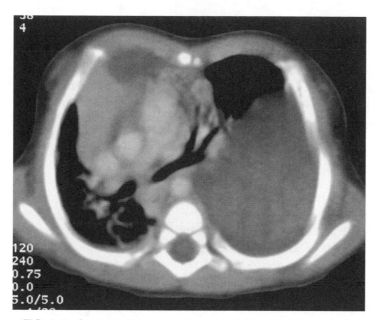

FIG. 1-5. Computed tomography scan of the chest (case 1-3).

liver was palpable 1 cm below the right costal margin. The spleen was not palpable. The Moro reflex, grasp, tone, and reflexes were normal. There were no rashes or petechiae.

IV. Diagnostic Studies

Arterial blood gas revealed the following: pH, 7.40; carbon dioxide tension (PaCO$_2$), 40 mm Hg; oxygen tension (PaO$_2$), 214 mm Hg; and bicarbonate, 26 mEq/L. The complete blood count demonstrated 37,900 WBCs/mm^3, including 3% band forms, 67% segmented neutrophils, and 30% lymphocytes. The platelet count was 520,000/mm^3, and hemoglobin was 9.4 g/dL. Serum electrolytes, blood urea nitrogen, and creatinine were normal. There were no WBCs, protein, or nitrites on urinanalysis. A blood culture was obtained. Lumbar puncture was not performed due to the patient's respiratory distress. Chest radiography demonstrated left lower lobe consolidation with an associated pleural effusion causing rightward shift of the mediastinal structures (Fig. 1-4).

V. Course of Illness

The patient was diagnosed with bacterial pneumonia and treated with vancomycin and cefotaxime. The blood culture was subsequently negative. A CT scan of the chest, performed to better delineate the pulmonary findings, suggested an alternative diagnosis (Fig. 1-5).

DISCUSSION: CASE 1-3

I. Differential Diagnosis

In this 5-week-old boy with respiratory distress and lobar consolidation, the most likely diagnosis is bacterial pneumonia with pleural empyema. Etiologic organisms in this age group include group B *Streptococcus*, *Listeria monocytogenes*, and gram-negative enteric bacilli. The radiographic appearance of the lung may suggest a congenital lung malformation such as pulmonary sequestration, bronchogenic cyst, or cystic adenomatoid malformation. Infantile lobar emphysema is unlikely because the lung, despite causing a mediastinal shift, does not appear to be overinflated. Other congenital considerations include enterogenic cysts and CDH. Acquired causes include mediastinal neoplasm (e.g., neuroblastoma) and chronic pulmonary infection distal to an aspirated foreign body or an area of bronchiectasis. Chronic pulmonary infection may result in neovascularization of the infected tissue by ingrowth of systemic arteries. Such acquired systemic vascularization typically consists of several small arteries rather than one or two large arteries that typically supply a pulmonary sequestration. It may be impossible to make the distinction between true pulmonary sequestration and so-called pseudosequestration secondary to chronic infection preoperatively.

II. Diagnosis

CT of the chest (Fig. 1-5) revealed a large (6 cm × 5 cm × 8 cm), heterogeneously enhancing mass with disorganized vasculature in the posterior aspect of the left hemithorax. These findings were most consistent with an **extralobar pulmonary sequestration.**

III. Incidence and Anatomy

The term *pulmonary sequestration* refers to a congenital malformation consisting of abnormally developed pulmonary parenchyma that is separate from the normal lung. The tissue is nonfunctioning, does not communicate with the tracheobronchial tree, and derives its blood supply from the aorta. There may be a single large anomalous artery, but occasionally multiple small anomalous arteries from above or below the diaphragm supply the sequestered lobe. The venous drainage may be pulmonary or systemic (inferior vena cava, azygous vein, or portal vein). Drainage into systemic veins produces a left-to-right shunt. In this case, the vessels appeared to drain into the azygous and hemiazygous veins.

The overall incidence of pulmonary sequestration is not well defined, but sequestrations have been found in 1% to 2% of all resected pulmonary specimens. Pulmonary sequestration occurs when an accessory lung bud originates during embryonic development. If the bud originates early, the sequestration is considered intralobar, because the normal and sequestered lung share a common pleural covering. If the bud originates later, the sequestration is considered extralobar, because the sequestered lung has its own pleura. About 75% of reported cases of pulmonary sequestration are intralobar; 1% have both an intralobar and an extralobar component.

Associated malformations occur in 60% of extralobar sequestrations and 10% of intralobar sequestrations. The most common associated malformations are duplications of the colon or terminal ileum, esophageal cysts or communications, vertebral or rib anomalies, diaphragmatic hernia, and congenital heart disease. Pulmonary sequestration is left-sided in 90% of cases and bilateral in fewer than 0.5% of cases. Approximately two thirds of all cases involve the left lower lobe.

IV. Clinical Presentation

Most children with extralobar pulmonary sequestration present during the first year of life. They may be discovered during the neonatal period while undergoing evaluation of other congenital anomalies. In such cases, the associated congenital anomalies usually dominate the clinical picture. A few children with extralobar sequestration present with respiratory distress when the sequestered lobe impairs ventilation by impinging on the surrounding lung. Cases not diagnosed in the neonatal period may be detected incidentally on chest radiographs obtained during a respiratory illness. Infection of an extralobar sequestration is uncommon.

Intralobar pulmonary sequestration is rarely detected during infancy; two thirds of patients present after 10 years of age. Common symptoms include productive cough, hemoptysis, recurrent pneumonia, fever, and chest pain. A few patients with large supplying arteries have worsening exercise tolerance or congestive heart failure due to a large systemic arterial-to-pulmonary venous shunt through the sequestration. Infection of the sequestration, usually due to a fistula between the sequestration and the respiratory or digestive tract, occurs more commonly with intralobar than with extralobar sequestrations.

Physical examination reveals dullness to percussion and decreased breath sounds in the area of the sequestration. Digital clubbing and cyanosis may be present. Skeletal abnormalities such as pectus excavatum, thoracic asymmetry, and rib anomalies are noted in some patients. Rarely, an intrathoracic bruit is heard in the region of the sequestration.

V. Diagnostic Approach

Prenatal ultrasound. Pulmonary sequestration may be diagnosed during routine obstetric screening or during investigation of polyhydramnios, which is reported in many cases.

Chest roentgenogram. It is difficult to distinguish between intralobar and extralobar sequestrations by chest roentgenogram alone. Both are typically found in the posteromedial aspect of the lower lobe, and calcifications are occasionally present. Intralobar sequestrations more often appear cyst-like. Air-fluid levels indicate a pulmonary communication. Extralobar sequestrations appear as a solid mass.

Chest computed tomography. CT allows differentiation of pulmonary sequestration from other lung abnormalities.

Angiography. Angiography of the thoracic and abdominal aorta will demonstrate both the systemic arterial blood supply and the venous drainage.

Nuclear scintigraphy. After intravenous injection, peak radioisotope activity occurs earlier in lung tissue with normal pulmonary blood supply than in the sequestration with systemic blood supply. Nuclear scintigraphy has been proposed as an alternative to traditional angiography.

Other studies. Magnetic resonance angiography (MRA) is a less invasive study that may eventually replace traditional angiography in the evaluation of pulmonary sequestration. An upper gastrointestinal barium study should be considered to exclude the possibility of a communication with the gastrointestinal tract.

VI. Treatment

Symptomatic intralobar and extralobar sequestrations require immediate resection. Asymptomatic sequestrations also require removal because of the risk of subsequent serious infection. Extralobar sequestrations, because of their separate pleural covering, can often be removed without disruption of the normal lung. Intralobar sequestrations require lobectomy for removal because of the inability to separate the sequestration from the normal lung. In cases of acute infection, preoperative antibiotic coverage should be directed against common respiratory pathogens, *Staphylococcus aureus*, and anaerobes. Ampicillin-sulbactam or the combination of clindamycin and cefotaxime are appropriate empiric antibiotic choices. The resected tissue should be sent for aerobic and anaerobic bacterial cultures, mycobacterial cultures, and fungal cultures.

Intraoperative mortality is highest in those with associated congenital anomalies. Intraoperative complications are usually caused by severance of a systemic artery. Postoperative complications include emphysema, hemothorax, and bronchopleural fistulas; the incidence of each is approximately 1%. The long-term prognosis in those patients without other debilitating congenital anomalies is excellent.

In this case, MRA was performed and the extralobar sequestration was removed without complications on the following day. Cultures of the resected sequestration were sterile. The patient recovered uneventfully.

VII.   References

1. Carter R. Pulmonary sequestration. *Ann Thorac Surg* 1969;7:68–88.
2. Collin PP, Desjardins JG. Pulmonary sequestration. *J Pediatr Surg* 1987;22:750–753.
3. Kravitz RM. Congenital malformation of the lung. *Pediatr Clin North Am* 1994;41: 453–472.
4. Lierl M. Congenital abnormalities. In: Hilman BC, ed. *Pediatric respiratory disease: diagnosis and treatment.* Philadelphia: WB Saunders, 1993:457–498.
5. Oliphant L, McFadden RG, Carr TJ, et al. Magnetic resonance imaging to diagnose intralobar pulmonary sequestration. *Chest* 1987;91:500–502.
6. Savic B, Birtel FJ, Tholen W, et al. Lung sequestration: report of seven cases and review of 540 published cases. *Thorax* 1979;34:96–101.
7. Stocker JT, Kagan-Hallet K. Extralobar pulmonary sequestration: analysis of 15 cases. *Am J Clin Pathol* 1979;72:917–925.

Case 1-4: 15-Month-Old Girl

I. History of Present Illness

The patient was a 15-month-old girl hospitalized for respiratory distress. She was well until 3 days before admission, when she began coughing during a meal. She had moderate respiratory distress initially but gradually improved. On the day of admission, she had a fever to 39.5°C and worsening tachypnea. She received albuterol with some improvement in her respiratory status.

II. Past Medical History

The patient was born at term after an uncomplicated pregnancy and delivery. She was diagnosed with reactive airways disease in infancy after three hospitalizations for wheezing. She received nebulized albuterol and prednisone for 5 days during each of those episodes. Mild GER was diagnosed by a pH probe study at 7 months of age; an upper gastrointestinal barium study performed at that time was normal. At 11 months of age, ranitidine and metoclopramide were started, after which her symptoms of chronic cough improved. She was treated with intravenous antibiotics for a right middle lobe pneumonia at 12 months of age. At the time of presentation, she was receiving metoclopramide for GER, as well as nebulized albuterol for wheezing approximately twice per week. A distant relative was diagnosed with cystic fibrosis a decade ago and died during infancy. There was no family history of atopy or asthma.

III. Physical Examination

T, 37.4°C; RR, 44/min; HR, 110 bpm; BP, 103/65 mm Hg; SpO_2, 96% in room air
Weight, 16.5 kg (10th percentile); height, 105 cm (25th percentile)

Physical examination revealed a thin child in mild respiratory distress. There was no conjunctival infection. The sinuses demonstrated symmetric transillumination. The oropharynx was clear. There was no cervical lymphadenopathy. There were mild intercostal retractions with good aeration and mild diffuse wheezing. Breath sounds were slightly diminished in the right lower lobe. The cardiac examination was normal. There were no rashes or skin lesions. The remainder of the examination, including the neurologic examination, was normal.

IV. Diagnostic Studies

Her WBC count was 18,300 mm³, with 9% band forms, 78% segmented neutrophils, and 13% lymphocytes. Her hemoglobin and platelet counts were normal. A blood culture was obtained and subsequently was found to be negative. Chest radiography revealed a right middle lobe density. There was no hyperinflation or peribronchial thickening.

V. Course of Illness

A repeat upper gastrointestinal barium study was performed (Fig. 1-6) while other diagnostic possibilities were considered.

DISCUSSION: CASE 1-4

I. Differential Diagnosis

The most common cause of recurrent wheezing in a young infant is GER with pulmonary aspiration. Other causes of recurrent aspiration include cricopharyngeal incoordination, submucosal cleft palate, seizures, neuromuscular disorders, and TEF. Esophageal obstruction due to webs or strictures may also predispose to recurrent aspiration.

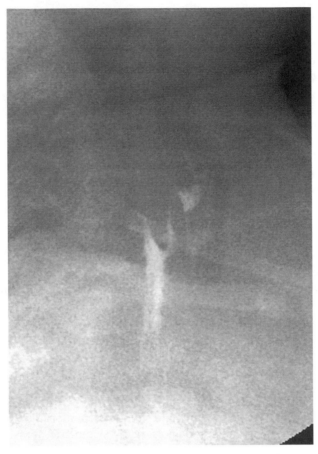

FIG. 1-6. Contrast esophagogram (case 1-4).

Although bronchiolitis and poorly controlled reactive airways disease remain a consideration, the frequency of wheezing episodes and the recurrent pneumonia warrant further investigation. Cystic fibrosis should be excluded, particularly in light of the family history. The differential diagnosis also includes extrinsic obstructing lesions such as mediastinal lymphadenopathy, diaphragmatic hernia, and vascular ring. Intraluminal obstructing lesions can occur in this age group and include aspirated foreign body, bronchial papilloma or lipoma, and segmental bronchomalacia. The history of recurrent pneumonia may be a sign of underlying primary immunodeficiency—for example, an agammaglobulinemia, a dysgammaglobulinemia, or a phagocytic defect such as chronic granulomatous disease, which occasionally exhibits autosomal recessive inheritance. Infectious causes of recurrent or persistent pneumonia, such as *Coxiella burnetii* (Q fever), *Histoplasma capsulatum*, and *Mycobacterium tuberculosis*, are less likely in this age group.

II.   Diagnosis

On very direct questioning, her mother stated that the child's cough, although chronic, seemed worse when she drank liquids. This information, combined with a history of right middle lobe pneumonia, chronic cough, and recurrent wheezing, suggested chronic aspiration. The sweat test was negative, but the contrast esophagogram (Fig. 1-6) revealed filling of the trachea through a small esophageal fistula. **The diagnosis is TEF without esophageal atresia (H-type fistula).** In retrospect, this patient's symptomatic improvement at 11 months of age coincided with her transition from a predominantly liquid to predominantly solid diet.

III. Incidence and Epidemiology

TEF with or without esophageal atresia occurs as a congenital pulmonary abnormality in 1 of every 3,000 to 5,000 live births. The most common form of TEF, proximal esophageal atresia with distal TEF, occurs in 85% of cases of TEF. Communication between the trachea and esophagus with an otherwise normal esophagus, known as an H-type TEF, occurs in 3% to 5% of cases. Approximately 10% of cases of esophageal atresia are not associated with TEF.

The anomalies arise from defective differentiation of the primitive foregut into trachea and esophagus. The role of genetic factors is unclear; TEF has been described in siblings and identical twins. Autosomal dominant transmission has been reported in a few kindreds. Approximately 40% of infants with a TEF have associated congenital anomalies, usually cardiac or gastrointestinal, including anal atresia, pyloric stenosis, duodenal obstruction, and malrotation. One cluster of congenital abnormalities, the VATER association (*V*ertebral anomalies, *A*nal anomalies, *T*racheoesophageal fistula with *E*sophageal atresia, and *R*enal and *R*adial limb anomalies), is seen most often among infants of diabetic mothers.

IV. Clinical Presentation

Infants with TEF and esophageal atresia are symptomatic from birth. They accumulate large amounts of oral secretions, which precipitate coughing, choking, emesis, and respiratory distress. Abdominal distention results from accumulation of intestinal air via the TEF. A flat, gasless abdomen suggests esophageal atresia either without a TEF or with an obliterated TEF that still requires surgical repair.

Infants with an H-type TEF do not present in the neonatal period. Instead, their symptoms are mild or moderate and persistent. Symptoms in infants with H-type fistulas include coughing, choking, and cyanosis with feedings. Because the tracheoesophageal connection is small, these symptoms usually occur with liquid or formula feedings. There is no dysphagia. Children with H-type TEF may have improvement of their symptoms when they make the transition from formula to more solid foods. Many children have recurrent episodes of pneumonia or pneumonitis due to aspiration of gastrointestinal contents through the fistula. On examination, abdominal distention occurs after crying as air traverses through the fistula into the stomach. Diffuse wheezing may be related to aspiration.

V. Diagnostic Approach

Nasogastric tube placement and chest radiography. Esophageal atresia with or without TEF is easily detected by attempted passage of a radiopaque 5 Fr or 8 Fr nasogastric tube. The tube will coil in the proximal pouch and can be seen on chest radiograph. H-type TEF is more difficult to detect. Chest radiography may show evidence of recurrent pulmonary aspiration, particularly in the right upper or right middle lobe.

Contrast esophagogram. H-type TEF can be visualized by this technique, although the study must be carefully performed. As in this case, an H-type TEF may be missed on the initial study; therefore, a high level of suspicion is required.

Endoscopy. Endoscopic visualization may reveal an H-type TEF not demonstrated on the esophagogram. The tracheal aspect of the fistula is located in the upper third of the posterior tracheal wall and appears as a pit or crescent-shaped hole. Dyes (e.g., methylene blue) instilled into the trachea may be detected in the esophagus by endoscopy.

VI. Treatment

An H-type TEF requires surgical ligation. Esophageal atresia is treated with end-to-end or end-to-side anastomosis of the esophagus.

Tracheoesophageal fistula with esophageal atresia. Immediate postoperative complications include leakage at the anastomotic site causing mediastinitis or sepsis. Strictures at the anastomotic site may develop at any time and require repeated esophageal dilatation. Tracheomalacia at the fistula site is common and results in a brassy cough and impaired clearance of secretions. Esophageal dysmotility and GER are common.

Recurrence of the TEF occurs in 4% to 10% of cases. The manifestations of a recurrent TEF are similar to the presentation of children with H-type TEF. Recurrent TEFs do not close spontaneously; therefore, they also require surgical ligation. The survival rate is 95% among those patients with good respiratory function and no major congenital anomalies. The survival rate among infants with moderate pneumonia or congenital anomalies in addition to the TEF is approximately 70%. In a series of 82 patients with TEF and esophageal atresia, Holder and Ashcraft found that 79% of patients were alive and taking food by mouth 3 to 15 years postoperatively.

H-type tracheoesophageal fistula. Postoperative complications such as tracheomalacia, strictures, and mediastinitis are uncommon after repair of an H-type fistula. The prognosis in children with H-type fistula is excellent. Morbidity and mortality are related to the extent of chronic pulmonary disease in infants diagnosed later in life. Infants with multiple anomalies and those with severe respiratory disease have greater morbidity.

VII. References

1. Berseth CL. Disorders of the esophagus. In: Taeusch HW, Ballard RA, eds. *Avery's diseases of the newborn.* Philadelphia: WB Saunders, 1998:908–913.
2. Holder TM, Ashcraft KW. Developments in the care of patients with esophageal atresia and tracheoesophageal fistula. *Surg Clin North Am* 1981;61:1051–1061.
3. Lierl M. Congenital abnormalities. In: Hilman BC, ed. *Pediatric respiratory disease: diagnosis and treatment.* Philadelphia: WB Saunders, 1993:457–498.
4. Quan L, Smith DW. The VATER association: vertebral defects, anal atresia, T-E fistula with esophageal atresia, radial and renal dysplasia, a spectrum of associated defects. *J Pediatr* 1973;7:104–107.
5. Touloukian RJ, Pickett LK, Spackman T, et al. Repair of esophageal atresia by end-to-side anastomosis and ligation of the tracheoesophageal fistula: a critical review of 18 cases. *J Pediatr Surg* 1974;9:305–310.

Case 1-5: 5-Week-Old Boy

I. History of Present Illness

A 5-week-old Caucasian boy presented to the emergency department with worsening cough and respiratory difficulty. Two weeks before admission, he was evaluated by his primary physician for poor weight gain and periodic emesis. His weight of 3,050 g was the same as his birth weight. He had Hemoccult-positive stool and was diagnosed with cow's milk protein allergy. His formula was changed to a protein hydrolysate formula. One week before admission, his weight had increased to 3,100 g. However, he began having more frequent episodes of emesis. Three days before admission he developed a cough, tachypnea, and audible wheezing. He was evaluated at a nearby hospital, diagnosed with bronchiolitis, and treated with nebulized albuterol. His tachypnea had not improved despite receiving nebulized albuterol every 4 hours. His cough had increased in frequency. He was evaluated in the emergency department for worsening cough and continued tachypnea. The parents mentioned that the infant had always appeared dusky with crying, but this color change has occurred more frequently over the past few days. He had also had numerous episodes of posttussive emesis. Over the past 3 days, he had taken only 2 ounces of formula every 4 hours. The parents denied ill contacts, diarrhea, and lethargy. Both parents smoked, but only outside the home. There were no pets.

II. Past Medical History

He was born at 37 weeks' gestation after an uncomplicated pregnancy. The mother's group B *Streptococcus* colonization status was not known, so she received two doses of ampicillin before delivery. The infant's Apgar scores were 7 and 8 at 1 and 5 minutes, respectively. He had not previously required hospitalization.

III. Physical Examination

T, 37.7°C; RR, 60/min; BP, 78/37 mm Hg; HR 160 bpm; SpO_2, 88% in room air
Weight, 3.0 kg (less than 5th percentile); length, 49 cm (less than 5th percentile)

Physical examination revealed a cyanotic infant in moderate respiratory distress. The anterior fontanelle was open and flat. There was no conjunctival injection. There were no oral mucosal ulcerations. Capillary refill was brisk. The heart sounds were normal. Femoral pulses were palpable. There were intercostal retractions. Rales and wheezes were present diffusely. The liver edge was palpable 3 cm below the right costal margin. The remainder of the examination was normal.

IV. Diagnostic Studies

Laboratory analysis revealed 10,200 WBCs/mm³, with 76% segmented neutrophils, 19% lymphocytes, and 3% monocytes. The hemoglobin was 13.0 g/dL, and there were 350,000 platelets/mm³. Hepatic function panel was as follows: total bilirubin, 0.3 mg/dL; alanine aminotransferase, 32 U/L; aspartate aminotransferase, 66 U/L. The prothrombin and partial thromboplastin times and fibrinogen split products were normal. Blood cultures were obtained. Chest radiography revealed diffuse interstitial pulmonary edema but a normal cardiothymic silhouette.

V. Course of Illness

The patient was treated with ampicillin and cefotaxime for presumed bacterial sepsis. He also received nebulized albuterol. His respiratory status progressively worsened. An arterial blood gas analysis revealed the following: pH, 7.22; $PaCO_2$, 65 mm Hg; PaO_2, 45 mm Hg. The patient required endotracheal intubation. Electrocardiographic studies suggested a possible diagnosis (Fig. 1-7).

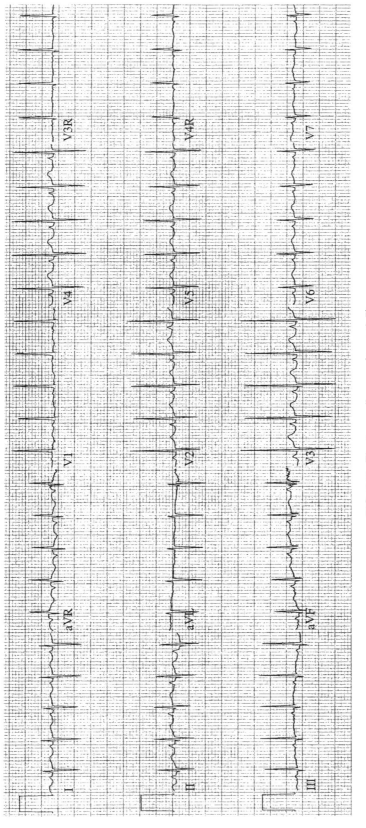

FIG. 1-7. Electrocardiogram (case 1-5).

DISCUSSION: CASE 1-5

I. Differential Diagnosis

In an infant with cyanosis and respiratory distress, bacterial or viral sepsis must be considered. Children with either viral bronchiolitis or pertussis may present with cyanosis, respiratory symptoms, and rapid deterioration. In this child, the history of periodic cyanosis with crying since birth provided a clue to the diagnosis. The differential diagnosis includes a large ventricular septal defect, patent ductus arteriosus, truncus arteriosus, atrioventricular canal, single ventricle without pulmonary stenosis, and total anomalous pulmonary venous connection (TAPVC). Except for TAPVC, these cardiac anomalies typically produce electrocardiographic evidence of left atrial or left ventricular hypertrophy. Children with TAPVC have right ventricular hypertrophy. The severity of illness warranted an echocardiogram, which provided the definitive diagnosis.

II. Diagnosis

The electrocardiogram (Fig. 1-7) revealed right axis deviation (QRS axis = 135°) and right ventricular hypertrophy. Echocardiography revealed a large and dilated right ventricle with a moderately hypoplastic left atrium and a patent foramen ovale. The pulmonary veins merged to form a common vein that drained into the portal venous system below the diaphragm (Fig. 1-8). No pulmonary veins entered the left atrium. There were no

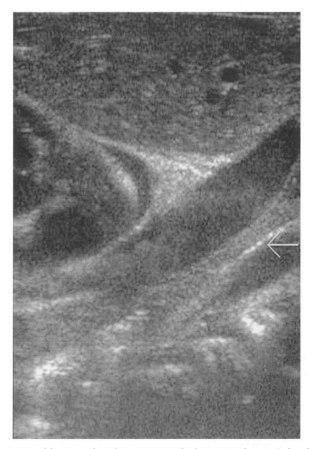

FIG. 1-8. Ultrasound image showing venous drainage to the portal vein (case 1-5).

other cardiac defects. **The echocardiographic findings confirmed the diagnosis of infradiaphragmatic TAPVC.**

III. Incidence and Epidemiology

TAPVC defines an anomaly in which there is no direct connection between the pulmonary veins and the left atrium. Instead, the pulmonary veins merge to form a common pulmonary vein that connects either to one of the systemic veins or directly to the right atrium. The malformation does not compromise fetal circulation during intrauterine life, because pulmonary arterial resistance is high and some blood flows to the systemic circulation through the patent foramen ovale. The combined systemic and pulmonary blood flow to the lungs is only mildly elevated. After birth, as pulmonary resistance falls, a progressively larger proportion of the mixed venous blood flows to the lungs, causing massive pulmonary overcirculation.

Several classification schemes have been proposed based on physiologic or prognostic implications of the anomalous connections. Generally, the connections are divided by whether the pulmonary veins merge with the coronary sinus of the right atrium (cardiac) or with the systemic venous circulation above the diaphragm (supracardiac) or below it (infradiaphragmatic). Approximately 75% of the connections are supracardiac, with the left innominate vein, coronary sinus, and superior vena cava serving as the most common anatomic sites of connection.

In TAPVC, because all venous blood ultimately returns to the right atrium, a communication between the right and left sides of the heart is necessary to sustain life. A patent foramen ovale or an atrial septal defect allows free communication between the two atria and, therefore, is considered part of the disorder. Other intracardiac anomalies occur in up to one third of cases and include common atrioventricular canal, transposition of the great arteries, tetralogy of Fallot, and hypoplastic left heart syndrome. TAPVC with drainage directly into the right atrium occurs in patients with visceral heterotaxy and polysplenia.

The incidence of TAPVC is not clear. TAPVC occurred in 2% of cases in an autopsy series of 800 children with congenital cardiac disease who died during the first year of life. TAPVC also occurred in 41 (1.5%) of 2,659 infants with cardiovascular malformations identified in the Baltimore-Washington Infant Study. Infradiaphragmatic TAPVC is more prevalent in boys (male:female ratio, 3:1). There is no sex prevalence in TAPVC with other sites of connection.

IV. Clinical Presentation

The clinical presentation of children with TAPVC depends on the presence or absence of pulmonary venous obstruction. Most children without obstruction present with tachypnea and failure to thrive, with gradually worsening cyanosis and congestive heart failure. Approximately 50% have symptoms during the first month of life, and the remainder during the first year. Cyanosis may be minimal initially, but it increases as congestive heart failure progresses. Cyanosis occurs because the pulmonary veins carry oxygenated blood to the systemic venous circulation instead of to the left atrium. Congestive heart failure occurs because of increased pulmonary blood flow and pulmonary hypertension. Hepatomegaly and peripheral edema often accompany cardiac failure. There is no cardiac murmur.

Obstruction is more common in children with infradiaphragmatic TAPVC because of venous compression as the common venous trunk passes through either the esophageal hiatus of the diaphragm or the portal venous circulation. Most children with infradiaphragmatic TAPVC, and one third of children with supracardiac TAPVC, present with pulmonary venous obstruction. These infants are usually asymptomatic at birth but develop symptoms within the first few weeks of life. Infants with pulmonary venous obstruction present with rapidly progressive dyspnea, pulmonary edema, cyanosis, and congestive heart failure.

Alteration in the character of the cry ("neonatal dysphonia") occurs in one fourth of infants with supracardiac TAPVC as a result of compression of the left recurrent laryngeal nerve as it passes the dilated common pulmonary vein. Infants with infradiaphragmatic TAPVC may have worsening cyanosis with swallowing, straining, and crying, as a consequence of interference with pulmonary venous outflow caused by increased intraabdominal pressure or impingement of the esophagus on the common pulmonary vein as it exits through the esophageal hiatus. The child in the presented case did not have pulmonary venous obstruction despite having infradiaphragmatic TAPVC. His history of cyanosis with crying is consistent with infradiaphragmatic TAPVC.

V. Diagnostic Approach

The diagnosis should be suspected on the basis of the clinical presentation.

Electrocardiogram. A tall peaked P wave in lead II or in the right precordial leads characterizes right atrial enlargement, a feature of TAPVC without obstruction. Right atrial enlargement is not usually present in TAPVC with obstruction, due to fulminant presentation very early in life. Right ventricular hypertrophy is manifested by high voltages in the right precordial leads. Right axis deviation is always present due to right-sided hypertrophy.

Chest roentgenogram. The lung fields reflect increased pulmonary blood flow. The cardiac silhouette may be normal, or right ventricular hypertrophy may be evident.

Echocardiography. The echocardiogram reveals signs of right ventricular volume overload. The right atrium is enlarged. The right ventricle is hypertrophied and dilated and compresses the intraventricular septum. The pulmonary arteries are dilated. The pulmonary veins are seen to form a common vein behind the heart. The size and orientation of the venous confluence are important for surgical planning. Associated intracardiac defects may be identified.

Cardiac catheterization. The accuracy of Doppler echocardiography precludes the routine need for diagnostic catheterization. Right ventricular pressures are usually equal to systemic pressures.

VI. Treatment

Complete surgical repair should be performed as early as possible. A large side-to-side anastomosis is created between the left atrium and the common pulmonary vein. Occasionally, the distal portion of the common pulmonary vein is ligated. The foramen ovale or atrial septal defect is closed. A hypoplastic left atrium may require surgical enlargement.

Residual stenosis at the left atrial-venous anastomosis created at operative repair develops in 10% of children. This stenosis requires reintervention and patch plasty. Postoperative pulmonary venous obstruction occurs 1 to 3 months after repair in 5% of patients. Late atrial arrhythmias develop in a small number of patients.

VII. References

1. Correa-Villasenor A, Ferencz C, Boughman JA, et al. Total anomalous pulmonary venous return: familial and environmental factors. The Baltimore-Washington infant study group. *Teratology* 1991;44:415–428.
2. Geva T, Van Praagh S. Anomalies of the pulmonary veins. In: Allen HD, Gutgesell HP, Clark EB, et al., eds. *Moss and Adams' heart disease in infants, children, and adolescents, including the fetus and young adult,* 6th ed. Philadelphia: Lippincott Williams & Wilkins, 2001:736–772.

3. Hyde JA, Stumper O, Barth MJ, et al. Total anomalous pulmonary venous connection: outcome of surgical correction and management of recurrent venous obstruction. *Eur J Cardiothorac Surg* 1999;15:735–740.

4. Michielon G, Di Donato RM, Pasquini L, et al. Total anomalous pulmonary venous connection: long-term appraisal with evolving technical solutions. *Eur J Cardiothoracic Surg* 2002;22:184–191.

5. Shankargouda S, Krishnan U, Murali R, et al. Dysphonia: a frequently encountered symptom in the evaluation of infants with unobstructed supracardiac total anomalous pulmonary venous connection. *Pediatr Cardiol* 2000;21:458–460.

Case 1-6: 4-Month-Old Boy

I. History of Present Illness

A 4-month-old African-American boy was well until 9 days before admission, when he developed fever to 38.9°C and a cough. Seven days before admission, he was evaluated by his primary physician and treated with ranitidine for suspected GER. Four days before admission, he developed tachypnea and grunting and received nebulized albuterol. On the day of admission he had continued fevers and worsening cough. His oral intake was poor. He had taken only 2 to 3 ounces of breast milk every 4 hours over the past day. His urine output was also decreased. Several family members had upper respiratory tract infections.

II. Past Medical History

He was born at 40 weeks' gestation after an uncomplicated pregnancy. He had received all of the appropriate immunizations for age, including the second dose of diphtheria-tetanus-alellular pertussis vaccine (DTaP). There was no family history of asthma or sickle cell disease.

III. Physical Examination

T, 37.0°C; RR, 76/min; HR, 120 bpm; BP, 102/72 mm Hg; SpO_2, 93% with 3 L O_2/min by nasal cannula

Weight, 10th to 25th percentile; length, 10th percentile; head circumference, 10th percentile

He was awake and alert. The anterior fontanelle was open and flat. He had flaring of the alae nasi. There were moderate intercostal, subcostal, and supraclavicular retractions. Scattered rhonchi were present, with diminished breath sounds at the bases bilaterally. There was no focal wheezing. The heart sounds were normal. The spleen was palpable just below the left costal margin. The remainder of the examination was normal.

IV. Diagnostic Studies

The WBC count was 10,200/mm³, with 15% band forms, 68% segmented neutrophils, and 12% lymphocytes. The hemoglobin was 10.3 g/dL, and the platelet count was 277,000/mm³. Arterial blood gas analysis revealed the following: pH, 7.42; $PaCO_2$, 30 mm Hg; and PaO_2, 90 mm Hg. Hepatic function panel revealed a total bilirubin of 0.3 mg/dL; alanine aminotransferase, 55 U/L; aspartate aminotransferase, 82 U/L, and lactate dehydrogenase, 3,280 U/L. No antigens to respiratory syncytial virus; parainfluenza types 1, 2, and 3; influenza A and B; or adenovirus were detected by immunofluorescence of nasopharyngeal aspirate. Serum immunoglobulin (Ig) results were as follows: IgA, 24 mg/dL (normal range, 27 to 73 mg/dL); IgM, 528 mg/dL (normal range, 37 to 124); and IgG, 650 mg/dL (normal range, 292 to 816 mg/dL).

V. Course of Illness

The patient was treated with nebulized albuterol and a racemic mixture of epinephrine without significant improvement in his respiratory status. An echocardiogram showed normal cardiac anatomy. The patient required endotracheal intubation for worsening respiratory distress. A chest radiograph suggested a diagnosis (Fig. 1-9).

DISCUSSION: CASE 1-6

I. Differential Diagnosis

The most common cause of progressive respiratory distress during infancy is bronchiolitis, which is most often caused by respiratory syncytial virus; adenovirus; influenza

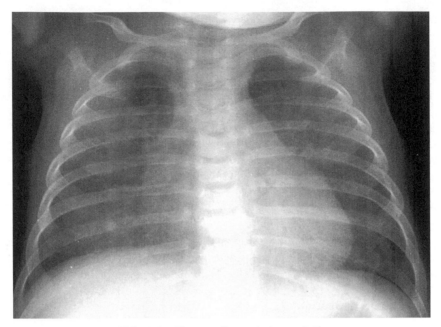

FIG. 1-9. Chest radiograph (case 1-6).

viruses A and B; or parainfluenza viruses types 1, 2, and 3. The differential diagnosis of perihilar or diffuse infiltrates includes *B. pertussis*, *C. trachomatis*, and *M. pneumoniae*. Herpes simplex virus and cytomegalovirus (CMV) can cause pneumonia in the young infant. CMV pneumonia is frequently associated with hepatosplenomegaly, thrombocytopenia, and lymphocytosis. PCP should be considered, particularly if there are maternal risk factors for HIV infection. Other conditions predisposing to PCP include primary B-cell defects, primary T-cell defects, and combined defects. The immune disorders most likely to result in PCP are severe combined immunodeficiency, DiGeorge anomaly, Wiskott-Aldrich syndrome, X-linked agammaglobulinemia, and hyper-IgM syndrome.

Noninfectious causes of pneumonia include GER associated with pulmonary aspiration. Occasionally, an anatomic defect such as TEF may predispose to aspiration. Primary cardiac abnormalities (e.g., ventricular septal defect), pulmonary vascular abnormalities, and impaired lymphatic flow (e.g., congenital lymphangiectasia) can cause tachypnea and progressive respiratory distress in a 4-month-old child. Cystic fibrosis can masquerade as any of these conditions.

II. Diagnosis

The chest radiograph (Fig. 1-9) revealed hazy, ground-glass opacities bilaterally. There was no pleural effusion. **The diagnosis of PCP was confirmed by Gomori methenamine silver staining of a specimen obtained by bronchoalveolar lavage (BAL).** The patient was treated with intravenous trimethoprim-sulfamethoxazole (TMP-SMX; 20 mg/kg per day trimethoprim component) and prednisone. He required ventilatory support for 5 days and made a gradual recovery. HIV DNA was detected in the patient's blood by polymerase chain reaction (PCR), confirming the underlying diagnosis of HIV.

III. Incidence and Epidemiology

P. carinii is an opportunistic parasite with some features of protozoa but greater genetic homology to fungi. Approximately 85% of immunocompetent children develop asymptomatic primary infection by 3 years of age. Severe PCP after primary infection occurs in immunocompromised infants and children.

The risk of PCP is related to the extent of immunosuppression and the use of chemoprophylaxis. PCP occurs in children with the acquired immunodeficiency syndrome (AIDS, 25% to 50%), severe combined immunodeficiency syndrome (25% to 50%), acute lymphocytic leukemia (10% to 20%), allogeneic bone marrow transplantation (5%), and organ transplantation (2% to 10%) if no chemoprophylaxis is given. Use of TMP-SMX prophylaxis reduces the PCP rate to less than 5% in HIV-infected children. Children receiving agents that impair cell-mediated immunity, including corticosteroids and cyclosporine, are at even greater risk of developing PCP. Patients with a history of PCP are at high risk for recurrence.

IV. Clinical Presentation

Infants with unrecognized HIV usually develop PCP between 2 and 6 months of age. A bronchiolitis-like illness occurs, with gradually worsening tachypnea and accessory muscle use. Physical examination reveals the absence of fever and a paucity of findings on auscultation. Rales and cyanosis develop as the illness progresses.

In older HIV-infected children, the spectrum of clinical manifestations varies. The symptoms may initially be mild and slowly progressive, delaying the diagnosis. High fevers are common. Findings on lung auscultation are often unimpressive compared with the degree of dyspnea, tachypnea (80 to 100/minute) and hypoxia. Scattered rales, rhonchi, or wheezes may be heard as the illness resolves. In children with an underlying non-AIDS immunodeficiency disorder such as leukemia or solid organ transplantation, the onset of symptoms occurs more abruptly than in HIV-infected children, but the physical examination findings are similar.

V. Diagnostic Approach

PCP should be considered in any immunocompromised patient with respiratory symptoms, fever, and an abnormal chest radiograph. The diagnosis should also be considered in any patient with risk factors for HIV infection. If the patient does not have a known predisposing condition, testing to exclude HIV and congenital immune deficiencies should be performed.

Chest roentgenogram. The chest radiograph typically shows bilateral alveolar disease, beginning in the perihilar region and progressing to the periphery. The chest radiograph may be normal in 10% of cases.

Examination of lower respiratory tract specimens. Definitive diagnosis requires demonstration of *P. carinii* in the pulmonary parenchyma or in lower respiratory tract secretions. Specimens should be stained with either Gomori silver or fluorescein-labeled antibody stains. The diagnostic yield of various procedures is as follows: induced sputum (in children older than 5 years of age), 20% to 40%; BAL, 75% to 95%; transbronchial biopsy, 75% to 95%; and open lung biopsy, 90% to 100%. The optimal procedure to obtain a specimen depends on many factors, including the age and clinical status of the patient. The traditional algorithm involves examination of induced sputum in those patients older than 5 years of age, followed by BAL if the sputum sample is negative. Open lung biopsy is reserved for patients with a nondiagnostic BAL. Children younger than 5 years of age should undergo BAL initially.

PCR, although still under investigation, may allow diagnosis with fewer invasive procedures. PCR analysis of oral washes shows a sensitivity of 80% compared with results of concomitant BAL.

Serum lactate dehydrogenase. Rising serum lactate dehydrogenase (LDH) reflects lung injury. Increased serum LDH, although common in children with PCP, is a nonspecific finding.

Other studies. Additional studies should be performed to diagnose alternative or concomitant respiratory conditions. Nasopharyngeal aspirates, sputum, or BAL specimens should be sent for immunofluorescent viral antigen detection (respiratory syncytial virus, influenza, parainfluenza, and adenovirus), viral culture, CMV shell vial culture, and *Mycoplasma* PCR.

Extrapulmonary involvement due to *P. carinii* is rare, but potential sites of dissemination include the lymph nodes, spleen, retina, thyroid, gastrointestinal tract, and adrenal glands. Routine radiologic imaging to exclude extrapulmonary manifestations of *P. carinii* is not necessary.

VI. Treatment

TMP-SMX remains the treatment of choice for PCP in children. The oral route may be used in mild cases, if the patient can reliably take and retain oral medication. Most children require intravenous treatment. The course of treatment is 14 to 21 days. If no improvement is demonstrated in 5 to 7 days, treatment should be changed to pentamidine. Pentamidine, atovaquone, or primaquine plus clindamycin may be used for children who are unable to tolerate TMP-SMX. Adjunctive therapy with corticosteroids reduces the occurrence of respiratory failure and improves oxygenation in moderately ill adults with PCP; limited data in children suggest similar benefits.

Children with an episode of PCP require posttreatment prophylaxis with TMP-SMX (5 mg/kg per day), either daily or three days per week for the duration of risk (indefinitely for those with HIV). Because of the high risk of acquiring PCP during the first year of life, all infants born to HIV-infected mothers require PCP prophylaxis from 4 weeks to 12 months of age, regardless of their CD4-positive T-lymphocyte count; prophylaxis may be discontinued sooner if HIV infection is excluded. After 12 months of age, prophylaxis is required if the percentage of CD4+ T cells is less than 15% or if the CD4+ count is less than 500 cells/μL (less than 200 cells/μL in those older than 5 years of age). Patients in other high-risk groups, including those with severe combined immune deficiency, lymphoproliferative malignancy, and organ transplantation, also require PCP prophylaxis.

VII.   References

1. Grubman S, Simonds RJ. Preventing *Pneumocystis carinii* pneumonia in human immunodeficiency virus-infected children: new guidelines for prophylaxis. *Pediatr Infect Dis J* 1996;15:165–168.
2. Hughes WT, Rivera GK, Schell MJ, et al. Successful intermittent chemoprophylaxis for *Pneumocystis carinii* pneumonia. *N Engl J Med* 1987;316:1627–1632.
3. Hughes WT. *Pneumocystis carinii* pneumonia. *Semin Pediatr Infect Dis* 2001;12: 309–314.
4. Kovacs JA, Gill VJ, Meshnick S, et al. New insights into transmission, diagnosis, and drug treatment of *Pneumocystis carinii* pneumonia. *JAMA* 2001;386:2450–2460.
5. Opravil M, Marincek B, Fuchs WA, et al. Shortcomings of chest radiography in detection *Pneumocystis carinii* pneumonia. *J Acquir Immune Defic Syndr Hum Retrovirol* 1994;7:39–45.
6. Vargas SL, Hughes WT, Santolaya ME, et al. Search for primary infection by *Pneumocystis carinii* in a cohort of normal, healthy infants. *Clin Infect Dis* 2001;32: 855–861.
7. Thea DM, Genevieve L, Weedon J, et al. Benefit of primary prophylaxis before 18 months of age in reducing the incidence of *Pneumocystis carinii* pneumonia and early death in a cohort of 112 human immunodeficiency virus-infected infants. *Pediatrics* 1996;97:59–64.

2

Decreased Activity Level

Phillip Spandorfer

APPROACH TO THE PATIENT WITH DECREASED ACTIVITY LEVEL

I. Definition of the Complaint

The term *decreased activity level* potentially describes a wide spectrum of existence ranging from boredom to coma. Encouraging parents to provide a detailed account, particularly with regard to the magnitude and time course of the changes, focuses the diagnostic evaluation. Clearly, the differential diagnosis of subtle behavioral changes developing over several months differs from that of changes occurring over several hours.

II. Complaint by Cause and Frequency

The cause of decreased activity level in children varies by age (Table 2-1). The etiology of decreased activity level can also be placed into several broad categories (Table 2-2). Additional issues to consider include whether there is depressed sensorium indicating an underlying central nervous system (CNS) disorder, weakness indicating a muscular disorder, or endurance problems suggesting a cardiac or pulmonary issue. Systemic illness may manifest with somnolence or lethargy.

III. Clarifying Questions

The patient who presents for evaluation of decreased activity level represents a broad differential. Several important historical questions can help to classify the etiology.

TABLE 2-1. *Differential Diagnosis of Decreased Activity by Age*

Prevalence	Neonate/infant	School age child	Adolescent
Common	Anemia Neonatal infection Hypoglycemia Ingestion Congenital heart defect	Anemia Lack of sleep Obesity Hypoglycemia Ingestion Boredom Depression	Anemia Lack of sleep Obesity Pregnancy Infectious mononucleosis Hypoglycemia Ingestion Boredom Depression
Uncommon	Intussusception Polycythemia Hypothyroidism CHF Pericarditis Uremia RTA	Intussusception CHF Pericarditis Uremia RTA JRA	Adrenal insufficiency Hypothyroidism CHF Pericarditis Uremia RTA Myasthenia gravis Chronic fatigue syndrome Inflammatory bowel disease JRA

CHF, congestive heart failure; JRA, juvenile rheumatoid arthritis; RTA, renal tubular acidosis.

TABLE 2-2. *Differential Diagnosis of Decreased Activity Level by Etiology*

Diagnostic category	Disease
Infectious	Mononucleosis
	Hepatitis
	Human immunodeficiency virus
	Lyme disease
	Cytomegalovirus
	Meningitis
	Encephalitis
	Bacteremia
	Histoplasmosis
	Toxoplasmosis
	Brucellosis
	Intestinal parasites
Neurologic	Seizure
	Stroke
	Intracranial injury
	Vasculitis
	Migraine
Muscular	Myasthenia gravis
Cardiac	Congenital heart disease
	Congestive heart failure
	Pericarditis
	Endocarditis
	Cardiomyopathy
Hematologic	Anemia
Gastrointestinal	Intussusception
	Inflammatory bowel disease
	Liver disease
Pulmonary	Asthma
	Cystic fibrosis
	Sleep apnea
	Primary pulmonary hypertension
Toxicologic	Lead poisoning
	Hypoglycemic agents
	Sedative/hypnotic agents
	Antihistamines
	Anticonvulsants
	Opiates
Psychologic	Depression
Rheumatologic	Systemic lupus erythematosus
	Juvenile rheumatoid arthritis
	Sarcoidosis
	Dermatomyositis
	Chronic fatigue syndrome
	Fibromyalgia
Allergic	Seasonal allergies
Endocrine	Diabetes mellitus
	Hypothyroidism
	Hyperthyroidism
	Adrenocortical insufficiency
	Cushing syndrome
	Primary aldosteronism
Metabolic	Hypoglycemia
	Inborn errors of metabolism
Renal	Uremia
	Renal tubular acidosis

- What time course has the decreased activity level presented?

  — Infectious etiologies typically manifest over a shorter time course than do other etiologies such as iron deficiency anemia or CNS malignancy.

- Is the patient febrile?

  — Fever frequently can cause a decreased level of activity. Often a fever raises the possibility of an infectious etiology. However, neonates younger than about 8 weeks of age do not always mount a fever in response to an infection. In fact, they can occasionally become hypothermic.

- What activities are involved?

  — If the decreased activity level is related to physical exertion, then cardiac or pulmonary disease might be the etiology. In neonates, feeding constitutes physical exertion. In older children, if the decreased activity level affects school attendance, one must assess whether there is secondary gain.

- Is there a history of decreased intake or increased output?

  — Children are at a high risk for hypoglycemia because they have an increased metabolic demand for glucose and decreased stores of glycogen. If they experience decreased oral intake or increased output caused by vomiting or diarrhea, they may become hypoglycemic.

- Has there been a change in school performance or other behaviors?

  — Depression can manifest with a decreased level of activity and is usually associated with decreased school performance and changes in behavior.

- Is there any history of trauma?

  — Intracranial bleeding precipitated by accidental or intentional trauma may be the cause of depressed mental status and hence a decreased level of activity.

- Is there any reason to suspect nonaccidental trauma?

  — Child abuse can manifest in many ways and is often unsuspected. If there has been a delay in seeking care for the child, or if the history does not correlate well with the physical examination findings, there should be concern for possible child abuse. Any obvious marks on the child should also raise the clinician's concern for child abuse.

- Is there a history of ingestion?

  — Toxins frequently alter mental status in children. The mechanism may be sedation (hypnotic agents, opiates) or hypoglycemia (oral hypoglycemic agents).

- Is there any history of abdominal pain or vomiting?

  — Intussusception can manifest with depressed mental status in a child between 6 months and 5 years of age.

Case 2-1: 15-Year-Old Girl

I. History of Present Illness

A 15-year-old girl presented to the emergency department with a 3-month history of increasing fatigue. She had gradually stopped participating in sports because of dizziness and palpitations. Her decreased level of activity had worsened to the point that as soon as she returned home from school in the afternoon she went to bed and slept the rest of the day. She had had an 18-pound weight loss over the 3-month period. In addition, for the past 5 days she had had a headache and occasional nonbloody, nonbilious emesis. For the past 4 days she had also had mild upper abdominal pain. The remainder of her history and review of systems were noncontributory.

II. Past Medical History

She was the product of a full-term delivery and had had no major medical illnesses. She had not required any surgeries.

III. Physical Examination

T, 37.2°C; RR, 16/min; HR, 110 bpm; BP, 100/60 mm Hg

Weight and height, 25th percentile

On examination, she appeared pale and tired but was not toxic-appearing. She answered questions appropriately. The head and neck examination revealed pale conjunctiva. She did not have any papilledema. Her lungs were clear to auscultation. Cardiac examination revealed tachycardia but no murmurs or other abnormal heart sounds. Her abdomen was soft with normal bowel sounds. There was no hepatosplenomegaly. Capillary refill was delayed at 3 seconds. Her neurologic examination was normal. Of particular interest, her cranial nerve examination and motor strength were normal.

IV. Diagnostic Studies

A complete blood count revealed a white blood cell (WBC) count of 2,100 cells/mm^3, including 3% bands, 45% segmented neutrophils, and 51% lymphocytes. Hemoglobin was 5.4 g/dL, and the platelet count was 173,000/mm^3. The mean corpuscular volume (MCV) was elevated at 98.7 fL.

V. Course of Illness

The patient was hospitalized for evaluation of her severe anemia. The peripheral blood smear provided a clue to the diagnosis (Fig. 2-1).

DISCUSSION: CASE 2-1

I. Differential Diagnosis

This patient had a significant anemia. There are several categories of anemia. The anemia could be caused by a nutritional deficit (e.g., iron, folic acid, vitamin B_{12}). It could be caused by a hemoglobinopathy (e.g., sickle cell anemia, thalassemia). The anemia could also be the result of a hemolytic process such as hereditary spherocytosis or glucose-6-phosphate dehydrogenase deficiency. Finally, the anemia could result from a hypoplastic or aplastic crisis.

When evaluating anemia, it is easiest to arrive at the correct diagnosis by assessing the hematologic indices, specifically the MCV. If the MCV is low, the anemia is a microcytic anemia and causes such as iron deficiency anemia, lead poisoning, anemia of chronic disease, and thalassemias should be considered. If the MCV is normal, chronic disease, hypoplastic or aplastic crisis, malignancy, renal failure, acute hemorrhage, and hemolytic

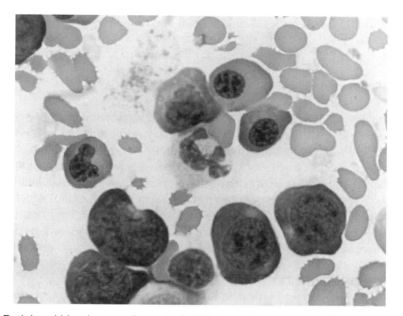

FIG. 2-1. Peripheral blood smear (case 2-1). (Photograph courtesy of Marybeth Helfrich, MT, ASCP.)

processes should be considered. Finally, if the MCV is high, the megaloblastic anemias should be evaluated, specifically folate deficiency and vitamin B_{12} deficiency, as well as some of the aplastic anemias.

II. Diagnosis

This patient had a macrocytic anemia, as indicated by an elevated MCV of 98.7 fL. A hypersegmented neutrophil is located in the center of the peripheral blood smear in Fig. 2-1. In the lower portion of the figure are several megaloblasts with a loose-appearing nuclear chromatin. Also noted are numerous misshapen mature erythrocytes, reflecting the mechanical fragility associated with megaloblastic anemias. As the appropriate next step, serum levels of folate and vitamin B_{12} were measured. The folate level was 8.2 ng/mL (normal range, 2 to 20 ng/mL). The vitamin B_{12} level was less than 100 pg/mL (normal range, 200 to 1,100 pg/mL). On further questioning, the patient stated that she had been a strict vegetarian for the past 2 years and had eaten no meat or animal-based products. Additionally, she did not take vitamin supplements and did not attempt to eat non-meat-based foods containing vitamin B_{12}, such as fortified cereal and fortified meat analogs (e.g., wheat gluten, soy products). **The diagnosis is dietary vitamin B_{12} deficiency.**

III. Incidence and Epidemiology

To be absorbed, dietary vitamin B_{12} must combine with a glycoprotein (intrinsic factor), which is secreted from the gastric fundus. The vitamin B_{12}–intrinsic factor complex then is absorbed at the terminal ileum via specific receptor mechanisms. Vitamin B_{12} is present in many foods, and a pure dietary deficiency is rare. However, it may be seen in patients who do not eat any milk, eggs, or animal products (vegans). Vitamin B_{12} deficiency can also result from lack of secretion of intrinsic factor in the stomach. When the cause of the lack of intrinsic factor is chronic atrophic gastritis, this condition is referred to as pernicious anemia. Other causes of vitamin B_{12} deficiency include surgical resection of the terminal ileum, regional enteritis of the terminal ileum, overgrowth of intestinal bacteria, disruption of the B_{12}–intrinsic factor complex, abnormalities or absence of the receptor site in the terminal ileum, and inborn errors in the metabolism of vitamin B_{12}.

IV.   Clinical Presentation

Vitamin B_{12} plays an important role as a cofactor for two metabolic reactions: methylation of homocysteine to methionine and conversion of methylmalonyl coenzyme A (CoA) to succinyl CoA. Vitamin B_{12} deficiency leads to accumulation of these precursors. Methionine is an important step in the synthesis of DNA. In individuals with vitamin B_{12} deficiency, RNA and cytoplasmic components are produced normally, and red blood cell (RBC) production in the bone marrow yields large cells and, hence, a macrocytic anemia. Methionine is also converted to S-adenosylmethionine, which is used in methylation reactions in the CNS; therefore, CNS effects are seen with vitamin B_{12} deficiency. Neurologic manifestations in children include abnormalities such as paresthesias, loss of developmental milestones, hypotonia, seizures, dementia, and depression. The neurologic changes are not always reversible.

V.   Diagnostic Approach

Complete blood count and folic acid and vitamin B_{12} levels. The term *megaloblastic anemia* refers to a macrocytic anemia usually accompanied by a mild leukopenia or thrombocytopenia. The presence of a macrocytic anemia with normal folic acid levels and low vitamin B_{12} levels is diagnostic for most vitamin B_{12} deficiencies. However, reliance on abnormal hemoglobin may miss up to 30% of adult cases of vitamin B_{12} deficiency. On peripheral blood smear, there are numerous schistocytes and misshapen mature RBCs due to the increased mechanical RBC fragility associated with this condition. Erythroid precursors have loose-appearing chromatin, giving them a characteristic appearance. Hypersegmented or multilobar neutrophils may also be noted. The appearance of at least one neutrophil with more than six lobes, or more than five neutrophils with more than five lobes, is considered significant. In vitamin B_{12} deficiency, serum levels of homocysteine and methylmalonyl CoA may be elevated, assisting in the diagnosis. Levels of methylmalonic acid (MMA), a precursor to methylmalonyl CoA, may be elevated as well.

Other studies. After the diagnosis of vitamin B_{12} deficiency has been made, further studies can be performed to identify the cause. Specifically, a comprehensive dietary assessment, evaluation for parasitic infections, a Schilling test (which measures the ability to absorb orally ingested vitamin B_{12}), amino acid analysis, measurement of the unsaturated B_{12} binding capacity and transcobalamin II levels, genetic evaluation, and measurement of antibodies to parietal cells and intrinsic factor may be performed. Subspecialty consultation is often required to assist with the diagnosis.

VI.   Treatment

Treatment of vitamin B_{12} deficiency depends on the cause. Frequently, vitamin B_{12} administration is necessary. If the anemia is severe, treatment should be instituted slowly and in a monitored environment. For malabsorptive causes, long-term treatment is indicated. The recommended treatment is monthly injections of 100 µg of vitamin B_{12}. Monitoring of the clinical response and laboratory values enables the clinician to titrate treatment to the patient's response. It is not known whether folic acid therapy in patients who have vitamin B_{12} deficiency will worsen the neurologic symptoms of the vitamin B_{12} deficiency; it may mask the hematologic symptoms of the megaloblastic anemia. In this case, the patient received a vitamin B_{12} injection and then began oral multivitamin and vitamin B_{12} supplementation. She also received nutritional counseling to help her create a nutritionally balanced vegan diet.

VII. References

1. O'Grady LF. The megaloblastic anemias. In: Keopke JA, ed. *Laboratory hematology*. New York: Churchill Livingstone, 1984:71–83.
2. Rasmussen SA, Fernhoff PM, Scanlon KS. Vitamin B_{12} deficiency in children and adolescents. *J Pediatr* 2001;138:10–17.
3. Snow CF. Laboratory diagnosis of vitamin B_{12} and folate deficiency: a guide for the primary care physician. *Arch Intern Med* 1999;159:1289–1298.
4. Toh BH, van Driel IR, Gleeson PA. Pernicious anemia. *N Engl J Med* 1997;337:1441–1448.
5. Whitehead VM, Rosenblatt DS, Cooper BA. Megaloblastic anemia. In: Nathan DG, Orkin SA, eds. *Nathan and Oski's hematology of infancy and childhood,* 5th ed. Philadelphia: WB Saunders, 1998:385–422.

Case 2-2: 2-Week-Old Boy

I. History of Present Illness

A 16-day-old male infant presented to the emergency department with a 24-hour history of decreased level of activity. Breast-feeding had not been going well since birth, but he had been breast-feeding even less than usual for the past several days. The infant received cow's milk-based formula supplementation 2 days before presentation because of the difficulty with breast-feeding. The incident that prompted the emergency department visit was a 2-second choking episode during a feed. The incident occurred at the beginning of the feed, and the infant's eyes appeared to "roll into the back of his head." The parents denied tonic-clonic or jerking activity and color change, although the child was less active after this episode. The infant had had decreased urine output, with only one wet diaper in the preceding 24 hours.

II. Past Medical History

This infant was born after 36 weeks of gestation, the fourth child of a 28-year-old mother. The pregnancy was complicated by preterm labor, and the mother received magnesium tocolysis. At 36 weeks, the magnesium was stopped and labor was allowed to progress. Delivery was uncomplicated. Maternal prenatal laboratory and culture results were reportedly normal. The child was discharged from the hospital on the second day of life.

III. Physical Examination

T, 37.5°C; RR, 32/min; HR, 142 bpm; BP, 95/65 mm Hg

Weight and height, 5th percentile

On examination, he appeared awake but hypotonic. He was thin-appearing and cried only with stimulation. His anterior fontanel was sunken, and his lips and mucous membranes were dry. He had decreased tear production. His lungs were clear. The cardiac examination revealed a normal rate and rhythm without any murmur or abnormal heart sounds. His abdomen was soft without any organomegaly. His extremities were cool, with a 2-second capillary refill time. Both testicles were descended. His neurologic examination revealed no focal abnormalities.

IV. Diagnostic Studies

The WBC count was 16,300 cells/mm^3, with 38% segmented neutrophils, 54% lymphocytes, and 6% monocytes. The hemoglobin was 18.2 g/dL. The platelet count was 658,000/mm^3. The results of the basic metabolic panel revealed the following: sodium, 115 mEq/L; potassium, 7.7 mEq/L; chloride, 81 mEq/L; bicarbonate, 16 mEq/L; blood urea nitrogen, 31 mg/dL; creatinine, 1.0 mg/dL; glucose, 89 mg/dL; and calcium, 10.7 mg/dL. The serum ammonia level was 39 μg/dL. Lumbar puncture revealed 1 WBC/mm^3. The cerebrospinal fluid (CSF) glucose and protein concentrations were normal. Cultures of CSF, blood, and urine were obtained.

V. Course of Illness

The infant was treated with ampicillin and cefotaxime empirically due to his ill appearance. He was admitted to the neonatal intensive care unit for further evaluation. Careful consideration of the laboratory findings suggested a diagnosis.

DISCUSSION: CASE 2-2

I. Differential Diagnosis

Hyponatremia with hyperkalemia in a 2-week-old infant is most concerning for congenital adrenal hyperplasia (CAH). Other causes of electrolyte abnormalities in a young infant include water intoxication, gastroenteritis, and inappropriate formula preparation. If an ill-appearing infant presents primarily with vomiting, pyloric stenosis and malrotation should be included in the differential diagnosis. The choking incident provided in the history could also indicate an episode of gastroesophageal reflux or a seizure.

II.   Diagnosis

The laboratory pattern was consistent with CAH. Additional laboratory evaluation revealed a markedly increased concentration of 17-hydroxyprogesterone (greater than 120,000 ng/dL; normal range, 4 to 200 ng/dL), which is a precursor for 21-hydroxylase enzyme. Additionally, the concentration of corticotropin (ACTH) was markedly elevated at 541pg/ml (normal range, 9 to 52). This child is a male infant who is presenting with a salt-wasting form of CAH. **The diagnosis is 21-hydroxylase deficiency.**

III.   Incidence and Epidemiology

The adrenal gland is responsible for the production of three categories of steroids: mineralocorticoids, glucocorticoids (cortisol), and androgens (dehydroepiandrosterone, androstenedione, 11-β-hydroxyandrostenedione, and testosterone). CAH is a category of autosomal recessive disorders that result in deficiency of an enzyme necessary for cortisol synthesis. Depending on the location of the blockade, excesses or deficiencies of the mineralocorticoids and androgens can occur.

Cortisol deficiency results in increased production of ACTH by the anterior pituitary gland and subsequent hyperplasia of the adrenal cortex. Severity of illness depends on the severity of the genetic mutation. The incidence of CAH ranges from 1 in 5,000 to 1 in 15,000 live births. Although several enzyme deficiencies can result in CAH, 90% to 95% of cases are due to lack of 21-hydroxylase, and 4% are due to 11-β-hydroxylase deficiency. Other rare enzyme defects that have been described include 3-β-hydroxysteroid dehydrogenase deficiency, 17-α-hydroxylase deficiency, and cholesterol side chain cleavage enzyme deficiency.

IV.   Clinical Presentation

There are several clinical forms of presentation for CAH. Androgen excess results in virilization. In the female, there is usually some degree of clitoromegaly and labial fusion, but the female internal genital organs are normal. Mineralocorticoid deficiency results in an inability to exchange potassium for sodium in the distal tubule of the nephron; hence, there is sodium loss in the urine and an inability to secrete potassium. This electrolyte abnormality is referred to as salt wasting. Patients with the salt-wasting type of CAH become symptomatic shortly after birth. They have progressive weight loss, dehydration, and vomiting. If the condition is not recognized, death occurs within a few weeks.

Girls with virilization tend to be diagnosed at birth due to their ambiguous genitalia. Boys may be diagnosed at 1 to 2 weeks of life if they present with a salt-wasting type of CAH or at about 4 years of age if they present with premature development of secondary sexual characteristics.

The two most common forms of CAH, 21-hydroxylase deficiency and 11-β-hydroxylase deficiency, result in virilization. Approximately 75% of the 21-hydroxylase deficiencies also cause salt wasting; however, 25% of patients present with virilization alone. Patients with 11-β-hydroxylase deficiency do not have salt wasting, but they develop hypertension after the first few years of life.

The 3-β-hydroxysteroid dehydrogenase defect causes salt wasting and mild virilization. Patients with the cholesterol side chain cleavage enzyme defect present with salt wasting and female phenotype.

V. Diagnostic Approach

There are several tests to assess for CAH.

Serum electrolytes. Hyponatremia and hyperkalemia, although not diagnostic, are often the laboratory abnormalities that prompt further investigation.

Other studies. In classic 21-hydroxylase deficiency, serum levels of 17-hydroxyprogesterone are markedly elevated. Interpretation of 17-hydroxyprogesterone levels in neonates is difficult, because this hormone may be increased in sick or premature infants and also in healthy infants during the first 2 days of life. Cortisol levels are typically low in patients with the salt-wasting variety and normal in patients with virilization. In 11-hydroxylase deficiency, the levels of 11-deoxycorticosterone and 11-deoxycortisol are increased. The 3-β-hydroxysteroid dehydrogenase defect causes levels of 17-hydroxypregnenolone as well as 17-hydroxyprogesterone to be elevated and hence may be confused with 21-hydroxylase deficiency.

VI. Treatment

Administration of glucocorticoids inhibits excessive production of androgens. The most frequently recommended glucocorticoid is hydrocortisone administered orally. Dosages should be individualized based on growth and hormone levels. The administration of exogenous glucocorticoids continues indefinitely. Children with CAH require higher doses of glucocorticoids during periods of stress, such as illness, infection, or surgery.

If the patient also has salt wasting, then mineralocorticoid replacement and sodium supplementation are also required. Florinef (9-α-fluorocortisol) is the currently recommended mineralocorticoid.

Determination of the sex of a neonate with ambiguous genitalia is important. If a girl has clitoromegaly, surgical correction can reposition the clitoris under the pubis to achieve a more normal appearance. Because CAH is an autosomal recessive disorder, it is important to test siblings of affected patients.

VII. References

1. Laue L, Rennert OM. Congenital adrenal hyperplasia: molecular genetics and alternative approaches to treatment. *Adv Pediatr* 1995;42:113–143.
2. Lim YJ, Batch JA, Warne GL. Adrenal 21-hydroxylase deficiency in childhood: 25 years' experience. *J Paediatr Child Health* 1995;31:222–227.
3. White PC, New MI, Dupont B. Congenital adrenal hyperplasia [first of two parts]. *N Engl J Med* 1987;316:1519–1524.
4. White, PC, New, MI, Dupont, B. Congenital adrenal hyperplasia [second of two parts]. *N Engl J Med* 1987;316:1580–1586.

Case 2-3: 3-Month-Old Girl

I. History of Present Illness

A 3-month-old female infant presented to the emergency department with a 1-week history of increasing fussiness. Three days before admission, the infant developed poor breast-feeding and weak suck. Although the number of wet diapers had not changed, they were less saturated after the poor feeding. The parents related that the child's cry was not as loud as usual. The child had had no bowel movement during the previous 4 days. The child was evaluated by her pediatrician and referred to the emergency department. There was no history of fever, vomiting, or diarrhea, and there had been no ill contacts.

II. Past Medical History

The child had been healthy until the past week. Pregnancy and delivery were uncomplicated. There was a family history of pyloric stenosis in the father. A 2-year-old sibling was healthy.

III. Physical Examination

T, 37.4°C; RR, 30/min; HR, 156 bpm; BP, 100/80 mm Hg

Weight and height, 50th percentile

On examination she was alert but had a weak cry. Her head and neck examination was remarkable for bilateral ptosis and decreased facial expression. Cardiac and pulmonary examinations were normal. Her abdomen was distended but soft. On neurologic examination, she had a weak gag and poor tone. Her deep tendon reflexes were intact.

IV. Diagnostic Studies

Laboratory testing revealed a WBC count of 10,100 cells/mm^3, with 33% segmented neutrophils, 56% lymphocytes, and 8% monocytes. Hemoglobin was 11.7 g/dL; platelets, 490,000/mm^3; sodium, 139 mmol/L; potassium, 4.9 mmol/L; chloride, 106 mmol/L; carbon dioxide, 18 mmol/L; blood urea nitrogen, 12 mg/dL; creatinine, 0.3 mg/dL; and glucose, 58 mg/dL. A negative inspiratory force was measured at 20 cm H$_2$O.

V. Course of Illness

Intravenous glucose and normal saline were administered in the emergency department. The patient ultimately required endotracheal intubation due to inability to protect her airway. Her appearance combined with historical features suggested a diagnosis that was confirmed by additional testing.

DISCUSSION: CASE 2-3

I. Differential Diagnosis

The diagnostic possibilities in this child with decreased activity and hypotonia include neurologic conditions that involve either the upper motor neuron (cerebral cortex and spinal cord) or the lower motor neuron (anterior horn cell, peripheral nerve, neuromuscular junction, or muscle). Upper motor neuron diseases, such as stroke, hemorrhage, trauma, oncologic processes, tethered cord, epidural abscess, and transverse myelitis, are possibilities. Lower motor diseases include poliomyelitis, spinal muscular atrophy, ascending Guillain-Barré syndrome, heavy metal poisoning, congenital myasthenia gravis, paralysis, botulism, organophosphate poisoning, inflammatory myopathy, and muscular dystrophies. Infectious etiologies such as overwhelming sepsis, meningitis, and metabolic encephalopathies should be considered. Ingestions can cause weakness, particularly ingestion of barbiturates. Inborn errors of metabolism should be considered as well. Chromosomal disorders such as Down syndrome, Prader-Willi syndrome, achondroplasia, familial dysautonomia, and trisomy 13 may manifest with hypotonia as an early clinical feature. The history of weakness, decreased feeding, weak cry, and constipation is a classic presentation of infant botulism.

II. Diagnosis

The infant had significant hypotonia but was not tachycardic or hypotensive. An electromyogram (EMG) was obtained to assist with confirmation of the suspected diagnosis of infantile botulism. The EMG revealed a 56% incremental response that is consistent with a presynaptic neuromuscular junction disorder. The pattern is consistent with infantile botulism. Furthermore, stool studies isolated the botulinum toxin, type B. **The diagnosis of infant botulism was made.**

III. Incidence and Epidemiology

Infantile botulism occurs after the ingestion of botulinal spores. Spores then germinate in the intestine, and the organism, *Clostridium botulinum*, produces toxin. The botulinal toxin prevents the release of acetylcholine at the neuromuscular junction. The acidity of the infant's stomach is not great enough to kill the ingested spores. Spores are frequently found in honey and soil. The adult form of the illness occurs after ingestion of preformed toxin. Although the disease has been reported in all 50 states, it is more common in Pennsylvania, Hawaii, California, Utah, and Arizona. A significant number of the infants with infant botulism are breast-fed infants. It is possible that breast-fed infants develop different intestinal microflora than formula-fed infants, making them more susceptible to disease.

IV. Clinical Presentation

The average age at onset is 10 weeks, with a range of 10 days to 7 months. Patients typically present to medical attention with constipation, poor feeding, irritability, and weakness. Approximately 1 week after the onset of symptoms, additional neurologic symptoms are seen, such as facial diplegia, weak suck, poor gag, and hypotonia. On physical examination, patients have progressive weakness, as manifested by ptosis, poor head control, and diminished suck, gag, and respiratory effort. The paralysis progresses in a descending fashion. Seventy percent of patients with infantile botulism have respiratory failure that necessitates mechanical ventilation. Patients also have autonomic dysfunction, manifested by decreased intestinal motility, distended urinary bladder, decreased tear production, decreased saliva production, periodic flushing and sweating, and fluctuations in heart rate and blood pressure. Reflexes are diminished. Other complications include syndrome of inappropriate secretion of antidiuretic hormone (SIADH) and urinary tract infections.

V. Diagnostic Approach

Typically, the diagnosis is made on a clinical basis from the history and physical examination findings.

Electromyography. EMG can be helpful in making the diagnosis, particularly if an incremental response is found. Brief, small-amplitude, overly abundant motor unit potentials suggest the diagnosis of infant botulism.

Stool studies. Although results of stool testing are not immediately available, the test is helpful to confirm the diagnosis by detection of botulinum toxin.

VI. Treatment

The mainstay of treatment is supportive care. Most children require nasogastric tube feedings. Anticipation of complications such as respiratory failure, urinary retention, and SIADH are critical. Although there may be a role for augmentation of intestinal motility to help remove botulinal spores, there is no clear role for antibiotics. Additionally, aminoglycosides may worsen the paralysis by potentiating the neuromuscular blockade.

A new development in the treatment of infantile botulism is the use of human botulism immune globulin (BIG). When given within 3 days of hospitalization, BIG was shown to decrease duration of hospitalization, length of mechanical ventilation, and length of nasogastric tube feedings. The cost of hospitalization was also reduced by half.

VII. References

1. Frankovich TL, Arnon SS. Clinical trial of botulism immune globulin for infant botulism. *West J Med* 1991;154:103.
2. Long SS, Gajewski JL, Brown LW, et al. Clinical, laboratory, and environmental features of infant botulism in southeastern Pennsylvania. *Pediatrics* 1985;75:935–941.
3. Wigginton JM, Thill P. Infant botulism: a review of the literature. *Clin Pediatr* 1993; 32:669–674.

Case 2-4: 11-Month-Old Boy

I. History of Present Illness

An 11-month old boy was brought to the emergency department because of decreased activity level. He had had a 3-day illness consisting of fever to 39°C and diarrhea. He had had approximately four episodes of nonbloody diarrhea per day. He had no history of emesis. On the day of presentation, he had been tired all day and wanted to lie down constantly. He had consumed four 8-ounce bottles of Pedialyte. His urine output was decreased. The mother called the paramedics when she felt that he was worsening.

II. Past Medical History

His prenatal and birth histories were normal. He had a history of wheezing, with an upper respiratory tract infection at 3 months of age. He had had no hospitalizations or surgeries. He was taking no medications and had no allergies. His immunizations were current.

III. Physical Examination

T, 40.3°C; RR, 46/min; HR, 183 bpm; BP, 99/41 mm Hg

Weight and height, 75th percentile

On examination, he was lethargic and minimally responsive to painful stimuli. The head and neck examination did not reveal any signs of external trauma. His gaze was dysconjugate, but pupils were reactive from 3 mm to 2 mm bilaterally. He had sunken eyes and dry mucous membranes. Respiratory examination revealed shallow, labored respirations with moderately increased work of breathing. He had intercostal and substernal retractions as well as abdominal breathing. Breath sounds were coarse to auscultation. Cardiac examination was significant for the tachycardia; there was no murmur or abnormal cardiac sounds. Abdominal examination revealed hypoactive bowel sounds but no tenderness or hepatosplenomegaly. There were no masses. Rectal examination revealed gross blood. Neurologic examination was significant for overall hyoptonia and unresponsiveness. Cranial nerves were intact and deep tendon reflexes were 2+ and symmetric. He had an intact gag reflex.

IV. Diagnostic Studies

In the emergency department, blood, urine, and CSF cultures were obtained. Additional laboratory studies revealed a WBC count of 13,400 cells/mm^3, with 11% bands, 63% segmented neutrophils, 34% lymphocytes, and 2% monocytes. Hemoglobin was 6.6 g/dL; platelets, 195,000/mm^3; sodium, 131 mmol/L; potassium, 5.8 mmol/L; chloride, 101 mmol/L; carbon dioxide, 18 mmol/L; blood urea nitrogen, 19 mg/dL; creatinine, 0.7 mg/dL; and glucose, 57 mg/dL. His prothrombin time (PT) was prolonged at 16.4 seconds, and his activated partial thromboplastin time (PTT) was 29.1 seconds. Serum and urine toxicology screens were negative.

V. Course of Illness

Immediate, life-threatening causes were initially addressed. Coffee-ground material was aspirated from the stomach after placement of a nasogastric tube. Pediatric surgery staff were consulted in the emergency department on suspicion of an intraabdominal catastrophe, particularly intussusception or volvulus. He received broad-spectrum antimicrobial agents and was immediately taken to the operating room for an exploratory laparotomy. In the intensive care unit, after the procedure, the patient developed a rash that suggested the diagnosis (Fig. 2-2).

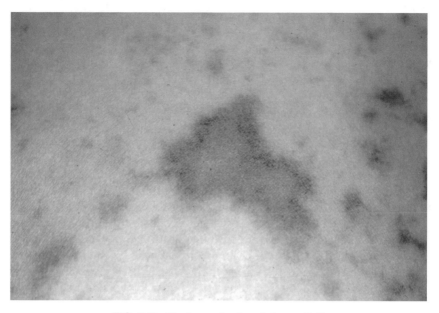

FIG. 2-2. Photograph of rash (case 2-4).

DISCUSSION: CASE 2-4

I. Differential Diagnosis

This child's critical appearance, in association with fever, made the clinician most concerned for an overwhelming systemic infection. The original source could have been a bacterial infection such as bacteremia, pneumonia, pyelonephritis, or meningitis. Aside from infectious causes, the history of bright red blood from the rectum is concerning for intestinal ischemia. Intussusception, malrotation with volvulus, or some other abdominal catastrophe could result in a similar clinical picture at presentation. Other causes of bleeding diathesis should be considered as well.

II. Diagnosis

Because of the concern for an abdominal catastrophe, the child was taken to the operating room for an exploratory laparotomy. The laparotomy findings were normal; there was no volvulus or intussusception. While the child was in the operating room, an alert laboratory technician noted gram-negative intracellular diplococci on the peripheral blood smear. In the intensive care unit, the patient developed diffuse purpuric lesions that suggested bacterial sepsis due to *Neisseria meningitidis* (see Fig. 2-2). His blood and CSF cultures ultimately grew *N. meningitidis.* **The diagnosis is meningococcal meningitis and sepsis.**

III. Incidence and Epidemiology

N. meningitidis (meningococcus) is a gram-negative diplococcus. It causes bacteremia and meningitis. There are 13 serogroups, but serogroups A, B, C, Y, and W-135 are most frequently implicated in the United States. Serogroups B, C, and Y each account for about 30% of systemic disease.

N. meningitidis is a component of the normal flora of the upper respiratory tract, which is the only reservoir for the organism. Transmission occurs via respiratory secretions and by person-to-person contact. Approximately 2.5% of children and 10% of the general population are asymptomatic carriers. In one study, 32.7% of persons between the ages of 20 and 24 years were found to be asymptomatic carriers. Peak rates of infection occur between November and March. The incubation period is most commonly less than 4 days but can be as long as 10 days. Fifty percent of cases of meningococcemia occur in children younger than 2 years of age; however, during epidemics, there is a shift in incidence toward older children, adolescents, and young adults.

IV.   Clinical Presentation

The disease caused by *N. meningitidis* varies from asymptomatic transient bacteremia to fulminant sepsis and death. Pathogenic *N. meningitidis* colonizes the respiratory tract and may invade the bloodstream. The patient becomes bacteremic and progressively sicker. The bacteremia may seed the meninges, causing meningitis. Those patients who present with meningitis have a better prognosis than do patients with bacteremia alone. Shortly after the administration of appropriate antibiotics, some patients have a marked clinical deterioration, ranging from hypotension to death. This deterioration is thought to be caused by stimulation of the host inflammatory pathway by endotoxin (a component of the gram-negative bacterial cell wall). Meningococcal disease can lead to death in as few as 12 hours. Invasive infection usually results in meningococcemia, meningitis, or both. However, the bacteria can infect any organ, including myocardium, adrenals, lungs, and joint spaces. Approximately 55% of patients with meningococcal disease have meningitis. Additionally, 50% of patients have positive blood cultures.

A history of a preceding upper respiratory tract infection can often be elicited from patients with meningococcemia. The onset of illness is abrupt, with fever, lethargy, and rash. The rash is typically petechial and occasionally urticarial or maculopapular. Some patients develop fulminant meningococcemia, with disseminated intravascular coagulopathy, shock, and myocardial dysfunction. Coagulopathy leads to the development of purpura. There is a 20% mortality rate in cases of fulminant disease.

V.   Diagnostic Approach

The prompt diagnosis of meningococcal disease requires a high index of clinical suspicion. Recovery of the organism from a normally sterile site provides the definitive diagnosis.

Appropriate cultures. The organism can be isolated from blood, CSF, and scrapings from the petechial rash. Blood cultures are positive in about 50% of patients with presumed meningococcal disease. Because the organism is a normal component of the nasopharynx, nasopharyngeal cultures are not helpful.

Other studies. Children with meningococcemia are often critically ill. Laboratory studies that may affect management include serum electrolytes, PT, and PTT.

VI.   Treatment

The initial antimicrobial coverage of meningococcal infections should be a third-generation cephalosporin such as cefotaxime or ceftriaxone. Chloramphenicol, although rarely used, is appropriate for patients who have anaphylactoid reactions to penicillins or cephalosporins. Although most isolates in the United States are sensitive to penicillin, penicillin-resistant isolates, first identified in Spain in 1987, are prevalent in Spain, Italy, and parts of Africa. In the United States, routine susceptibility testing is not indicated. Therapy for 5 to 7 days is adequate for most cases of invasive meningococcal disease. There does not appear to be a role for steroid use. Treatment with heparin and other anticoagulants remains controversial.

Chemoprophylaxis is indicated for individuals who were exposed to the index case within 7 days before the onset of illness. Particularly, all household contacts, all daycare or nursery school contacts (children and adults), and health care workers who had intimate exposure to secretions (e.g., mouth-to-mouth resuscitation, secretions that came in contact with the health care worker's mucous membranes) should be treated prophylactically. Family members of the index case have a 400 to 800 times higher risk for invasive disease. If the index patient received only penicillin for therapy, then the patient should also be treated with chemoprophylaxis to eradicate the organism. School age classmates do not need chemoprophylaxis because they are not at increased risk of disease. The drug of choice for chemoprophylaxis is rifampin, but ceftriaxone (intravenous or intramuscular) and single-dose ciprofloxacin or azithromycin are reasonable alternatives. All cases must be reported to the local public health department.

Additionally, a polysaccharide vaccine that is effective against serogroups A, C, Y, and W-135 is available. This vaccine should be routinely administered to children who are functionally or anatomically asplenic, children who have terminal complement deficiencies, college students living in the dormitories, and military recruits. A conjugate meningococcal vaccine is being evaluated in clinical trials.

VII. References

1. American Academy of Pediatrics. Meningococcal infections. In: Pickering LK, ed. *2000 Red Book: Report of the Committee on Infectious Diseases,* 25th ed. Elk Grove Village, IL: American Academy of Pediatrics; 2000:396–401.

2. Anderson MS, Glode MP, Smith AL. Meningococcal disease. In: Feigin RD, Cherry JD, eds. *Textbook of pediatric infectious diseases,* 4th ed. Philadelphia: WB Saunders, 1998:1143–1156.

3. Cohen J. Meningococcal disease as a model to evaluate novel anti-sepsis strategies. *Crit Care Med* 2000;28:s64–s67.

4. Herf C, Nichols J, Fruk S, et al. Meningococcal disease: recognition, treatment, and prevention. *The Nurse Practitioner* 1998;23:30–46.

5. Kirsch EA, Barton RP, Kitchen L, et al. Pathophysiology, treatment and outcome of meningococcemia: a review and recent experience. *Pediatr Infect Dis J* 1996;15:967–979.

6. Periappuram M, Taylor M, Keane C. Rapid detection of meningococci from petechiae in acute meningococcal infection. *J Infect* 1995;31:201–203.

7. Rosenstein NE, Perkins BA, Stephens DS, et al. Meningococcal disease. *N Engl J Med* 2001;344:1378–1388.

Case 2-5: 9-Year-Old Boy

I. History of Present Illness

A 9-year-old boy developed emesis about 5:00 p.m. one evening and afterward went to sleep. A few hours later, the parents had a difficult time arousing him, and subsequently brought him to an emergency department. In the emergency department, the child was able to relate that he fell at school and hit his head against the wall. He did not lose consciousness at the time. He complained of a headache. He denied any potential ingestion.

II. Past Medical History

He was a healthy child with no significant past medical history. He did not take any medications and was not allergic to any medications. His immunizations were appropriate for age.

III. Physical Examination

T, 37.5°C; RR, 26/min; HR, 86 bpm; BP, 120/70 mm Hg; SpO$_2$, 97% in room air

On examination he was asleep but was easily arousable. His head was atraumatic, but he had occipital pain with forward neck flexion. His occiput was diffusely tender, but no bony defects were palpated. Pupils were 4 mm and reactive to 2 mm. A funduscopic examination was attempted but was unsuccessful. Kernig's and Bruzinski's tests were negative. The remainder of his head and neck examination was normal. His lungs, cardiac, and abdominal examination findings were normal as well. His neurologic examination revealed that the cranial nerves were intact. He was able to follow commands and to respond appropriately.

IV. Diagnostic Studies

A head computed tomographic (CT) study was obtained and revealed a left-sided parietal intracranial hemorrhage, mild hydrocephalus, asymmetric ventricles with the left ventricle being larger than the right, and blood in the fourth ventricle. A complete blood count and serum electrolytes were normal. Serum and urine toxicology screens were negative.

V. Course of Illness

Shortly after his CT scan results were returned, the patient had a 5-minute generalized tonic-clonic seizure. He was loaded with phenytoin intravenously after the seizure activity ceased. An angiogram was performed after the patient was stable and revealed the diagnosis (Fig. 2-3).

DISCUSSION: CASE 2-5

I. Differential Diagnosis

This case illustrates a patient who has an intracranial hemorrhage. Although these lesions are not as common in children as in adults, they can occur, particularly after head trauma. The differential diagnosis includes any cause of intracranial hemorrhage, including accidental and nonaccidental trauma and nontraumatic causes such as an aneurysm, arteriovenous malformation (AVM), bleeding disorders, arachnoid cysts, hypernatremia, galactosemia, glutaric aciduria, and meningitis.

II. Diagnosis

Magnetic resonance imaging (MRI) scan of the head revealed a left-sided medial parieto-occipital hemorrhage with significant intraventricular extension. The findings suggested an AVM, but no AVM was detected on the MRI. **The patient was then sent for cranial angiography, which revealed an AVM that arose from the left posterior cere-**

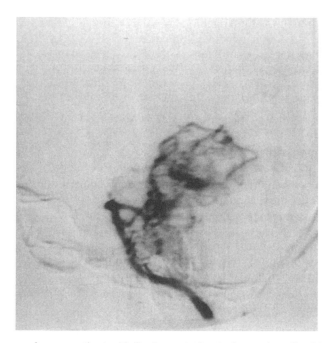

FIG. 2-3. Angiogram from a patient with findings similar to those described in case 2-5. (From Kanaan IN, Al-Watban J. Cerebrovascular disease in children. In: Elzouki AY, Harfi HA, Nazer H, eds. *Textbook of clinical pediatrics.* Philadelphia: Lippincott Williams & Wilkins, 2001:1482, with permission.)

bral artery and the superior cerebellar artery (see Fig. 2-3). He subsequently underwent operative drainage of the hematoma and resection of the AVM.

III. Incidence and Epidemiology

Cerebral AVMs are congenital vascular malformations. They most likely result from failed differentiation of the embryonic vessels into separate arterial and venous systems, which occurs between 3 and 12 weeks of fetal age. AVMs are arteriovenous shunts that consist of feeding arteries, a mass of coiled vessels (the nidus), and draining veins without a capillary network. Usually, there is no brain tissue between the two sides of the AVM, which allows a high-flow shunt from the arterial side to the venous side. The AVM, in essence, is stealing blood from the neighboring parts of the brain. Spontaneous thrombosis and subsequent recanalization may occur and may account for the change in size of an AVM over time. Ten percent of cerebral AVMs are in the posterior fossa, 10% in the midline, and the remainder in the cortex. They may be located superficially or deep. The incidence of cerebral AVMs is 1 per 100,000 persons. Fewer than 12% of cerebral AVMs are symptomatic. They are frequently diagnosed between the ages of 20 and 40 years. About one fifth of AVMs that become symptomatic do so before 15 years of age. Hemorrhage is the most frequent complication associated with AVMs, and it is more commonly seen in children than in adults.

IV. Clinical Presentation

Hemorrhage is the initial manifestation in up to 80% of cases of cerebral AVMs. Seizures, which occur in about one third of the cases, may result from an acute hemorrhage or from an epileptogenic focus from a previous hemorrhage. Infants may present with congestive heart failure and hydrocephalus. Stroke and seizures are more commonly seen in older children. Intracranial hemorrhage may occur after an episode of trivial head trauma. Headache is a frequent symptom in patients with AVMs, although it is not a very specific clinical sign. Patients with untreated AVM who have had previous hemorrhages are at a higher risk for rebleeding. The presentation varies with the location of the AVM: superficial AVMs cause seizures more frequently, and deep AVMs tend to manifest with hemorrhage.

AVMs usually continue to increase in size, with increasing risk of hemorrhage and ischemia, resulting in seizures, gliosis, and neurologic deficits. However, some AVMs remain the same size, and some even regress.

Two thirds of adults with AVMs have documented learning disorders. The implication is that there are functional brain deficits that may arise before other signs and symptoms that ultimately lead to the diagnosis of a cerebral AVM.

V.   Diagnostic Approach

Brain imaging. The diagnosis of an AVM can be made with CT, MRI, or cerebral angiography. CT frequently is obtained after the first hemorrhage and reveals only that a hemorrhage has occurred. If an intravenous contrast agent is administered for the CT, the AVM nidus typically can be seen; however, if it is a small AVM, it may be missed on CT scanning. MRI is very helpful in diagnosing AVMs. Additionally, MRI is useful in the planning of the surgical correction of the AVM. MRI and magnetic resonance angiography (MRA) are also used to monitor patients after their AVM has been treated. Angiography provides an excellent view of the vascular anatomy of the AVM.

VI.   Treatment

The aim of treatment is complete removal of the AVM, because there is a high mortality rate from untreated AVMs. The options for removal include neurosurgical excision, embolization of the AVM, and radiotherapy obliteration using the gamma knife, proton beam, or linear accelerator. The therapeutic option that is most appropriate for the patient depends on the location and size of the AVM. If the location of the AVM is deep within the brain or on the motor cortex, excision might not be the best option. The effect of radiotherapy takes months or years to manifest, whereas surgical excision and embolization are immediately effective.

VII.   References

1. Di Rocci C, Tamburrini G, Rollo, M. Cerebral arteriovenous malformations in children. *Acta Neurochirurgica* 2000;142:142–158.
2. Hofmeister C, Stapf C, Hartmann A, et al. Demographic, morphological, and clinical characteristics of 1289 patients with brain arteriovenous malformation. *Stroke* 2000; 31:1307–1310.
3. Menovsky T, van Overbeeke JJ. Cerebral arteriovenous malformations in childhood: state of the art with special reference to treatment. *Eur J Pediatr* 1997;156:741–746.
4. The Arteriovenous Malformation Study Group. Arteriovenous malformations of the brain in adults. *N Engl J Med* 1999;340:1812–1818.

Case 2-6: 20-Month-Old Boy

I.   History of Present Illness

A 20-month-old boy was brought to the emergency department with decreased activity level. He had been vomiting for the previous 3 days and had had two or three episodes of nonbloody, nonbilious emesis per day. On the day of presentation, he had been acting listless all day and appeared pale to the family. There had been no diarrhea. He had just recovered from coxsackievirus hand-foot-mouth disease 1 week before development of these symptoms. The family denied any trauma or ingestions. There had been no fever, rhinorrhea, or cough.

II.   Past Medical History

One month before this presentation, the patient's serum lead level was found to be 31 µg/dL. His past medical history was otherwise unremarkable. He had not undergone any surgical procedure. He was not taking any medications and was not allergic to any medications. His immunization status was up to date.

III.   Physical Examination

T, 37.0°C; RR, 27/min; HR, 75 bpm; BP, 100/68 mm Hg

Weight, 10th percentile; height, 50th percentile

On examination, he was somnolent but arousable. He fell asleep as soon as he was no longer being stimulated. His head was normocephalic and atraumatic. His tympanic membranes were pearly gray bilaterally, without hemotympanum. His mucous membranes were moist. His neck was supple, and there was full range of motion. His lung and cardiac examinations were normal. His abdomen was soft. There was no abdominal tenderness, masses, or organomegaly. His extremities were warm and well perfused. His neurologic examination revealed a Glasgow coma score of 13 but was otherwise normal.

IV.   Diagnostic Studies

A complete blood count revealed 12,100 WBCs/mm^3 (86% segmented neutrophils, 9% lymphocytes, and 5% monocytes). Hemoglobin was 7.4 g/dL, and the platelet count was 851,000/mm^3. The MCV was low at 55 fL. Basophilic stippling was noted on the peripheral blood smear. Samples were sent for a serum lead determination and hemoglobin electrophoresis. Serum electrolytes and transaminases were normal. A lumbar puncture revealed WBCs, 4/mm^3; RBCs, 4,365/mm^3; glucose, 82 mg/dL; and protein, 31 mg/dL. A urine toxicology screen was negative. Additional laboratory evaluation revealed a PT of 13.0 seconds and a PTT of 36.6 seconds.

V.   Course of Illness

The child was hospitalized. Over the next several days, he awakened and began to act normally. A head MRI performed at the time of admission suggested the diagnosis (Fig. 2-4).

DISCUSSION: CASE 2-6

I.   Differential Diagnosis

Several diagnoses are possible for this child. Given the microcytic anemia, basophilic stippling noted on the smear, and history of increased lead levels, lead encephalopathy is a possibility. However, intracranial hemorrhage is not characteristic of lead encephalopathy. Other causes of intracranial bleeding, such as accidental and nonaccidental trauma, must be considered as well. Causes of intracranial bleeding in children include inten-

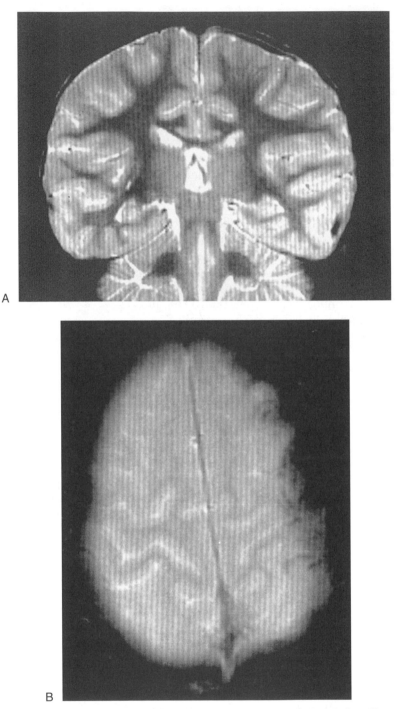

FIG. 2-4. Head magnetic resonance images (case 2-6). **A,** Coronal view. **B,** axial view.

tional injury, major trauma (e.g., motor vehicle collision, substantial fall), aneurysms, arachnoid cysts, cerebral infections, hematologic disorders, metabolic disorders such as glutaric aciduria or galactosemia, and hypernatremia.

II. Diagnosis

The serum lead level was normal. The hemoglobin electrophoresis revealed normal hemoglobin (AA2). The iron level was low, at 5 µg/dL. The head MRI revealed extensive left subdural hemorrhage that extended over the frontal convexity, down to the temporal lobe, and posteriorly to the occipital lobe (see Fig. 2-4). Dilated retinal examination performed by an ophthalmologist revealed multiple bilateral retinal hemorrhages. No fractures, either new or healing, were detected on a radiographic skeletal survey (radiographs of all bones in his body). **The final diagnosis was child abuse and iron deficiency anemia.** Social services were consulted and determined that a relative who lived in the house had caused the nonaccidental trauma in this child.

In this child, basophilic stippling of RBCs was noted on the peripheral blood smear. Basophilic stippling represents aggregated ribosomes and can be a prominent feature in children with thalassemia syndromes, iron deficiency, syndromes accompanied by ineffective erythropoiesis, pyrimidine-5'-nucleotidase deficiency, or lead poisoning.

III. Incidence and Epidemiology

The recognition of child abuse is difficult and requires a high index of suspicion. The exact incidence of child abuse is not known, but it is more common than many think: estimates range from 500,000 to 4 million cases per year in the United States. Homicide is the fifth leading cause of death in children age 1 to 4 years. Although the exact incidence of abuse may be in question, the number of child abuse reports filed has increased, partially due to increased awareness, increased ease of reporting, and perhaps an increase in abuse.

IV. Clinical Presentation

The presentation of child abuse varies according to the type of injury inflicted, and medical personnel should be alert to any sign that may indicate abuse. The child may have been the victim of a one-time abuse or of multiple previous episodes of abuse. The abuse may be physical, sexual, emotional, or neglect. The child may have marks and bruises on the body from the abuse, there may be a change in mental status, the child may present with an intracranial hemorrhage, the child may present in full arrest or there may be no obvious signs that the abuse occurred. The perpetrator may not have intended to harm the child but may have overdisciplined or punished the child, resulting in abuse. Physical abuse represents 25% of the cases of abuse in the United States.

Risk factors that place a child at increased risk for abuse include parental/caretaker factors, child factors, and situational factors. Caretaker factors that increase the risk of abuse include caretakers who are not prepared to perform their role, have unrealistic expectations of the child, have a poor role model, use corporal punishment, have inconsistent discipline skills, have an unsupportive partner, have psychological issues such as impulse disorder or depression, have been victims of abuse themselves, or have a substance abuse problem. Children who are handicapped, have developmental delays, or have behavioral problems are at increased risk. Economic difficulties, poor housing, crowding, illness, and unemployment are situations that increase the likelihood of abuse. Injuries that have occurred without any history, inconsistent histories, "magical" injuries, and a delay in seeking care after injury are concerning for abuse. Physical examination findings of patterned marks, pathognomonic injuries, multiple injuries, injuries at various stages of healing, and unexplained injuries are concerning for abuse.

It is important to be able to determine what constitutes abuse and what does not. Being able to differentiate osteogenesis imperfecta from fractures due to child abuse, Mongolian spots from bruising, and ecthyma from cigarette burns are important skills that health care professionals should learn. Normal bruising is common in children older than 1 year of age; it typically occurs on the lower extremities and is not associated with petechiae, purpura, or mucosal bleeding. It is difficult to determine which injuries were sustained accidentally and which were caused by nonaccidental trauma. If doubt exists, a social services report should be filed.

V.   Diagnostic Approach

Several studies are frequently obtained when abuse of a child is suspected.

Radiographic skeletal survey. A radiographic skeletal survey (radiographs of all the bones in the child's body) is indicated for children younger than 2 years of age.

Radionuclide bone scan. A bone scan is helpful in detecting fractures that did not show up on the skeletal survey.

Dilated retinal examination. An ophthalmology consultation is frequently helpful in detecting retinal hemorrhages.

Other studies. Laboratory studies are often indicated as well. A complete blood count, PT, and PTT should be obtained if the child presents with bruising. Liver function tests with amylase and lipase should be obtained if abdominal injury is suspected. Urinalysis is appropriate for abdominal trauma and for the detection of myoglobin if muscle injury has occurred. Screening for sexually transmitted diseases and semen may be appropriate if a child presents within 24 to 72 hours after a sexual assault. Toxicologic testing is indicated if the child presents with altered mental status. Head CT or MRI may be indicated if the child has a large head, to look for chronic subdural bleeds, or if there is reason to suspect intracranial injury.

VI.   Treatment

The approach to the abused child is to first treat the medical issues. Anyone involved in the care of a child is a mandated reporter of suspected child abuse. It is not the job of the medical team to prove abuse and then report it, but rather to report suspected abuse and allow the social services to perform further investigations. The criteria for reporting child abuse vary in regard to the history, physical examination, and diagnostic results. Occasionally, physical examination findings alone are enough to trigger the filing of a social services report. At other times, it is the cumulative effect of the history, physical examination, laboratory results and caretaker interactions that trigger the filing of a report. If it is not safe for the child to be discharged, hospitalization is warranted.

VII.   References

1. Christian CW. Child Abuse. In: Schwartz MW, ed. *Clinical handbook of pediatrics,* 2nd ed. Philadelphia: Williams & Wilkins, 1999:179–189.
2. Kemp AM. Investigating subdural haemorrhage in infants. *Arch Dis Child* 2002;86: 98–102.
3. Ludwig S. Child abuse. In: Fleisher GR, Ludwig S, eds. *Textbook of pediatric emergency medicine,* 4th ed. Philadelphia: Lippincott Williams & Wilkins, 2000: 1669–1704.
4. Vora A, Makris M. An approach to investigation of easy bruising. *Arch Dis Child* 2001;84:488–491.

3

Vomiting

James P. Cavanagh

APPROACH TO THE PATIENT WITH VOMITING

I. Definition of the Complaint

Vomiting is defined as the forceful contraction of abdominal muscles and the diaphragm in a coordinated fashion that expels the gastric contents through an open gastric cardia into the esophagus and out of the mouth. The medullary vomiting center coordinates this process of vomiting via efferent pathways of the vagus and phrenic nerves. Stimulation of the medullary vomiting center occurs either directly or through the chemoreceptor trigger zone (CTZ). Direct stimulation may occur through afferent vagal signals from the gastrointestinal tract or other sites including, but not limited to, the vestibular system, the cerebral cortex, and the hypothalamus. The CTZ in the area postrema of the fourth ventricle can be activated by noxious sights and smells or by chemical stimuli in the blood secondary to medications, metabolic abnormalities, or certain toxins.

Gastroesophageal reflux (GER) is not vomiting but rather regurgitation. Although GER can be projectile at times, it is an effortless return of gastric contents into the mouth without nausea or coordinated muscular contractions.

II. Complaints by Cause and Frequency

Vomiting is not a diagnosis but rather a symptom of an underlying pathologic process that requires a thorough evaluation. The causes of vomiting can be grouped according to age at presentation (Table 3-1) or according to etiology (Table 3-2): (a) obstructive gas-

TABLE 3-1. *Causes of Vomiting and Regurgitation in Childhood by Age*

Disease prevalence	Newborn	Infant/child	Adolescent
Common	Gastroesophageal reflux	Gastroesophageal reflux	Gastroenteritis
	Gastroenteritis	Systemic infections	Toxic ingestion
	Pylorospasm	Pulmonary infections	Medications
	Systemic infections	CNS infections	Crohn's disease
	Pulmonary infections	Toxic ingestion	Appendicitis
	CNS infections	Medications	Pregnancy
	Obstructive lesions		Bulimia
			Migraine
Less common	Increased ICP	Increased ICP	Increased ICP
	Obstructive uropathy	Peptic ulcers	Peptic ulcer
	Renal insufficiency	Pancreatitis	Pancreatitis
		Hepatitis	Hepatitis
		Pancreatitis	Pancreatitis
			Psychogenic
Uncommon	Inborn errors of metabolism	Inborn error of metabolism	Adrenal insufficiency
	CAH	Reye syndrome	Cyclical vomiting
	Neonatal tetany	Adrenal insufficiency	Reye syndrome
	Kernicterus	Duodenal hematoma	Duodenal hematoma

CAH, congenital adrenal hyperplasia; CNS, central nervous system; ICP, intracranial pressure.

TABLE 3-2. *Causes of Vomiting and Regurgitation in Childhood by Etiology*

Diagnostic category	Cause
Obstructive gastrointestinal	Esophageal atresia or stenosis
	Lactobezoar
	Intestinal atresia or stenosis
	Pyloric stenosis
	Annular pancreas
	Congenital diaphragmatic hernia
	Hiatal hernia
	Malrotation
	Volvulus
	Foreign body
	Ascariasis
	Duplication
	Intussusception
	Adhesions
	Intramural hematoma
	Meconium ileus
	Meconium plug
	Meckel diverticulum
	Hirschsprung's disease
	Imperforate anus
	Incarcerated hernia
	Chronic intestinal pseudo-obstruction
Nonobstructive gastrointestinal	Gastroesophageal reflux disease
	Necrotizing enterocolitis
	Cow's milk protein allergy
	Eosinophilic gastropathy
	Crohn's disease
	Peritonitis
	Achalasia
	Food poisoning
	Peptic or duodenal ulcer
	Celiac disease
	Superior mesenteric artery syndrome
	Viral gastroenteritis
	Bacterial enteritis
	Gastritis
	Pancreatitis
	Hepatitis
	Appendicitis
	Peritonitis
Neurologic	Increased intracranial pressure
	Meningitis/Encephalitis/Abscess
	Seizure
	Migraine
	Hypertensive encephalopathy
	Motion sickness
	Postconcussive syndrome
	Kernicterus
Metabolic	Amino acid and organic acid defects
	Urea cycle defects
	Congenital adrenal hyperplasia
	Neonatal tetany
	Hypercalcemia
	Diabetic ketoacidosis
	Acidosis
	Galactosemia
	Fructosemia
	Phenylketonuria
	Adrenal insufficiency
	Reye syndrome
	Porphyria

TABLE 3-2. *Continued.*

Diagnostic category	Cause
Renal	Obstructive uropathies
	Hydronephrosis
	Renal insufficiency
	Renal tubular acidosis
	Urinary calculi
	Urinary tract infections/pyelonephritis
Pulmonary	Postnasal drip
	Asthma
	Pneumonia
	Foreign body aspiration
	Acute otitis media
	Labyrinthitis
Toxicologic	Salicylate poisoning
	Theophylline toxicity
	Digoxin toxicity
	Ipecac
	Iron ingestion
	Lead poisoning
Miscellaneous	Pregnancy
	Psychogenic
	Cyclic vomiting
	Sepsis

trointestinal lesions, (b) nonobstructive gastrointestinal disorders, (c) neurologic causes, (d) metabolic causes, (e) renal causes, (f) pulmonary causes, (g) toxicologic causes, and (h) miscellaneous causes.

III. Clarifying Questions

Thorough history taking is imperative for formulating an accurate differential diagnosis and eventually discovering the correct etiology of vomiting. Consideration of the vomiting duration and pattern, the content of the emesis, and associated symptoms provides a framework for creating a differential diagnosis. The following questions may help provide clues to the correct diagnosis:

- What is the duration of vomiting?

  — Acute episodes of vomiting, chronic vomiting, and cyclic vomiting carry very different differential diagnoses. Acute vomiting is mostly caused by transient, self-limited infectious or metabolic conditions. Chronic vomiting tends to have a gastrointestinal origin and may be caused by a partial mechanical obstruction (e.g., hiatal hernia, achalasia, duplications, webs). Other conditions causing prolonged vomiting include peptic and duodenal ulcers, dysmotility syndromes, increased intracranial pressure, psychogenic disturbance, pregnancy, and lead poisoning. Cyclic vomiting tends to be extraintestinal and is usually caused by migraine or migraine equivalents, cardiac arrhythmias, or ureteropelvic junction (UPJ) obstruction.

- Is there any timing pattern to the vomiting?

  — Episodes of vomiting that occur with a regular diurnal pattern also provide helpful clues. Early-morning vomiting can be very ominous if it is caused by increased intracranial pressure, but it could also occur secondary to morning sickness from pregnancy. Vomiting after eating of specific foods may be the result of a food allergy. Vomiting patterns may also become apparent if secondary gain is achieved (e.g., absence from school or tests), or vomiting may be associated with school phobia. Vomiting that occurs shortly after eating is consistent with psychogenic vomiting as well as gastric outlet obstruction or peptic ulcer disease.

- Is the vomiting effortless?

  — GER occurs in almost all newborns, but by 6 months of age fewer than 5% of children are symptomatic. GER tends to be effortless and is not associated with pain or morbidity. Rarely, reflux is severe enough to cause discomfort and arching, Sandifer syndrome, or poor weight gain, at which point medical therapy may be necessary. True vomiting tends to be a more noxious event, often causing pain and retching.

- Is there bilious emesis?

  — The presence of bilious emesis suggests an obstruction distal to the ampulla of Vater but may also be present in nonobstructed patients after prolonged episodes of vomiting due to a relaxed pylorus. Bilious vomiting in a newborn infant should be treated as a surgical emergency until proved otherwise. Newborn infants with bilious emesis may have intestinal obstruction associated with duodenal atresia or intestinal malrotation and midgut volvulus. The absence of bilious emesis is also important, because in that case any obstruction that was present would be located proximal to the ampulla of Vater (e.g., pyloric stenosis).

- Is there any blood in the vomitus?

  — The presence of blood in emesis must first be confirmed by either a Gastroccult or a Hematest test. If blood is present, then hematemesis must be distinguished from hemoptysis. The blood in hematemesis ranges in color from bright red to coffee-ground, depending on its length of time in contact with gastric contents, but compared with hemoptysis it tends to be darker red, acidic, and associated with retching or gastrointestinal complaints. The blood in hemoptysis is bright red, frothy, alkaline, and associated with respiratory symptoms. Hematemesis may be a result of peptic ulcers, Mallory-Weiss tears, esophagitis, esophageal varices, acute iron ingestion, gastritis, bleeding diathesis, or vascular malformations.

- Is undigested food present in the vomitus?

  — The presence of undigested food material is very common in children with GER who present with episodes of effortless, postprandial regurgitation. Other conditions that predispose to undigested food in emesis include esophageal atresia or strictures, esophageal or pharyngeal (Zenker's) diverticulum, and achalasia. Old food present in the emesis may signify a gastric outlet obstruction or a gastric motility disorder.

- Is fecal material present in the emesis?

  — The presence of fecal material in the emesis suggests a distal intestinal obstruction, peritonitis, a gastrocolic fistula, or bacterial overgrowth in the stomach or small intestine.

- Is diarrhea occurring with the vomiting?

  — The presence of diarrhea and vomiting suggests a gastrointestinal disorder, of which an infectious gastroenteritis is the most common. Isolated vomiting tends to have a far greater differential, involving many other organ systems. Isolated vomiting may occur in serious conditions such as increased intracranial pressure, lower-lobe pneumonias, ingestions, and diabetic ketoacidosis.

- Is there any abdominal pain?

  — When vomiting is associated with abdominal pain, the location of the abdominal pain and the descriptive nature of the pain can be clues as to the etiology. Pain in the right lower quadrant may be caused by an acute appendicitis, whereas right upper quadrant pain is more likely to be of gall bladder or hepatic in origin. The most common cause of diffuse abdominal pain is constipation. Colicky pain tends to occur with an obstructed hollow viscous, whereas well-localized, sharp pain tends to occur when parietal peritoneum is inflamed. Flank or lateral pain signifies a renal etiology. Pain from peptic ulcer disease is often alleviated by vomiting, whereas pain secondary to pancreatitis or biliary tract disease is not improved with vomiting.

- Is fever present?

  — The presence of fever in a patient with vomiting is very common. It may signify an infectious gastrointestinal process, such as acute viral gastroenteritis, bacterial enteritis, appendicitis, hepatitis, pancreatitis, peritonitis, or an acute extraintestinal infection, such as sepsis, meningitis, acute otitis media, pharyngitis, or urinary tract infection. Other causes of fever include inflammatory conditions such as inflammatory bowel disease.

- Are any associated symptoms present?

  — Other information that may help in narrowing the differential includes the presence of weight loss, headache, lethargy, poor school performance, or environmental or infectious exposures.

The following cases present less common causes of vomiting in children.

Case 3-1: 7-Week-Old Boy

I. History of Present Illness

A 7-week-old African-American male infant presented with a 2-day history of frequent vomiting. The vomiting was nonprojectile, nonbilious, and, on one occasion, streaked with blood. Oral intake was poor. He had urinated once over an 18-hour period. On the day of admission, he had profuse, watery diarrhea. No one in the family had had vomiting or diarrhea.

II. Past Medical History

The patient was born at term and weighed 3,300 g. He was delivered via cesarean section due to arrested descent. Because of feeding difficulties in the nursery, he was discharged home on a lactose-free formula. Since then, his oral intake had been appropriate. He had not previously been hospitalized. He had received his first hepatitis B immunization.

III. Physical Examination

T, 38.1°C; RR, 50/min; HR, 170 bpm; BP, 86/38 mm Hg; SpO$_2$, 88% in room air

Weight, 4.0 kg (10th percentile); length, 25th percentile; head circumference, 10th percentile

Examination revealed a well-nourished infant who was crying but consolable (Fig. 3-1). The anterior fontanelle was open and slightly sunken. The mucous membranes were moist, and the sclerae were nonicteric. The lungs were clear to auscultation, and the cardiac examination was normal without any murmurs. The abdomen was soft and mildly distended, without hepatomegaly or splenomegaly. The extremities were cool. He had no rashes, good tone, and a symmetric neurologic examination.

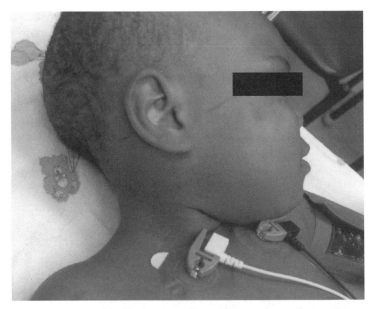

FIG. 3-1. Photograph of a slightly older child with findings similar to those of the patient in case 3-1.

IV. Diagnostic Studies

Laboratory evaluation revealed 24,500 white blood cells(WBCs)/mm^3, with 9% band forms, 24% segmented neutrophils, 40% lymphocytes, 20% monocytes, and 5% atypical lymphocytes. The hemoglobin was 15.2 g/dL, and the platelet count was 577,000 cells/mm^3. On red blood cell morphologic analysis, mild anisocytosis, poikilocytosis, and burr cells were noted. Serum chemistries and cerebral spinal fluid analysis were normal. His urine was dark yellow and turbid, with a specific gravity of 1.038, a pH of 5.5, 3+ protein, and 5 to 10 granular casts without bacteria, nitrites, or WBCs. On chest radiography, the cardiac silhouette and lung fields were normal.

V. Course of Illness

The patient's oxygen saturation on pulse oximeter increased to 93% when oxygen was administered by nasal cannula. Four extremity blood pressures were obtained as follows: right arm, 90/32 mm Hg; left arm, 88/42 mm Hg; right leg, 80/40 mm Hg; left leg, 76/35 mm Hg. On arterial blood gas (ABG) analysis, the pH was 7.01; partial pressure of carbon dioxide (PaCO$_2$), 18 mm Hg; partial pressure of oxygen (PaO$_2$), 232 mm Hg; bicarbonate level, 4.7 mEq/L; and base deficit, 24.7. The patient received multiple normal saline boluses and bicarbonate in an attempt to correct his metabolic acidosis. The appearance of the patient (see Fig. 3-1) in conjunction with the ABG results suggested a diagnosis.

DISCUSSION: CASE 3-1

I. Differential Diagnosis

Vomiting in early infancy can be a very worrisome symptom. The most common cause of emesis in this age group is GER, either physiologic or due to overfeeding. Anatomic obstruction should always be considered. Obstructive lesions include malrotation with a volvulus, intestinal or esophageal atresia, pyloric stenosis, congenital adhesions or bands, incarcerated hernia, intussusception, and Hirschsprung's disease. The level of the obstruction determines whether the vomitus is bilious and whether the abdomen is distended. Infectious causes include gastroenteritis, urinary tract infection, meningitis, pneumonia, and pericarditis. Bloody streaks in the emesis could be the result of a milk protein allergy, gastroenteritis, necrotizing enterocolitis, or achalasia.

Metabolic disorders must be considered in this child who presents with vomiting and a significant metabolic acidosis. Etiologies such as congenital adrenal hyperplasia (CAH), adrenal hypoplasia, inborn errors of metabolism including both amino acid and organic acid disorders, and galactosemia must also be considered.

II. Diagnosis

The patient was cyanotic, a feature best visualized by noting the contrast of his lips with the white portion of the blanket (see Fig. 3-1). An ABG analysis with co-oximetry measurements revealed acidosis, with a pH of 7.01; PaCO$_2$, 18 mm Hg; and PaO$_2$, 232 mm Hg. **Co-oximetry readings revealed an oxyhemoglobin of 78.2%; methemoglobin, 21.8%; and lactate, 2.7 mmol/L, confirming the diagnosis of methemoglobinemia.**

III. Incidence and Epidemiology of Methemoglobinemia

Although methemoglobinemia is a rare condition in pediatrics, it can cause significant cyanosis and even death. Methemoglobin is a derivative of normal hemoglobin in which the iron component has been oxidized from the ferrous (Fe^{2+}) to the ferric (Fe^{3+}) state. The oxidized iron (Fe^{3+}) is unable to reversibly bind oxygen. Therefore, the oxidation of hemoglobin to methemoglobin produces a functional anemia by impairing the ability of the blood to transport oxygen. Methemoglobin occurs regularly in the body but rarely exceeds levels of 2% of the total hemoglobin because of antioxidant reactions in the body that reduce methemoglobin back to hemoglobin. The most important of these antioxidant reactions uses either reduced nicotinamide adenine dinucleotide (NADH)–cytochrome b5 reductase or NADH phosphate (NADPH)–methemoglobin reductase. NADPH-methemoglobin reductase also reduces methylene blue, an action that has important therapeutic implications, as described in the treatment section below.

Methemoglobin levels increase when there is a disturbance in the balance between the oxidation and reduction of heme iron. Infants are at an increased risk for methemoglobinemia for two main reasons: (a) young infants have a lower level of the reductase enzymes, and (b) fetal hemoglobin is more easily oxidized than adult hemoglobin. Methemoglobinemia can be caused by exposure to oxidant drugs, development of acidosis, or inherited conditions. The most common oxidizing agents in acquired methemoglobinemia are sulfonamides, aniline dyes, chlorates, quinones, benzocaine, lidocaine, metoclopramide, and phenytoin. Ingestion of well water nitrates can also cause methemoglobinemia. Gastroenteritis with acidosis can cause methemoglobinemia in infants, especially when nitrite-forming bacteria such as *Escherichia coli* and *Campylobacter jejuni* are present. Less common causes are inherited deficiencies of erythrocyte methemoglobin reductase or the presence of M hemoglobin.

IV.   Clinical Presentation

The clinical presentation of patients with methemoglobinemia depends on the serum concentrations of both hemoglobin and methemoglobin. Increasing methemoglobin levels are associated with progressively worsening symptoms. Patients with lower serum hemoglobin concentrations are affected at lower levels of methemoglobin. Patients with methemoglobin concentrations lower than 10% rarely have symptoms unless they are already anemic. Most patients with concentrations of methemoglobin between 10% and 25% have cyanosis but few other symptoms. Depending on the degree of cyanosis, metabolic acidosis may also develop. Levels from 30% to 50% are associated with confusion, dizziness, fatigue, headache, tachypnea, and tachycardia. Levels greater than 50% are associated with severe acidosis, arrhythmias, seizures, lethargy, and coma. Lethal levels occur at methemoglobin concentrations of about 70%.

V.   Diagnostic Approach

Diagnosis of a rare pediatric condition like methemoglobinemia depends on having a high index of suspicion. Clinical clues include a cyanotic child without evidence of cardiac or pulmonary disease.

Bedside examination of blood. In a cyanotic patient, differentiating methemoglobin from deoxyhemoglobin is important. On white filter paper, blood containing a high level of methemoglobin turns chocolate brown; blood containing deoxygenated hemoglobin appears dark red or purple initially but turns bright red on exposure to atmospheric oxygen.

Potassium cyanide test. This test distinguishes between methemoglobin and sulfhemoglobin. Methemoglobin reacts with cyanide to form cyanomethemoglobin. The formation of cyanomethemoglobin turns the blood from chocolate brown to bright red. Sulfhemoglobin appears dark brown initially and does not change color after the addition of potassium cyanide.

Pulse oximetry. Oxygen saturation, as measured by pulse oximetry, is falsely elevated in the presence of methemoglobinemia. By using two wavelengths of light, the pulse oximeter determines "functional oxygen saturation," which is the ratio of oxyhemoglobin to all hemoglobin capable of carrying oxygen. Normally, all hemoglobin present can potentially carry oxygen, so that *functional* and *true* oxygen saturation are equal. Because methemoglobin does not carry oxygen, it does not register as functional hemoglobin on the pulse oximeter. At normal methemoglobin levels (less than 2%), this exclusion is not important, but at high methemoglobin levels (greater than 10%), the functional and true oxygen saturations differ substantially. Pulse oximeter readings may be abnormal with methemoglobinemia. Because of the light absorption characteristics of methemoglobin, the pulse oximetry readings will not drop below 82% unless there is an accompanying increased level of deoxyhemoglobin.

Arterial blood gases. Children with methemoglobinemia have a normal or an abnormally elevated PaO_2, as calculated by a blood analyzer, in the presence of cyanosis. PaO_2 refers to *dissolved* oxygen molecules, not oxygen molecules *bound to hemoglobin.* In ABG measurements, the PaO_2 is a value that is *calculated* from the measured pH and $PaCO_2$ values. The calculation of PaO_2 is based on the assumption that the hemoglobin function is normal. A dyshemoglobin such as methemoglobin cannot carry oxygen but does not interfere with pulmonary oxygen diffusion. Therefore, the PaO_2 calculated by the blood gas analyzer is falsely elevated.

Co-oximetry. Co-oximeters are spectrophotometers that measure light absorbance at different wavelengths, including the wavelengths for methemoglobin, oxyhemoglobin, deoxyhemoglobin, and carboxyhemoglobin. Co-oximeters accurately distinguish methemoglobin from oxyhemoglobin and provide a definitive diagnosis. Interpretation of results from a blood gas analyzer without co-oximetry may lead to misdiagnosis, because the blood gas analyzer calculates the PaO_2 and the co-oximeter measures it directly.

VI. Treatment

Treatment regimens for methemoglobinemia depend on the level and the patient's symptoms. In general, only symptomatic patients with methemoglobin levels greater than 20% or asymptomatic patients with methemoglobin levels greater than 30% require specific therapy. Patients with concurrent problems that impair oxygen delivery, such as anemia, cardiac disease, or pulmonary disease, should be treated even if they have low methemoglobin levels. Symptomatic patients must receive proper airway management and supplemental oxygen as needed. Intravenous methylene blue, after reduction to leukomethylene blue by NADPH-methemoglobin reductase, aids in the reduction of methemoglobin back to hemoglobin. It is the treatment of choice and should reduce methemoglobin levels significantly within 1 hour after administration. Exchange transfusions are necessary for those patients who have extremely high levels of methemoglobin that do not respond to methylene blue therapy.

Glucose-6-phosphate dehydrogenase (G6PD) is the first enzyme in the hexose monophosphate shunt, which is the sole source of NADPH in the red blood cell. Patients with G6PD deficiency may not produce sufficient NADPH to reduce methylene blue to leukomethylene blue. Therefore, methylene blue therapy may not be effective in patients with G6PD deficiency. In such patients, methylene blue may also induce hemolysis.

VII. References

1. Lukens J. Methemoglobinemia and other disorders accompanied by cyanosis. In: Lee RG, Foerster J, Lukens J, et al., eds. *Wintrobe's clinical hematology,* 10th ed. Baltimore: Williams & Wilkins, 1998:1046–1055.
2. Pollack ES, Pollack CV. Incidence of subclinical methemoglobinemia in infants with diarrhea. *Ann Emerg Med* 1994;24:652–656.
3. Ralston AC, Webb RK, Runciman WB. Potential errors in pulse oximetry: effects of interference, dyes, dyshemoglobins and other pigments. *Anaesthesia* 1991;46: 291–294.
4. Wright RO, Lewander WJ, Woolf AD. Methemoglobinemia: etiology, pharmacology, and clinical management. *Ann Emerg Med* 1999;34:646–656.

Case 3-2: 9-Month-Old Girl

I. History of Present Illness

A 9-month-old girl presented with a 12-day history of poor feeding, decreased activity, irritability, and frequent nonbloody, nonbilious emesis with feeds. Ten days earlier she was initially diagnosed with a viral gastroenteritis, and 6 days before admission she was treated with amoxicillin for an acute otitis media. She presented with continued emesis and decreased urine output, having had only two wet diapers in the previous 18 hours. She had a history of poor feeding and frequent episodic bouts of emesis lasting 2 to 3 days. The parents denied any fever, diarrhea, cough, gagging with feeds, rash, bloody stools, ill contacts, recent travel, or animal exposure. Her diet consisted of Nutramigen formula and various infant foods.

II. Past Medical History

The patient was born at full term from an uncomplicated pregnancy, labor, and delivery and was well until 3 months of age, when she developed episodic vomiting. The emesis was nonbloody and nonbilious, lasted 1 to 3 days, and was associated with decreased activity. It began during the transition from breast milk- to cow's milk-based formula and was therefore attributed to a "feeding intolerance." At 4 months, she was changed to a soy- protein based formula, and then finally, at 6 months, Nutramigen was started, without any relief in her symptoms. She was treated with ranitidine starting at 7 months for suspected GER. A sweat test performed at 8 months of age was normal. The family history was noncontributory.

III. Physical Examination

T, 37.3°C; RR, 22 to 25/min; HR, tachycardic; BP, 85/53 mm Hg

Weight, 6.5 kg (less than 5th percentile; 50th percentile for a 5-month-old child); length, 66.5 cm (less than 5th percentile); head circumference, 43.5 cm (25th percentile)

The patient was fussy but not toxic-appearing, with scant nasal discharge and dry oral mucosa. Her lungs were clear bilaterally, and she had a soft systolic murmur at the lower left sternal border with a prominent S3 gallop. The liver edge was palpated 1 cm below the right costal margin, and her spleen tip was also palpable. The extremities were warm and well perfused. There were no rashes, and her neurologic examination was normal for age.

IV. Diagnostic Studies

Laboratory analysis revealed 10,200 WBCs/mm^3, with 41% segmented neutrophils, 53% lymphocytes, and 6% monocytes. The hemoglobin was 11 g/dL, and the platelet count was 232,000 cells/mm^3. Serum electrolytes were as follows: sodium, 128 mmol/L; potassium, 4.5 mmol/L; chloride, 100 mmol/L; and bicarbonate, 20 mEq/L. Blood urea nitrogen (BUN) was 19 mg/dL, creatinine was 0.3 mg/dL, glucose was 84 mg/dL, and calcium was 9.2 mg/dl. Her ABG analysis showed pH, 7.43; $PaCO_2$, 31 mm Hg; and PaO_2, 270 mm Hg.

V. Course of Illness

A chest radiograph revealed mild cardiomegaly and a small right pleural effusion. An electrocardiogram (ECG) (Fig. 3-2) was diagnostic.

DISCUSSION: CASE 3-2

I. Differential Diagnosis

This patient presented with recurrent episodes of emesis and intermittent asymptomatic periods, consistent with cyclic vomiting. Quantitative criteria for the diagnosis of cyclic vomiting include at least four episodes of vomiting per hour during the peak inten-

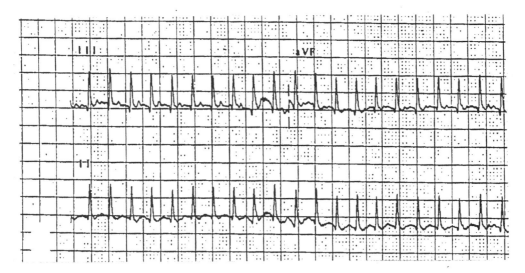

FIG. 3-2. Patient's initial electrocardiogram (case 3-2).

sity and a frequency of no more than nine episodes per month. In contrast, the patient with chronic vomiting has less frequent episodes and fewer symptom-free days.

Cyclic vomiting frequently has a nongastrointestinal etiology. Common causes include migraine headaches, abdominal migraines, metabolic disorders including adrenal insufficiency, amino acidurias, and organic acidurias. Renal disorders such as UPJ obstruction and renal calculi, as well as intermittent cardiac arrhythmias, can also cause cyclic vomiting. Familial dysautonomia (Riley-Day syndrome) and Munchausen syndrome by proxy must also be considered. Gastrointestinal etiologies include pancreatitis, malrotation with intermittent volvulus, and intestinal duplications.

In patients with significant tachycardia and cyclic vomiting, an intermittent cardiac tachyarrhythmia must be strongly considered. The source of the tachyarrhythmia may be sinus, supraventricular, or ventricular. Differentiation of supraventricular tachycardia from sinus tachycardia may be difficult at times. Sinus tachycardia rarely exceeds 230 bpm, has a normal P wave and P-wave axis, and results in a varying HR due to changes in vagal and sympathetic tone.

Antidromic supraventricular tachycardia (SVT) or SVT with a preceding bundle branch block (see later discussion) may result in a widened QRS complex that resembles ventricular tachycardia. The absence of P waves and the presence of a wide QRS complex that is dissimilar to the QRS complex observed during sinus rhythm are more diagnostic of ventricular tachycardia.

II. Diagnosis

The EKG in this patient revealed a narrow-complex tachycardia of 250 bpm, consistent with SVT (see Fig. 3-2). After ice was applied to the patient's face without success, she was cardioverted to a normal sinus rhythm with the use of intravenous adenosine. She was treated with digoxin and over the next 2 days had normalization of her cardiac examination and resolution of her hepatomegaly. An echocardiogram revealed mild left ventricular dilation, mild mitral valve regurgitation, and a small pericardial effusion but good cardiac function without any structural defects. A repeat EKG before discharge showed mild right atrial enlargement and a normal sinus rhythm without signs of preexcitation (shortened PR interval and delta wave) (Fig. 3-3). After 2 months on digoxin, her weight had increased to the

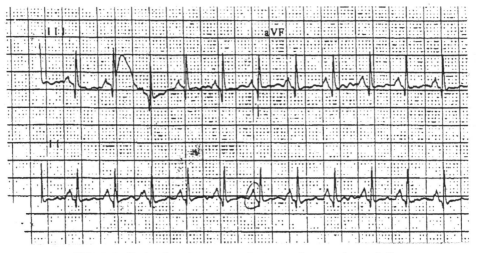

FIG. 3-3. Patient's subsequent electrocardiogram (case 3-2).

25th percentile. In retrospect, her history of episodic feeding intolerance, with each episode lasting 1 to 2 days, may have been episodes of supraventricular tachycardia.

III.   Incidence and Epidemiology of Supraventricular Tachycardia

SVT is a generic term encompassing a group of cardiac arrhythmias that originate above the atrioventricular (AV) node. It is the most common sustained accelerated nonsinus tachyarrhythmia, with an incidence of 1 per 250 to 1,000 children. SVT can be diagnosed by EKG during an episode. Episodes can be captured by means of a diagnostic EKG, a 24-hour Holter monitor, or transtelephonic monitoring. Two mechanisms account for virtually all cases of SVT: (a) an abnormal or enhanced normal automatic rhythm and (b) a reentrant rhythm. Approximately 75% of patients with a reentrant rhythm exhibit findings of preexcitation, with a shortened PR interval and initial slurred upstroke of the QRS (delta wave). Children younger than 12 years of age are more likely to have an accessory AV connection in adolescence, nodal reentry tachycardia increases in frequency.

Reentrant rhythms account for 90% of all cases of SVT. Two separate conducting pathways must be present, either AV or within the atrium, that lead to a cyclic pattern of excitation resulting in SVT. Atrial reentry rhythms may lead to either atrial fibrillation or atrial flutter. AV reentrant rhythms may be either through the AV node (nodal) or associated with an accessory AV pathway termed the bundle of Kent. Tachycardia may result from transmission of the impulse antegrade through the AV node-His-Purkinje system, through the myocardium retrograde, and through the accessory pathway completing the circuit. This orthodromic reciprocating tachycardia (ORT) is the most common pattern seen in Wolf-Parkinson-White syndrome and results in the typical narrow-complex QRS tachycardia. Rarely, the antegrade impulse travels via the accessory pathway and retrograde through the AV node-His-Purkinje system, resulting in antidromic reciprocating tachycardia (ART).

Preexcitation occurs in 75% of individuals with accessory pathways. This implies that the accessory pathway can conduct the impulse in antegrade fashion, from the atria to the ventricle. Bypassing the intrinsic delay of the AV node results in a shortened PR interval and a slurred upstroke of the QRS, the so-called delta wave. Twenty-five percent of accessory pathways transmit impulses only in retrograde fashion, from the ventricle to the atrium, resulting in a normal resting EKG (i.e., with no evidence of preexcitation).

SVT secondary to increased automaticity or atrial and junctional ectopic tachycardias occurs more commonly in children with postoperative congenital heart disease or cardiomyopathies.

IV. Clinical Presentation

Signs and symptoms of SVT depend on the age at presentation and the duration of the tachycardia. Episodes of SVT may last only a few seconds or may persist for hours. Many children tolerate these episodes extremely well, and it is unlikely that short paroxysms are dangerous. Infants with SVT often present with heart failure after the tachycardia goes unrecognized for a prolonged period. Episodes lasting longer than 6 to 24 hours may result in an acutely ill child with evidence of cardiopulmonary distress, with tachypnea, poor feeding, vomiting, lethargy, ashen color, restlessness, and irritability. Physical findings in such cases include pallor, tachypnea, diaphoresis, and hepatomegaly.

Older children may complain of lightheadedness, chest tightness, palpitations, and fatigue. Chest pain or discomfort is less common. The patient may become faint, dizzy, or even syncopal. If the HR is exceptionally rapid or if the attack is prolonged, heart failure may ensue.

V. Diagnostic Approach

Electrocardiogram. An EKG should be performed on any patient with tachycardia that is not thought to be normal sinus tachycardia. Patients with SVT have a very rapid and regular ventricular rate, usually about 240 bpm. The P waves are usually absent; when present, they have an abnormal axis and may precede or follow the QRS. Pending the results of the ECG, a chest radiograph or even an echocardiogram may need to be performed.

VI. Treatment

Treatment of SVT depends on the etiology and the duration of symptoms. Automatic rhythms are difficult to treat medically but respond well to ablation surgery.

Acute treatment of reentrant tachycardias depends on the age and stability of the patient. In hemodynamically stable children, vagotonic maneuvers such as straining, breath-holding, applying ice to the face, or adopting a particular posture should be attempted first. For patients who do not respond to simple vagal maneuvers, medical cardioversion should be attempted. Adenosine, a nucleoside derivative that blocks the orthodromic conduction at the AV node, is the medication of choice. Intravenous verapamil and propranolol can break an SVT but are contraindicated in infants and children because of the risk of bradycardia, hypotension, and cardiac arrest. If these modalities fail or if the patient is hemodynamically unstable, then synchronized electrical cardioversion should be performed immediately.

Once a patient has been successfully converted to a normal sinus rhythm, maintenance therapy is selected depending on the age of the patient and the cause of the SVT. In newborns and infants, digoxin remains the primary medication for prevention of SVT, which is usually self-limited. Medications that target the specific area of reentry (nodal or accessory) tend to work better. In patients with a hidden accessory pathway, digoxin or β-blockers are the mainstay of therapy. In children with evidence of preexcitation syndrome (e.g., Wolff-Parkinson-White syndrome), digoxin and calcium channel blockers are contraindicated, and β-blockers are usually used.

Radiofrequency ablation of the accessory pathway is one choice for definitive treatment. Success rates range from approximately 80% to 95%, depending on the location of the bypass tract or tracts. Surgical ablation of bypass tracts can also be successful in selected patients.

VII. References

1. Case CL. Diagnosis and treatment of pediatric arrhythmias. *Pediatr Clin North Am* 1999;46:351–352.
2. O'Connor B, Dick M. What every pediatrician should know about supraventricular tachycardia. *Pediatr Ann* 1991;20:368–376.
3. Park M, ed. *Pediatric cardiology for practitioners,* 3rd ed. St. Louis: Mosby, 1996.

Case 3-3: 6-Year-Old Girl

I.   History of Present Illness

The patient, a 6-year-old Caucasian girl with a 1-year history of intermittent vomiting, presented with a 2-week history of increased vomiting frequency. Her emesis was nonbilious, nonbloody, and not associated with eating or any specific time of day. Occasionally she had been awakened from sleep with vomiting. She denied abdominal pain, diarrhea, and rashes. She complained of intermittent headaches. The mother reported that her daughter had lost 2 pounds over the past month. On the previous day, the child had presented to her primary care physician with a 3-day history of cold symptoms and fever of 38.8°C, and the physician had begun treatment with cefixime for sinusitis.

II.   Past Medical History

The patient's past medical history was significant for severe failure to thrive, and she continued to grow below the 5th percentile for weight and height. Her family history was significant for a mother with Graves' disease and two maternal cousins on dialysis for unknown reasons.

III.   Physical Examination

T, 36.8°C; RR, 24/min; HR, 118 bpm; BP, 98/55 mm Hg

Weight (12.4 kg) and height (102 cm) both well below the 5th percentile

Examination revealed a thin, pale female in no acute distress. She had moist mucous membranes and clear nasal discharge, but her optic discs could not be visualized. Her neck was supple with full range of motion, the lungs were clear, and heart sounds were normal. Her abdomen was soft with good bowel sounds, nontender, nondistended, and without any masses, hepatomegaly, or splenomegaly. She had no rashes, and her neurologic evaluation was normal.

IV.   Diagnostic Studies

Laboratory evaluation revealed a normal complete blood count. Serum chemistry analysis showed the following: sodium, 128 mmol/L; potassium, 2.0 mmol/L; chloride, 93 mmol/L; bicarbonate, 21 mEq/L; BUN, 37 mg/dL; creatinine, 2.2 mg/dL; glucose, 89 mg/dL; calcium, 7.9 mg/dL; phosphorus, 4.1 mg/dL; and magnesium, 2.0 mg/dL. Liver function tests showed total protein, 6.5 g/dL; albumin, 3.3 g/dL; total bilirubin, 0.71 mg/dL; aspartate aminotransferase (AST), 68 U/L; lactate dehydrogenase, 1220 U/L; cholesterol, 265 mg/dL; and uric acid, 5.8 mg/dL. Urinalysis showed a specific gravity of 1.010, pH 6.5, trace blood, 3+ protein, 1+ glucose, and hyaline casts. Urine electrolytes were as follows: sodium, 38 mmol/L; potassium, 22 mmol/L; and chloride, 37 mmol/L. ABG analysis showed pH, 7.58; $PaCO_2$, 27 mm Hg; PaO_2, 115 mm Hg; and bicarbonate, of 22 mmol/L. A chest radiograph was normal, and an ECG demonstrated normal sinus rhythm with ST-segment depression. A renal ultrasound examination displayed small, echogenic kidneys.

V.   Course of Illness

The patient received intravenous potassium and normal saline and was admitted with a diagnosis of chronic renal failure of unknown etiology. After her electrolytes normalized, she was prescribed oral calcium and sent home, but she returned 2 days later with persistent vomiting. Metoclopramide therapy was started for delayed gastric emptying. Magnetic resonance imaging (MRI) of her brain was normal. Two months later she presented with photophobia; an ophthalmologic evaluation at that time provided the diagnosis (Fig. 3-4).

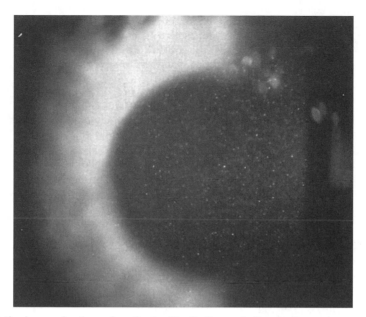

FIG. 3-4. Retinal examination of patient with findings similar to those in case 3-3. (From Oppenheim RA, Mathers WD. The eye in endocrinology. In: Becker KL, ed. *Principles and practice of endocrinology and metabolism.* Philadelphia: Lippincott Williams & Wilkins, 2001:1968, with permission.)

DISCUSSION: CASE 3-3

I. Differential Diagnosis

Differential diagnosis of a child with renal failure depends on whether the condition is prerenal, intrinsic renal, or postrenal in etiology. With a BUN/creatinine ratio lower than 20, a specific gravity of less than 1.020, and small, echogenic kidneys on ultrasound, the renal failure in this case was most likely caused by an intrinsic process. Intrinsic renal failure could be a result of vascular, glomerular, or tubular injury. This patient had tubular dysfunction or Fanconi syndrome, and the differential diagnosis includes tyrosinemia, hereditary fructose intolerance, vitamin D dependency (type I), galactosemia, Wilson disease, and Lowe syndrome.

II. Diagnosis

The ophthalmologic evaluation at the time of diagnosis revealed corneal crystals suggesting cystine deposits (see Fig. 3-4). **Subsequently, an elevated leukocyte cystine concentration was found, confirming the diagnosis of cystinosis.**

III. Incidence and Epidemiology of Cystinosis

Cystinosis, a rare lysosomal storage disorder, is associated with the accumulation of cystine in many cells of the body. Deletion or mutation of the gene that codes for the cystine transport protein, cystinosin, causes an accumulation of intracellular cystine to toxic levels. This gene has been mapped to chromosome 17p13. Cystinosis is inherited as an autosomal recessive disorder and occurs in 1 of every 200,000 live births in North America. The carrier frequency has been estimated to be 1 in 225 people. The disease predominately affects individuals of European descent with blond hair and fair complexion, but it has been diagnosed in most ethnic groups.

IV. Clinical Presentation

Three classic presentations of cystinosis exist; they differ based on the age of the patient at presentation. Cystine accumulation in cells accounts for the symptoms that include Fanconi syndrome, kidney failure, corneal opacities and photophobia, linear growth failure, hypothyroidism, and hypohidrosis.

The early or infantile nephropathic form is the most common form; it occurs in patients 3 to 18 months of age. These patients present with Fanconi syndrome, severe failure to thrive, rickets, corneal crystals, and hypohidrosis.

Fanconi syndrome is a disorder characterized by dysfunctional proximal tubule transport, which impairs resorption of amino acids, glucose, phosphate, citrate, urate, and bicarbonate. It is also associated with a vitamin D-resistant rickets or osteopenia. The resultant polyuria, extracellular fluid volume depletion, hypokalemia, impaired growth, and rickets begin in the first years of life. End-stage renal failure occurs by 10 years of age in untreated patients.

Ocular findings in cystinosis consist of corneal crystals that appear in the first year but do not impair vision at that time. The crystals may lead to photophobia, and 15% of patients develop corneal ulcerations. Thirty percent of patients develop decreased visual acuity by the end of the first decade of life, and some patients develop blindness due to retinal deterioration. Other manifestations include a generalized patchy depigmentation around the periphery of the retina that is evident very early in life.

Other findings associated with cystinosis include hypothyroidism secondary to cystine accumulation in the thyroid follicles. Levels of thyroid-stimulating hormone are increased before symptom onset, and the average age for initiation of thyroid replacement therapy is 10 years. Cystine accumulation in the gonads results in hypogonadism and sterility. Most patients fail to develop secondary sexual characteristics. Diabetes mellitus and pancreatic exocrine insufficiency can develop. Neurologic complications include progressive neurologic involvement with encephalopathy and dementia.

The second category of cystinosis is very similar to the infantile form except that the initial presentation occurs later, during the second decade of life, and there is a slower rate of progression to end-stage renal failure.

The third and final category is the benign adult type. This condition is not associated with renal damage or Fanconi syndrome. Intracellular cystine levels are only modestly elevated, to 30 to 50 times normal, but cystine crystals may still form in the corneas, bone marrow, leukocytes, and skin fibroblasts.

V. Diagnostic Approach

Diagnosis of a rare pediatric condition such as cystinosis depends on maintaining a high index of suspicion.

Urine studies. Findings are consistent with a Fanconi syndrome and include aminoaciduria, glycosuria, and phosphaturia.

Cysteine levels. Increased fibroblast or leukocyte cystine levels (30 to 50 times the normal concentration in the benign adult form, and 100 to 1,000 times greater in the homozygous infantile form) are diagnostic of cystinosis. These levels are abnormal in both symptomatic children and asymptomatic children with a family history of cystinosis.

Ophthalmology. Ocular slit-lamp examination may reveal birefringent, hexagonal or rectangular crystals as well as depigmentation of the retina.

Tissue biopsy. Microscopic examination of kidney cells, thyroid follicles, or reticuloendothelial cells reveals crystal formation.

Prenatal testing. Prenatal diagnosis is possible by measurement of elevated cystine levels in cells obtained through either chorionic villus sampling at 9 weeks' gestation or amniocentesis at 16 weeks' gestation.

VI. Treatment

Two treatment regimens exist for cystinosis. One focuses on correction of electrolyte abnormalities, rickets, and other systemic problems, and the other is aimed at reducing the overall cystine load. Symptomatic relief for Fanconi syndrome and rickets includes replacement therapy with bicarbonate, potassium, phosphorus, and 1,25-dihydroxyvitamin D. Severe growth failure is treated with growth hormone therapy, and both endocrine and exocrine pancreatic deficiency are treated as required.

Almost all patients progress to renal failure by 10 years of age if their cystine level is not reduced. Cysteamine, a sulfhydryl binder, binds to cystine and utilizes another transport protein for removal from the lysosome. Cysteamine significantly lowers the cystine level and if it is started early in life, and it has been shown to slow the rate of progression to renal failure. Hemodialysis and renal transplantation have also proved effective. Although renal transplantation does not stop the accumulation of cystine in all other cells of the body, cystine does not accumulate in the tubules of the transplanted kidney, and therefore Fanconi syndrome and renal failure do not occur. Cysteamine eye drops are also available and may decrease the formation of ocular crystals.

VII. References

1. Almond PS, Matas AJ, Nakhleh RE, et al. Renal transplantation for infantile cystinosis: long-term follow-up. *J Pediatr Surg* 1993;28:232–238.
2. Gahl WA. Cystinosis. *N Engl J Med* 2002;347:111–121.
3. Norman M. Cystinosis. In: Behrman RE, Kliegman RM, Jenson HB, eds. *Nelson textbook of pediatrics,* 16th ed. Philadelphia: WB Saunders, 2000:1599–1600.
4. Simon JW, Kaw P. Commonly missed diagnoses on the childhood eye examination. *Am Family Physician* 2001;64:623–628.
5. Thoene JG. Cystinosis. *J Inherit Metab Dis* 1995;18:380–386.

Case 3-4: 10-Year-Old Girl

I. History of Present Illness
A 10-year-old Caucasian girl presented with vomiting. She had been in her usual state of good health until 5 days ago, when she developed nonbloody but occasionally bilious emesis. She also complained of a 2-day history of worsening weakness, dizziness, and lethargy. She had a poor appetite, decreased urine output, and weight loss. She denied diarrhea, fever, rash, joint pain, dysuria, and cough.

II. Past Medical History
The patient has a history of mild intermittent asthma but denied any hospitalizations or family history of autoimmune diseases.

III. Physical Examination
T, 37.8°C; RR, 28/min; HR, 138 bpm; BP, 108/53 mm Hg

Weight, 22.9 kg (5th percentile); height, 150 cm (95th percentile)

Examination revealed a thin female in no acute distress. She had moist mucous membranes, but there were numerous hyperpigmented macules scattered about the buccal surface and on the tongue. The lung and heart sounds were normal. Her abdomen was soft with good bowel sounds, nontender, and nondistended without any palpable masses.

IV. Diagnostic Studies
Laboratory evaluation revealed a normal complete blood count. Serum chemistry values were as follows: sodium, 123 mEq/L; potassium, 6.6 mEq/L; chloride, 95 mEq/L; bicarbonate, 14 mEq/L; BUN, 55 mg/dL; creatinine, 2.4 mg/dL; glucose, 40 mg/dL; calcium, 8.1 mg/dL; phosphorus, 5.2 mg/dL; and urinary sodium, 30mEq/L. Urinalysis was notable for a specific gravity of 1.020 and the presence of ketones. The venous blood gas had a pH of 7.25.

V. Course of Illness
On questioning, the mother reported that her daughter had had a 1-year history of salt craving and recently had developed dark spots on her body. The patient received a rapid intravenous infusion of normal saline followed by dextrose. Based on the history, clinical examination, and laboratory studies, she was given a presumptive diagnosis and appropriate therapy was started.

DISCUSSION: CASE 3-4

I. Differential Diagnosis
Patients who present with acute renal failure should first be categorized as having prerenal, renal, or postrenal disease. Prerenal acute renal failure is caused by decreased renal perfusion from hypovolemia, hypotension, and hypoxia of various etiologies. Intrinsic acute renal failure could be secondary to a vascular, glomerular, or tubular dysfunction. Vascular lesions include renal vein thrombosis, hemolytic uremic syndrome, and various vasculitides. Glomerular pathology includes glomerulonephritis from multiple causes (including poststreptococcal glomerulonephritis) and nephritis from lupus and Henoch-Schönlein purpura. Tubular injury may occur secondary to acute tubular necrosis, interstitial nephritis, or certain medications. Finally, postrenal causes include obstructive uropathies, renal calculi, blood clots, and urinary tract infections.

This patient's history of fluid loss, decreased intake, and weight loss, as well as the physical examination findings, support a prerenal etiology. Laboratory data also support a prerenal etiology, with a high urine specific gravity, the presence of ketonuria and the absence of proteinuria, hematuria and hyaline casts, and a BUN/creatinine ratio greater than 20.

Because the patient is not hypoxic or hypotensive, the most probable cause of prerenal renal failure is hypovolemia. Causes of hypovolemia include hemorrhage, vomiting and diarrhea, hypoproteinemia, third spacing from burns, and renal or adrenal disease with salt wasting. Given the patient's history and the laboratory results of hyperkalemia and hyponatremia, the most likely etiology is either renal or adrenal. An adrenal etiology is supported by the increased urinary sodium concentration in the face of hyponatremia and by the normal urinalysis and lack of laboratory evidence of an intrinsic renal pathology.

II. Diagnosis

Evidence that suggests the diagnosis of adrenal insufficiency in this case includes the history of vomiting, anorexia, weight loss, salt craving, and mucosal hyperpigmentation. Laboratory data that support the diagnosis include low serum sodium, glucose, and bicarbonate and increased potassium and BUN. Definitive diagnosis of a patient with adrenal insufficiency depends on whether the condition is primary, secondary, or tertiary. Addison's disease is usually synonymous with primary adrenal insufficiency. Evaluation of the patient's blood obtained before the administration of hydrocortisone confirmed an elevated serum pituitary corticotropin (ACTH) level and a low serum cortisol level. Subsequently, the patient failed to mount an adequate response to the ACTH stimulation test, confirming the diagnosis of primary adrenal insufficiency. Normalization of all laboratory values and the clinical course occurred after appropriate glucocorticoid and mineralocorticoid replacement therapy was started. She was prescribed fludrocortisone acetate and discharged home.

III. Incidence and Epidemiology of Adrenal Insufficiency

Adrenal insufficiency is a rare and often underdiagnosed condition with significant morbidity and mortality. It may be caused by destruction of the adrenal cortex (primary adrenal insufficiency), deficient pituitary ACTH secretion (secondary adrenal insufficiency), or deficient hypothalamic secretion of corticotropin-releasing hormone (CRH) or other ACTH secretagogues (tertiary adrenal insufficiency).

Addison's disease is a vague term used to describe primary adrenal insufficiency. Because there are numerous causes of adrenal insufficiency, it is more appropriate to diagnose adrenal insufficiency based on its etiology. In the last century, the most common cause of primary adrenal insufficiency was tuberculosis infection of the adrenal gland. Currently, autoimmune idiopathic and congenital adrenal insufficiency account for most of the cases of primary adrenal insufficiency diagnosed in children.

The specific causes of adrenal insufficiency are also age dependent. At birth adrenal hemorrhage from perinatal events is the most common cause, and adrenal insufficiency from CAH usually manifests in the first few weeks of life. Older children and adults often suffer from an autoimmune process that may be part of a larger autoimmune polyglandular syndrome (APS). Type I autoimmune polyendocrinopathy, an autosomal recessive disorder, consists of chronic mucocutaneous candidiasis initially followed by hypoparathyroidism and then Addison's disease. Type II autoimmune polyendocrinopathy consists of Addison's disease associated with autoimmune thyroid disease or insulin-dependent diabetes. Autoimmune disease coordinates antibodies with a cell-mediated process resulting in lymphocytic infiltration of the cortex. In adults, adrenal infections and metastatic cancer to the adrenal gland become more common. Adrenoleukodystrophy should also be considered in male patients.

IV. Clinical Presentation

The presentation of a child with adrenal insufficiency depends on the age of the child, the etiology, and the acuity of symptoms. Newborns who present with adrenal insufficiency from a perinatal event or from CAH often are in shock. In patients with CAH, signs and symptoms begin shortly after birth and are characteristic of the salt-losing nature of the illness. They include failure to thrive, vomiting, lethargy, anorexia, and dehydration with eventual shock, which may be fatal.

Clinical evidence of adrenal insufficiency in older children is often more insidious, inapparent until at least 90% of the adrenal cortex is destroyed. Normally the adrenal medulla is preserved. Signs and symptoms of both glucocorticoid and mineralocorticoid deficiency are present and include persistent vomiting, poor weight gain or weight loss, weakness, fatigue, anorexia, hypotension, hyponatremia, hyperkalemia, abdominal pain, and hyperpigmentation. Initial manifestations of mild glucocorticoid deficiency result in inadequate cortisol increase in response to stress or episodic postprandial hypoglycemia. Initial mineralocorticoid deficiency manifests as mild postural hypotension, with progression to hypotension, hyperkalemia, and dehydration if not corrected.

Hyperpigmentation associated with chronic primary adrenal insufficiency occurs mostly in sun-exposed areas and in the flexor creases of the knees, elbows, knuckles, and genitalia. It is caused by increased levels of ACTH and melanocyte-stimulating hormone (MSH) secondary to a stimulated hypothalamic-pituitary axis. Abdominal pain may simulate an acute abdominal process, and there may be an intense craving for salt. If the condition is not recognized early and treated, adrenal crisis may develop.

The most worrisome presentation of primary adrenal insufficiency in a child is adrenal crisis. Adrenal crisis is caused primarily to a lack of mineralocorticoid activity. However, glucocorticoid deficiency also contributes to the hypotension as a result of decreased vascular sensitivity to angiotensin II and norepinephrine, decreased synthesis of renin substrate, and increased prostaglandin I_2 production. These patients present in a shock-like state with cyanosis, labored breathing, hypotension, confusion, lethargy, and coma. Adrenal crisis is typically precipitated by an antecedent infection or stress to which the body is unable to mount an adequate glucocorticoid response. This may occur in undiagnosed patients, including newborns, or in previously diagnosed patients who are taking inadequate amounts of mineralocorticoid replacement. In the absence of immediate and intensive therapy, the course is rapidly fatal.

In patients with secondary adrenal insufficiency due to a decreased secretion of ACTH, the presentation is slightly different. Hypoglycemia occurs much more commonly, but, because the mineralocorticoid and androgen secretion is normal, these patients do not present with hyperkalemia or hypotension. Hyperpigmentation does not occur, because ACTH levels are not elevated and plasma renin activity is also usually normal. Hyponatremia still exists, because the lack of cortisol secretion causes an increase in arginine vasopressin (AVP).

Mineralocorticoid deficiency causes hyperkalemia by (a) decreased renal potassium and hydrogen ion excretion and (b) a mild acidosis that contributes to the hyperkalemia by permitting potassium to shift from the intracellular to the extracellular space. Potassium retention leads to high serum potassium levels, which can cause cardiac dysrhythmias such as peaked T waves, low P waves, wide QRS complexes, atrial asystole, intraventricular block, ventricular asystole, and death.

Hyponatremia and hypotension are the result of reduced mineralocorticoid and glucocorticoid activity. Low aldosterone levels cause increased urinary excretion of sodium and chloride and therefore decreased serum levels, causing volume depletion. This volume depletion is compounded by reduced peripheral vascular adrenergic tone, which is caused by glucocorticoid deficiency and can lead to vascular collapse and shock. AVP secretion is increased in response to volume depletion, which impairs free water clearance to increase intravascular volume. Plasma renin activity is also increased to offset volume depletion.

V. Diagnostic Approach

Accurate and quick diagnosis of a rare medical condition depends on having a high index of suspicion. Patients who present in adrenal crisis typically have hyponatremia (88%) and hyperkalemia (64%), and unusual episodes of hyperpigmentation should be considered adrenal insufficiency until proved otherwise.

Serum cortisol. The most definitive test for adrenal insufficiency is measurement of serum cortisol levels before and after administration of ACTH. A short ACTH stimulation test reveals partial adrenal insufficiency that may be missed by the standard test. A normal response in the short ACTH stimulation test excludes primary adrenal insufficiency but does not eliminate secondary adrenal insufficiency of recent onset. The overnight metyrapone test should be used for definitive diagnosis if this is a consideration. An impaired response confirms adrenal insufficiency, but additional studies are necessary to establish its type and cause.

Other studies. In primary adrenal insufficiency, resting cortisol levels are low and there is no increase after administration of ACTH. Secretion of aldosterone, dehydroepiandrosterone (DHEA), and dehydroepiandrosterone sulfate (DHEAS) is low. The serum testosterone level is normal in men but low in women, in whom it is mostly derived from peripheral conversion of adrenal androgens. Plasma ACTH is elevated but exhibits a normal diurnal rhythm. Normal resting levels that do not increase after administration of ACTH indicate an absence of adrenocortical reserve.

A low initial level followed by a significant response to ACTH may indicate either secondary or tertiary adrenal insufficiency. Further testing with metyrapone, an inhibitor of 11-hydroxylase, helps differentiate secondary from tertiary causes of adrenal insufficiency.

Serum electrolytes. Hypernatremia and hypokalemia occur as described earlier.

VI. Treatment

Acute adrenal insufficiency—adrenal crisis—is a life-threatening emergency that requires immediate treatment for shock and electrolyte abnormalities. After the airway and breathing have been secured, intravenous or intraosseous access must be obtained immediately. Resuscitation continues with normal saline to correct hypotension and hyponatremia and glucose to correct hypoglycemia. Glucocorticoid therapy must be given if the diagnosis of adrenal insufficiency is entertained. Dexamethasone is the preferred treatment for adrenal crisis because it is long-lasting and does not interfere with cortisol assays or subsequent ACTH stimulation tests. Alternatively, hydrocortisone could be given, but extra blood specimens should be obtained before hydrocortisone therapy is initiated for determination of the levels of ACTH, cortisol, aldosterone, plasma renin activity, 17-α-hydroxyprogesterone, and adrenal androgens. Mineralocorticoid is not useful acutely, because it takes several days for its sodium-retaining effects to become manifest and because adequate sodium replacement can be achieved by intravenous saline administration. After the patient is stabilized, the precipitating cause of the crisis must be identified and treated if possible. Chronic therapy consists of daily replacement with hydrocortisone and fludrocortisone acetate (Florinef).

Long-acting synthetic glucocorticoids such as dexamethasone or prednisone provide a more physiologic effect, and the replacement dose is adjusted based on symptoms of adrenal insufficiency, decreased hyperpigmentation, and morning cortisol levels. Excess replacement results in cushingoid characteristics such as excessive weight gain, facial plethora, and a suppressed morning cortisol level.

Mineralocorticoid replacement is required for all patients with primary adrenal insufficiency and is considered optimal if the patient is without symptoms of postural hypotension and has normal pulse and blood pressure readings, potassium level, and plasma renin activity. Excessive replacement is suggested if the patient has hypertension, edema, and hypokalemia.

As with most chronic diseases, education about normal activities, medications, and when to increase the hydrocortisone dose during periods of bodily stress is paramount. Every patient should wear a medical alert bracelet at all times and should always carry and be prepared to administer dexamethasone via a prefilled syringe.

VII. References

1. Coursin DB, Wood KE. Corticosteroid supplementation for adrenal insufficiency. *JAMA* 2002;287:236–240.
2. Laron Z. Hypoglycemia due to hormone deficiencies. *J Pediatr Endocrinol* 1998;11: s117–s120.
3. Melby JC. Assessment of adrenocortical function. *N Engl J Med* 1971;285:735–739.
4. Schatz DA, Winter DE. Autoimmune polyglandular syndrome: clinical syndrome and treatment. *Endocrinol Metab Clin North Am* 2002;31:339–352.
5. Ten S, New M, Maclaren N. Clinical review 130: Addison's disease. *J Clin Endocrinol Metab* 2001;86:2909–2922.

Case 3-5: 4-Year-Old Girl

I. History of Present Illness

A 4-year-old girl presented to the outpatient oncology clinic with vomiting. She was receiving interim maintenance chemotherapy for a history of acute lymphoblastic leukemia (ALL). Three days earlier, she began to have decreased activity and decreased appetite, taking only liquids. Over the past 2 days, she had developed nonbloody, nonbilious vomiting that occurred about every 2 hours. She had had two bloody stools the previous morning but had not stooled since that time. On the day of admission, her frequency of vomiting increased to six times per hour and she became listless. She had been afebrile.

II. Past Medical History

The patient was diagnosed with ALL four months ago, and her last chemotherapy treatment was 1 month ago. She had had two recent hospitalizations, 1 month ago for a viral pneumonia and 1 week ago for fever and a central line with negative blood cultures.

III. Physical Examination

T, 37.7°C; RR, 28/min; HR, 160 bpm; BP, 100/60 mm Hg

Weight, 14.2 kg (5th percentile), down from 16.6 kg one week ago; height, 150 cm (95th percentile)

General examination revealed a lethargic, disoriented child responding only to voice and painful stimuli. She had sunken eyes, dry mucous membranes without mucositis, normal lung examination findings, and tachycardia with good peripheral perfusion. Her abdomen was slightly distended, but there was no tenderness, rebound, or guarding. Bowel sounds were hypoactive. There was a small amount of gross blood on rectal examination.

IV. Diagnostic Studies

Laboratory evaluation revealed 10,200 WBCs/mm^3, with 6% band forms, 64% segmented neutrophils, 8% lymphocytes, and 20% monocytes. The hemoglobin was 10 g/dL, and the platelet count was 240,000 cells/mm^3. Serum chemistry results were as follows: sodium, 133 mmol/L; potassium, 3.2 mmol/L; chloride, 78 mmol/L; bicarbonate, 22 mEq/L; BUN, 105 mg/dL; creatinine, 1.4 mg/dL; glucose, 100 mg/dL; phosphorus, 7.2 mg/dL; uric acid, 20.6 mg/dL; bilirubin, 1.2 mg/dL; alanine aminotransferase (ALT), 342 U/L; AST, 96 U/L; lactate dehydrogenase, 1,432 U/L; amylase, 36 U/L; lipase, 82 U/L; and ammonia, 24 μmol/L.

Abdominal radiographs showed multiple dilated loops of small bowel, with no air in the distal large bowel and no free air in the abdominal cavity.

V. Course of Illness

The patient's altered mental status did not improve with fluid resuscitation. She had normal MRI of the head. The abdominal radiograph showed dilated loops of small intestine, suggestive of an ileus. She was treated with intravenous fluids and broad-spectrum antibiotics. A nasogastric tube was placed to decompress the abdomen. On the following day, she developed increasing abdominal pain and distention. She was now tympanitic, with absent bowel sounds but still without signs of peritoneal inflammation. A nuclear medicine imaging study revealed the diagnosis.

DISCUSSION: CASE 3-5

I. Differential Diagnosis

The patient presented with a history and physical and radiographic evidence of intestinal obstruction. She presented suddenly with abdominal distention, vomiting, pain, and failure to pass stool. On physical examination, she was found to have a distended, tympanitic abdomen. The abdominal radiograph showed dilated loops of small bowel, with a paucity of air in the large bowel. These findings are consistent with a distal small bowel obstruction requiring surgical exploration. The cause of intestinal obstruction could be intraluminal or extraluminal. Intraluminal disorders consist of foreign bodies, bezoars, fecaliths, chronic constipation, parasites, intraluminal tumors, inflammatory bowel disease, Hirschsprung's disease, and imperforate anus. Extraluminal disorders include incarcerated hernias, intussusception, a Meckel diverticulum, malrotation with volvulus, duplications, extraluminal tumor or lymph node compressing the intestine, superior mesenteric artery syndrome, and postoperative adhesions.

II. Diagnosis

A technetium 99m (^{99m}Tc)–pertechnetate scan was positive, suggesting a Meckel diverticulum. In the operating room, she was found to have a distal small bowel obstruction related to a Meckel diverticulum. The diverticulum was resected without any evidence of bowel wall infarction.

III. Incidence and Epidemiology of a Meckel Diverticulum

Occurring in 2% of the population, the Meckel diverticulum is the most common congenital anomaly of the gastrointestinal tract. The diverticulum is an embryonic remnant of the vitelline duct, which connects the intestine to the yolk sac and provides nutrition until 8 weeks' gestational age, at which time the placenta provides complete nutrition. When the aspect of the duct that is closest to the intestine remains open, it forms a Meckel diverticulum.

The Meckel diverticulum is consistently located within 2 feet of the ileocecal valve and always arising from the antimesenteric border of the ileum. Half of all Meckel diverticula contain ectopic gastric, pancreatic, or duodenal tissue.

IV. Clinical Presentation

Only 5% of all patients with a Meckel diverticulum become symptomatic. Despite an equal incidence in both sexes, males tend to have a higher rate of complications. Painless rectal bleeding, the most common presentation, occurs in almost half of all symptomatic patients. Stool may be either red or maroon in color but is not tarry. Anemia may develop, but the bleeding does not usually cause hemodynamic compromise. The bleeding is intermittent and usually is caused by ulcers adjacent to the ectopic gastric acid–secreting tissue in the diverticulum. Other common symptoms include abdominal pain, nausea, vomiting, and abdominal distention.

In a study by St.-Vil et al., 49 (42%) of 117 children with symptomatic presentation of Meckel diverticulum developed complete or partial bowel obstruction. In older children, especially boys, this obstruction was usually caused by the diverticulum's becoming a lead point for intussusception into the ileum. The other common mechanism was residual fibrous bands of the duct, which served as a fulcrum causing volvulus, or an internal hernia with subsequent bowel obstruction. An inflamed diverticulum, diverticulitis, in the right lower quadrant often manifests as an acute abdomen mimicking an acute appendicitis that may progress to perforation and peritonitis.

V. Diagnostic Approach

A Meckel diverticulum should be considered in any patient with painless rectal bleeding.

Meckel scan. A Meckel scan is performed using the radiopharmaceutical ^{99m}Tc-pertechnetate, which is administered intravenously. Gastric uptake of the tracer progressively increases during the first 30 minutes of the study. Patients with ectopic gastric mucosa also have increasing activity in that area, usually the right lower quadrant. Images are obtained in multiple projections to prevent missing a focus obscured by other structures. The Meckel scan has a high sensitivity, because even though ectopic gastric tissue is present in only 30% to 50% of all Meckel diverticula, it is present in almost 100% of those responsible for rectal bleeding. Administration of histamine$_2$ (H_2)–receptor antagonists (e.g., cimetidine) before the study decreases luminal gastric acid secretion and thus luminal ^{99m}Tc-pertechnetate secretion, allowing better visualization of the ectopic focus. The sensitivity of the Meckel scan with cimetidine is greater than 90%, and the specificity is as high as 95%. Intravenous glucagon, by delaying gastric emptying, may also allow better visualization of the ectopic gastric mucosa. False-negative Meckel scans can be caused by inadequate tracer uptake (e.g., hypofunctioning or absent gastric mucosa within the diverticulum, mucosal ischemia or necrosis), rapid tracer washout (e.g., active bleeding, hyperperistalsis), or interference by overlying structures such as the kidneys or bladder. False-positive scans are caused by misinterpretation of normal background activity in the testes, kidneys, bladder, or uterus as ectopic gastric mucosa.

Laparotomy and laparoscopy. An inflamed Meckel diverticulum may be implicated as the cause of right lower-quadrant abdominal pain during surgical exploration. It may also be an incidental finding when surgery is performed for another reason.

Abdominal radiographs. Radiographs may reveal obstruction.

Upper gastrointestinal contrast study. An upper gastrointestinal contrast study with small bowel followthrough occasionally demonstrates the diverticulum. This study is not recommended if a Meckel diverticulum is suspected.

Barium enema. A barium enema may reduce an associated intussusception, but it is not usually diagnostic for Meckel diverticulum.

VI. Treatment

Treatment begins with ensuring hemodynamic stability. Definitive therapy includes surgical resection of the Meckel diverticulum on an emergency or semi-elective basis. Associated intussusception usually requires surgical rather than hydrostatic reduction; partial bowel resection with primary anastomosis is occasionally required. The management of a Meckel diverticulum found incidentally during laparotomy is not clear. Because the risk of a serious complication of Meckel diverticulum is low, many surgeons recommend removal only in the presence of suspected ectopic mucosa or if the diverticulum is attached to the umbilicus or mesentery by fibrous bands—situations that increase the risk of subsequent bowel obstruction.

VII. References

1. Brown RL, Stevenson RJ. Meckel diverticulum. In: Rudolph CD, Rudolph AM, eds. *Rudolph's pediatrics,* 21st ed. New York: McGraw-Hill, 2003:1405–1407.
2. D'Agostino J. Common abdominal emergencies in children. *Emerg Med Clin North Am* 2002;20:139–153.
3. Gainey MA. Radionuclide diagnosis. In: Walker WA, Durie PR, Hamilton JR, et al., eds. *Pediatric gastrointestinal disease: pathophysiology, diagnosis, management,* 3rd ed. Hamilton, Ontario: BC Decker, 2000:1655–1675.
4. St.-Vil D, Brandt ML, Panic S, et al. Meckel's diverticulum in children: a 20-year review. *J Pediatr Surg* 1991;26:1289–1292.
5. Valla JS, Steyaert H, Leculee R, et al. Meckel's diverticulum and laparoscopy of children: what's new? *Eur J Pediatr Surg* 1998;8:26–28.

Case 3-6: 10-Month-Old Girl

I. History of Present Illness
A 10-month-old girl presented with a 1-day history of vomiting and fever to 38.3°C. The emesis was nonbloody and nonbilious. She had a history of constipation and failure to thrive starting at 4 months of age. She had had no recent changes in her stooling pattern of once a week. Stooling was painful, but there was no blood or mucus. Her mother used prune juice, Karo syrup, and laxatives to aid the patient's bowel movements. Her mother also claimed that her daughter had always had a distended abdomen.

II. Past Medical History
The patient had a history of constipation, failure to thrive (she was growing at the 50th percentile until 4 months of age), anemia, hypotonia, and developmental delay.

III. Physical Examination
T, 38.7°C; RR, 56/min; HR, 150 bpm; BP, 92/50 mm Hg

Weight, 6.2 kg; length, 66 cm; head circumference, 40.5 cm—all significantly less than the 5th percentile for age

General examination revealed a pale, crying infant with a distended abdomen. Her heart and lungs were normal, but her abdomen was distended and tender, with hypoactive bowel sounds and a palpable mass in the right lower quadrant. There was no hepatomegaly or splenomegaly. Her neurologic examination was notable for general hypotonia.

IV. Diagnostic Studies
Laboratory evaluation revealed 25,000 WBCs/mm^3, with 81% segmented neutrophils, 10% lymphocytes, and 6% monocytes. The hemoglobin was 8.7 g/dL with hypochromia, occasional schistocytes, and burr cells. The mean corpuscular volume (MCV) was 74.6 fL, the red blood cell distribution width index (RDW) was 23.2; and the reticulocyte count was 2.2%. The platelet count was 649,000 cells/mm^3. Serum chemistry results were as follows: sodium, 137 mEq/L; potassium, 4.9 mEq/L; chloride, 115 mEq/L; bicar-

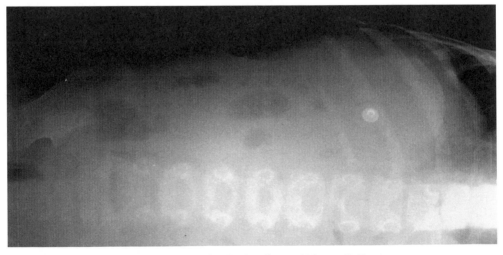

FIG. 3-5. Abdominal radiograph (case 3-6).

bonate, 18 mEq/L; BUN, 3 mg/dL; creatinine, 0.2 mg/dL; glucose, 98 mg/dL; alkaline phosphatase, 77 U/L; total bilirubin, 0.8 mg/dL; ALT, 98 U/L; and AST, 156 U/L.

V.   Course of Illness

The chest radiograph was normal. An abdominal radiograph revealed findings that led to an immediate therapeutic procedure (Fig. 3-5).

DISCUSSION: CASE 3-6

I.   Differential Diagnosis

Vomiting in a child with a distended, tender abdomen; a palpable mass in the right lower quadrant; and an abdominal radiograph revealing a large pneumoperitoneum is considered a ruptured hollow viscus until proved otherwise and requires immediate surgical exploration. Once the perforation has been identified and resected, the cause of the perforation must be discovered and corrected.

Vomiting in an infant with a history of chronic constipation could be caused by mechanical obstruction resulting from tumors, malrotation with volvulus, congenital bands, strictures, or duplications. Intestinal problems that can cause constipation include neuropathies, myopathies, and Hirschsprung's disease. Extraintestinal problems include endocrine disorders, hypothyroidism, hypokalemia, hypercalcemia, infant botulism, certain medications, familial dysautonomia, and spinal cord lesions. Finally, functional disorders caused by a slow transit time or by dietary abnormalities can also cause constipation.

II.   Diagnosis

The abdominal radiograph showed a moderate amount of free air in the abdomen, suggesting bowel perforation (see Fig. 3-5). The patient was taken to the operating room, where a large rush of air was felt when the abdominal cavity was entered. A massively dilated colon was discovered, and an 18-cm segment of the colon was resected after a 3-mm perforation was found in the sigmoid colon. **Pathologic review of the resected segment confirmed the diagnosis of Hirschsprung's disease.**

III.   Incidence and Epidemiology of Hirschsprung's Disease

Hirschsprung initially reported this condition in 1888, but it was not until the 1920s that the absence of ganglion cells in the distal gastrointestinal tract was discovered. Hirschsprung's disease has an incidence of 1 in 5,000 live births, with a male predominance of almost 4:1. Ninety percent of cases occur in full-term infants, and it is the most common cause of lower intestinal obstruction in neonates. A family history is noted in 7%, and if the cecum is involved the proportion rises to 21%. Hirschsprung's disease occurs in up to 10% of patients with Down syndrome and is associated with other conditions such as Smith-Lemli-Opitz syndrome, Waardenburg syndrome, congenital deafness, Laurence-Moon-Biedl-Bardet syndrome, and Ondine's curse.

Hirschsprung's disease is caused by the failed cephalocaudal migration of neural crest cells during the 5th through 12th week of gestation. The absence of neurons begins at the anus and extends proximally. This defect is limited to the rectal and sigmoid area in 75% of patients and includes the total colon in only 8%. Absence of these neural crest cells interrupts the inhibitory parasympathetic nerves in the myenteric plexus, thereby inhibiting relaxation and causing unopposed contraction.

IV.   Clinical Presentation

The clinical presentation of patients with Hirschsprung's disease depends on the length of the aganglionic segment. Ninety-four percent of all patients with Hirschsprung's disease fail to pass meconium within the first 24 hours of life. Other symptoms include constipation (93%), vomiting (64%), diarrhea (25%), rectal fissures with bleeding (5%), and bowel perforation (3%). Abdominal distention occurs in 83%, and rectal examination reveals an empty rectal vault in 60% (especially with long-segment Hirschsprung's disease) or rectal impaction in 7% (especially with short-segment Hirschsprung's disease).

V. Diagnostic Approach

Only 15% of patients are diagnosed in the first month of life, 65% by 3 months, and 80% by 1 year of age; almost 10% are diagnosed after 3 years of age. Early diagnosis is associated with a decreased incidence of enterocolitis and mortality.

Abdominal radiographs. Plain abdominal radiographs show a paucity of air in the distal rectum.

Barium enema. Barium enema is diagnostic in 80% of cases but may be inconclusive or falsely negative in cases of short-segment disease and in patients who are younger than 1 month of age. The colon must be unprepared; in inconclusive cases, follow-up films 24 hours later that show retained barium suggest the disease.

Anal manometry. If barium enema is inconclusive, anal manometry can rule out Hirschsprung's disease by the demonstration of normal relaxation.

Rectal biopsy. The most accurate diagnosis is acetylcholinesterase staining of a suction rectal biopsy specimen that shows thick acetylcholinesterase-positive nerve fibers in the muscularis mucosa. This finding is pathognomonic for Hirschsprung's disease. If the diagnosis is still in doubt, the demonstration of aganglionosis in the myenteric and submucosal plexuses of full-thickness biopsy specimens identifies 98% of all cases.

VI. Treatment

Medical treatment with fluids and antibiotics, if necessary, is used to stabilize the patient before surgery. Surgical treatment includes resection of the aganglionic segment, with the creation of a stoma until 6 to 12 months of age. Ninety percent of patients return to a normal stooling pattern, and the remaining 10% have a continuing problem with either constipation or incontinence. Death occurs in one third of those patients presenting with enterocolitis.

VII. References

1. Curran TJ, Raffensperger JG. Laparoscopic endorectal pull-through: a comparison with the open procedure. *J Pediatr Surg* 1996;31:1155–1157.
2. Milla PJ. Hirschsprung disease and other neuropathies. In: Rudolph CD, Rudolph AM, eds. *Rudolph's pediatrics,* 21st ed. New York: McGraw-Hill, 2003:1461–1463.
3. Sherman JO, Snyder ME, Weitzman JJ, et al. A 4-year multinational retrospective study of 880 Swenson procedures. *J Pediatr Surg* 1989;24:833–838.
4. Swenson O. Hirschsprung's disease: a review. *Pediatrics* 2002;109:914–918.

Case 3-7: 2-Year-Old Boy

I. History of Present Illness

A 2-year-old boy presented with a 2-day history of vomiting and abdominal pain. The emesis was bilious but nonbloody, and the pain was periumbilical. He had had decreased urine output over the previous day, although his oral intake had been good. His mother denied any history of fever or diarrhea.

II. Past Medical History

The patient had been evaluated in the emergency department for nonbilious emesis three times in the past month. At each evaluation, electrolyte values were normal. A urinalysis performed at the last visit was within normal limits. The child was born at term by spontaneous vaginal delivery. The prenatal evaluation was unremarkable according to the parents. There was no family history of malignancy.

III. Physical Examination

T, 37.8°C; RR, 24/min; HR, 88 bpm; BP, 120/64 mm Hg

Weight and length, 75th percentile for age

The patient was comfortable in no acute distress. His cardiac and pulmonary examination findings were normal. His abdomen was soft and nontender, with absent bowel sounds and fullness in the left lower quadrant. There was no hepatomegaly or splenomegaly. His rectal examination showed normal sphincter tone with hard guaiac-negative stool in the rectal vault.

IV. Diagnostic Studies

Laboratory evaluation revealed 23,000 WBCs/mm^3, with 1% band forms, 47% segmented neutrophils, 45% lymphocytes, and 7% monocytes. The hemoglobin was 12.2 g/dL, and the platelet count was 300,000 cells/mm^3. Serum chemistry values were normal.

V. Course of Illness

Abdominal radiographs showed a left lower quadrant mass displacing the bowel to the right. Further studies indicated the diagnosis.

DISCUSSION: CASE 3-7

I. Differential Diagnosis

Vomiting associated with an abdominal mass is always an emergency, and early imaging is imperative. The typical causes of an abdominal mass vary with the age of the patient and the location of the mass. A newborn is most likely to have an obstructive renal lesion (about 80% of cases). Other, nonobstructive causes of genitourinary masses include ureteral duplications and multicystic kidneys. Abdominal masses in young children are more likely to be neoplastic, most commonly neuroblastoma, Wilms tumor, or hepatoblastoma. Older children are more likely to have non-Hodgkin's lymphoma, rhabdomyosarcoma, or ovarian tumors. Signs of inflammation in an older child are more likely to indicate an infectious etiology, such as an abscess from a ruptured hollow viscus, or an inflammatory process, such as inflammatory bowel disease. The location of the mass in the left lower quadrant to flank area is more consistent with a renal mass, adrenal mass, lymphoma, or fecal impaction.

II. Diagnosis

The patient was admitted to the hospital and underwent an abdominal sonogram that revealed a large, cystic renal lesion. A follow-up radionuclide scan helped confirm the diagnosis. **The radionuclide scan showed delayed emptying in an enlarged kidney with evidence of obstruction at the proximal ureter, suggesting the diagnosis of UPJ obstruction.** A nephrostomy tube was placed, and the patient was discharged home with follow-up in 3 weeks for either pyeloplasty or nephrectomy if kidney function remained poor.

The patient who presents with vomiting and an abdominal mass deserves immediate imaging. Initial radiographs may determine whether a mass is extraluminal, displacing bowel loops, or an intraluminal cause of obstruction. Calcifications in lesions such as neuroblastomas can be detected on radiographs. Ultrasonography is beneficial to distinguish solid from fluid-filled masses and location within or adjacent to an organ. Computed tomographic scans provide more precise anatomic information, demonstrating lymph nodes and metastasis.

III.   Incidence and Epidemiology of Ureteropelvic Junction Obstruction

UPJ obstruction is the most common obstructive uropathy in infancy and childhood, with an annual incidence of 5 cases per 100,000. More than 50% of patients with UPJ obstruction are diagnosed after 20 years of age. Familial forms do exist. Two thirds of all cases occur in males, and 60% occur on the left side. Twenty percent of the cases are bilateral in children younger than 1 year of age, and 15% of all patients have an associated high-grade vesicoureteral reflux (VUR).

UPJ obstruction is thought to result from an aperistaltic segment of the ureter that cannot propel urine away from the renal pelvis. This dysfunctional segment is usually caused by intrinsic factors associated with abnormal intrinsic musculature, increased collagen content, or alterations in peristalsis. Extrinsic compression via aberrant or accessory vessels is a controversial etiology and may be a result rather than a cause of the obstruction. Commonly found is a narrow segment of the upper ureter (ureteral hypoplasia) accompanied by a variable amount of tortuosity and periureteral fibrosis. Ureteral valves and fibroepithelial polyps are rare causes of obstruction.

IV.   Clinical Presentation

Most cases of hydronephrosis due to UPJ obstruction are discovered by fetal ultrasonography. Neonates commonly present with a painless abdominal or flank mass. Older children may present with episodes of colicky abdominal or flank pain mimicking an acute abdomen, whereas adults usually present with flank pain. In any age group, UPJ obstruction may be associated with hematuria after minor trauma, recurrent urinary tract infections, renal failure, failure to thrive, kidney stones, or hypertension. Isolated vomiting is another common presentation of UPJ obstruction, especially after ingestion of large amounts of liquid. Renal calculi and hypertension also may be presenting manifestations of a UPJ obstruction.

V.   Diagnostic Approach

Ultrasonography. Ultrasonography is usually the preferred primary study. In the first 1 to 3 days of life, renal sonography may underestimate or completely overlook renal dilatation because of the oliguric state of the healthy newborn. Later, the degree of dilatation observed in UPJ obstruction may vary with the state of hydration and the degree of bladder fullness. Ureteral dilation detected more proximally, or behind the bladder, argues against UPJ obstruction.

Voiding cystourethrography. Controversy exists as to whether a voiding cystourethrogram (VCUG) to rule out VUR should be performed on all patients diagnosed with UPJ obstruction. Twenty-five percent of children with UPJ obstruction have associated VUR unrelated to the obstruction accompanying ureteral dilatation. Recent studies have shown that low-grade VUR resolves spontaneously after pyeloplasty, whereas high-grade VUR is easily diagnosed by the demonstration of dilated ureters on ultrasonography.

VI. Treatment

Treatment regimens for UPJ obstruction depend on the age of the patient and the degree of obstruction and hydronephrosis. If the hydronephrosis is bilateral, severe, or progressive, neonatal evaluation with percutaneous drainage (nephrostomy tube placement) and intravenous antibiotics must proceed without delay. The initial sonogram may underestimate the degree of hydronephrosis, and the serum creatinine concentration in the first few days of life reflects maternal levels. If the prenatal hydronephrosis is unilateral and not severe, the evaluation can be performed during the first month of life, after discharge from the hospital.

In a patient with severe hydronephrosis or contralateral hypertrophy, early pyeloplasty is indicated, because the contralateral kidney's hypertrophy is half completed by 4 months of age and finished by 1 year. Despite the safety of this procedure, to date no studies have shown that early pyeloplasty preserves renal function. If the patient is asymptomatic and the differential function of the affected kidney is greater than 40% on renal scans, then observation is preferred, because some patients show improvement and actual resolution with time.

VII. References

1. Figenshau RS, Clayman RV. Endourologic options for management of ureteropelvic junction obstruction in the pediatric patient. *Urol Clin North Am* 1998;25:199–209.
2. Gonzalez R, Schimke C. Ureteropelvic junction obstruction in infants and children. *Pediatr Clin North Am* 2001;48:1505–1518.
3. Gupta DK, Chandrasekharam M, Srinivas M, et al. Percutaneous nephrostomy in children with ureteropelvic junction obstruction and poor renal function. *Urology* 2001; 57:547–550.
4. Kim YS, Do SH, Hong CH, et al. Does every patient with ureteropelvic junction obstruction need voiding cystourethrography? *J Urol* 2001;165:2305–2307.

Case 3-8: 2-Year-Old Girl

I. History of Present Illness

A 2-year-old African-American girl presented with a history of vomiting for 1 week. The emesis was nonbloody and nonbilious and occurred daily. Each time, after vomiting, the patient refused to eat for the rest of the day. She had a normal activity level and normal urine and stool output. The patient's mother believed that the child's face was swollen but denied any history of fever, diarrhea, abdominal pain, or weight loss.

II. Past Medical History

She was born at 36 weeks via cesarean section secondary to fetal distress. She remained in the neonatal intensive care unit for 8 days, but had had no residual problems. She had not required any surgery.

III. Physical Examination

T, 36.5°C; RR, 22/min; HR, 111 bpm; BP, 94/67 mm Hg

Weight, 14.8 kg (75th percentile); length, 91 cm (50th percentile)

General examination revealed an alert child in no acute distress. Her cardiac and pulmonary examinations were normal. She had no hepatomegaly and no splenomegaly or costovertebral angle tenderness. Her physical examination was notable only for periorbital swelling and pitting edema of both lower extremities.

IV. Diagnostic Studies

Laboratory evaluation revealed 14,600 WBCs/mm^3, with 6% band forms, 34% segmented neutrophils, 55% lymphocytes, 6% eosinophils, and 5% monocytes. The hemoglobin was 14.7 g/dL, and the platelet count was 383,000 cells/mm^3. Serum chemistry results were as follows: sodium, 130 mmol/L; potassium, 3.5 mmol/L; chloride, 103 mmol/L; bicarbonate, 24 mEq/L; BUN, 9 mg/dL; creatinine, 0.4 mg/dL; glucose, 103

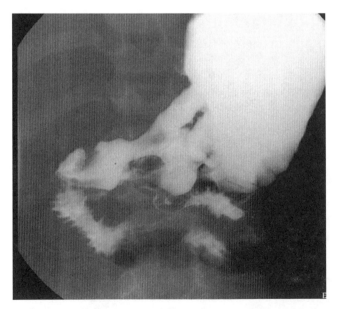

FIG. 3-6. Upper gastrointestinal barium study (case 3-8).

mg/dL; bilirubin, 0.1 mg/dL; ALT, 36 U/L; AST, 49 U/L; albumin, 1.4 g/dL; cholesterol, 122 mg/dL; erythrocyte sedimentation rate (ESR), 0 mm/hour and urinalysis, negative (no protein). Chest and abdominal radiographs were normal.

V. Course of Illness

The patient was evaluated for a protein-losing enteropathy because of hypoalbuminemia without proteinuria. An upper gastrointestinal contrast procedure and endoscopy were performed and confirmed the diagnosis (Fig. 3-6).

DISCUSSION: CASE 3-8

I. Differential Diagnosis

The patient was noted to have generalized edema associated with vomiting. Generalized edema can be caused by four mechanisms: (a) increased capillary permeability, (b) decreased oncotic pressures, (c) increased hydrostatic pressures, or (d) impaired lymphatic drainage. Once cardiovascular disease has been ruled out as the cause of generalized edema, it is usually found to be secondary to hypoproteinemia of renal origin. This patient's generalized edema was attributed to decreased oncotic pressure due to hypoproteinemia. Hypoproteinemia is caused by either decreased production of proteins by the liver or increased renal or gastrointestinal losses. A negative urinalysis for protein and no evidence of hepatic disease makes a protein-losing enteropathy much more likely. Differential diagnosis of a protein-losing enteropathy includes celiac disease, Crohn's disease, cystic fibrosis, intestinal lymphangiectasia, gastritis, eosinophilic gastritis, and Ménétrier's disease.

II. Diagnosis

After it was determined that the patient most likely had a protein-losing enteropathy, she underwent an upper gastrointestinal barium study that showed evidence of hypertrophic gastric folds (thumb-printing and enlarged folds within the gastric antrum) (see Fig. 3-6). **The upper endoscopy performed the next day showed normal anatomy with histologic proof of Ménétrier's disease, including hyperplasia of foveolae (pits) and marked loss of oxyntic glands with accompanying cystic changes.** Cytomegalovirus (CMV) serum immunoglobulin M was positive, and CMV was isolated from the urine by rapid shell vial testing.

III. Incidence and Epidemiology of Ménétrier's Disease

Ménétrier's disease is an extremely rare condition, with about 60 reported cases in the pediatric population. Initially described in 1888, it is characterized by a protein-losing gastropathy, gastric rugae hyperplasia, and hypoproteinemia. More than one third of all pediatric cases show acute evidence of CMV infection. The condition usually occurs in children younger than 10 years of age, with a mean age of 5½ years and a 3:1 male predominance. The cause is believed to be increased production of transforming growth factor-α (TGF-α) that triggers abnormal regulation of gastric epithelial growth factors.

IV. Clinical Presentation

The onset of clinical symptoms is abrupt and usually occurs 1 to 2 weeks after a viral prodrome. Gastrointestinal symptoms predominate, with almost 80% of patients having emesis, 50% having abdominal pain or anorexia, and 10% having frank upper gastrointestinal bleeding. Almost all patients present with generalized edema, and one third have pleural effusions. Characteristic laboratory abnormalities include low levels of serum albumin and total serum protein.

V. Diagnostic Approach

Diagnosis of Ménétrier's disease when the clinical presentation is supportive depends on a combination of laboratory evaluation, radiographic findings, and endoscopic results.

Complete blood count. Laboratory findings include a mild normochromic, normocytic anemia in 20% of patients and eosinophilia in 60%.

Miscellaneous studies. A low serum albumin concentration, usually less than 2 g/dL, and an elevated α_1-antitrypsin level are supportive.

Upper gastrointestinal barium study. Contrast radiographs show swollen gastric rugae of the fundus and body, with antral sparing. Diagnosis by ultrasonography has also been described.

Endoscopy. Endoscopy shows swollen, convoluted rugae. Histologic features include tortuous pits with cystic dilatations that may extend into the muscularis mucosa and submucosa and an edematous lamina propria with increased numbers of eosinophils, lymphocytes, and round cells. Mucosal thickening, glandular atrophy, and hypochlorhydria occur.

VI.   Treatment

Treatment for Ménétrier's disease is mostly supportive and includes a high-protein diet, acid blockers to treat gastric inflammation, and diuretics to reduce edema. Appropriate therapy should be instituted in cases associated with *Helicobacter pylori* infection. The condition is self-limited and usually resolves within weeks to months without recurrence or sequelae. Cases in adults tend to be more chronic, commonly require surgery, and are also associated with an increased risk of gastric cancer.

VII.   References

1. Weinstein WM. Other types of gastritis and gastropathies, including Ménétrier's disease. In: Feldman M, Scharschmidt BF, Sleisenger MH, eds. *Sleisenger and Fordtran's gastrointestinal and liver disease,* 6th ed. Philadelphia: WB Saunders, 1998:711–737.
2. Hassall E. Peptic diseases. In: Rudolph CD, Rudolph AM, eds. *Rudolph's pediatrics,* 21st ed. New York: McGraw-Hill, 2003:1429–1435.
3. Meuwissen SG, Ridwan BU, Hasper HJ. Hypertrophic protein-losing gastropathy: a retrospective analysis of 40 cases in the Netherlands (The Dutch Menetrier Study Group). *Scand J Gastroenterol* 1992;194:s1–s7.
4. Zenkl B, Zieger MM. Menetrier disease in a child of 18 months: diagnosis by ultrasonograph. *Eur J Pediatr* 1988;147:330–331.

4

Cough

Debra Boyer

APPROACH TO THE PATIENT WITH COUGH

I. Definition of the Complaint

Cough is one of the most common presenting complaints to pediatricians. Cough is not a disease itself, but rather a manifestation of underlying pathology. A cough is a protective action, and it can be initiated both voluntarily and via stimulation of cough receptors located throughout the respiratory tract (ear, sinuses, upper and lower airways to the level of the terminal bronchioles, pleura, pericardium, and diaphragm). A cough may serve to remove irritating substances or excessive or abnormal secretions, or it may be secondary to intrinsic or extrinsic airway compression. •

A cough is divided into three distinct phases: a deep inspiration, closure of the glottis with contraction of expiratory muscles, and glottic opening. Thus, one can see how some patients with glottic disease or neuromuscular disease may have ineffective cough.

Classification should initially involve differentiating an acute from a chronic cough. A chronic cough is one that lasts longer than 3 weeks. Furthermore, the clinical description of the cough can often be helpful in suggesting an etiology: staccato (pertussis, chlamydia), barking (croup), grunting (asthma), or honking (psychogenic). Timing of the cough, its relationship to daily activities, and the age of the patient are important factors in further defining the etiology.

II. Complaint by Cause and Frequency

Overall, the most common causes of chronic cough are viral upper respiratory tract infection and asthma (Table 4-1). Beyond these etiologies, age is very important in creating a differential diagnosis for the patient with chronic cough (Table 4-2). Causes of cough may also be divided by diagnostic category, including infectious and allergic/inflammatory causes, congenital malformations, irritants, aspiration, psychogenic cough, and other categories (Table 4-3).

III. Clarifying Questions

In most cases of a child who presents with a cough, the diagnosis is obtained with a thorough history and physical examination. The following questions may help to define the diagnosis.

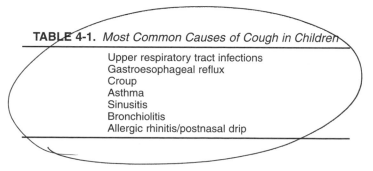

TABLE 4-1. *Most Common Causes of Cough in Children*

Upper respiratory tract infections
Gastroesophageal reflux
Croup
Asthma
Sinusitis
Bronchiolitis
Allergic rhinitis/postnasal drip

TABLE 4-2. *Causes of Cough in Childhood by Age*

Disease prevalence	Infant	Preschool age child	School age child/adolescent
Common	Infectious 　Viral (RSV) 　*Chlamydia 　　trachomatis* 　Pertussis GER	Infectious 　Viral 　*Mycoplasma 　　pneumoniae* 　Pertussis 　Bacterial Asthma Foreign body aspiration	Infectious 　Viral 　*Mycoplasma 　　pneumoniae* 　Pertussis Asthma Psychogenic 　Habit cough 　Vocal cord 　　dysfunction
Less common	Congenital 　Tracheoesophageal 　　fistula 　Tracheobronchomalacia 　Vascular ring 　Lobar emphysema 　Bronchogenic cyst 　Pulmonary sequestration 　Laryngeal cleft 　Airway hemangiomas 　Cystic adenomatoid 　　malformation Infectious 　Bacterial pneumonia 　HIV 　Measles 　Tuberculosis 　Fungal Cystic fibrosis Aspiration 　GER 　Swallowing dysfunction Congestive heart failure Toxic exposure 　Passive smoke 　Fumes Bronchopulmonary 　dysplasia	Congenital 　Tracheoesophageal 　　fistula 　Tracheobronchomalacia 　Vascular ring 　Lobar emphysema 　Bronchogenic cyst 　Pulmonary sequestration 　Laryngeal cleft 　Airway hemangiomas 　Cystic adenomatoid 　　malformation Infectious 　Bacterial pneumonia 　HIV 　Measles 　Tuberculosis 　Fungal Cystic fibrosis Allergic rhinitis Sinusitis Aspiration 　GER 　Swallowing dysfunction Croup Toxic exposure 　Passive smoke 　Fumes	Infectious 　Bacterial 　　pneumonia 　HIV 　Measles 　Tuberculosis 　Fungal Allergic rhinitis Cystic fibrosis Sinusitis Aspiration 　GER 　Swallowing 　　dysfunction Smoking Foreign body 　aspiration
Uncommon	Ciliary dyskinesia Swyer-James syndrome Interstitial pneumonitis Congenital 　immunodeficiency	Ciliary dyskinesia Pneumonitis 　Hypersensitivity 　Interstitial Congenital 　immunodeficiency Bronchiectasis Malignancy Airway papillomas Granulomatous disorders	Ciliary dyskinesia Pneumonitis 　Hypersensitivity 　Interstitial Congenital 　immunodeficiency Bronchiectasis Malignancy Airway papillomas Granulomatous 　disorders

GER, gastroesophageal reflux; HIV, human immunodeficiency virus; RSV, respiratory syncytial virus.

TABLE 4-3. *Cause of Cough in Childhood by Etiology*

Diagnostic category	Cause
Infectious	Viral
	Chlamydia sp.
	Pertussis
	Tuberculosis
	Fungal
	Sinusitis
	Human immunodeficiency virus
	Bacterial pneumonia
	Croup
	Mycoplasma pneumoniae
Allergy/Inflammatory	Allergic rhinitis/postnasal drip
	Reactive airways disease/asthma
	Hypersensitivity pneumonitis
Congenital malformations	Tracheoesophageal fistula
	Tracheobronchomalacia
	Vascular rings
	Lobar emphysema
	Bronchogenic cysts
	Pulmonary sequestration
	Laryngeal cleft
	Cystic adenomatoid malformation
Irritants	Active/passive smoking
	Fumes
Aspiration	Gastroesophageal reflux
	Neuromuscular diseases
	Foreign body aspiration
Psychogenic	Habit cough
	Vocal cord dysfunction
Miscellaneous	Cystic fibrosis
	Malignancy
	Bronchopulmonary dysplasia
	Congestive heart failure
	Interstitial pneumonitis
	Primary ciliary dyskinesia
	Granulomatous disorders

- Did the cough begin with an upper respiratory tract infection?

  — The most common cause for a cough is a viral upper respiratory tract infection. This can occur with or without reactive airways disease or asthma. Without other significant generalized signs of illness or respiratory distress, often no significant initial evaluation or therapy is necessary. Many young children have frequent viral infections (six to eight per year) accompanied by a cough, giving the appearance of chronic cough.

- Are there systemic signs or symptoms that may suggest a particular etiology?

  — Fever, sinus tenderness, and headache may be present with sinusitis. Weight loss and night sweats may indicate tuberculosis or malignancy. Dysphagia suggests an esophageal foreign body, and dysphonia indicates laryngeal or glottic pathology.

- In young infants, is there any history of conjunctivitis in association with a cough and tachypnea?

  — Conjunctivitis and pneumonitis in a young infant may suggest infection due to *Chlamydia trachomatis*.

- Are there environmental stimuli that may irritate the airway?

  — Passive smoking in infants and young children and active smoking in adolescents can trigger a chronic cough. Solvent fumes as well as recreational drug use can exacerbate a chronic cough.

- How is the cough related to time of day and to daily activities?

  — A cough that is most prominent during or after eating is suggestive of aspiration or gastroesophageal reflux (GER). If exposure to cold air and exercise precipitates the cough, reactive airways disease should be considered. Seasonal coughing suggests an allergic component. Similarly, a nighttime cough may indicate postnasal drip secondary to either allergies or sinusitis.

- Does the cough resolve with sleep?

  — Coughs that disappear when the patient is asleep or appear only when an adult is present may be psychogenic.

- Is there a history of a choking episode?

  — Often, a significant choking episode occurs at the time of foreign body ingestion. For this reason, a thorough history is essential. Foreign body aspiration is most common in toddlers, and older siblings may place inappropriate objects in the mouth of infants. If foreign body aspiration is suspected, one should obtain either lateral decubitus or inspiratory and expiratory chest roentgenograms.

- Is there a history of recurrent pneumonias or other infections?

  — Recurrent infections should cause one to consider immune dysfunction such as human immunodeficiency virus (HIV) infection and congenital immunodeficiencies. Recurrent pneumonias associated with sinusitis, multiple otitis medias, bronchiectasis, and situs inversus suggest primary ciliary dyskinesia.

- How is the patient's growth?

  — Failure to thrive, steatorrhea, and recurrent pneumonias can occur with cystic fibrosis (CF). Other features suggestive of CF are nasal polyps, recurrent sinusitis, and rectal prolapse.

- Is there any history of hemoptysis?

  — Hemoptysis can be seen with a viral or bacterial pneumonia. However, it is also present in many other conditions, including fungal disease, autoimmune diseases, granulomatous disorders, CF, congenital heart disease, and pulmonary hemosiderosis.

IV. References

1. Pasterkamp H. The history and physical examination. In: Chernick V, Boat TF, eds. *Kendig's disorders of the respiratory tract in children.* Philadelphia: WB Saunders, 1998:98–101.
2. Durbin WA. Cough. In: Hoekelman RA, Friedman SB, Nelson NM, et al., eds. *Primary pediatric care.* St. Louis: Mosby, 1997:895–897.
3. Cough. In: Tunnessen WW, ed. *Signs and symptoms in pediatrics.* Philadelphia: Lippincott Williams & Wilkins, 1999:375–382.
4. Bachur R. Cough. In: Fleisher GR, Ludwig S, eds. *Textbook of pediatric emergency medicine.* Philadelphia: Lippincott Williams & Wilkins, 2000:183–186.
5. Morgan WJ, Taussig LM. The child with persistent cough. *Pediatr Rev* 1987;8:249–253.
6. Kamie RK. Chronic cough in children. *Pediatr Clin North Am* 1991;38:593–605.

The following cases represent less common causes of cough in childhood.

Case 4-1: 16-Year-Old Girl

I.   History of Present Illness

A 16-year-old black female presented with a 2-week history of a dry cough. She described shortness of breath, which was worse when she was lying down. She had been sleeping on three pillows since her cough began. Her cough and shortness of breath were waking her at night, and symptoms were somewhat relieved with sitting up. She had chest tightness with deep inspiration as well as pain when lying on her left side. She had had intermittent fevers (38.0°C) over the last few weeks, as well as drenching night sweats.

She was initially treated with albuterol for her cough without significant relief. One week into her illness, she was seen by an allergist, who noted decreased breath sounds on the left side. A chest roentgenogram was obtained, and the patient was admitted for further evaluation.

Review of systems revealed decreased appetite with early satiety. She had had some weight loss over the last 12 months. She denied headaches, sore throat, or changes in her voice. She reported an episode of diffuse pruritus 2 months before admission.

II.   Past Medical History

Her past history was remarkable for no prior significant illnesses and no hospitalizations. She had had a fibroadenoma excised from her right breast 3 months before this admission. Her family history was significant for a maternal grandmother with uterine cancer, an aunt with breast cancer, and a maternal great-grandmother with thyroid cancer.

III.   Physical Examination

T, 38.1°C; RR, 20/min; HR, 127 bpm; BP, 139/73 mmHg

Weight, 50th percentile; height, 95th percentile

Initial examination revealed an alert young woman, sitting forward, with noticeable shortness of breath and cough. Physical examination was remarkable for decreased breath sounds on the left, most significantly at the base. She had two small, subcutaneous nodules on her left superior chest wall. The remainder of her physical examination was normal.

IV.   Diagnostic Studies

Laboratory analysis revealed a peripheral blood count with 21,200 white blood cells (WBCs)/mm^3, including 94% segmented neutrophils, 3% lymphocytes, and 3% monocytes. The hemoglobin was 8.4 gm/dL, and the mean corpuscular volume was 63 fL. Platelets were 386,000/mm^3. Electrolytes, blood urea nitrogen, creatinine, and liver function tests were normal. The erythrocyte sedimentation rate (ESR) was elevated at 60 mm/hour.

V.   Course of Illness

Computed tomographic (CT) scans of the chest were obtained to further assess abnormalities seen on chest radiography (Fig. 4-1). The patient was admitted to the intensive care unit with concerns of impending respiratory failure.

DISCUSSION: CASE 4-1

I.   Differential Diagnosis

The most common causes of cough in adolescents are infections and asthma. Whereas viral infections are certainly most common, other agents include *Mycoplasma pneumoniae, Bordetella pertussis,* and bacterial species. Patients with asthma are most likely to

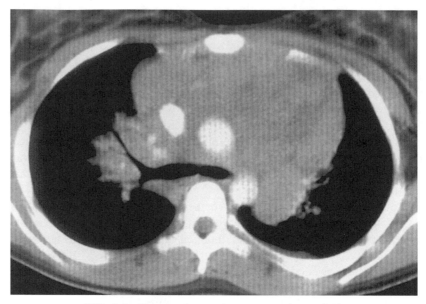

FIG. 4-1. Chest computed tomogram (case 4-1).

have had a prior history of some wheezing and possibly atopy. Less common infectious causes include HIV and related infections, measles, tuberculosis, and fungal infections. Other diagnoses that should be considered in an adolescent with a chronic cough include allergic rhinitis, sinusitis, GER, and smoking, among others. Rare causes include primary ciliary dyskinesia, interstitial pneumonitis, granulomatous disorders, and malignancies.

The concerning features of this case involve the patient's significant shortness of breath and orthopnea. These are not common complaints with simple viral infections or asthma exacerbations. Her persistent fevers and night sweats suggest a systemic disorder warranting further investigation. Finally, her pleural fluid was bloody and appeared to be transudative, further limiting her differential diagnosis.

II. Diagnosis

A chest roentgenogram revealed a large anterior mediastinal mass with rightward tracheal deviation. Chest CT revealed a large, bulky, infiltrating, anterior mediastinal mass that extended from above the level of the clavicle to near the level of the diaphragm (see Fig. 4-1). It also extended posteriorly to involve the middle mediastinum. There was also bilateral axillary adenopathy and a right pleural effusion. Chest tube placement yielded 1,200 mL of pleural fluid with red blood cells, 3,900/mm^3; WBCs, 772/mm^3 (including 22% segmented neutrophils and 78% lymphocytes); pH, 7.44; glucose, 100 mg/dL; lactate dehydrogenase, 386 U/L; and amylase, less than 30 U/L. **A lymph node biopsy performed in the operating room revealed nodular sclerosing Hodgkin's lymphoma.** Bone marrow biopsy did not reveal hematologic involvement. With a negative abdominal CT scan, she was considered to have a stage IIB lymphoma and commenced a course of chemotherapy according to the COPP protocol.

III. Incidence and Epidemiology

Hodgkin's disease has a bimodal age distribution in industrialized countries, with an early peak between 20 and 30 years of age and a second peak after age 50 years. There appear to be three separate forms of the disease, affecting children (up to 14 years of age), young adults (15 to 34 years), and older adults (55 to 74 years). The incidence is slightly higher in males.

Hodgkin's disease develops when a single transformed B cell is clonally expanded. The malignant cells consist of Reed-Sternberg cells, lymphocytic cells, and histiocytic cells. Only 1% of the tumor consists of malignant cells; the greatest proportion of cells are inflammatory cells resulting from a significant cytokine release. Based on histology, there are four subtypes of Hodgkin's disease: lymphocytic predominance, mixed cellularity, lymphocytic depletion, and nodular sclerosing. Epstein-Barr virus (EBV) has been associated with some cases of Hodgkin's disease, with virus reactivation as a possible causative factor. This appears to be more common in younger children.

IV. Clinical Presentation

Often, a patient present with a firm but painless lymphadenopathy. Approximately 60% of patients have mediastinal involvement as part of their initial presentation. It is rare to have primary disease present in subdiaphragmatic locations. Constitutional symptoms are common and include fatigue, weight loss, anorexia, fevers, and night sweats. Pruritus is often a complaint of patients with Hodgkin's disease, as in this case.

Abnormal laboratory findings may include leukocytosis, lymphopenia, eosinophilia, monocytosis, anemia, and thrombocytopenia. In contrast to many affected adults, most children have a normal lymphocyte count at diagnosis. Autoimmune disorders that can accompany Hodgkin's disease include nephrotic syndrome and autoimmune hemolytic anemia, neutropenia, and thrombocytopenia. Nonspecific markers of inflammation (e.g., ESR, ferritin level) may be elevated.

V. Diagnostic Approach

A large pleural effusion and an anterior mediastinal mass were concerning findings in this adolescent patient. Initial evaluation included a chest roentgenogram as well as aspiration of the pleural fluid.

Chest roentgenogram. Discovery of a large pleural effusion requires further diagnostic studies. Initially, lateral decubitus chest roentgenograms may be used to determine whether the fluid is free flowing or loculated. Loculated pleural fluid suggests infection, whereas free-flowing pleural fluid may be seen in many conditions. As in this patient, mediastinal masses, hilar lymphadenopathy, and pleural effusions may be noted in cases of malignancy.

Ultrasound. Chest ultrasound can facilitate management decisions by rapidly determining whether a pleural effusion is loculated or free flowing.

Computed tomography of the chest. CT of the chest may also be useful to analyze a pleural effusion for loculations. Chest CT is very useful to view the lung parenchyma in depth, revealing subtle lung disease not apparent on the chest roentgenogram. In addition, a chest CT can further delineate masses, including mediastinal lesions and lymphadenopathy, that may have been suggested on chest roentgenogram. With Hodgkin's disease specifically, the most common extranodal disease sites are lung parenchyma, chest wall, pleura, and pericardium.

Aspiration of pleural fluid. Ultimately, with a significant pleural effusion, the pleural fluid should be aspirated. This is important from a diagnostic standpoint and in many cases from a therapeutic view as well. Pleural fluid should be sent for pH, culture, Gram staining, cell count with differential, glucose, protein, and lactate dehydrogenase determinations. These studies can help to divide pleural effusions into exudates and transudates (Table 4-4). Exudates are most common in parapneumonic effusions, neoplasms, and connective tissue disease, whereas transudates are more common in congestive heart failure, nephrotic syndrome, and cirrhosis. If the pleural fluid pH is greater than 7.4, the effusion is unlikely to be an exudative process. Malignant pleural effusions, such as those from Hodgkin's lymphoma, are exudative in nature, and most often the glucose level is quite reduced. On occasion, malignant cells themselves are noted in the pleural fluid.

TABLE 4-4. *Pleural Fluid Analysis*

Test	Transudate	Exudate
pH	7.4–7.5	<7.4
Protein (g/dL)	<3.0	>3.0
Lactate dehydrogenase (IU)	<200	>200
Pleural/serum lactate dehydrogenase	<0.6	>0.6
Glucose	Same as serum	Decreased
Red blood cells (/mm^3)	<5000	>5000
White blood cells (/mm^3)	<1000	>1000

Tissue biopsy. The key to diagnosis of Hodgkin's disease is pathologic confirmation of disease. This can be obtained from mass lesions or from affected lymph nodes.

Computed tomography of the neck, chest, abdomen, and pelvis. Once the diagnosis of Hodgkin's disease is established, these studies are performed in addition to a chest CT to stage the degree of disease.

Magnetic resonance imaging (MRI). In selected cases, MRI may be helpful in further delineating lymph node involvement and therefore in staging of the disease.

Lymphography. Although lymphography is rarely used today, it can detect abnormal lymph nodes not seen on CT or MRI. However, the procedure is technically difficult.

Bone marrow biopsy. This procedure is useful for staging.

Gallium scan. This procedure may be helpful with the initial staging workup, and it is used on occasion to monitor response to therapy.

VI. Treatment

Determination of staging is essential in choosing the course of therapy for Hodgkin's disease. Stages are based on the Ann Arbor staging classification and include the following:

- Stage I—Involvement of a single lymph node region or a single extralymphatic organ or site
- Stage II—Involvement of two or more lymph node regions on the same side of the diaphragm or localized involvement of an extralymphatic organ or site and one or more lymph node regions on the same side of the diaphragm
- Stage III—Involvement of lymph node regions on both sides of the diaphragm
- Stage IV—Diffuse or disseminated involvement of one or more extralymphatic organs or tissues with or without associated lymph node involvement

Standard therapy for Hodgkin's disease includes risk-adapted involved-field radiation combined with a multiagent chemotherapy protocol. Patients with favorable presentations (i.e., localized nodal involvement with no constitutional symptoms and without "bulky disease") have been treated with fewer cycles of chemotherapy and lower radiation doses. In contrast, those patients with unfavorable presentations (i.e., constitutional symptoms, "bulky mediastinal or peripheral lymphadenopathy," and advanced stage IIIB/IV disease) undergo much more intense protocols.

VII. References

1. Hudson MM, Donaldson SS. Treatment of pediatric Hodgkin's lymphoma. *Semin Hematol* 1999;36:313–323.
2. Hudson MM, Donaldson SS. Hodgkin's disease. In: Pizzo PA, Poplack DG, eds. *Principles and practice of pediatric oncology,* 4th ed. Philadelphia: Lippincott Williams & Wilkins, 1998:637–656.
3. Potter R. Paediatric update: paediatric Hodgkin's disease. *Eur J Cancer* 1999;35: 1466–1476.
4. Montgomery M. Air and liquid in the pleural space. In: Chernick V, Boat TF, eds. *Kendig's disorders of the respiratory tract in children,* 6th ed. Philadelphia: WB Saunders, 1998:389–411.

Case 4-2: 7-Week-Old Boy

I. History of Present Illness

A 7-week-old boy presented to his pediatrician with a 3-week history of rhinorrhea, congestion, and cough; previously he was in good health. He had no history of fever. A chest roentgenogram demonstrated a left lower lobe infiltrate, and a 10-day course of erythromycin for treatment of pneumonia was started. At the completion of this antibiotic course, the boy's mother felt that his respiratory status had improved to some extent, but his work of breathing was still increased from baseline. Furthermore, his cough was persistent in nature. One week later, a repeat chest roentgenogram revealed persistence of the left lower lobe infiltrate, and he was referred for further evaluation. The review of symptoms revealed good oral intake and normal urine output.

II. Past Medical History

He was born at 41 weeks' gestation with a birth weight of 3,000 g. There were no pregnancy- or birth-related complications. He had no history of cyanosis or feeding difficulties. He was feeding on formula, taking 2 ounces every 2 hours. He had two older siblings who were both healthy.

III. Physical Examination

T, 37.3°C; RR, 54/min; HR, 153 bpm; BP in right upper extremity, 93/59 mm Hg; BP in left upper extremity, 87/62 mm Hg; BP in right lower extremity, 94/63 mm Hg; SpO$_2$, 95% in room air

Weight, 4.5 kg

Initial examination revealed a well-developed infant in moderate respiratory distress. The physical examination was remarkable for nasal flaring, intercostal retractions, and intermittent grunting. He had good aeration and scattered rales at both lung bases. Cardiac examination revealed a normal first heart sound (S$_1$) and a prominent second pulmonary sound (P$_2$). A II-III/VI systolic murmur was appreciated at the left sternal border. The liver edge was palpated 4 cm below the right costal margin. The remainder of the physical examination was normal.

IV. Diagnostic Studies

Laboratory analysis revealed a peripheral blood count of 8,400 WBCs/mm^3, with 35% segmented neutrophils, 60% lymphocytes, and 5% eosinophils. The hemoglobin was 11.4 g/dL, and there were 203,000 platelets/mm^3. Electrolytes, blood urea nitrogen, and creatinine were all within normal limits. Antigens of respiratory viruses were not detected by immunofluorescence of nasopharyngeal washings.

V. Course of Illness

An electrocardiogram (ECG) was performed that suggested a diagnosis (Fig. 4-2).

DISCUSSION: CASE 4-2

I. Differential Diagnosis

The causes of a chronic cough in an infant are diverse, but the most common causes are viral infections. In infants with a history of conjunctivitis, *C. trachomatis* should be considered. *B. pertussis* can occur in infants and produce a chronic cough. Most often, infants are unable to generate the force necessary for the classic "whoop." Certainly, other bacterial pneumonias should be considered with the lobar infiltrate noted on chest roentgenogram in this case. Finally, GER must always be considered a common cause for cough in infancy. Other, less common causes of cough in this age group include congen-

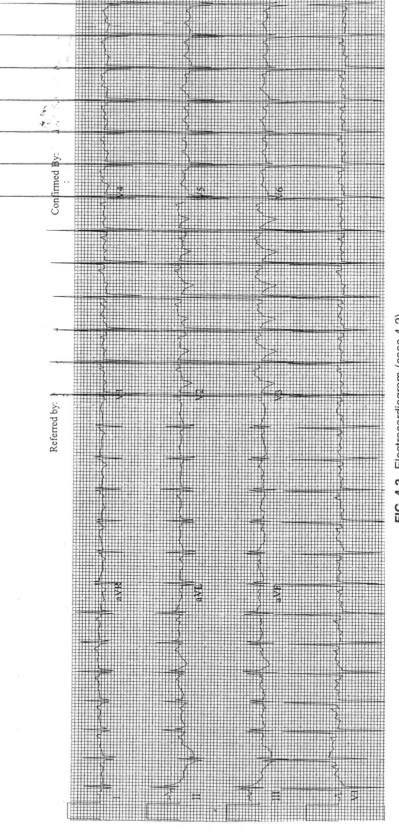

FIG. 4-2. Electrocardiogram (case 4-2).

ital malformations including tracheoesophageal fistulas, tracheobronchomalacia, vascular rings, lobar emphysema, bronchogenic cyst, pulmonary sequestration, laryngeal cleft, and airway hemangiomas.

Congestive heart failure should always be considered, with common etiologies in infancy being volume overload (patent ductus arteriosus, truncus arteriosus, ventricular septal defect, common atrioventricular canal, total anomalous pulmonary venous return), myocardial dysfunction (myocarditis, Kawasaki syndrome, anomalous left coronary artery), arrhythmias (supraventricular tachycardia), pressure overload (coarctation of the aorta, aortic stenosis), and secondary causes (hypertension, sepsis).

The features of this case that prompted additional evaluation were cardiomegaly and increased vascular markings noted on the chest roentgenogram, presence of a heart murmur, and biventricular hypertrophy seen on the ECG.

II. Diagnosis

The ECG revealed a ventricular rate of 150 bpm and dramatic biventricular hypertrophy. An echocardiogram revealed a large perimembranous ventricular septal defect (VSD) with left-to-right shunting. It also demonstrated moderately depressed biventricular function, with a shortening fraction of 29%. **The diagnosis is perimembranous VSD.**

III. Incidence and Epidemiology

VSDs are the most common cardiac malformation seen in children. Recent studies have shown the incidence of VSD in newborns to be 5 to 50 per 1,000 children, with a slight female predominance. VSDs are the most common form of congenital heart disease associated with chromosomal disorders.

VSDs are classified into four types: perimembranous (80%), outlet (5% to 7%), inlet (5% to 8%), and muscular (5% to 20%). Muscular defects have the greatest likelihood of undergoing spontaneous closure. Approximately 75% to 80% of all VSDs close spontaneously, most often by 2 years of age.

IV. Clinical Presentation

Pulmonary vascular resistance determines the extent of the left-to-right shunt. Pulmonary vascular resistance is elevated at birth and declines to adult levels over the first week of life. Therefore, with small VSDs, usually no heart murmur is heard at birth. Most often, the murmur is heard at about 1 to 6 weeks of age; it is usually holosystolic, harsh, and located along the left sternal border. Most infants with small VSDs have no significant symptoms and thrive.

In those infants with moderate or large VSDs, symptoms may develop at about 2 weeks of age and can include tachypnea, irritability, diaphoresis or fatigue with feeding, and failure to thrive. These symptoms develop secondary to progressive heart failure and pulmonary edema. Not uncommonly, symptoms come to attention immediately after a respiratory infection, which stresses the infant's small reserve. With large defects, infants often have a hyperactive precordium with a palpable thrill. Large VSDs, like small ones, produce an associated harsh, holosystolic murmur located along the left sternal border.

V. Diagnostic Approach

Chest roentgenogram. With small VSDs, the chest roentgenogram may be normal. In contrast, a large VSD may lead to significant cardiomegaly and increased vascular markings.

Electrocardiography. The ECG, like the chest roentgenogram, may be normal with small VSDs. However, with moderate-sized VSDs, left ventricular hypertrophy is likely to be present secondary to volume overload of the left ventricle, and right ventricular hypertrophy secondary to pressure overload of the right ventricle. Importantly, these changes are not always evident on the ECG of infants with moderate-sized VSDs.

Echocardiography. Doppler echocardiography is essential to pinpoint the size and location of a VSD. Ventricular, pulmonary artery, and interventricular pressure differences can be determined. Echocardiography also identifies associated cardiac defects.

Magnetic resonance imaging. Cardiac MRI can be used if echocardiography does not reveal sufficient detail. On occasion, MRI may be needed to evaluate extracardiac vascular anomalies.

Cardiac catheterization. Cardiac catheterization is necessary only for patients with complicated cardiovascular anatomy or physiology and need not be performed in all cases of VSD. Pulmonary blood flow and vascular resistance may be evaluated in more detail with this procedure than with Doppler echocardiography.

VI. Treatment

As mentioned, infants with small VSDs usually do not require any intervention. They do require careful surveillance during the first 6 months of life, to assess growth and respiratory status. Many of these small VSDs close spontaneously. Importantly, these patients still require endocarditis prophylaxis.

Usually, those infants with moderate or large VSDs develop some degree of congestive heart failure. Medical management is often the initial therapy and may include furosemide, chlorothiazide, spironolactone, and digoxin. On occasion, afterload reduction with captopril is also required. In those patients with persistent failure to thrive, caloric augmentation may be required. If the patient's congestive heart failure and growth failure are not controlled with medical management, surgical intervention is required.

VII. References

1. Fink BW. Ventricular septal defect. In: Fink BW, ed. *Congenital heart disease: a deductive approach to its diagnosis,* 3rd ed. St. Louis: Mosby, 1991:13–30.
2. Gersony WM. Ventricular septal defect and left sided obstructive lesions in infants. *Curr Opin Pediatr* 1994;6:596–599.
3. Gumbiner CH. Ventricular septal defect. In: Oski FA, DeAngelis CD, Feigin RD, et al., eds. *Principles and practice of pediatrics,* 2nd ed. Philadelphia: JB Lippincott, 1994:1561–1564.
4. Lee HR. Congestive heart failure. In: Schwartz MW, ed. *The 5 minute pediatric consult,* 2nd ed. Philadelphia: Lippincott Williams & Wilkins, 2000:276–277.
5. McDaniel NL, Gutgesell HP. Ventricular septal defects. In: Allen HD, Gutgesell HP, Clark EB, et al., eds. *Moss and Adams' heart disease in infants, children, and adolescents,* 6th ed. Philadelphia: Lippincott Williams & Wilkins, 2001:636–650.

Case 4-3: 7-Month-Old Girl

I. History of Present Illness

A 7-month-old girl was well until 4 days before presentation, when she developed a cough with fevers to 40.5°C. On the day of presentation, she developed wheezing and a rash on her trunk and face. This rash began on her chest and spread to her face. Over the 4 days, her cough had increased significantly. She received nebulized albuterol twice at home without relief. Her oral intake and urine output were poor.

II. Past Medical History

She was the full-term product of an uncomplicated vaginal delivery. She had been to the emergency department three times for wheezing episodes. She was currently receiving only nebulized albuterol. At the time of presentation, the patient and her family were living in a shelter. A roommate at the shelter was recently hospitalized with a rash, fever, and pneumonia.

III. Physical Examination

T, 40.6°C; RR, 60/min; HR, 168 bpm; BP, 102/55 mm Hg; SpO$_2$, 99% in room air

Weight, 50th percentile; height, 75th to 90th percentile

Initial examination revealed an alert baby who was crying but consolable. She appeared slightly pale. Physical examination was notable for an erythematous right tympanic membrane and bilaterally injected conjunctiva with yellow discharge. She had moderate rhinorrhea and some notable buccal thrush. Her oropharynx was mildly erythematous. The chest examination was remarkable for an elevated respiratory rate, but there were no retractions. She had fine expiratory wheezes bilaterally, with decreased breath sounds at both bases. Her skin exhibited a fine, erythematous, blanching maculopapular rash on her face and torso (Fig. 4-3) and, to a lesser degree, on her extremities. Her palms and soles were spared. The rash appeared confluent in her perineal area and torso. The remainder of her physical examination was unremarkable.

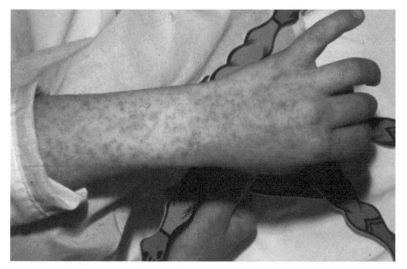

FIG. 4-3. Example of rash.

IV. Diagnostic Studies

Laboratory analysis revealed a peripheral blood count of 10,900 WBCs/mm^3, with 41% segmented neutrophils, 50% lymphocytes, 8% monocytes, and no band forms. The hemoglobin was 10.6 g/dL, and there were 290,000 platelets/mm^3. A urinalysis was normal, and a chest roentgenogram revealed mild hyperinflation and right middle lobe atelectasis with some peribronchial cuffing.

V. Course of Illness

The patient received two nebulized albuterol treatments without significant change in her respiratory rate. Blood and urine cultures were sent and revealed no growth. Her fever resolved over the next 2 days, and her respiratory status began to normalize. Her rash also began to fade, and she was discharged back to the shelter after a 4-day hospitalization. Examination of the rash (see Fig. 4-3) suggested a diagnosis that was confirmed by studies on blood samples sent during her hospitalization.

DISCUSSION: CASE 4-3

I. Differential Diagnosis

Viral infections are the most common cause of a cough in infancy, with respiratory syncytial virus, adenovirus, and influenza and parainfluenza viruses among the leading agents. In infancy, these viruses also commonly produce lower airways disease, so that bronchiolitis quite often accompanies the cough. Infants with bronchiolitis have decreased aeration with diffuse rales and wheezing appreciated on auscultation. Fever is common, as is profuse rhinorrhea.

Other infectious etiologies are possible and should always be considered in the differential diagnosis; they include *C. trachomatis,* pertussis, and bacterial pneumonia. Less commonly, infants present with pulmonary tuberculosis or a fungal infection. Rarely, infectious entities such as measles or parasitic infections manifest with cough.

Although cough can be the presenting symptom in many cases of congenital malformations, this case strongly suggests an infectious etiology. The features of this case that prompted additional evaluation included the rash and the associated respiratory findings.

II. Diagnosis

The rash was characteristic of measles (see Fig. 4-3). Antibody titers to measles were sent on admission and were negative. Repeat titers were sent before her discharge on hospital day 4. Immunoglobulin M (IgM) antibodies specific for measles were found to be positive. **The diagnosis is measles.**

III. Incidence and Epidemiology

Measles is the infectious condition caused by the rubeola virus, an RNA virus of the family Paramyxoviridae. Before the introduction of the measles vaccine in 1963, some 200,000 to 300,000 cases of measles were seen each year in the United States. Since then, this has decreased by 99%. Currently, measles is reported rarely in preschool children, some of whom are too young to be vaccinated. Infrequently, cases of primary vaccine failure are reported.

Measles is spread as an airborne virus, and infection results from direct contact with droplets from the respiratory secretions of infected patients. The typical incubation period is 10 days. Children are most infectious when cough and coryza are at their peak, which occurs during the late prodromal phase. Children are considered contagious from several days before until 5 days after the onset of the rash. The mortality rate for measles in the United States is 1 in 3,000 cases.

IV.   Clinical Presentation

The prodromal phase begins with 3 to 5 days of malaise, fever, cough, coryza, and conjunctivitis. These symptoms increase over the course of the prodromal phase. Fevers vary from 39.4° to 40.6°C and usually peak as the exanthem begins. Just before the development of the exanthem, Koplik's spots are noted. These are bluish spots on a red base that are found on the buccal mucosa. Koplik's spots are pathognomonic of measles. The exanthem begins as Koplik's spots begin to slough. The rash typically begins on the face and then moves in a caudal direction. The rash is initially erythematous and maculopapular but then becomes confluent. The rash usually lasts 5 to 7 days.

Other symptoms can include pharyngitis, lymphadenopathy, splenomegaly, diarrhea, vomiting, and abdominal pain. With typical measles, patients are ill for 7 to 10 days. However, complications can occur and include pneumonia, encephalitis, myocarditis, pericarditis, appendicitis, and corneal ulcerations. Subacute sclerosing panencephalitis (SSPE) is an uncommon neurologic complication of measles infection. SSPE consists of a degenerative central nervous system process that is associated with a persistent measles infection.

V.   Diagnostic Approach

The diagnosis of measles is based on the classic clinical criteria. The following studies may be used to confirm a suspected diagnosis.

Viral culture. Viral isolation is not commonly used, because it is difficult to perform. However, this study may be important in the immunocompromised patient.

Immunofluorescence. Immunofluorescent staining for measles antigen may be performed on nasopharyngeal washings.

Serologic titers. If there is a question about the diagnosis from a clinical standpoint, one can look for a serologic response to the viral infection. Antibodies can initially be seen on days 1 to 3 of the exanthem and reach their peak levels in 2 to 6 weeks. Therefore, if serologic confirmation is necessary, patients should have both acute and convalescent titers sent. A four-fold rise in the measles titer over time, or the presence of measles-specific IgM antibodies, establishes the diagnosis.

VI.   Treatment

In uncomplicated measles, patients require only supportive care, including antipyretics and fluids. Antibiotics are necessary only in cases of bacterial superinfection, particularly pneumonia. Typical organisms causing a superinfected bacterial pneumonia include *Streptococcus pneumoniae, Staphylococcus aureus, Haemophilus influenzae,* and *Streptococcus pyogenes.*

VII.   References

1. Gerson AA. Measles virus (rubeola). In: Mandell GL, Bennett JE, Dolin R, eds. *Mandell, Douglas, and Bennett's principles and practice of infectious diseases,* 5th ed. Philadelphia: Churchill Livingstone, 2000:1801–1807.
2. Rosa C. Rubella and rubeola. *Semin Perinatol* 1998;22:318–322
3. Taber LH, Demmier GJ. Measles (rubeola). In: Oski FA, DeAngelis CD, Feigin RD, McMillan JA, et al., eds. *Principles and practice of pediatrics,* 2nd ed. Philadelphia: JB Lippincott, 1994:1340–1343.
4. West CE. Vitamin A and measles. *Nutr Rev* 2000;58:S46–S54.

Case 4-4: 3-Year-Old Boy

I. History of Present Illness

A 3-year old boy with a past history of asthma presented with cough and chest pain. His illness began 2 weeks earlier, with left-sided chest pain with inspiration. The family had recently misplaced his baseline asthma medications. He was seen in the emergency department and was believed to have musculoskeletal pain. His pain improved somewhat, but he was brought back to the emergency department 8 days later with wheezing and rhinorrhea. He was described as having increased work of breathing and a significant cough. There was no fever. In the emergency department, he was believed to be in mild respiratory distress and was treated with prednisone and albuterol and then discharged. However, the following day, he developed blood-streaked sputum evolving into possible hemoptysis and was brought back to the emergency department. There was no evidence of fever, chills, or weight loss.

II. Past Medical History

The patient had a history of asthma, for which he has been hospitalized three times. His last admission was 3 years before this current presentation. His medications were albuterol, which he received twice a day, and fluticasone in a metered-dose inhaler, which he had not received in several weeks.

III. Physical Examination

T, 37.2°C; RR, 30/min; HR, 70 bpm; BP, 108/52 mm Hg; SpO$_2$, 99% in room air

In general, he was a well-appearing young boy in no acute distress. His physical examination was significant for a clear lung examination with no evidence of wheezes, rales, or rhonchi. The remainder of his physical examination was unremarkable.

IV. Diagnostic Studies

A chest roentgenogram was obtained (Fig. 4-4). A tuberculin skin test reaction was less than 5 mm.

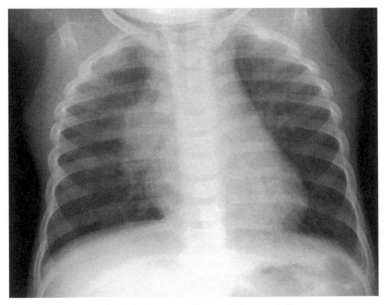

FIG. 4-4. Chest radiograph (case 4-4).

V. Course of Illness

He was initially started on a course of azithromycin for a presumed *M. pneumoniae* infection. His chest pain continued, but his hemoptysis resolved. With concern for his chest roentgenogram findings, a further diagnostic test was performed, which revealed the diagnosis.

DISCUSSION: CASE 4-4

I. Differential Diagnosis

With this patient's past medical history, the most likely cause for his cough was asthma with a superimposed infectious process. His symptoms did appear to improve somewhat with standard asthma therapy (bronchodilators and steroids). Allergic or sinus symptoms can also cause a significant cough in this age group. One should also inquire about a history of smoking in the family or possible foreign body aspiration.

The hemoptysis in this case is not unusual in many of the processes described. It is important to try to establish that this is true hemoptysis and not hematemesis or bleeding from the nasal passages. With true hemoptysis, the most common causes are CF, pneumonia, bronchiectasis, congenital heart disease, and tracheobronchitis. Finally, the hilar adenopathy noted on the chest roentgenogram should alert the physician to pursue a more thorough investigation, with consideration of mycobacterial infections and granulomatous disorders.

II. Diagnosis

The chest radiograph revealed a right middle lobe infiltrate with right hilar adenopathy (see Fig. 4-4). Nasogastric aspirates were sent for acid-fast bacilli (AFB) stain and cultures. The AFB stain was negative, but AFB culture revealed growth of *Mycobacterium avium-intracellulare*. **The diagnosis is a pulmonary infection with *Mycobacterium avium-intracellulare*.**

III. Incidence and Epidemiology

Nontuberculous mycobacteria (NTM) are ubiquitous in the environment. They are found in soil, water, food, house dust, and domestic and wild animals. Human infection most likely occurs with aspiration of aerosolized particles. Human-to-human transmission is not believed to occur.

It is difficult to determine the incidence of NTM infections, because they are not a reportable disease to health authorities. Furthermore, symptoms may be confused with those of *Mycobacterium tuberculosis* infections. It is also challenging to properly differentiate asymptomatic colonization from true infection. A positive culture for NTM does not always represent invasive disease.

The most common NTM organisms form the *Mycobacterium avium* complex (MAC), which consists of both *Mycobacterium avium* and *Mycobacterium intracellulare*. Aside from patients with HIV infection, the patients at greatest risk of becoming infected with pulmonary MAC are those with underlying lung disease. This includes chronic obstructive pulmonary disease, chronic bronchitis, bronchiectasis, recurrent aspiration, and CF. However, there are reports of patients with no underlying lung disease and MAC infection. The southeastern United States appears to have a higher incidence of MAC infections.

Rarely, a patient presents with disseminated NTM infection. Such patients should be investigated for an underlying immune deficiency, because individuals with certain disorders such as interferon-γ receptor defects and interleukin-12 defects are highly susceptible to infections with NTM.

IV. Clinical Presentation

Four major clinical syndromes of NTM infection that are most commonly seen in children: lymphadenitis, pulmonary infections, skin and soft tissue infections, and disseminated disease.

Pulmonary infections with NTM are rare in children; they are more often seen in elderly individuals. MAC is the most common NTM to cause pulmonary infections, but cases have been reported with *Mycobacterium kansasii* and *Mycobacterium fortuitum* as well. Symptoms are very similar to those of tuberculosis, with a productive cough, fevers, and weight loss. Hemoptysis is seen in fewer than 25% of patients with pulmonary MAC infection. It is rare for disease to disseminate beyond a pulmonary infection if the host is immunocompetent.

Wheezing is a common presenting symptom, and often hilar adenopathy leads to signs and symptoms of bronchial obstruction. It is common for these children to be evaluated for possible foreign body aspiration before the discovery of their NTM infection. On occasion, a child has repeated illnesses with fever and cough and is diagnosed as having recurrent pneumonias.

V. Diagnostic Approach

Diagnosis of NTM infections requires a high degree of clinical suspicion. Diagnosis is based on isolation of the organism in conjunction with appropriate clinical disease. The following tests can be useful.

Blood tests. Complete blood count, ESR, urinalysis, and serum chemistry test results are usually normal with NTM infections.

Mycobacterial culture and acid-fast stain of sputum or gastric aspirate. Acid-fast stains of sputum and gastric aspirates are often negative in cases of NTM, because the number of organisms may be quite small. Therefore, a negative AFB stain does not exclude the diagnosis of NTM infection. NTM can be grown from sputum or gastric aspirate culture, but the results must be interpreted with caution, because asymptomatic patients may be colonized with NTM. For this reason, clinical criteria have been developed that require either radiographic evidence of disease and more than one positive sputum sample, or reproducibility of positive cultures over the course of 1 year.

Purified protein derivative (PPD) skin testing. Patients with MAC usually have reactions of 0 to 10 mm; larger reactions are rare. A positive PPD result should never be considered diagnostic for NTM infection, and a negative PPD should never eliminate the diagnosis.

Chest roentgenogram. This may reveal findings similar to those seen with tuberculosis. Cavitary lesions are not uncommon, but they are often smaller than with *M. tuberculosis* infection. Other possible radiographic presentations include patchy, nodular infiltrates or even isolated pulmonary nodules. Hilar adenopathy may also be seen.

Bronchoscopy. Inadequate sputum samples are often obtained from children, and bronchoscopy may be indicated to obtain useful cultures. Adenopathy large enough to cause bronchial obstruction can occur, and often bronchoscopy is performed in an attempt to rule out an anatomic cause for the bronchial compression.

VI. Treatment

Because the majority of NTM organisms are resistant in vitro to single-drug therapy, combination therapy is generally the rule. Treatment often includes isoniazid, rifampin, rifabutin, ethambutol, streptomycin, amikacin, azithromycin, or clarithromycin. For many patients, treatment regimens extend for 18 to 24 months, and specifically for at least 12 months after sputum cultures have become negative. Many of these medications have significant side effects, and patients must be monitored closely for signs of ototoxicity and gastrointestinal toxicity.

VII. References

1. Ferfie JE, Milligan TW, Henderson BM, et al. Intrathoracic *Mycobacterium avium* complex infection in immunocompetent children: case report and review. *Clin Infect Dis* 1997;24:250–253.

2. Havlir DV, Ellner JJ. *Mycobacterium avium* complex. In: Mandell GL, Bennett JE, Dolin R, eds. *Mandell, Douglas, and Bennett's principles and practice of infectious diseases,* 5th ed. Philadelphia: Churchill Livingstone, 2000:2616–2630.

3. Osorio A, Kessler RM, Guruprasad H, et al. Isolated intrathoracic presentation of *Mycobacterium avium* complex in an immunocompetent child. *Pediatr Radiol* 2001;31:848–851.

4. Starke JR. Nontuberculous mycobacterial infections in children. *Adv Pediatr Infect Dis* 1992;7:123–159.

5. Starke JR, Correa AG. Management of mycobacterial infection and disease in children. *Pediatr Infect Dis J* 1995;14:455–470.

6. Stone AB, Schelonka RL, Drehner DM, et al. Disseminated *Mycobacterium avium* complex in non-human immunodeficiency virus-infected pediatric patients. *Pediatr Infect Dis J* 1992;11:960–964.

Case 4-5: 2-Year-Old Girl

I. History of Present Illness

A 2-year-old girl presented with a history of fevers and a nonproductive cough. She was well until approximately 6 weeks before presentation, when she developed fevers and a dry cough. Soon afterward, she was admitted to the hospital with the diagnosis of an otitis media and pneumonia. After a 2-day hospitalization, during which she received intravenous antibiotic therapy, she was discharged home. However, her parents believed that her symptoms had not improved. Her fevers continued to occur every few days, with maximum temperatures of 39.4° to 41.1°C. She was treated with albuterol nebulizers without improvement in her cough.

She had had a decreased appetite for the last month before presentation, with a 2-kg weight loss. She also had had nonbloody, nonbilious emesis occurring three to four times each day. Her parents reported three to four loose bowel movements each day. In her doctor's office, a stool sample was obtained and was found to be heme-positive.

II. Past Medical History

She was born at full term, with a birth weight of 2,800 g. She had had four episodes of otitis media and two episodes of sinusitis in the past. Her only medications were albuterol nebulizers as needed. Her family history included two aunts with asthma.

III. Physical Examination

T, 40.0°C; RR, 44/min; HR, 140 bpm; BP, 98/60 mm Hg; SpO_2, 90% to 92% in room air
Weight, 5th to 10th percentile

In general, she was a young girl with very mild increased work of breathing. Her chest examination revealed good aeration throughout, with bilateral end-expiratory wheezes in the left upper lobe and on the right anteriorly. No rales or rhonchi were noted. The remainder of her physical examination was within normal limits.

IV. Diagnostic Studies

The complete blood count revealed 8,800 WBCs/mm³, with 66% segmented neutrophils, 27% lymphocytes, and 7% monocytes. Her hemoglobin was 12.2 gm/dL, and her platelet count was 268,000/mm³. ESR was 24 mm/hour. Electrolytes and liver function tests were within normal limits. Prothrombin and partial thromboplastin times were elevated at 15.1 and 33.5 seconds, respectively. Blood and urine cultures did not reveal any growth.

V. Course of Illness

A chest roentgenogram was performed and revealed diffuse peribronchial thickening as well as subsegmental atelectasis in the right middle lobe. A CT scan of her sinuses revealed extensive maxillary sinus disease with some ethmoidal opacification. A chest CT revealed subcarinal and hilar adenopathy.

Ultimately, a diagnostic procedure was performed that revealed the diagnosis.

DISCUSSION: CASE 4-5

I. Differential Diagnosis

As with all other age groups, the most common cause for a cough in a toddler is an infectious process. Viruses, *M. pneumoniae*, and pertussis should all be considered as possible infectious causes. However, almost equally as important in the toddler is inquiry about the possibility of a foreign body ingestion. Appropriate history taking can often be quite revealing in diagnosing a foreign body ingestion. Other clues include a focal finding on chest auscultation, as was seen in this patient, and localized wheezing. If there is a concer[n of for]eign body ingestion, inspiratory and expiratory chest roentgenograms should b[e taken.] If the child is too young for these maneuvers, bilateral decubitus chest roentgen[ograms can] be substituted. In the case of foreign body ingestion, these films would reveal hyperinflation on the side on which the foreign body had lodged.

Other concerning findings in this patient's history are her relatively poor growth, her diffuse sinus disease, and her history of frequent stooling. With this constellation of symptoms, some rarer causes of cough should be included in the differential diagnosis, such as congenital immunodeficiencies, HIV infection, and CF.

II. Diagnosis

Based on her poor growth, sinus disease, chronic cough, and frequent stooling, a sweat test was performed. The results revealed sweat chloride levels of 96 mEq/L and 88 mEq/L (normal, less 40 mEq/L.) **Therefore, the diagnosis is CF.**

III. Incidence and Epidemiology

CF is the most common lethal inherited disease in the Caucasian population. The worldwide incidence is 1 in 2,500 in Caucasians, 1 in 17,000 African-Americans, and 1 in 90,000 in Asians. It is inherited in an autosomal recessive pattern with a carrier rate of 1 in 25 individuals. Life expectancy for patients with CF has improved dramatically over the last 50 years. In the 1950s, median survival time was less than 5 years. Children born in the year 2000 with CF should expect a median survival time of 40 to 50 years.

The gene for CF was discovered in 1989 and is located on chromosome 7. The gene product is a cyclic adenosine monophosphate (cAMP)–activated chloride channel called the cystic fibrosis transmembrane conductance regulator (CFTR.) CFTR is expressed in many organs including the pancreas, sweat glands, gastrointestinal tract, reproductive tract, and respiratory tract.

IV. Clinical Presentation

With such diffuse expression of CFTR, it is understandable that the clinical presentation of CF is quite diverse. The most common and life-threatening manifestations are respiratory disease, although extrapulmonary manifestations of CF are also common (Table 4-5).

Individuals with CF can present initially in a variety of ways. In infancy, meconium ileus, failure to thrive, rectal prolapse, and chronic cough can provide the clue to the initial diagnosis. Other presenting features in childhood can include nasal polyps, cough, frequent episodes of wheezing, frequent respiratory infections, liver disease, and recurrent sinusitis or pancreatitis (or both).

TABLE 4-5. *Extrapulmonary Manifestations of Cystic Fibrosis*

Diagnostic category	Cause
Pancreatic	Exocrine pancreatic insufficiency
	Pancreatitis
	Diabetes mellitus
Hepatobiliary	Biliary obstruction
	Biliary cirrhosis
	Portal hypertension
	Cholelithiasis
Gastrointestinal	Meconium ileus
	Distal intestinal obstruction syndrome
	Intussusception
	Rectal prolapse
Genitourinary	Aspermia
Hematologic	Bleeding diathesis

The respiratory complications are the greatest cause of morbidity and mortality. Patients commonly have nasal polyps and recurrent sinusitis. The recurrent pulmonary infections lead to bronchiectasis and commonly involve organisms such as *S. aureus, H. influenzae, Burkholderia cepacia,* and *Pseudomonas aeruginosa.* Complications in patients with CF can include allergic bronchopulmonary aspergillosis, hemoptysis, and pneumothorax.

Because gastrointestinal disease often includes pancreatic insufficiency, failure to thrive is a common presentation. Other gastrointestinal complications can include liver disease, CF-related diabetes, GER, and rectal prolapse. Fertility is commonly affected in both men and women with CF. Ninety percent of men with CF have congenital bilateral absence of the vas deferens. Women have significantly decreased fertility due to nutritional, respiratory, and cervical mucous abnormalities.

V.   Diagnostic Approach

Sweat test. Quantitative pilocarpine iontophoresis is the gold standard in diagnosing CF. The chloride levels in collected sweat are measured. Levels ranging from 0 to 40 mEq/L are considered normal, values of 40 to 60 mEq/L are borderline, and levels greater than 60 mEq/L are considered positive. Elevated sweat chloride concentrations have been reported with other entities (untreated adrenal insufficiency, hypothyroidism, nephrogenic diabetes insipidus, ectodermal dysplasia, mucopolysaccharidosis, and panhypopituitarism), but most of those other conditions differ clinically from CF.

Genetic mutation analysis. Currently more than 1,000 different mutations in the CFTR gene have been identified. Standard genetic screening usually covers 20 to 70 of these mutations. Testing can be performed on blood or even on a buccal swab.

Chest roentgenogram. Although a chest roentgenogram cannot be used to diagnose CF, it can certainly have suggestive features. These may include significant peribronchial thickening, hyperinflation, and bronchiectasis. Progressive pulmonary disease in patients with CF leads to nodular pulmonary infiltrates and apical cystic lesions that predispose to pneumothoraces.

Sputum culture. Initially, most patients with CF are colonized with *S. aureus* and *H. influenzae.* By young adulthood, almost 80% of patients are colonized with *P. aeruginosa.*

VI.   Treatment

Therapy for CF has both therapeutic and preventative aspects. Patients with pancreatic insufficiency are treated with supplemental pancreatic enzymes and fat-soluble vitamins (i.e., vitamins A, D, E, and K). From a respiratory standpoint, patients have poor clearance of their thick mucous. Therefore, mucolytics such as *N*-acetylcysteine and chest physiotherapy are prescribed, as well as antibiotics directed at the offending organisms.

In terms of prevention, antiinflammatory medications have been tried with some success. Macrolide antibiotics may be important, more often for their antiinflammatory rather than their antimicrobial properties. Vaccines against influenza, respiratory syncytial virus, and pneumococcus are all believed to be important to prevent further damage to an already compromised host.

The ultimate therapy entails a cure with gene therapy. Much research has been devoted to this endeavor, but it is currently in the early experimental stages. Lung transplantation is available to patients with end-stage lung disease; the 3-year survival rate averages 50%.

VII.   References

1. Colin AA, Wohl MEB. Cystic fibrosis. *Pediatr Rev* 1994;15:192–200.
2. Davis, PB, Drumm M, Konstan MW. Cystic fibrosis. *Am J Respir Crit Care Med* 1996;154:1229–1256.
3. Doull IJM. Recent advances in cystic fibrosis. *Arch Dis Child* 2001;85:62–66.
4. MacLusky I, Levison H. Cystic fibrosis. In: Chernick V, Boat TF, eds. *Kendig's disorders of the respiratory tract in children,* 6th ed. Philadelphia: WB Saunders, 1998:838–882.

Case 4-6: 4-Month-Old Boy

I. History of Present Illness

A 4-month-old boy, who was born prematurely at 28 weeks' gestation, presented with a 1-week history of a cough. Over the next 4 days, his mother reported an increasing cough with no history of fever or rhinorrhea. He had decreased oral intake and decreased urine output. He had some posttussive emesis and no diarrhea. His uncle had been sick for the previous 3 weeks with rhinorrhea and a cough.

II. Past Medical History

He was born at 28 weeks' gestation and required endotracheal intubation for a short period after birth. While in the newborn intensive care unit, he had course of necrotizing enterocolitis that did not require surgery. He was ultimately discharged home with an apnea monitor and oral caffeine. However, his mother had recently run out of this medication, and he was no longer receiving it. He had two siblings who were healthy.

III. Physical Examination

T, 37.2°C; RR, 27 to 40/min; HR, 138 bpm; BP, not obtained; SpO$_2$, 96% in room air and decreasing to 93% with feeds

Weight, 25th percentile

On examination, he was alert with moderate respiratory distress and frequent episodes of coughing. His chest examination was significant for grunting with substernal, intercostal, and supraclavicular retractions. Rales were appreciated on the right with good aeration throughout. No wheezes were heard. The remainder of his physical examination was within normal limits.

IV. Diagnostic Studies

The complete blood count revealed 25,400 WBCs/mm^3, with 51% lymphocytes, 17% atypical lymphocytes, 25% segmented neutrophils, and 6% monocytes. The hemoglobin was 12.3 gm/dL, and the platelet count was 494,000/mm^3.

VI. Course of Illness

The patient received an albuterol nebulizer treatment, with no significant relief. While in the emergency department, he had frequent episodes of coughing, with two episodes complicated by bradycardia to 60 bpm and desaturations to 80%. A chest radiograph was obtained (Fig. 4-5). A presumptive diagnosis was made, and the appropriate test was sent for confirmation of the diagnosis.

DISCUSSION: CASE 4-6

I. Differential Diagnosis

A cough in infancy is most likely related to an infectious process, with viral processes the leading causes. Respiratory syncytial virus is a common cause of cough. However, other infectious etiologies should always be considered. Even with good adherence to vaccine regimens, bacterial infections such as *B. pertussis* are possible in infants. *M. pneumoniae* infections also occur rarely in infants.

Reactive airways disease, most often secondary to viral infection, is also a common cause of cough in infancy. GER should be considered as well, even if gastrointestinal symptoms are few.

Less common causes for cough in infancy include congenital malformations such as tracheoesophageal fistula, tracheobronchomalacia, vascular rings, lobar emphysema,

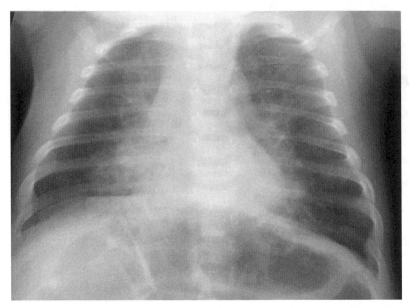

FIG. 4-5. Chest radiograph (case 4-6).

bronchogenic cysts, pulmonary sequestration, laryngeal cleft, and cystic adenomatoid malformation. Furthermore, one should attempt to elicit a history for any possible swallowing disorder that might lead to recurrent aspiration.

Other, less common causes of cough in infancy include CF, congestive heart failure, interstitial pneumonitis, and congenital immunodeficiencies.

This patient's history is suggestive of an infectious etiology, because he was in good health until approximately 1 one week before presentation. However, his history of prematurity should add one more disease to the differential diagnosis: bronchopulmonary dysplasia. Such patients are also more likely to develop reactive airways disease in response to a viral infection.

II. Diagnosis

Chest radiography revealed bilateral perihilar infiltrates (see Fig. 4-5). Given the combination of the radiographic findings, worsening cough, dramatic leukocytosis, lymphocytosis with a substantial number of atypical lymphocytes, and contact with an adult with prolonged cough, a presumptive diagnosis of *B. pertussis* infection was made. A nasopharyngeal specimen was sent for *B. pertussis* polymerase chain reaction (PCR) analysis and was positive. **Therefore, the diagnosis is infection with *B. pertussis*.**

III. Incidence and Epidemiology

B. pertussis, a gram-negative bacillus, is the causative organism for what is commonly referred to as whooping cough. A whooping cough syndrome can also be seen with *Bordetella parapertussis, M. pneumoniae, C. trachomatis, Chlamydia pneumoniae,* and some adenoviruses.

Pertussis is considered one of the most highly communicable diseases, with transmission occurring via contact with respiratory tract secretions of an infected patient. With waning immunity from childhood vaccination, adults and adolescents are commonly the source of infection in infants and young children.

The true incidence of pertussis is unknown, because many cases in adolescents and adults are unrecognized. However, it is known to be a worldwide threat, with an estimated 40,000,000 cases and 360,000 deaths per year. In general, the disease is endemic, but there are 3- to 5-year cycles of epidemics that occur in addition to the endemic levels. For unknown reasons, girls are affected at much higher rates and with higher morbidity than boys.

IV.   Clinical Presentation

The incubation period is 1 to 3 weeks. Infection is divided into three stages. The catarrhal stage begins with symptoms of a mild upper respiratory tract infection and lasts a few days to 1 week. The paroxysmal stage follows, with the characteristic inspiratory whoop. Posttussive emesis is common, and fever is infrequent. The whoop is typically absent in infants, because they are unable to generate the force needed for this maneuver.

Increased intrathoracic and intraabdominal pressures during coughing may lead to conjunctival and scleral hemorrhages, petechiae on the upper body, epistaxis, and retinal hemorrhages. In infancy, apnea is a common complication of *B. pertussis* infections. Even young adults can have episodes of laryngospasm. Seizures result from either hypoxia or hyponatremia due to inappropriate secretion of antidiuretic hormone.

In most cases, a pertussis infection lasts 6 to 10 weeks, but it is not uncommon for infants and children to have persistent coughs for 3 to 4 months. Respiratory distress between paroxysms of coughing suggests superinfection with various viruses (adenovirus, respiratory syncytial virus, cytomegalovirus) or bacteria (*S. pneumoniae, S. aureus*). Other complications include pneumothorax, encephalopathy, and feeding difficulties in infancy. The disease is most severe in infants younger than 1 year of age, especially premature infants.

V.   Diagnostic Approach

Blood counts. Leukocytosis (WBC count greater than $15,000/mm^3$), usually due to an absolute lymphocytosis, is present in more than 75% of unvaccinated children during the late catarrhal and paroxysmal stages. The degree of lymphocytosis typically parallels the severity of illness. Lymphocytosis is less common and less extreme in previously vaccinated children who develop pertussis. Eosinophilia is uncommon.

Chest roentgenogram. Pulmonary infiltrates are often seen and are most commonly perihilar. Classically, a "shaggy" right heart border is seen, but the finding is nonspecific. Chest radiography should be performed to exclude other causes of cough or respiratory distress, such as pneumonia or congestive heart failure.

***Bordetella pertussis* culture.** Growing the organism in culture is certainly the gold standard for diagnosis. However, during the paroxysmal phase, the ability to grow the organism decreases significantly.

Direct immunofluorescent assay. This is performed on nasopharyngeal secretions and has a variable sensitivity and low specificity. Furthermore, it requires a significant level of skill and is therefore not very reliable or reproducible.

Polymerase chain reaction. PCR has been used to document *B. pertussis* infections even after the organism will no longer grow in culture. Therefore, it is able to detect disease even in the late paroxysmal stage. This is the preferred method to confirm the diagnosis of pertussis.

VI.   Treatment

Because young infants with pertussis have a high risk for complications, there should be a low threshold for admitting these patients. Many of these infants require admission to the intensive care unit to monitor for apneic episodes and neurologic sequelae.

Infants should be treated with a macrolide antibiotic, and erythromycin is the most common choice. The length of therapy is generally recommended to be 14 days. Azithromycin and clarithromycin appear to be effective as well. There is some controversy as to whether antibiotics given during the catarrhal stage decrease disease severity. However, antibiotics should still be given, even in the paroxysmal stage, because they limit the spread of the disease to others. Studies are underway to assess the efficacy of pertussis immune globulin as an adjunctive therapy in extremely ill infants.

Antibiotic prophylaxis is recommended for all household members and close contacts and usually consists of 10 to 14 days of erythromycin. Prevention is essential to limit the morbidity and mortality from pertussis, and the acellular pertussis vaccine is currently the recommended form. It is given in combination with diphtheria and tetanus toxoids (DTaP). It is recommended that children receive five doses before school entry.

VII.   References

1. American Academy of Pediatrics. Pertussis. In: Pickering LK, Peter, G, Baker CJ, et al., eds. *2000 Red Book: report on infectious diseases,* 25th ed. Elk Grove Village, IL: American Academy of Pediatrics; 2000:448.
2. Hewlett EL. *Bordetella* species. In: Mandell GL, Bennett JE, Dolin R, eds. *Mandell, Douglas, and Bennett's principles and practice of infectious diseases,* 5th ed. Philadelphia: Churchill Livingstone, 2000:2414–2419.
3. Hoppe JE. Neonatal pertussis. *Pediatr Infect Dis J* 2000;19:244–247.
4. Long SS, Edwards KM. *Bordetella pertussis* (pertussis) and other species. In: Long SS, Pickering LK, Prober CG, eds. *Principles and practice of pediatric infectious diseases,* 2nd ed. New York: Churchill Livingstone, 2003:880–888.
5. Senzilet LD, Halperin SA, Spika JS, et al. Pertussis is a frequent cause of prolonged cough illness in adults and adolescents. *Clin Infect Dis* 2001;32:1691–1697.
6. Sprauer MA, Cochi SL, Zell ER, et al. Prevention of secondary transmission of pertussis in households with early use of erythromycin. *Am J Dis Child* 1992;146: 177–181.

5

Back, Joint, and Extremity Pain

Samir S. Shah, Jacqueline Owusu-Antwi, and Lisa B. Zaoutis

APPROACH TO THE PATIENT WITH BACK, JOINT, AND EXTREMITY PAIN

I. Definition of the Complaint

Back, extremity, and joint pain are worrisome symptoms in children. The inability of young children to clearly describe the location and nature of the pain contributes to diagnostic difficulties. Because the diverse complaints of back, extremity, and joint pain frequently share a common etiology, a uniform approach to such symptoms facilitates accurate diagnosis.

II. Complaint by Cause and Frequency

Back pain, or discomfort anywhere along the spinal and paraspinal area, reflects potential pathology in a wide range of organ systems, including musculoskeletal, central nervous system (CNS), pulmonary, vascular, and intraabdominal or retroperitoneal structures (Table 5-1). Young children who cannot accurately localize pain require indirect symptom assessment. For example, refusal to walk, irritability with repositioning, or reluctance to participate in specific activities often provides the earliest clues to underlying infectious, inflammatory, or neoplastic disorders.

Alteration in gait or changes in the use of a limb also suggest an underlying extremity or joint disorder (Table 5-2). Examination of one joint above and one below the site of the chief complaint can prevent missing a diagnosis in cases of referred pain. For example, knee pain may be the presenting symptom for hip pathology. Joint and extremity symptoms can also represent referred pain from a spinal or paraspinal process. The radicular symptoms of nerve root entrapment in the lumbar spine may manifest as foot pain.

TABLE 5-1. *Causes of Back Pain in Childhood by Etiology*

Diagnostic category	Cause
Infectious/Inflammatory	Vertebral ostemyelitis
	Spinal epidural abscess
	Diskitis
Orthopedic	Scheuermann disease
	Spondylolysis
	Intravertebral disk herniation
	Trauma
	Muscle strain
Rheumatologic	Juvenile ankylosing spondylitis
	Juvenile rheumatoid arthritis
Neoplastic	Neuroblastoma
	Ganglioneuroma
	Lymphoma
	Leukemia
	Eosinophilic granuloma

TABLE 5-2. *Causes of Joint or Extremity Pain in Childhood by Etiology*

Diagnostic category	Cause
Infectious/Inflammatory	Bacterial arthritis
	Lyme arthritis
	Disseminated *Neisseria gonorrhoeae*
	Osteomyelitis
	Pyomyositis
	Acute rheumatic fever
	Reactive/Postinfectious arthritis
	Immunization
Orthopedic	Trauma
	Osteochondritis dessicans
	Chondromalacia patella
	Overuse syndromes
	Osgood-Schlatter disease
Rheumatologic	Systemic juvenile arthritis
	Systemic lupus erythematosus
	Dermatomyositis
Neoplastic	Leukemia
	Lymphoma
	Bone/soft tissue tumors
	Metastatic malignancy
Hematologic	Sickle cell disease
	Hemophilia
Miscellaneous	Kawasaki disease
	Serum sickness
	Behçet disease
	Sarcoidosis
	Henoch-Schönlein purpura
	Guillain-Barré syndrome

The evaluation of back, extremity, and joint pain requires an understanding that extensive interplay of symptoms, findings, and etiologies exists among these diagnostic groups.

III. Clarifying Questions

Routine inquiry into the onset, location, duration, character, radiation, and intensity of the pain may clarify the diagnosis. Caretaker observations may supplement the history, especially in nonverbal patients. Special mention should be made regarding the onset of pain in relation to trauma. Many children with nontraumatic abnormalities first notice a previously underappreciated symptom after an insignificant injury. For example, a child with a spinal tumor may fall off a bicycle and complain of leg pain, when in fact the tumor had been present for weeks and it was the progressive paresis that caused the child to fall from the bike. Incidental injuries are present in almost all children's recent history; they may be associated with the underlying problem, but they may not necessarily be the primary cause. Beware of the red herring of trauma.

The following questions can be particularly helpful.

• What is the age of the patient?

— In younger children, especially those younger than 5 years of age, back pain is often a manifestation of a serious underlying disorder. In contrast, older adolescents are more likely to have nonspecific musculoskeletal disorders, similar to adults with back pain.

- What is the timing of the pain?

  — Mechanical strains and stresses are often improved at night and resolve within several weeks. However, spondylolysis, spondylolisthesis, and Scheuermann disease may also improve with rest. Pain that worsens at night is more typical of tumors or infections.

- Are there systemic symptoms?

  — Fever, malaise, and weight loss are more suggestive of an inflammatory, neoplastic, or infectious etiology.

- Are there any neurologic findings?

  — Bowel or bladder dysfunction and skin lesions such as café-au-lait spots, sacral dimples, or hairy patches may be useful clues to spinal pathology. Some examples are syringomyelia, tethered cord, ruptured disc, spinal cord tumor, or unrecognized spinal dysraphism.

- Is there decreased range of motion of the back?

  — Stiffness of the spine is an unusual finding in young children and may indicate infection, inflammation, or tumor. In adolescents, muscle spasm from overuse injuries can limit the range of motion, but this resolves quickly.

- Is a deformity of the back noticeable?

  — Deformity of the normal spinal curvature may represent primary spinal pathology, a congenital or idiopathic process, or muscular abnormalities that contribute to progressive scoliosis or kyphosis. Splinting during acute pneumonia leads to transient abnormal lateral curvature of the thoracic spine.

Case 5-1: 2-Year-Old Boy

I. History of Present Illness

A 2-year-old boy presented to the emergency department for evaluation of back pain. Three days before admission, he began to complain of abdominal pain, refused to eat lunch that day, and spent most of the afternoon watching television rather than playing outside with his siblings. At that time, he was taken to a nearby hospital for evaluation. On examination, he had mild, diffuse abdominal tenderness but no rebound tenderness or involuntary guarding. Abdominal radiographs showed significant stool in the rectum and distal colon. He was diagnosed with constipation, was given a glycerin suppository, and was discharged home after producing a moderate amount of stool.

On the day of admission, he returned to the hospital with persistent abdominal pain and new complaints of low back pain. His oral intake had been poor over the past few days. There had been minimal response to a glycerin suppository earlier that day. He also seemed particularly uncomfortable while his diaper was being changed. There was no fever, cough, hematemesis, hematochezia, dysuria, or urinary frequency. There were no ill contacts and no known trauma. The only pet was an elderly dog that had been euthanized earlier in the week.

II. Past Medical History

Tympanostomy tubes had been placed at 15 months of age for recurrent otitis media. He had only one episode of otitis media after the tubes were placed. He did not have a previous history of constipation. He does not take any medications. The family history was remarkable for a paternal uncle who had a myocardial infarction at 55 years of age.

III. Physical Examination

T, 38.9°C; RR, 36/min; HR, 130 bpm; BP, 115/55 mm Hg; SpO_2, 99% in room air

Weight, 18.0 kg (greater than the 95th percentile)

The child appeared uncomfortable and refused to stand. The eyes, nose, and oropharynx were clear. The neck was supple. The abdomen was mildly distended and diffusely tender, particularly in the right lower quadrant. However, there was no rebound tenderness or involuntary guarding. There was no costovertebral angle tenderness. There was discomfort with passive flexion of the right hip. There was mild edema and tenderness to percussion along the right paraspinous muscle at the level of the L1 vertebra. There was no kyphosis, scoliosis, or abnormal lordosis. There were no apparent sensory or motor neurologic deficits, although the degree of back and abdominal pain made assessment of muscle strength in the lower extremities difficult. There was no muscle atrophy. Rectal tone was normal. The deep tendon reflexes were symmetric and appropriately brisk. The remainder of the examination was normal.

IV. Diagnostic Studies

Complete blood count revealed the following: 19,700 white blood cells (WBCs)/mm^3, with 67% segmented neutrophils, 29% lymphocytes, and 3% monocytes; hemoglobin, 11.4 g/dL; and platelets, 390,000/mm^3. Serum electrolytes were remarkable for a bicarbonate level of 19 mEq/L, a blood urea nitrogen level of 7 mg/dL, and a creatinine level of 0.3 mg/dL. Urinalysis revealed a specific gravity of 1.020 and 3+ ketones but the microscopic examination was normal. Serum albumin and transaminases were normal. C-reactive protein (CRP) and the erythrocyte sedimentation rate (ESR) were elevated at 7.9 mg/dL and 65 mm/hour, respectively. Abdominal obstruction series revealed scattered air–fluid levels and a small amount of stool in the rectum.

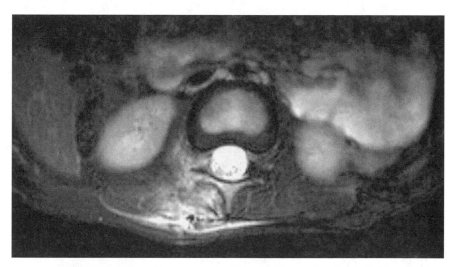

FIG. 5-1. Magnetic resonance image of the spine (case 5-1).

V.   Course of Illness

Magnetic resonance imaging (MRI) of the spine localized the abnormality (Fig. 5-1), and the definitive diagnosis was made by an interventional study.

DISCUSSION: CASE 5-1

I.   Differential Diagnosis

Back pain is a relatively common complaint among children, although fewer than 2% of older children with back pain require specific medical evaluation. In a young child, neoplastic, infectious, and inflammatory disorders should be considered. Malignant causes may be primary or metastatic and include osteoid osteoma, neuroblastoma, Wilms tumor, and leukemia. Infectious or inflammatory causes include pyelonephritis, vertebral osteomyelitis, spinal epidural abscess, and pyomyositis. Diskitis in children usually involves the lower thoracic or lumbar spine. The presence of fever, if related to the back pain, makes diskitis less likely. Local tenderness and elevated CRP and ESR can be seen with many infectious and neoplastic causes. MRI of the spine readily differentiates diskitis, vertebral osteomyelitis, and spinal epidural abscess. Rheumatologic conditions include systemic juvenile rheumatoid arthritis. Mechanical disorders such as muscle strains and intervertebral disk herniation are less likely in this age group. The absence of neurologic findings, although reassuring, does not permit exclusion of any of these entities.

II.   Diagnosis

MRI of the spine revealed an abnormal heterogeneous enhancing mass (7 × 4 cm) involving the right psoas muscle and extending to the epidural space at the L1–L3 vertebral level (see Fig. 5-1). There was associated compression of the thecal sac. Urine homovanillic acid and vanillylmandelic acid levels were normal, making neuroblastoma less likely. Gram staining of purulent material drained during biopsy of the mass revealed many WBCs and gram-positive cocci. Group A *Streptococcus* subsequently grew from culture. **The diagnosis is spinal epidural abscess due to group A *Streptococcus.*** The demise of the pet dog did not appear to be related to this patient's diagnosis.

III.   Epidemiology and Incidence of Spinal Epidural Abscess

Spinal epidural abscesses occur rarely in children. Auletta and John reported an incidence of 0.6 per 10,000 hospital admissions. Most patients are boys that were previously healthy, but predisposing factors include sickle cell disease (SCD), hematologic malignancy, and spinal surgery. Spinal epidural abscess occasionally complicates serial lumbar puncture and varicella infection. *Staphylococcus aureus* causes more than two-thirds of cases but infections due to group A *Streptococcus*, group B *Streptococcus*, *Salmonella* species, *Escherichia coli*, and *Pseudomonas aeruginosa* have also been reported. Rare fungal causes include *Candida* species and *Aspergillus flavus*. *Mycobacterium tuberculosis* may be seen more commonly in areas with a high prevalence of tuberculosis.

The infection is usually acquired by hematogenous spread and occasionally by direct extension from an adjacent site of infection. Associated osteomyelitis is present in approximately 50% of patients. In the study by Auletta and John, seven of eight children with spinal epidural abscess had an associated psoas or paraspinal abscess.

IV.   Clinical Presentation

Most children develop fever early during the course of infection. Common presenting complaints include back pain, limp, and refusal to walk. Hip pain is an unusual presenting complaint, although it may be difficult to differentiate back from hip pain in an ill and irritable child. Depending on the level of involvement, progression of infection can cause spinal cord compression, muscle weakness, and bowel and bladder incontinence followed by paralysis. On examination, there may be tenderness over the vertebrae or paraspinal tissues. Some children develop protective paraspinal muscle spasm. There may also be loss of normal curvature of the spine (usually decreased lumbar lordosis) and limited lumbosacral mobility. Abdominal pain is relatively common and can indicate radicular pain or associated psoas abscess.

V.   Diagnostic Approach

Spinal epidural abscesses can result in a range of clinical and laboratory findings, and a high level of suspicion is required to make the diagnosis early in the course of infection. Surgical aspiration should always be performed, because identification of a specific pathogen permits optimal antibiotic selection. Other studies may increase the level of suspicion for spinal epidural abscess.

Complete blood count. The peripheral WBC count is elevated in approximately 50% of cases. Thrombocytosis may be present.

C-reactive protein and erythrocyte sedimentation rate. These markers of inflammation are usually elevated, especially when there is an associated vertebral osteomyelitis. They may be elevated also in noninfectious conditions such as malignancy.

Blood culture. Organisms are isolated from blood culture in approximately 10% of cases. If positive, the blood culture is invaluable in guiding specific antibiotic therapy.

Tuberculin skin testing. Tuberculin skin testing should be performed if no bacterial organism is isolated from blood or abscess culture, because *M. tuberculosis* can cause spinal epidural abscesses.

Spine radiographs. Radiographs of the spine exclude other causes of back pain. Associated vertebral osteomyelitis may be evident in children with a prolonged duration of symptoms.

Magnetic resonance imaging of the spine. MRI of the spine demonstrates the abscess, although definitive diagnosis requires biopsy. MRI reveals concomitant vertebral osteomyelitis in 20% to 50% of cases.

Other studies. At the time of diagnostic biopsy, specimens should be sent for stains and cultures of aerobic and anaerobic bacteria, fungi, and mycobacteria. Radionuclide bone scans to detect osteomyelitis at sites distant from the abscess should be considered in cases in which the abscess occurred as a consequence of hematogenous seeding. Cerebrospinal fluid (CSF) abnormalities are common with spinal epidural abscesses. In a review by Rubin et al., 33 (78%) of 42 children with spinal epidural abscess had findings consistent with meningeal infection (mild to moderate pleocytosis or hypoglycorrachia). In 12%, elevated CSF protein was the only CSF abnormality. Examination of the CSF was completely normal in 10% of children with spinal epidural abscess. Lumbar puncture should not be performed if the abscess is located in the lumbar region.

VI. Treatment

Standard management of epidural abscesses includes antibiotic therapy and surgical drainage. Sporadic cases reported in the literature have been treated with antibiotics alone. Candidates for antibiotic therapy without surgical drainage may include patients without neurologic deficits and those with numerous abscesses that would be technically difficult to drain. In those children who are treated with antibiotics without surgical drainage, diagnostic surgical aspiration to identify the infecting organism should be strongly considered. This decision usually is made in consultation with infectious disease and neurosurgical specialists. The empiric antibiotic regimen should include agents with activity against *S. aureus,* such as oxacillin or vancomycin. Vancomycin should be the initial antibiotic if (a) methicillin-resistant *Staphylococcus aureus* (MRSA) accounts for more than 10% to 15% of local *S. aureus* isolates, (b) a household member works in a nursing home or other facility with high rates of MRSA colonization, and (c) the patient lives with someone known to be colonized with MRSA. Cefotaxime and metronidazole should be added if gram-negative or anaerobic organisms are suspected. Ultimate antibiotic selection depends on the results of blood and abscess culture. The duration of antibiotic treatment usually is determined by improvements in clinical findings (e.g., improved pain and function), laboratory results (e.g., normalization of ESR and CRP levels), and radiologic imaging studies (e.g., resolved epidural fluid collection on MRI). Most children require approximately 6 weeks of parenteral antibiotic therapy.

Mortality rates for adults with spinal epidural abscesses range from 5% to 25%. Mortality rates in children are substantially lower. There were no deaths among the 34 children reviewed in one series. Approximately 75% to 85% of children treated for spinal epidural abscess have normal neurologic function at the completion of therapy. Risk factors for persistent deficits include multiple medical problems, previous spinal surgery, and severe neurologic deficit at presentation.

VII. References

1. Auletta JJ, John CC. Spinal epidural abscesses in children: a 15-year experience and review of the literature. *Clin Infect Dis* 2001;32:9–16.
2. Bair-Merritt MH, Chung C, Collier A. Spinal epidural abscess in a young child. *Pediatrics* 2000;106:e39. Available at: http://www.pediatrics.org/cgi/content/full/106/3/e39 (accessed July 20, 2003).
3. Herold BC, Immergluck LC, Maranan MC, et al. Community-acquired methicillin-resistant *Staphylococcus aureus* in children with no identified predisposing risk. *JAMA* 1998;279:593–598.
4. Mason DE. Back pain in children. *Pediatr Ann* 1999;28:727–738.
5. Rubin G, Michowiz DS, Ashkenasi A, et al. Spinal epidural abscess in the pediatric age group: case report and review of the literature. *Pediatr Infect Dis J* 1993;12:1007–1011.
6. Yogev R. Focal suppurative infections of the central nervous system. In: Long SS, Pickering LK, Prober CG, eds. *Principles and practice of pediatric infectious diseases,* 2nd ed. New York: Churchill Livingstone, 2003:302–312.

Case 5-2: 2-Year-Old Boy

I. History of Present Illness

A 2-year-old boy presented with a 2-week history of difficulty walking. The parents had noticed that he would no longer run while playing with his siblings. Over the past week, he had begun walking with a limp and refusing to climb stairs. His pediatrician detected splenomegaly and tenderness over the right hip. There was no fever, cough, rhinorrhea, throat pain, diarrhea, or trauma. There had been no ill contacts. A pet dog was acquired 1 week earlier. Hip radiographs and several laboratory studies were obtained, after which the patient was immediately referred to the emergency department.

II. Past Medical History

The patient was born at term without complications. He had been hospitalized with wheezing at 4 months of age and required oral antibiotics at 12 months of age for outpatient treatment of pneumonia. He was not receiving any medications and had no allergies. Family history was remarkable for a maternal aunt with rheumatic heart disease.

III. Physical Examination

T, 37.3°C; RR, 34/min; HR, 104 bpm; BP, 98/43 mm Hg

Height and weight, both 25th percentile for age

On examination, the child was pale and tired-appearing. His sclerae were anicteric. The heart and lung sounds were normal. The spleen tip was palpable just below the left costal margin. The liver edge was palpable 3 cm below the right costal margin. There was mild discomfort with passive flexion of the right hip, but the range of motion was normal. There was no overlying erythema or warmth. Examination of the left hip was unremarkable. The testes were in normal position and were not enlarged, swollen, or tender. Numerous petechial lesions were scattered on his lower extremities bilaterally. Small lymph nodes were palpable in the anterior cervical and inguinal regions.

IV. Diagnostic Studies

The complete blood count revealed 4,300 WBCs/mm^3, with 3% band forms, 8% segmented neutrophils, and 85% lymphocytes, giving an absolute neutrophil count of 473/mm^3. The hemoglobin was 8.0 g/dL, with a reticulocyte count of 1.3%. The platelet count was 31,000/mm^3. CRP and ESR were 2.6 mg/dL and 60 mm/hour, respectively. Serum lactate dehydrogenase (LDH), uric acid, transaminases, and electrolytes were normal. The hip radiographs performed earlier were reviewed (Fig. 5-2A).

V. Course of Illness

Results of the hip radiography, combined with results of the peripheral blood smear (see Fig. 5-2B), suggested a diagnosis.

DISCUSSION: CASE 5-2

I. Differential Diagnosis

Infectious causes of hip pain in a young boy include septic arthritis of the hip, osteomyelitis of the femur or pelvis, and psoas abscess. The prolonged duration of symptoms with recent worsening, in conjunction with an elevated CRP and ESR, may indicate osteomyelitis of the femur with extension of infection into the hip joint. However, the relatively unimpressive amount of pain on hip examination, combined with pancytopenia, makes infectious causes unlikely. Toxic synovitis can cause hip pain in this age group but also is not typically associated with pancytopenia.

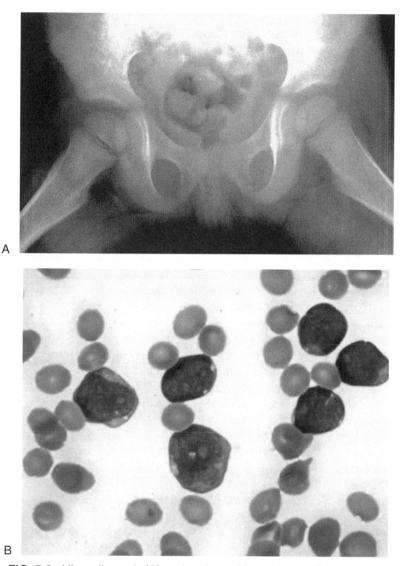

FIG. 5-2. Hip radiograph **(A)** and peripheral blood smear **(B)** for case 5-2.

Causes of pancytopenia, hepatosplenomegaly, and bone pain include leukemia, epiphyseal tumors, neuroblastoma, infectious mononucleosis, and hemophagocytic syndrome. The normal uric acid and LDH do not exclude malignancy.

II. Diagnosis

The hip radiographs revealed dense metaphyseal lines bilaterally with adjacent metaphyseal lucency, a finding suggestive of leukemia (see Fig. 5-2A). The peripheral blood smear revealed numerous cells with scant cytoplasm and finely dispersed to variably condensed chromatin, morphologically consistent with lymphoblasts (see Fig.5-2B). Morphologic, cytochemical, and immunophenotypic features of the bone marrow aspirate were diagnostic of acute lymphocytic leukemia. The child was initially treated with vincristine, dexamethasone, and intrathecal ara-C.

III. Epidemiology

Leukemia results from malignant transformation and clonal expansion of hematopoietic cells that have stopped at a particular stage of differentiation and are unable to progress to more mature forms. Leukemias are divided into acute and chronic subtypes and are further classified on the basis of leukemic cell morphology into lymphocytic leukemias (lymphoid lineage cell proliferation) and nonlymphocytic leukemias (granulocyte, monocyte, erythrocyte, or platelet lineage cell proliferation). Acute leukemias constitute more than 95% of all childhood leukemias and are subdivided into acute lymphocytic leukemia (ALL) and acute nonlymphocytic leukemia, also known as acute myelogenous leukemia (AML). The following discussion focuses on ALL.

ALL, the most common pediatric malignancy, accounts for approximately 25% of all childhood cancers and 75% of all childhood leukemias. Most children are diagnosed between 2 and 5 years of age. In the United States, the incidence of ALL is higher in whites than in blacks and in boys than in girls. Genetic factors also affect the risk of ALL. ALL develops in siblings of children with ALL two to four times more often than in unrelated children. The concordance of ALL in monozygotic twins is approximately 25%. Children with chromosomal abnormalities, including trisomy 21, and syndromes characterized by chromosomal fragility, such as Bloom's syndrome and Fanconi anemia, also have a substantially higher risk of leukemia.

IV. Clinical Presentation

The presenting symptoms and signs of children with ALL reflect the degree of bone marrow infiltration with leukemic cells and the extent of extramedullary disease spread. Symptoms may be present for days or months and include fever, anorexia, fatigue, and pallor. Bone pain occurs with leukemic involvement of the periosteum and bone. Young children often develop a limp or refuse to walk. Headache, vomiting, and seizures suggest CNS involvement. Rarely, children present with oliguria due to acute renal failure precipitated by hyperuricemia.

On examination, painless lymphadenopathy (50%) and hepatosplenomegaly (68%) result from extramedullary spread of the disease. Petechiae and purpura are more common, but some children also have subconjunctival and retinal hemorrhages. Children may have focal bone tenderness. Testicular enlargement due to leukemic infiltration is present in 5% of boys with ALL.

V. Diagnostic Approach

Complete blood count. The WBC count is between 10,000 and 50,000 cells/mm^3 in 30% of children with ALL and greater than 50,000 cells/mm^3 in approximately 20%. Neutropenia, defined as an absolute neutrophil count less than 500 cells/mm^3, is common at presentation. Other findings include moderate to severe anemia and an inappropriately low reticulocyte count. The platelet count is less than 100,000 cells/mm^3 in approximately 75% of patients, but isolated thrombocytopenia rarely occurs. The severity of bleeding correlates with the degree of thrombocytopenia. Leukemic cells may be noted on the peripheral blood smear, particularly if the WBC count is normal or high.

Bone marrow aspirate or biopsy. A bone marrow aspirate or biopsy definitively establishes the diagnosis of ALL, because the morphology of blasts seen on peripheral smear may not reflect the true bone marrow morphology. Monoclonal antibody testing of the bone marrow for specific cell surface antigens identifies lymphocytes and granulocytes at different stages of development. When this immunophenotyping is combined with cytochemical staining and molecular genotyping, the diagnostic classification, treatment, and prognosis become more specific.

Other laboratory studies. Other laboratory abnormalities reflect either leukemic cell infiltration or excessive proliferation and destruction of leukemic cells. Serum transaminases may be mildly abnormal with liver infiltration, but coagulation abnormalities are uncommon. Hypercalcemia results from leukemic infiltration of bone. Increased serum phosphorus levels occur as a result of leukemic cell lysis and may induce hypocalcemia. Cell lysis also leads to elevated serum uric acid concentrations, reflecting increased purine catabolism, and elevated LDH.

Radiographs. Long bone radiograph abnormalities include transverse radiolucent metaphyseal growth arrest lines, periosteal elevation with reactive subperiosteal cortical thickening, and osteolytic lesions.

Computed tomography. Computed tomography may reveal diffuse lymphadenopathy and hepatosplenomegaly. Approximately 5% to 10% of newly diagnosed patients have an anterior mediastinal mass detected on chest imaging.

VI. Treatment

Although specific treatment strategies vary from center to center, all modern approaches treat the complications of ALL at presentation, treat the leukemia, and manage treatment-related complications. Acute management involves blood product transfusions and treatment of infection, hyperviscosity, compressive symptoms, and metabolic abnormalities. The term *tumor lysis syndrome* describes the constellation of metabolic abnormalities resulting from spontaneous or treatment-induced tumor necrosis. Acute tumor cell destruction releases intracellular contents into circulation, leading to hypocalcemia, hyperphosphatemia, hyperkalemia, and hyperuricemia. Management of tumor lysis syndrome includes vigorous hydration, urine alkalinization, uric acid reduction, and diuretic therapy.

Specific therapy for ALL is instituted in three distinct phases. *Remission induction* therapy lasts approximately 4 weeks, during which most children have a complete remission (defined as the absence of clinical signs and symptoms of disease), recovery of normal blood cell counts, and recovery of normocellular bone marrow. Agents currently used for remission induction include dexamethasone or prednisone, vincristine, and L-asparaginase. Other agents may be used if the patient is considered to be at high risk or has CNS involvement. *Consolidation therapy* aims to kill additional leukemic cells with further systemic therapy and to prevent CNS relapse with intrathecal chemotherapy. *Maintenance therapy* aims to continue remission achieved by the first two phases; it is required because shorter treatment protocols are associated with a high rate of relapse. Methotrexate and 6-mercaptopurine are often used for consolidation and maintenance therapy.

Children with high WBC counts (greater than $50,000/mm^3$) and those who are younger (less than 2 years of age) or older (greater than 10 years of age) at diagnosis have the worst prognosis. However, between 95% and 98% of children diagnosed with ALL achieve complete remission after induction therapy. Relapse occurs in 20% to 30%, either during subsequent treatment or within the first 2 years after its completion. Relapse can affect virtually any site of the body, although bone marrow relapse is most common. Since the introduction of effective CNS-directed therapy, the frequency of CNS relapse has decreased to approximately 5%. Isolated testicular relapse occurs in 1% of boys. Bone marrow relapse is often treated with intense chemotherapy combined with bone marrow transplantation. The event-free survival rate after relapse ranges from 30% to 60%.

Late sequelae of ALL therapy include second neoplasms, neuropsychologic effects, endocrine dysfunction, and other organ-specific complications. Second neoplasms occur in 2.5% of patients; CNS tumors are the most common second neoplasm. Children who are younger than 5 years of age at ALL diagnosis and those who receive cranial irradiation are at highest risk. Short stature occurs due to cranial irradiation–induced growth hormone deficiency. Some late complications are related to specific chemotherapeutic agents, such as cardiomyopathy from anthracycline or bladder fibrosis from cyclophosphamide therapy. Chemotherapy may also have long-term effects on the child's immune system. Recovery of the immune system usually occurs within 1 to 2 years after the completion of chemotherapy. However, some children have low antibody titers of clinically significant viruses to which they have been previously immunized.

VII.   References

1. Hermiston ML, Mentzer WC. A practical approach to the evaluation of the anemic child. *Pediatr Clin North Am* 2002;49:877–891.
2. Margolin JF, Poplack DG. Acute lymphoblastic leukemia. In: Pizzo PA, Poplack DG, eds. *Principles and practice of pediatric oncology,* 3rd ed. Philadelphia: Lippincott–Raven, 1997:409–462.
3. Meister LA, Meadows AT. Late effects of childhood cancer therapy. *Curr Probl Pediatr* 1993;23:102–131.
4. Neglia JP, Meadows AT, Robison LL, et al. Second neoplasms after acute lymphoblastic leukemia in childhood. *N Engl J Med* 1991;325:1330–1336.
5. Pui CH, Crist WM. Biology and treatment of acute lymphoblastic leukemia. *J Pediatr* 1994;124:491–503.
6. Rubnitz JE, Look AT. Molecular genetics of childhood leukemias. *J Pediatr Hematol Oncol* 1998;20:1–11.
7. Sanders JE. Bone marrow transplantation for pediatric leukemia. *Pediatr Ann* 1991; 20:671–676.

Case 5-3: 14-Year-Old Boy

I. History of Present Illness

A 14-year-old boy presented to the emergency department complaining of left knee pain. Three days before this visit, he noted left knee pain after playing basketball and began to limp. This knee pain improved over the next few days. While walking across a wooden floor on the evening of his emergency department presentation, he slipped and fell. As soon as he stood up, he noted pain in his left knee again that occasionally radiated to the left hip. He did not strike his head. There was no other bone pain. There was no headache, blurry vision, or loss of consciousness. There was no fever, weight loss, myalgias, or malaise.

II. Past Medical History

The patient had required hospitalization at 8 years of age for disorientation after a car accident; his symptoms resolved, and he was discharged the next day. At 10 years of age, he developed poststreptococcal glomerulonephritis. He had been treated with a short course of corticosteroids but had not required specific therapy since that time. He did not report taking any medications. There was no family history of endocrine or autoimmune disorders.

III. Physical Examination

T, 37.1°C; RR, 24/min; HR, 105 bpm; BP, 125/80 mm Hg

Weight, 101 kg

Physical examination revealed an obese boy without visible evidence of head trauma. He was alert and cooperative. Heart and lung sounds were normal. The abdomen was soft without organomegaly. There was no deformity of either lower extremity. Passive flexion of the left hip accompanied by internal and external rotation significantly worsened the left knee pain. Internal rotation of the left hip was limited compared with that of the right hip. There was no tenderness, swelling, or erythema of the left knee. There was full range of motion of the left knee without discomfort when this joint was tested in isolation. There was no sign of knee ligament instability. The right lower extremity was normal. He was able to ambulate but clearly preferred not to place too much weight on the left leg.

IV. Diagnostic Studies

The complete blood count revealed the following: 8,600 WBCs/mm^3 (65% segmented neutrophils, 30% lymphocytes, and 5% monocytes); hemoglobin, 13.1 g/dL; and 204,000 platelets/mm^3. The CRP concentration was 0.7 mg/dL, and the ESR was 12 mm/hour. Serum electrolytes and calcium were normal.

V. Course of Illness

Radiographs of the left knee were normal. Hip radiographs revealed the diagnosis (Fig. 5-3).

DISCUSSION: CASE 5-3

I. Differential Diagnosis

Diagnosing the cause of knee pain in an adolescent can be difficult. Because knee pain may actually be pain referred from the hip via the obturator nerve, diagnostic considerations should include problems involving either the knee or the hip. In this case, although the patient was adamant in his complaint of pain localized to the knee, examination of

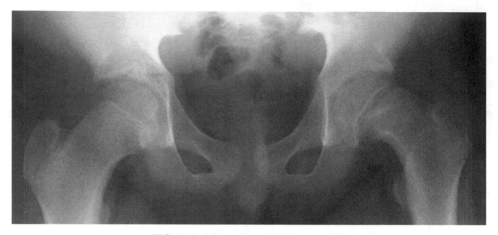

FIG. 5-3. Hip radiograph (case 5-3).

the knee was normal. The lack of physical findings localized to the knee made septic arthritis of the knee and fracture of the distal femur, patella, proximal tibia, or fibula unlikely. Antecedent trauma raised the possibility of knee hyperextension or patellar dislocation, but the normal knee examination placed these possibilities lower on the differential diagnosis. Osgood-Schlatter disease typically manifests with localized tenderness and swelling over the tibial tuberosity, findings that were absent in this case.

Hip disorders to consider in an adolescent boy include avascular necrosis of the femoral head, septic arthritis of the hip, femoral or pelvic osteomyelitis, femoral neck fracture, chronic developmental hip dysplasia, inguinal hernia, slipped capital femoral epiphysis, Ewing sarcoma, and osteogenic sarcoma. Avascular necrosis of the femoral head can be caused by corticosteroid use and also occurs in children with SCD and idiopathically (Legg-Calvé Perthes disease). The absence of fever, combined with normal CRP and ESR values, makes acute septic arthritis and osteomyelitis unlikely. In this case, radiographs of the hip narrowed the differential diagnosis even further.

II. Diagnosis

Anteroposterior radiographs of the hip (see Fig. 5-3) demonstrated inferior displacement of the left femoral head relative to the femoral neck. On the lateral frog leg view, this displacement appeared posterior and medial relative to the femoral neck. **These findings confirmed the diagnosis of slipped capital femoral epiphysis (SCFE).** The patient underwent percutaneous screw fixation (Fig. 5-4). Prophylactic screw fixation of the contralateral hip was also performed.

III. Incidence and Epidemiology of Slipped Capital Femoral Epiphysis

The term *SCFE* refers to displacement of the femoral head relative to the femoral neck through the physis (growth plate). This displacement results from either cumulative normal stresses acting on a weakened physis or the effect of an acute traumatic event on a normal or previously weakened physis. SCFE occurs with an annual incidence of 2 to 3 cases per 100,000 persons. It typically develops during the adolescent growth spurt, occurring in boys 10 to 16 years of age and girls 10 to 13 years of age. The incidence is approximately 2.5 times greater in boys than in girls. The incidence is also higher in African-Americans than in Caucasians. Obesity is a clear predisposing factor. One-half to two-thirds of children with SCFE have weight-for-height profiles greater than the 95th percentile. Obesity may contribute by creating increased shear forces across the weak-

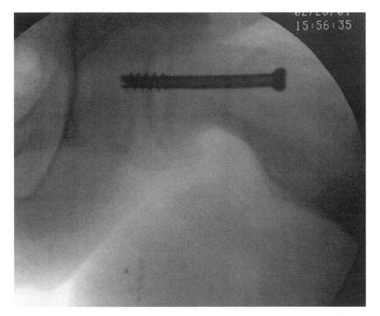

FIG. 5-4. Intraoperative fluoroscopy of the hip (case 5-3).

ened physis during ambulation. Underlying endocrine or metabolic disorders that delay skeletal maturation, such as primary or secondary hypothyroidism, panhypopituitarism, or hypogonadism, should be suspected in children who are outside the typical age or weight range for SCFE. In this case, the corticosteroids the patient received at 10 years of age were not thought to be a contributing factor in the development of SCFE.

IV. Clinical Presentation

Several studies have documented considerable delays in the diagnosis of SCFE. Patients frequently complain of symptoms for 3 to 4 months before the diagnosis is made. Therefore, clinicians should have a high level of suspicion for the diagnosis of SCFE even in adolescents with vague complaints of hip, thigh, or knee pain.

Patients with SCFE usually complain of pain in the affected hip or groin. Pain perceived in the medial thigh and knee is caused by referred hip pain along the sensory distribution of the femoral and obturator nerves. Isolated knee pain is the sole presenting feature in up to 15% of children diagnosed with SCFE. Early in the course, pain is usually associated with exercise, but as the slip progresses, the symptoms become more persistent and severe.

On physical examination, patients complain of pain with rotation of the hip. The pain is most prominent at the extremes of rotation. Internal rotation may be noticeably decreased. Furthermore, as the hip is flexed, the thigh rotates externally. This finding, when present, is almost pathognomonic for SCFE in an obese adolescent. Thigh or gluteal muscle atrophy occurs with long-standing symptoms and disuse.

V. Diagnostic Approach.

Anteroposterior and frog leg lateral hip radiographs. On the anteroposterior view, a line drawn along the superior femoral neck (Klein's line) normally intersects a portion of the femoral head. In SCFE, the femoral head is located below this line. On the frog leg lateral view, the femoral head is displaced posterior and medial to the femoral neck. In the early stages of SCFE, the only finding may be a widened and blurred physis. In chronic cases (symptom duration, longer than 3 weeks), radiographs may reveal bony remodeling along the posterior and medial aspects of the femoral neck. Both hips should be examined, because SCFE is bilateral in 25% of cases. Approximately 20% to 50% of those patients with known unilateral involvement ultimately develop SCFE in the contralateral hip. Radiographs also allow exclusion of conditions with similar manifestations, such as femoral neck fracture.

Additional imaging. Hip ultrasound, computed tomography, and MRI have been used to confirm the diagnosis in radiographically equivocal cases.

Other studies. Consider evaluating thyroid and pituitary function in children outside the typical age range for SCFE. Loder et al. reviewed 85 patients with endocrine disorders and SCFE. Only those with previously undiagnosed hypothyroidism or growth hormone deficiency presented before 10 years of age. Complete blood count, CRP, and ESR determinations should be obtained if the diagnosis of osteomyelitis or septic arthritis is being considered.

VI.   Treatment

The goals of treatment are to prevent further slippage and to restore function. The patient should not be allowed to bear weight on the affected extremity once the diagnosis has been confirmed. An untreated stable slip may progress to a more severe unstable slip, leading to increased morbidity. The most common surgical treatment involves percutaneous fixation of the displaced femoral head with one or more metallic pins or screws.

Prophylactic treatment of the asymptomatic contralateral hip is controversial. Given the high incidence of eventual bilateral involvement (20% to 50% of cases), some surgeons have advocated treatment of the contralateral hip at the time of initial surgery. Other orthopedic surgeons recommend fixation of an asymptomatic contralateral hip only in those patients who are at highest risk of developing SCFE of the contralateral hip, such as those with known endocrine or metabolic disorders.

Outcome after repair is generally good but depends on the degree of abnormality before repair. Subsequent avascular necrosis of the femoral head complicates 15% of cases. Avascular necrosis is most often a consequence of vascular injury associated with initial femoral head displacement rather than a consequence of the repair. Patients with a moderate or severe degree of femoral head displacement at presentation are also more likely to develop associated osteoarthritis. Chondrolysis or destruction of cartilage may occur after pin placement but has also occurred in patients without any surgical therapy. Leg length discrepancy may result from incomplete reduction, avascular necrosis, or chondrolysis. Early recognition and treatment of SCFE prevents many of these complications.

VII.   References

1. Kehl DK. Slipped capital femoral epiphysis. In: Morrissy RT, Weinstein SL, eds. *Lovell and Winter's pediatric orthopaedics,* 5th ed. Philadelphia: Lippincott Williams & Wilkins, 2001:999–1033.
2. Ledwith CA, Fleisher GR. Slipped capital femoral epiphysis without hip pain leads to missed diagnosis. *Pediatrics* 1992;89:660–662.
3. Loder RT, Wittenberg B, DeSilva G. Slipped capital femoral epiphysis associated with endocrine disorders. *J Pediatr Orthop* 1995;15:349–356.
4. Matava MJ, Patton CM, Luhmann S, et al. Knee pain as the initial symptom of slipped capital femoral epiphysis: an analysis of initial presentation and treatment. *J Pediatr Orthop* 1999;19:455–460.
5. Perron AD, Miller MD, Brady WJ. Orthopedic pitfalls in the ED: slipped capital femoral epiphysis. *Am J Emerg Med* 2002;20:484–487.

Case 5-4: 16-Year-Old Girl

I. History of Present Illness

A 16-year-old girl was admitted with joint pain and a 35-pound weight loss over the preceding 7 months. After completion of her gymnastics season 7 months before admission, she had noticed decreased energy and stiff, slightly swollen peripheral joints bilaterally, including elbows, wrists, knees, and ankles. She was diagnosed with juvenile rheumatoid arthritis and treated with naproxen, a nonsteroidal antiinflammatory drug (NSAID). Her pain improved slightly. Shortly after starting naproxen, she began having daily episodes of epistaxis that required four to five facial tissues to control the bleeding. Five months before admission, she changed from naproxen to ibuprofen without significant change in the degree of joint pain.

Three months before admission, she noticed a change in her bowel habits, from two to three stools per week to daily stools that were frequently mixed with blood. One month before admission, she developed intermittent cramping abdominal pain. She continued to have episodes of epistaxis and was treated with fluticasone nasal spray and an oral antihistamine for presumed allergic rhinosinusitis. Her weight decreased from 148 pounds to 113 pounds. She complained of decreased appetite and decreased activity level over the preceding few months. There were no fevers, flank tenderness, dysuria, urgency, or frequency. There was no change in mood or intentional weight loss. There was no change in her menstrual cycle. She had not traveled recently.

II. Past Medical History

She had not previously required hospitalization. Menarche occurred at 11 years of age. Her periods were regular. There were no other medical problems. Her only medications were ibuprofen, fluticasone nasal spray, and oral antihistamines as previously mentioned. There was a family history of hypertension in older relatives.

III. Physical Examination

T, 35.8°C; RR, 18/min; HR, 93 bpm; BP, 123/66 mm Hg

Weight, 40 kg; Height, 162 cm (50th percentile); weight-for-height ratio, less than 5th percentile

Physical examination revealed a thin girl. Her palpebral conjunctivae were slightly pale. There were several superficial but actively bleeding erosions on the left medial nasal septum. There were no oral ulcers. Heart and lung sounds were normal. The abdomen was soft with mild right lower-quadrant tenderness to palpation. There were no peritoneal signs. Bright red blood mixed with stool was detected on rectal examination. There was a small left knee effusion and bilateral ankle effusions. All joints had a normal range of motion.

IV. Diagnostic Studies

Complete blood count revealed 8,900 WBCs/mm³; hemoglobin, 9.6 mg/dL; and 463,000 platelets/mm³. MCV was 70 fL. The reticulocyte count was 1.5%. ESR was 89 mm/hour. Prothrombin time, partial thromboplastin time, and serum transaminases were normal. Serum albumin was 3.0 mg/dL. Urine pregnancy test was negative. There were no red blood cells (RBCs) or WBCs on urinanalysis. Stool was sent for bacterial culture, ova and parasite examination, and *Clostridium difficile* toxin detection. Abdominal radiography revealed stool in the rectal vault.

V. Course of Illness

An upper gastrointestinal barium study with small-bowel follow-through of contrast revealed the diagnosis (Fig. 5-5).

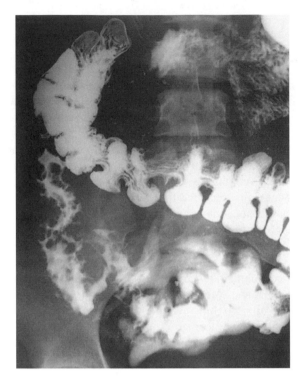

FIG. 5-5. Upper gastrointestinal barium study (case 5-4).

DISCUSSION: CASE 5-4

I. Differential Diagnosis

In an adolescent, hematochezia with cramping abdominal pain has several potential causes. Patients with chronic NSAID use often develop gastrointestinal tract ulceration, although gastric and duodenal ulcers typically result in melena rather than bright red blood. Infectious enterocolitis may be caused by *Salmonella* spp., *Shigella* spp., *Campylobacter jejuni*, enteroinvasive and enterohemorrhagic *E. coli* (including *E. coli* O157:H7), *Yersinia enterocolitica*, and *C. difficile*. Parasitic causes include *Entamoeba histolytica*, *Cryptosporidium parvum*, *Schistosoma*, and *Strongyloides stercoralis*. Exposure to undercooked meat and clusters of patients with similar symptoms suggest a common infectious source. Although 35% to 90% of patients with *E. coli* O157:H7 infection develop bloody diarrhea, only 10% progress to hemolytic-uremic syndrome. The absence of a pertinent travel history makes some of the parasitic diseases less likely. Proctitis can be caused by *Neisseria gonorrhoeae*, herpes simplex virus, or *Treponema pallidum*. Henoch-Schönlein purpura (HSP) may manifest with bloody diarrhea. Vascular malformations of the gastrointestinal tract often manifest with recurrent melena or hematochezia. Eosinophilic gastroenteropathy, a chronic, relapsing disorder characterized by eosinophilic inflammatory gastrointestinal tract infiltrate, often manifests with abdominal pain and rectal bleeding. Abdominal complaints, including abdominal pain due to ileocecal ulcerations, are seen in up to 15% of patients with Behçet's disease. Both Crohn's disease and ulcerative colitis commonly present with abdominal pain and lower gastrointestinal tract bleeding.

Joint involvement occurs in some of the previously mentioned conditions. Reactive arthritis can be associated with *Campylobacter* enteritis as well as with *Salmonella*,

Shigella, and *Yersinia* enteritis. However, the arthritis usually begins 1 to 6 weeks after the onset of diarrhea and resolves within 3 weeks. Arthritis or arthralgias occur in 65% to 85% of children with HSP. Though HSP may recur, prolonged, unremitting symptoms without rash or nephritis are unusual. Children with Behçet's disease usually have recurrent oral ulcers, genital ulcers, and iritis or uveitis in addition to the joint findings. Arthritis may be seen in 10% to 15% of children with Crohn's disease or ulcerative colitis.

II. Diagnosis

Colonoscopy revealed linear ulcerations and luminal edema in the ascending colon. During the gastrointestinal barium study, the contrast agent pursued a normal course through the duodenum, jejunum, and proximal ileum. However, only a thin line of barium connected the ileum to the cecum (Kantor string sign), indicating significant terminal ileal edema (see Fig. 5-5). Severe mucosal irregularity was noted in the distal ileum and ascending colon. **These radiologic findings, combined with the presence of bloody stool, arthritis, nasal ulceration, anemia, and elevated ESR, strongly suggested Crohn's disease.** She was treated with oral sulfasalazine, intravenous methylprednisolone, bowel rest, and parenteral nutrition support. Her symptoms improved over the course of 1 week. Three months later, her weight had increased to 140 pounds.

III. Incidence and Epidemiology of Crohn's Disease.

Crohn's disease, a major form of chronic intestinal inflammation, can segmentally involve any part of the gastrointestinal tract, from the esophagus to the colon. The inflammation involves the terminal portion of the ileum in approximately 90% of cases. Inflammation occurs in the ileum and colon together in 60% of cases, and the upper portion of the gastrointestinal tract is involved in approximately 30% of cases. In contrast, inflammation in ulcerative colitis begins in the rectum and extends continuously into the colon but does not involve more proximal portions of the gastrointestinal tract. Isolated colonic involvement occurs in 10% of cases of Crohn's disease, making distinction from ulcerative colitis difficult in some cases.

The prevalence of Crohn's disease in North America ranges from 26 to 198 cases per 100,000 persons, with higher rates occurring in the more northern latitudes. Crohn's disease is most common among Caucasians and least common among Hispanics and Asian-Americans. Peak incidence occurs in young adulthood, and a second, smaller peak occurs during the sixth decade of life. Approximately 15% of patients with Crohn's disease are diagnosed during childhood. The etiology of Crohn's disease is not known but probably involves a combination of environmental, genetic, and immunoregulatory factors. When the diagnosis of either Crohn's disease or ulcerative colitis is made, the likelihood of finding inflammatory bowel disease in a first-degree relative is 10% to 25%.

IV. Clinical Presentation

Approximately 80% of children with Crohn's disease present with abdominal pain, diarrhea, anorexia, and weight loss with or without extraintestinal manifestations. Recurrent oral ulcers are common. Abdominal pain in the right lower quadrant suggests ileocecal involvement, epigastric pain suggests gastroduodenal involvement, and periumbilical pain suggests generalized small-bowel disease. Fifty percent of children have gross or microscopic blood in the stool. Perirectal disease (e.g., fissures, fistulas, skin tags, abscesses) are present in up to 40% of patients.

Extraintestinal manifestations predominate in 8% to 10% of patients and are likely to be associated with diagnostic confusion and delay (Table 5-3). Although more than 100 localized extraintestinal manifestations have been described, the most common are joint complaints (including arthritis), which occur in 15% to 30% of cases. Approximately 50% of children with Crohn's disease and peripheral arthritis develop

TABLE 5-3. *Extraintestinal Manifestations of Crohn's Disease*

Site of involvement	Manifestation
Eye	Uveitis
	Episcleritis
	Orbital myositis
Hepatobiliary system	Sclerosing cholangitis
	Chronic active hepatitis
	Cholelithiasis
Pancreas	Pancreatitis
Renal system	Nephrolithiasis
	Entervesical fistula
Skin	Erythema nodosum
	Pyoderma gangrenosum
Vascular system	Thrombophlebitis
	Vasculitis
	Deep vein thrombosis
	Pulmonary emboli
	Cerebrovascular disease
Bones and joints	Arthritis—peripheral (knees, ankles, hips, wrists, elbows)
	Arthritis—axial (ankylosing spondylitis, sacroiliitis)
	Arthralgias
	Osteopenia
	Aseptic necrosis

ocular or skin findings (see Table 5-3). Sclerosing cholangitis develops in 1% of children with Crohn's disease. Symptoms of sclerosing cholangitis include jaundice, generalized pruritus, and abdominal pain. Pancreatitis occurs as an extraintestinal manifestation of Crohn's disease but can also occur as a complication of duodenal involvement, sclerosing cholangitis, or drug therapy. Renal stones complicating Crohn's disease may be due to calcium oxalate, calcium phosphate, or uric acid. Erythema nodosum tends to occur when intestinal disease is active, but it does not correlate with disease severity. Rashes due to trace mineral deficiencies may occur as a consequence of malabsorption.

   V.   **Diagnostic Approach**

Initial screening tests should include a complete blood count, ESR, liver function tests, and stool testing for blood, bacteria, and parasites. The results of the initial screening determine the need for further testing.

Complete blood count. Anemia is present in 40% to 70% of patients. MCV may be low due to the combination of iron deficiency and chronic inflammation. Vitamin B_{12} and folate deficiencies also contribute to the anemia. The WBC count is typically normal. Thrombocytosis occurs in more than half of patients.

Erythrocyte sedimentation rate. ESR, an acute phase reactant, is elevated in up to 70% of patients, but a normal ESR does not preclude the diagnosis of Crohn's disease.

Tests of liver function. Serum transaminases and γ-glutamyltransferase (GGT) may be mildly elevated in the absence of complications. Crohn's-related complications, such as sclerosing cholangitis and chronic active hepatitis, lead to more significant elevation of the transaminases and GGT. Hypoalbuminemia reflects compromised nutritional status and diffuse inflammation.

Stool studies. Stool bacterial culture, ova and parasite examination, and *C. difficile* detection should be performed in all children with bloody diarrhea and suspected Crohn's disease, to exclude other causes.

Endoscopic evaluation. Endoscopic evaluation of the colon should precede barium radiography in the presence of bloody diarrhea. Colonic mucosa biopsy, even if the mucosa appears normal, is required, because microscopic inflammation with granuloma formation may be present. If possible, the examination should extend to the terminal ileum. Esophagogastroduodenoscopy may be required to assess upper gastrointestinal tract symptoms.

Upper gastrointestinal tract barium study with small-bowel follow-through. This study is important early in the evaluation, because the terminal ileum is involved in 90% of patients with Crohn's disease. Features suggestive of Crohn's include terminal ileal thickening (Kantor string sign), nodularity, ulcers, and fistulous connections.

Other studies. The following studies may be useful in assessing the patient's nutritional status: folic acid, vitamin B_{12}, fat-soluble vitamins (especially vitamin D), prothrombin time, partial thromboplastin time, zinc, iron, total iron-binding capacity, calcium, magnesium, phosphorus, and prealbumin.

VI.   Treatment

Therapeutic strategies include a combination of medical and surgical interventions. Medical therapy includes 5-aminosalicylates, corticosteroids, immunomodulators, and antibiotics. Oral sulfasalazine consists of 5-aminosalicylic acid (5-ASA) bound to sulfapyridine. The sulfa moiety functions as a carrier, facilitating delivery of the agent to the colon, where it is cleaved by resident bacteria into therapeutically active 5-ASA. The 5-ASA decreases colon inflammation by inhibiting leukotriene synthesis via the lipoxygenase pathway of arachidonic acid metabolism. It also decreases neutrophil-mediated tissue damage by interfering with myeloperoxidase activity and scavenging reactive oxygen species. Newer oral 5-ASA analogues (e.g., mesalamine) function by either pH-dependent or timed-release mechanisms that allow the drug to be distributed throughout the small bowel.

Corticosteroids continue to be the mainstay of treatment. They exert antiinflammatory effects by decreasing cytokine release, capillary permeability, and neutrophil and monocyte function. Newer corticosteroids have a strong affinity for intestinal steroid receptors, leading to high topical antiinflammatory potency. Because they are rapidly transformed into inactivated metabolites by the liver after absorption, they cause fewer systemic side effects. For example, budesonide binds to intestinal receptors 15 times more efficiently than prednisolone but undergoes rapid hepatic metabolism, so systemic bioavailability is only 10%, compared with 80% for prednisolone. Delayed-release (time- and pH-dependent) formulations of budesonide permit more effective delivery of the drug to the terminal ileum and proximal colon.

Immunomodulators are being used to target the inflammatory response more selectively. For example, tumor necrosis factor-α (TNF-α), a cytokine, activates components of the immune system involved in Crohn's disease. Infliximab, a chimeric (mouse-human) anti-TNF-α immunoglobulin G antibody, binds to TNF-α and neutralizes its activity. Infliximab infusions administered at 4- to 12-week intervals induce remissions in patients with moderate to severe Crohn's disease and facilitate healing of fistulas. Infliximab also permits significant reduction in steroid use in children.

The antibiotic metronidazole may reduce Crohn's disease activity. It has also been used to treat perianal fistulas and abscesses. Indications for bowel resection include intractable disease, severe fistula formation, uncontrolled hemorrhage, and bowel perforation. More than 50% of children with Crohn's disease require intestinal surgery within 10 to 15 years after diagnosis. The disease is not usually limited to one portion of the gastrointestinal tract, so surgery is not curative. Recurrent disease after bowel resection is common.

The course of Crohn's disease is characterized by periods of symptom exacerbation and remission. Only 1% of children with well-documented Crohn's disease will have no relapses after diagnosis and initial therapy. Many children with Crohn's disease also suffer from medication- and central venous catheter–related complications. In the long term, impaired height velocity is common. Approximately 8% of patients with severe Crohn's disease develop colorectal cancer. Death from Crohn's disease in childhood is rare; however, the risk of death is 1.5 times higher in affected adults compared with age-matched controls.

VII. References

1. Hyams JS. Inflammatory bowel disease. *Pediatr Rev* 2000;21:291–295.
2. Hyams JS. Extraintestinal manifestations of inflammatory bowel disease in children. *J Pediatr Gastroenterol Nutr* 1994;19:7–21.
3. Hyams JS. Inflammatory bowel disease. In: Altschuler SM, Liacouras CA, eds. *Clinical pediatric gastroenterology.* Philadelphia: Churchill Livingstone, 1998:213–221.
4. Mamula P, Telega GW, Markowitz JE, et al. Inflammatory bowel disease in children 5 years of age and younger. *Am J Gastroenterol* 2002;97:2005–2010.
5. Stephens MC, Shepanski MA, Mamula P, et al. Safety and steroid-sparing experience using infliximab for Crohn's disease at a pediatric inflammatory bowel disease center. *Am J Gastroenterol* 2003;98:104–111.
6. Thomas DW, Sinatra FR. Screening laboratory tests for Crohn's disease. *West J Med* 1989;150:163–164.

Case 5-5: 13-Year-Old Boy

I. History of Present Illness

A 13-year-old African-American boy without significant past medical history presented to the emergency department with a 2-day history of worsening back pain. The pain was located in his upper and lower back, and, although he was uncomfortable in any position, standing upright made his back pain significantly worse. His pain was not relieved with cyclobenzaprine, a muscle relaxant. The patient had no history of trauma and denied weakness, sensory loss, and bowel or bladder dysfunction as well as recent fevers, upper respiratory symptoms, cough, nausea, vomiting, weight loss, and night sweats.

II. Past Medical History

His past medical history was remarkable for one previous episode of back pain 2 years earlier that required use of a wheelchair for 2 weeks. He had received iron supplements for treatment of anemia at that time. Additional details of that episode were not available. He had never been hospitalized and had no surgical problems. He was not sexually active and had no history of cigarette or drug use. Family history was significant for a sister with sickle cell trait.

III. Physical Examination

T 37.7°C; RR 24/min; HR 110 bpm; BP 105/70 mm Hg; Weight 35kg.

The patient was a well-developed, well-nourished male crying in pain. Head, eyes, ears, nose, and throat were normal. There was no lymphadenopathy. There was no thoracic wall tenderness. The heart and lung sounds were normal. His abdomen was soft and nontender without hepatomegaly or splenomegaly. He had no point tenderness of his back; however, he complained of "inside pain" over his sacrum. The rectal examination revealed normal sphincter tone and no palpable masses. His extremities were warm with good peripheral pulses, and he had full range of motion of all four extremities.

IV. Diagnostic Studies

Complete blood count revealed 8,400 WBCs/mm³ (81% segmented neutrophils, 17% lymphocytes, 2% basophils, 1% eosinophils, and no bands); hemoglobin, 10.4 g/dL; MCV, 72fL; mean corpuscular hemoglobin content (MCHC), 23.4 g/dL; red cell distribution width (RDW), 15.1; platelets 241,000/mm³; and a reticulocyte count of 3%. Blood smear showed anisocytosis, poikilocytosis, and polychromasia. Electrolytes, blood urea nitrogen, creatinine, and glucose were normal. ESR was 20 mm/hour. Urinalysis revealed small amounts of urobilinogen.

V. Course of Illness

The patient was treated with morphine and ketorolac without much relief. He became febrile to 38.7°C, and blood and urine cultures were obtained. The pain became localized to his sacral/coccygeal region; however, he had no numbness or tingling, and his reflexes remained normal. Abdominal radiography did not reveal bowel obstruction; however, it suggested a likely underlying condition (Fig. 5-6) that was later confirmed by specific testing. An MRI of the lumbosacral spine was negative for an abscess or a locally infiltrative process.

DISCUSSION: CASE 5-5

I. Differential Diagnosis

Back pain is less common in children than in adults, but in children is more often the result of a serious underlying pathology. In adolescents, traumatic or overuse injuries such

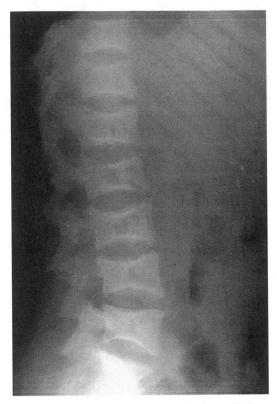

FIG. 5-6. Abdominal radiograph (case 5-5).

as compression fractures, musculoskeletal strain, spondylolysis, spondylolisthesis, and lumbar disc herniation should be considered. Most of these injuries manifest during the adolescent growth spurt and are associated with repeated lifting and back extension, especially in sports. Infections of the vertebral column that cause back pain include osteomyelitis and diskitis especially in toddlers and young children. Less common but serious causes include spinal epidural, paraspinal, or psoas abscess; transverse myelitis; and pyomyositis. Urinary tract infections and pneumonia can cause back pain but are less likely in the absence of urinary or respiratory symptoms. Neoplastic diseases such as leukemia and lymphoma should be considered, especially in the presence of progressive, indolent pain. Malignancies are usually accompanied by constitutional symptoms including weight loss, fatigue, fever, and loss of appetite. Rare causes of back pain include spinal hematoma, spinal tuberculosis (Pott's disease), and brucellosis, a zoonotic infection transmitted from animals to humans that causes flu-like symptoms including back pain. Back pain secondary to acute bone infarction often occurs in adolescents with SCD. Patients usually have normal or mildly elevated temperature and ESR. However, in some cases this condition is indistinguishable from acute osteomyelitis. SCD should be included in the differential diagnosis of an African-American child with back pain, anemia, and a family history of sickle cell trait. In this case, the acute fall in the patient's hemoglobin level, splenomegaly, vertebral abnormalities, and the persistence and severity of the symptoms prompted further evaluation, which led to the diagnosis. Although most patients are diagnosed by newborn screening tests, some patients may inadvertently not be screened or may be lost to follow-up.

II. Diagnosis

Biconcave vertebral depressions, known as the "fish-mouth" deformity, suggested the diagnosis of SCD (see Fig. 5-6), a group of conditions characterized by the presence of hemoglobin S (HbS) in the absence of normal hemoglobin A (HbA) or in a quantity greater than that of HbA. Hemoglobin electrophoresis confirmed the diagnosis of sickle–beta[+]-thalassemia (Sbeta[+]): HbA (18.4%), HbS (63%), HbF (8.1%), HbA2 (7.7%). Sbeta[+], a less severe form of SCD, results from inheritance of the sickle hemoglobin (HbS) and beta[+] thalassemia genes. In Sbeta[+], some normal beta chains are produced, and therefore some HbA is present. A similar hemoglobin profile may be seen in homozygous (HbSS) disease after transfusion; however, in this case, the patient never received a RBC transfusion. **The diagnosis was a vaso-occlusive event secondary to underlying Sbeta[+] thalassemia.** In retrospect, the anemia diagnosed during his previous episode of back pain was probably caused by SCD rather than isolated iron deficiency anemia.

III. Incidence and Epidemiology of Sickle Cell–Beta[+] Thalassemia

SCD is an autosomal recessive genetic disorder that is characterized by the presence of HbS in RBCs. The most common forms of SCD are homozygous SCD (HbSS), sickle cell–hemoglobin C disease (HbSC), and two types of sickle cell–beta-thalassemia, Sbeta[+] and Sbeta[0] (Table 5-4). Individuals who inherit the genes for both HbA and HbS have sickle cell trait, a generally benign and asymptomatic carrier state.

HbS results from an inherited abnormality of hemoglobin function caused by substitution of valine for glutamine at the sixth position of the beta-globin gene. Deoxygenated HbS polymerizes, distorting the shape of the RBC. RBC distortion leads to hemolysis and vaso-occlusion, the two dominant features of sickle cell disease. Beta-thalassemia is caused by single point mutations that result in decreased (beta[+]) or absent (beta[0]) synthesis of beta-globin. This commonly results in microcytic and hypochromic anemia.

The occurrence of sickle cell–beta-thalassemia is determined by the distribution and prevalence of two abnormal genes. The HbS gene occurs in high frequency among populations in equatorial Africa, the Mediterranean area, the Middle East, and India—populations that were exposed during evolution to selection pressure from falciparum malaria. The distribution of beta-thalassemia tends to be sporadic, with high frequencies in the Mediterranean and in southeast Asia. The combination of beta-thalassemia with the sickle mutation results in the combined heterozygous condition known as sickle cell–beta-thalassemia. The clinical problems are quite variable depending on the amount of HbA produced. Sbeta[0] produces no normal beta-chains and therefore no HbA. Sbeta[0] resembles HbSS electrophoretically, hematologically, and clinically. In contrast, the spectrum of severity in Sbeta[+] varies, ranging from very little HbA production to near-normal amounts, depending on the particular beta-thalassemia mutation.

IV. Clinical Presentation

Universal screening for SCD has been widely available in most states in the United States since 1986, and most children with SCD are diagnosed as newborns. A few infants,

TABLE 5-4. *Genotypes of the Most Common Types of Sickle Cell Disease in the United States*

Genotype	Full name	Frequency (%)
betaS/betaS	Homozygous sickle cell disease (SS)	65
betaS/betaC	Sickle cell–hemoglobin C disease (SC)	25
betaS/beta[0]	Sickle cell–sbeta[0] thalassemia disease (Sbeta[0])	3
betaS/beta[+]	Sickle cell–sbeta[+] thalassemia disease (Sbeta[+])	7

even in states with universal screening, may not be screened; in others, the diagnosis may be missed because of extreme prematurity, blood transfusions before screening, or inadequate follow-up after discharge. In some patients with Sbeta$^+$, the levels of HbA are high enough to impair polymerization of HbS and reduce intravascular sickling of the RBCs. The early clinical course in these patients is mild, with significant symptoms appearing later in life.

Acute and chronic complications of SCD involve multiple organ systems (Table 5-5). Bones and joints are major sites of pain in vaso-occlusive events. Acute bone pain is caused by marrow ischemia, which results in necrosis and inflammation. Pain is widespread and migratory during the acute painful crisis. Local tenderness, warmth, swelling, and impaired motion occur with a severe pain episode as the generalized pain improves. As seen in this patient, vertebral infarction may lead to collapse of the end-plates, known as "fish-mouth" vertebrae. No single clinical feature can reliably distinguish osteomyelitis from bone infarction. Acute painful events are the most common cause of emergency department visits and hospitalizations among patients with SCD. These events may be precipitated by weather extremes or temperature changes, dehydration, infection, stress, or menstruation; however, the majority of painful events have no identifiable trigger. Painful episodes vary from mild to debilitating. Pain is usually self-limited, lasting from a few hours to a few days, although inadequate treatment may prolong the episode for weeks.

V.   Diagnostic Approach

Hemoglobin electrophoresis. This is the most popular method used in clinical laboratories to determine hemoglobin phenotype.

Complete blood count with differential. At baseline in patients with Sbeta$^+$, the hemoglobin values, reticulocyte count, and WBC count are near-normal, with the major difference being modestly low MCV and MCHC values. This is in contrast to HbSS disease, in which the steady-state WBC and reticulocyte counts are higher than in an unaf-

TABLE 5-5. *Important Clinical Complications of Sickle Cell Disease during Childhood and Adolescence*

Type	Complication
Acute	Bacterial sepsis or meningitis
	Vaso-occlusive pain (musculoskeletal pain or abdominal pain, dactylitis)
	Splenic sequestration
	Aplastic crisis
	Acute chest syndrome
	Stroke
	Priapism
	Hematuria, papillary necrosis
Chronic	Anemia
	Jaundice
	Splenomegaly
	Functional asplenia
	Cardiomegaly and functional murmurs
	Proteinuria
	Cholelithiasis
	Delayed growth and sexual maturity
	Restrictive lung disease
	Pulmonary hypertension
	Avascular necrosis
	Proliferative retinopathy
	Leg ulcers
	Hyposthenuria and enuresis

fected person. The WBC count is often elevated with both bone infarcts and infection; however, a shift in the differential toward neutrophil predominance is more likely with osteomyelitis than with infarction.

Peripheral blood smear. Microcytosis, hypochromia, anisocytosis, and poikilocytosis characterize Sbeta$^+$. Sickled cells are not always seen, especially if high levels of non-S hemoglobin are present, making the diagnosis less obvious in some cases.

Blood Cultures. Blood cultures should be obtained before antibiotics are administered. Blood cultures are negative in bone infarction and frequently are positive in osteomyelitis.

Sequential radionuclide bone marrow and bone scan. Diminished radionuclide uptake on the bone marrow scan, indicative of decreased blood flow in the bone marrow, and abnormal uptake on the bone scan at the site of pain are seen with bone infarction. In contrast, acute osteomyelitis results in normal activity on bone marrow scans and increased activity on bone scans.

Plain radiography. This is useful in monitoring the progression of established changes of infection, infarction, and osteomyelitis but not in diagnosing acute infections or infarctions. In older children and adolescents, plain radiographs may show deossification due to marrow hyperplasia and flattened, widened vertebral bodies with biconcave depressions of the end-plates, known as "H-shaped" or "fish-mouth" vertebrae.

VI. Treatment

Severe bone pain should be considered a medical emergency that prompts timely and aggressive management until the pain decreases to a tolerable level. Major barriers to effective management of pain are inadequate assessment of pain and biases against opioid use. Most of the time, these biases are based on clinician uncertainty regarding opioid tolerance and physical dependence, and confusion with addiction.

As previously mentioned, bone infarction resembles osteomyelitis. Fever in cases of bone infarction is due to necrosis and inflammation associated with marrow ischemia. Blood cultures must be obtained if empiric antibiotics are initiated. Appropriate antibiotics should cover *Salmonella* spp. and *S. aureus*, the most common causes of osteomyelitis in children with SCD.

Patients with signs of moderate to severe dehydration should receive 10 to 20 mL/kg of intravenous normal saline, followed by intravenous fluid at or slightly above (1.0 to 1.5 times) the daily fluid requirement. It is important to assess the severity of pain at presentation and at frequent intervals, using age-appropriate pain-measuring scales. Pain should be reevaluated every 15 minutes until pain starts to decrease, then every 30 to 60 minutes as needed. Severe acute pain requires intravenous medication such as morphine sulfate, hydrocodone, or fentanyl, with or without NSAIDs such as ketorolac and ibuprofen. Patient-controlled analgesia (PCA) devices restore patient control over pain and may be used for patients in severe pain. PCA pumps provide analgesic medication continuously at a low baseline rate and allow patients to self-administer an additional dose of opioid whenever they feel a need for more pain relief. Continuous epidural analgesia has been used in patients with pain below the 4th thoracic dermatome for whom intravenous PCA opioids and nonopioid analgesics have failed; however, not much information is available about its use in patients with SCD.

Patient and parental preferences for pain medication should be considered, because individual variations in drug metabolism determine the dose-response to analgesia. The use of parental meperidine should be avoided because of CNS toxicity related to its metabolite normeperidine. Patients receiving opioids for longer than 1 or 2 weeks should be weaned slowly over several days to prevent withdrawal symptoms.

Side effects of opioids, including respiratory depression and sedation, should be monitored closely. Antiemetics such as Compazine (prochlorperazine) or metachlorpropamide effectively treat symptoms of opioid-related nausea. Stool softeners to prevent constipation should be taken daily if patients continue to take opioids for longer than a few days.

VII.   References

1. Benjamin LJ, Dampier CD, Jacox AK, et al. *Guidelines for the management of acute and chronic pain in sickle-cell disease.* APS Clinical Practice Guidelines Series, No. 1. Glenview, IL: American Pain Society, 1999.
2. Embury SH, Hebbel RP, Mohandas N, et al., eds. *Sickle cell disease: basic principles and clinical practice.* New York: Raven, 1994
3. Lane PA. Sickle cell disease. *Pediatr Clin North Am* 1996;43:639–664.
4. Serjeant GR, Sergeant BE. *Sickle cell disease,* 2nd ed. Oxford, England: Oxford University Press, 2001.
5. Yaster M, Kost-Byerly S, Maxwell LG. The management of pain in sickle cell disease. *Pediatr Clin North Am* 2000;47:699–710.

Case 5-6: 9-Year-Old Boy

I. History of Present Illness

In the winter of his 9th year of life, a very active young boy presented to his pediatrician with left ankle pain of approximately 5 days' duration. The boy's mother reported that her son had complained of various muscle injuries over the previous month. Three weeks earlier, he began limping, and explained that he had hurt his right hip playing basketball. After a few days of "taking it easy," he reported complete resolution. Shortly thereafter, he complained of left elbow pain, and his mother speculated that the injury occurred while the boy was wrestling with his older brother. He received ibuprofen, and after a few days of treatment he was able to play video games without discomfort. In the last few days, the mother had observed the boy limping again, but he denied any problems until the coach of his indoor soccer team sat him out for the first time all season. The boy confessed that his left ankle had been hurting him, but he had not wanted to miss any games. The coach had called the boy's mother and told her that her son would not be allowed back to practice until he had been checked by a doctor. The boy described the hip and elbow symptoms as vague pains that worsened with movement of the specific limbs. He denied swelling or redness of the elbow or hip when they were bothering him but thought that his ankle was "little puffy" now.

The mother reported that he has felt warm on occasion and had not been eating well. She believed that he had lost weight, and she had found his sheets damp on a few mornings after she had awakened him for school. The boy denied headache, rash, sore throat, nausea, vomiting, diarrhea, palpitations, or fatigue and asked if he could still make it to a practice scheduled for later that day.

II. Past Medical History

The patient had received all required immunizations, and, aside from a broken nose sustained from a batted softball 3 years earlier, he had no significant past medical history. He did not require any regularly scheduled medications. He had no known medication allergies.

His family history was significant for a mother and maternal grandmother with migraine headaches and trisomy 21 in his youngest brother. There is no family history of arthritis or malignancy. His recent travel had consisted of 2 weeks at the New Jersey shore over the summer and 1 month of "sleep-away" camp in northeastern Pennsylvania.

III. Physical Examination

T, 38.6°C; RR, 18/min; HR, 112 bpm; BP, 112/60 mm Hg

Weight, 60th percentile (down 3 kg from his preparticipation physical examination 4 months earlier); height, 75th percentile (up by 1.0 cm from the earlier measurements)

The patient was a cooperative boy in no acute distress. He was slender, and his clothes hung loosely from his frame. Eyes, nose, ears, and oropharynx were not inflamed. His tonsils were 3+ and symmetric without erythema or exudates. His neck was supple with only shotty anterior cervical adenopathy. His thyroid was not enlarged. His lungs were clear with good aeration. His heart had a regular rhythm but was tachycardic, with a soft systolic murmur at the apex that was audible throughout systole. His abdomen was soft, nontender, nondistended, and without hepatosplenomegaly. The left ankle demonstrated a small effusion with increased warmth and mild erythema. There was exquisite pain with active and passive range of motion and with gentle palpation of the joint. All other joints were normal on examination.

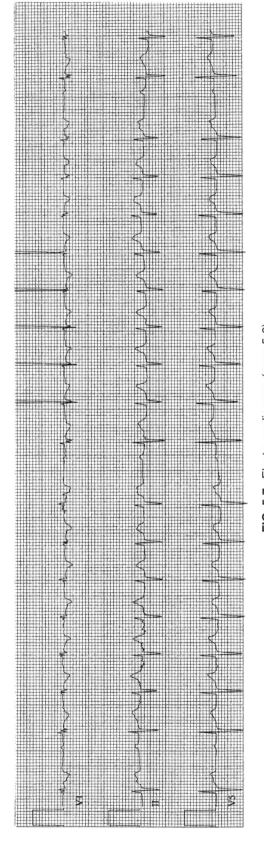

FIG. 5-7. Electrocardiogram (case 5-6).

IV.   Diagnostic Studies

A complete blood count revealed 12,200 WBCs/mm^3 (74% neutrophils, 20% lympho-cytes, 5% monocytes, and 1% eosinophils); hemoglobin, 9.5 g/dL; and a platelet count of 556,000/mm^3. A basic metabolic panel was normal, but inflammatory markers were elevated, with an ESR of 120 mm/hour and a CRP concentration of 8.3 mg/dL. A rapid streptococcal test and culture of his throat were both negative. Radiographs of both ankles were obtained and were normal.

V.   Course of Illness

The patient was treated with doxycycline for presumed Lyme arthritis. He also received regularly scheduled naproxen, with good symptomatic relief of his joint pain. Several days later, the Lyme antibody titers by Western blot were found to be negative. An electrocardiogram (ECG) suggested another possible etiology (Fig. 5-7). Additional testing confirmed the diagnosis that mandated definitive ongoing treatment.

DISCUSSION: CASE 5-6

I.   Differential Diagnosis

This previously healthy young man presented with a 1-month history of joint pains, with true arthritis of the ankle demonstrated at the office visit. The arthritis involved relatively large joints affected in a nonsimultaneous sequence. This pattern is referred to as a migra-tory pattern, one in which new joint inflammation occurs after previous joint inflammation resolves. The fever, weight loss, elevated inflammatory markers, and mild anemia were also noteworthy and suggested an infectious, rheumatologic, or malignant process.

Joint or extremity pain, with fever and weight loss, can certainly raise the suspicion of a malignancy. True arthritis (joint effusion, calor, rubor, and pain with range of motion) is not a typical presentation of musculoskeletal tumors but may be part of a paraneoplas-tic syndrome with reactive arthritis. Disseminated malignancies, such as neuroblastoma or leukemia, may also involve joints or the skeletal system through direct bony destruc-tion in close proximity to a joint. Abnormalities may or may not be detected by plain radi-ographs of the involved limb.

Infectious etiologies of arthritis include primary infection of a joint space or infection of bone or soft tissue in close proximity to a joint, with or without direct communication of the infection with the joint. These infections are more likely to involve a single site, but multifocal infections may be seen, with ongoing or intermittent bacteremia leading to multiple, hematogenously seeded sites. If more than one joint is involved, postinfectious arthritis should be considered. These inflammatory joint reactions are sequelae of pre-ceding infections and are usually considered to be sterile and mediated through an immune response. Epstein-Barr virus and parvovirus B19 are among the common viral agents associated with this reaction, and meningococcus is a notorious bacterial cause. Arthritis characterizes late-stage Lyme disease and develops 6 to 12 weeks after the bite of an infected tick. Large joints, especially the knees, are involved and recurrence of arthritis mimics a migratory pattern. Each bout of arthritis lasts 1 to 2 weeks but may become prolonged if left untreated. The involved joint often appears remarkably swollen, with little or no erythema, and ambulation is often maintained despite impressive effu-sion in the involved lower-extremity joint. Carditis, presenting as heart block, can also complicate the picture, but it is more common in the early disseminated stage of the dis-ease, which occurs a few weeks to months after infection.

The involvement of multiple joints and stigmata of acute inflammation make rheuma-tologic conditions an important consideration. Systemic-onset juvenile rheumatoid arthritis can manifest initially with or without arthritis, but chronic arthritis of at least 6 weeks duration is required for diagnosis. Systemic lupus erythematosus (SLE) most often manifests with joint involvement with constitutional complaints of fatigue, weight loss, fever, and a typical rash, and there is almost always an elevation in the antinuclear antibody (ANA) titer. Progressive muscle weakness is characteristic of dermatomyositis; patients may present with extremity complaints, and infrequently with true arthritis. Back pain eventually develops in ankylosing spondylitis, which is much more common in boys than in girls and is associated with the human leukocyte antigen HLA-B27 in 90% of cases.

Mixed connective tissue diseases can have overlapping features of many of these conditions, but the arthritis often involves small joints. Vasculitis syndromes may also cause arthritis, with HSP being the most common vasculitis of children. The characteristic palpable petechial or purpuric rash, especially evident on the lower extremities, in the absence of thrombocytopenia, is key in the diagnosis of this immunoglobulin A–mediated vasculitis. Other inflammatory conditions, including Crohn's disease, ulcerative colitis, Reiter syndrome, Behçet's disease, and Sjögren syndrome, may also result in arthritis, constitutional symptoms, and elevated ESR, but other features of the illnesses are usually present or eventually manifest themselves.

II. Diagnosis

The ECG revealed a ventricular rate of 110 bpm, sinus arrhythmia, first-degree atrioventricular block (P-R interval, 0.2 seconds), and a Mobitz II atrioventricular block (occasional atrial beats not conducted to the ventricle) (see Fig. 5-7). Echocardiography revealed mild aortic insufficiency and moderate mitral regurgitation. The ANA titer was less than 1:40. The anti-streptolysin O (ASO) and anti-DNase B titers were positive at 1:1955 and 1:680, respectively. The negative Lyme serology and the elevated titers to streptococcal antigens made acute rheumatic fever (ARF) an important diagnostic consideration in this case.

The Jones criteria are used to make the diagnosis of ARF (Table 5-6). The presence of two major criteria, or one major plus two minor criteria, along with evidence of preceding group A β-hemolytic streptococcal (GABHS) infection make the diagnosis of ARF highly probable. This young boy demonstrated several features of ARF, including ausculatory evidence of valvular heart disease, a migratory polyarthritis (two major criteria) and fever, prolongation of the PR-interval on ECG, and elevated ESR and CRP (three minor criteria). Echocardiography revealed mild aortic valvular insufficiency and moderate mitral valve regurgitation with thickening of the mitral valve.

Response to aspirin and other NSAIDs is typical and is perhaps a diagnostic clue. Children given aspirin for the arthritis of ARF have responded so well as to go from bed-rid-

TABLE 5-6. *The Jones Criteria for Diagnosis of an Initial Attack of Rheumatic Fever[a]*

Major criteria	Minor criteria
Carditis	Fever
Arthritis	Arthralgia
Erythema marginatum	Elevated acute phase reactants (erythrocyte sedimentation rate, C-reactive protein)
Chorea	Prolonged PR-interval on electrocardiogram
Subcutaneous nodules	

[a]The presence of two major criteria (or one major plus two minor criteria), plus evidence of a preceding group A β-hemolytic streptococcal infection by culture, rapid antigen, or antistreptococcal antibody titers, makes the diagnosis of acute rheumatic fever highly probable.

den to running down the halls within hours after the first dose. Current liberal use of ibuprofen for fever or analgesia may obscure the classic migratory pattern of arthritis in ARF due to the symptomatic relief this agent may provide.

III. Incidence and Epidemiology

Although ARF was common in the United States until the 1960s, its incidence decreased in the 1970s in developed nations. Regional outbreaks occurred throughout the United States in the 1980s and 1990s, and this resurgence may be related to the increased prevalence of strains of GABHS that are thought to be more "rheumatogenic." Populations at greatest risk for ARF mirror the populations with increased incidence of GABHS pharyngitis: children age 5 to 15 years, and older individuals living in close quarters (e.g., military recruits). In developing countries and in the United States before 1970, poorer socioeconomic communities had higher rates of GABHS pharyngitis and ARF. However, over the last two decades of the 20th century, outbreaks of ARF in the United States have occurred predominantly in suburban and rural middle-class communities and among military recruits.

IV. Clinical Presentation

Acute rheumatic fever is a nonsuppurative sequela of GABHS pharyngitis. The symptoms begin approximately 1 to 3 weeks after the throat infection, but in many cases a sore throat is not reported, even in retrospect. GABHS infections that do not include pharyngitis are not initiators of ARF.

Approximately 80% of patients present with arthritis, and it typically is a migratory polyarthritis with predilection for large joints. In contrast to Lyme arthritis, the subjective pain of ARF arthritis often is much more severe than the objective findings visible to the examiner. Analysis of fluid from an acutely inflamed joint reveals an elevated WBC count in the range of 20,000 to 40,000 cells/mm^3 with a neutrophil predominance.

Carditis can involve any part of the heart but most typically is an endocardial process with particular affinity for the mitral and aortic valves. Acutely the valves demonstrate insufficiency, but the lesions progress to stenosis over time. Involvement of the myocardium can be seen especially with the more severe presentations of congestive heart failure. Pericarditis and epicarditis can also complicate the picture, but they rarely occur in isolation. Carditis develops in approximately half of patients, but it has been reported in up to 80% of patients in the more recent U. S. outbreaks. Clinical signs accepted for evidence of carditis include appropriate murmurs, cardiomegaly, congestive heart failure, or pericardial friction rub. The most recent update of the Jones criteria (1992) did not consider echocardiographic evidence of valvulitis without auscultatory findings to be sufficient to establish the presence of carditis for ARF.

Erythema marginatum and subcutaneous nodules are seen infrequently. When erythema marginatum is fully developed, it has an indistinct serpiginous red border with central clearing and is nonpruritic. It is specific for ARF, but its usefulness is limited by the fact that the rash is evanescent and is present in fewer than 10% of patients. Subcutaneous nodules are usually a late finding of ARF and may correlate with more severe or prolonged carditis. The lesions are pea-sized and nontender, and they tend to be located over extensor tendons at the elbows, knees, or Achilles.

Sydenham's chorea is a late manifestation of ARF; it can manifest after resolution of the other features, or in isolation if the other features were never clinically apparent. This movement disorder may start with subtle deteriorations of handwriting before evolving into the involuntary, uncontrollable, and purposeless choreiform movements. Due to the late onset of this feature, the presence of Sydenham's alone can be considered diagnostic of ARF if other causes of chorea have been excluded.

Some of the minor criteria for ARF in some ways overlap with major criteria. Arthralgias, painful joints without objective findings of arthritis, should be considered only if arthritis is not used as a major criterion. However, PR prolongation by ECG can be considered in addition to ausculatory evidence of carditis. The ESR and CRP are significantly elevated with the acute illness, with the ESR usually greater than 50 mm/hour and often approaching or exceeding 100 mm/hour. The fever has no characteristic pattern; it usually resolves within 3 weeks, even without treatment.

V.   Diagnostic Approach

Establishing the diagnosis of ARF involves assessing for the presence of major and minor criteria, documenting a preceding GABHS infection, and excluding disorders that mimic ARF. The four major criteria were discussed in the preceding section. The minor criteria include clinical assessment (fever, arthralgias), laboratory assessment (ESR, CRP), and evidence of atrioventricular conduction delay by ECG (PR-interval prolongation). Evidence of preceding GABHS infection can be obtained by any of the following:

1. Throat swab yielding a positive antigen (rapid test) or culture for GABHS at the time of presentation or documented in the preceding weeks. Most patients do not demonstrate a positive throat swab when presenting with ARF, having cleared the infection during the latent period. Furthermore, a positive throat swab at the time of ARF presentation my represent colonization, which does not necessarily indicate a preceding GABHS pharyngitis.

2. History of scarlet fever in the preceding weeks. Scarlet fever does not occur during the presentation of ARF, but it is sufficiently specific for GABHS infection that it can serve as evidence of a preceding infection.

3. Elevated serum GABHS antibodies (ASO, anti-DNAase B, anti-hyaluronidase, anti-streptokinase). A commercial agglutination assay that tests for several streptococcal antigens is rapid and widely available, but it is less standardized and less reproducible than quantitative titers of specific antibodies. Quantitative ASO is positive in 80% of patients with ARF; when three antibodies are tested quantitatively, at least one will be elevated in 95% of ARF patients.

Other clinical findings of ARF are less specific but are often part of the clinical picture (Table 5-7).

If joint pain is the salient complaint, the differential diagnosis for ARF includes septic arthritis, juvenile rheumatoid arthritis, SLE, Lyme disease, postinfectious reactive arthritis, serum sickness, and malignancies. If carditis is the main manifestation, infective endocarditis and viral myocarditis/pericarditis should be considered.

VI.   Treatment

There are three distinct aspects to the treatment of ARF: eradication of the GABHS, secondary prophylaxis, and treatment of the ARF manifestations.

At the time of ARF diagnosis, patients require treatment for acute streptococcal pharyngitis regardless of the results of a throat culture or rapid antigen test. The treatment

TABLE 5-7. *Clinical Features Associated with Acute Rheumatic Fever*

Symptoms	Signs	Laboratory test findings
Fatigue, malaise Abdominal pain Epistaxis Palpitations	Pallor Tachycardia out of proportion to fever	Anemia Thrombocytosis

is not thought to alter the course of the active ARF illness, but it removes the inciting agent. After completion of this therapeutic regimen, secondary prophylaxis is begun.

Recurrence of ARF from a subsequent GABHS infection is a well-recognized phenomenon, and the degree of cardiac involvement increases with each episode of ARF. Both asymptomatic and symptomatic GABHS throat infections can cause recurrences of ARF, so prevention of these infections is vital. For this reason, continuous antibiotic prophylaxis is necessary for all patients with ARF. The American Heart Association has provided guidelines regarding choice of antibiotic, route and schedule of administration, and duration of prophylaxis. The risk for recurrence is greatest within the first 5 years after the initial attack, but in some cases lifelong prophylaxis is indicated.

After ARF, patients with valvular heart disease, require protection against infective endocarditis in addition to their ongoing secondary prophylaxis. A short course of additional antibiotics is required to protect the valves during certain procedures, such as dental procedures, cystoscopy, and intestinal surgery.

Antiinflammatory medications such as aspirin are effective treatment for the carditis and arthritis symptoms of ARF. Corticosteroids are reserved for the treatment of more severe carditis, where their use may more promptly suppress the inflammation, which may be critical in patients with life-threatening cardiac symptoms. Aspirin is highly effective for symptomatic treatment of the arthritis of ARF, and failure to respond to this therapy should bring the diagnosis of ARF into question. Congestive heart failure is managed with diuretics and inotropic support as indicated by the severity of the symptoms.

VII.   References

1. Special Writing Group of the Committee on Rheumatic Fever, Endocarditis, and Kawasaki Disease of the Council on Cardiovascular Disease in the Young of the American Heart Association. Guidelines for the diagnosis of rheumatic fever: Jones criteria, 1992 update. *JAMA* 1992;268:2069–2073.
2. Behrman RE, Kliegman RM, Jensen HB. *Nelson's textbook of pediatrics,* 16th ed. Philadelphia: WB Saunders, 2000.
3. Ruddy S, Harris ED, Sledge CB. *Kelley's textbook of rheumatology,* 6th ed. Philadelphia: WB Saunders, 2001.
4. Homer C, Shulman ST. Clinical aspects of acute rheumatic fever. *J Rheumatol* 1991; 18[Suppl 29]:2–13.

6

Poor Weight Gain

Stephen Ludwig

APPROACH TO THE PATIENT WITH POOR WEIGIIT GAIN

I. Definition of the Complaint

Poor weight gain, growth failure, and failure to thrive (FTT) are complaints that involve a vast array of potential causes. At the root of the problem there may be (a) failure to ingest an appropriate number of calories, (b) failure to metabolize the ingested food, (c) abnormal loss of calories, or (d) abnormal need for calories. Whatever the cause, a child's weight is a sensitive barometer of his or her health. In the case of weight gain, health must be defined broadly and includes family and psychosocial causes as well as consideration of disease states. Homer and Ludwig, in a review of FTT cases, found three broad etiologies: organic, nonorganic, and mixed.

Organic causes involve a physical condition or disease that leads to failure to gain weight. Nonorganic causes involve a breakdown in the relationship between parent and child and the feeding process. Mixed FTT is a condition in which the child has some organic problem (e.g., gastroesophageal reflux), which, in the context of the child's family, becomes a major obstacle to growth, although perhaps another family would have the capability to manage it. Another scenario for mixed FTT is a family whose ability to raise a child is marginal, in which the child's illness brings them into a dysfunctional state.

Many cases of growth failure are diagnostically solved without the need for hospitalization. But in some cases, either because the growth delay is so marked or because the child is at a vulnerable age, hospitalization is required. At times the indication for hospitalization (Table 6-1) is a complex or obscure problem that requires a more intensive diagnostic evaluation.

II. Complaint by Cause and Frequency

Growth failure is not a diagnosis on its own. It is a symptom whose root cause must be discovered in order to apply the correct therapies, whether they are medical, psychosocial, or a combination.

III. Clarifying Questions

* What is the child's pattern of growth over time?

TABLE 6-1. *Indications for Hospitalization of Children with Failure to Thrive*

Infant younger than 6 months of age
Below birth weight at 6 weeks
Head circumference falling below normal growth curve before 6 months of age
Signs of abuse
Signs of gross physical neglect
Failure at outpatient therapy
Organic diagnosis being pursued
Home unsafe
Caretaker deemed inadequate

TABLE 6-2. *Causes of Inadequate Weight Gain*

Inadequate intake
  Lack of appetite
    Chronic disease (e.g., central nervous system pathology, gastrointestinal disorders, chronic
      infections)
    Anemia (e.g., iron deficiency)
    Psychosocial problems (e.g., apathy)
  Difficulty with ingestion
    Feeding disorder
    Psychosocial problems (e.g., apathy, rumination)
    Neurologic disorders (e.g., cerebral palsy, hypertonia, hypotonia, generalized muscle
      weakness/pathology)
    Craniofacial anomalies (e.g., choanal atresia, cleft lip and palate, micrognathia)
    Dyspnea (e.g., congenital heart disease, pulmonary diseases)
    Generalized muscle weakness/pathology (e.g., myopathies)
    Tracheoesophageal fistula
    Genetic syndromes
    Congenital syndromes (e.g., fetal alcohol syndrome)
  Unavailability of food
    Inappropriate feeding technique
    Insufficient/inadequate volume of food
    Inappropriate food for age
    Withholding of food (abuse, neglect)
Altered growth potential regulation
  Prenatal insult
  Chromosomal abnormality/genetic syndrome
  Endocrinopathies
Calorie wasting
  Vomiting
    Central nervous system pathology (increased intracranial pressure)
    Intestinal tract obstruction (e.g., pyloric stenosis, malrotation)
    Gastrointestinal reflux
    Metabolic problems
    Drugs/toxins
  Malabsorption
    Primary gastrointestinal diseases: biliary atresia/cirrhosis, celiac disease
    Inflammatory bowel disease, enzymatic deficiencies, food (protein) sensitivity/intolerance,
      Hirschsprung's disease
    Cystic fibrosis
  Renal losses
    Diabetes
    Renal tubular acidosis
Increased caloric requirements
  Increased metabolism/increased use of calories
    Congenital/acquired heart disease
    Chronic respiratory disease (e.g., bronchopulmonary dysplasia)
    Neoplasms
    Chronic/recurrent infection
    Endocrinopathies (e.g., hyperthyroidism, hyperaldosteronism)
    Chronic anemia
    Drugs/toxins (e.g., lead, levothyroxine)
  Defective use of calories
    Metabolic disorders (e.g., aminoacidopathies, inborn errors of carbohydrate metabolism)
    Renal tubular acidosis

Adapted from Zenel JA: Failure to thrive: a general pediatrician's perspective. *Pediatr Rev* 1997;18:
371–378.

— This question seeks to establish a timing issue. Has this condition existed for weeks or months? Review of the child's growth chart created over time is helpful. This information often resides with the primary care physician.

• What aspects of growth have been affected?

— A comparison of the measurements of weight, length, and head circumference may provide clues to the etiology. With an acquired condition, the weight is affected first and most, the length next, and finally the head circumference. If the condition is congenital, genetic, or endocrinologic, the growth failure may be more symmetric, or there may be a recognizable pattern of growth failure.

• Has the child demonstrated any symptoms?

— Are there symptoms of vomiting or diarrhea, indicating loss of nutritional intake? Are there symptoms of cardiac or pulmonary disease, indicating an increased requirement for calories or an increased metabolic rate? The history is much more important than laboratory screening tests in determining the cause of growth failure.

• What has the child's diet and eating pattern been?

— There is a developmental sequence to the kind of foods given to a child and the way they are presented. For example, toward the end of the first year, children typically want to eat some table foods and to manipulate the foods into their own mouths. A parent who insists in giving strained foods by parenteral spoon-feeding at this stage may find their child resistant and therefore failing to gain weight. It may be instructive to watch a feeding encounter or mealtime to get a sense of the process. Meal-

TABLE 6-3. *Classification of Nonorganic Causes of Failure to Thrive*

Lack of education/preparation for parenting
    Missing information
    Lack of experience
Lack of family resources
    Food
    Money
    Housing
    Health care
    Alternate caretakers
Parental dysfunction
    Postpartum depression
    Parental substance abuse
    Parental psychosis
    "Apathy futility" syndrome (Polansky)
Difficult infant
    Temperamental differences
    Feeding difficulties
    Minor organic disorder
Parent-child interaction problems
    Bonding failure
    Vulnerable child
    Unwanted child/pregnancy
    Overinvolvement—enmeshment
Family system dysfunction
    Isolated family
    Marital stress
    Chaotic home

time may be pleasurable for child and parent or an exercise in frustration and stress for both.

• What is the state of the family unit and their lifestyle?

— This question gets at the many psychosocial causes of growth failure. Is this family functioning in other ways? Are there support systems for the parents? Often it is helpful to ask the parent to review a typical day. Some families have a well-traveled pathway through each day. For other families, each day is a new adventure from beginning to end. Just as there is a differential diagnosis for organic causes of growth failure (Table 6-2), there are a host of nonorganic causes (Table 6-3), including problems relating to the parents (e.g., postpartum depression) and problems with the entire family system (e.g., substance abuse).

IV.   References

1. Miller LA, Grunwald GK, Johnson SL, et al. Disease severity at time of referral for pediatric failure to thrive and obesity: time for a paradigm shift? *J Pediatr* 2002;141: 121–124.
2. Schwartz ID. Failure to thrive: an old nemesis in the new millennium. *Pediatr Rev* 2000;21:257–264.
3. Shah MD. Failure to thrive in children. *J Clin Gastroenterol* 2002;35:371–374.
4. Gordon EF, Vasquez DM. Failure to thrive: an expanded conceptual method. In: Drotar D, ed. *New directions in failure to thrive.* New York: Plenum Press, 1986:69.
5. Homer C, Ludwig S. Categorization of etiology for failure to thrive. *Am J Dis Child* 1981;135:848–851.
6. Bithoney WG, Dubowitz H, Egan H. Failure to thrive/growth deficiency. *Pediatr Rev* 1992;13:453–460.
7. Zenel JA. Failure to thrive: a general pediatrician's perspective. *Pediatr Rev* 1997;18: 371–378.

The following cases represent less common causes of poor weight gain or FTT in children.

Case 6-1: 16-Month-Old Boy

I. History of Present Illness

A 16-month-old African-American boy was seen in an outpatient clinic and admitted because of concern for FTT. He had also been noted by his parents to have lost some of his previously acquired developmental skills. Over the week before admission, he had had tactile fever and two to three loose stools per day. The stools were not bloody. He had no vomiting. He had a slight cough but no rhinitis, rash, or ear pain. From a developmental standpoint, he was always delayed, compared with his twin. He first rolled over at 10 months. He was not walking or sitting. He recently had been noted to be smiling less and interacting less. He had been receiving early intervention services for occupational and physical therapy. It had been recommended to the family that he start nutritional supplements, but the family has not been able to get any.

II. Past Medical History

He was the first born of a twin pregnancy. His birth weight was 5 pounds 10 ounces. He was delivered of a 20-year-old mother by cesarean section for breech presentation. He had been bottle-fed and had had no previous hospitalizations. He had pneumonia at 7 months of age that was treated in the outpatient setting. At 9 months of age, he was treated for thrush that responded promptly to oral nystatin. Otitis media had been recently diagnosed and treated at the clinic.

He had no allergies and was receiving no medication. He had not traveled outside the United States. The only pet was an older cat. One month earlier, the mother was hospitalized with a cerebrovascular accident. In process of evaluation, she was found to be human immunodeficiency virus (HIV)-antibody positive.

III. Physical Examination

T, 37.8°C; RR, 40/min; HR 130 bpm; BP 96/60 mm Hg; RR 40/min SpO$_2$, 100% in room air

Weight, 7.94 kg (less than 5th percentile for an 8-month-old); height, 75.5 cm (10th percentile; 50th percentile for an 11-month-old); head circumference, 47 cm (25th percentile)

In general, the child was apathetic and irritable, but consolable in his mother's arms. Frontal prominence and bitemporal wasting were noted. The tympanic membranes were normal in appearance and mobility. The oropharynx was clear; there was no thrush. Multiple small cervical, occipital, axillary, epitrochlear, and inguinal lymph nodes were palpable. The cardiac examination revealed normal first and second heart sounds (S1 and S2, respectively), with no murmurs, rubs, or gallops. The chest was clear to auscultation bilaterally. The abdomen was soft without tenderness or guarding. The liver edge was palpable 3 cm below the right costal margin, and the spleen was palpable 2 cm below the left costal margin. The child was globally hypotonic, but deep tendon reflexes were symmetrically increased. Plantar reflexes were downgoing.

IV. Diagnostic Studies

A complete blood count revealed the following: 37,900 white blood cels (WBCs)/mm^3, including 8% segmented neutrophils, 47% lymphocytes, and 38% atypical lymphocytes; hemoglobin, 11.0 g/dL; platelet count, 195,000/mm^3. Serum electrolytes, blood urea nitrogen, and creatinine were normal. Additional laboratory findings included the following: lactate dehydrogenase, 1,586 U/L alanine aminotransferase (ALT), 98 IU/L; aspartate aminotransferase (AST), 139 IU/L; alkaline phosphatase, 108 U/L; triglycerides, 212 mg/dL; and albumin, 3.4 mg/dL.

IV. Course of Illness

HIV antibody testing was performed at the time of admission, given the mother's recent diagnosis, and was positive. Initial evaluation focused on determining the child's HIV status (in utero exposure versus true infection), because maternal HIV antibodies may be present for the first 18 months of life. Additional testing by HIV polymerase chain reaction (PCR) was positive, confirming this child's diagnosis of HIV infection.

Given his HIV exposure, there was concern that his developmental regression could be secondary to HIV encephalopathy. A noncontrast computed tomography (CT) scan was done, which showed diffuse cerebral atrophy. Soon after hospitalization, the child began to have high spiking fevers to 40.1°, accompanied by tachycardia and tachypnea. His oxygenation remained adequate. A few days into the fever spikes, he began to have persistent tachypnea, with mild increased work of breathing and occasional rales at the left lower lung field. A chest radiograph showed mild volume loss at the right upper lobe and streaky atelectasis in the left lower and right upper lobes. An abdominal ultrasound study was performed to look for increased retroperitoneal adenopathy, because of the possibility that disseminated *Mycobacterium avium* may have caused his fevers. The ultrasound study showed hepatomegaly with an increase in the echotexture of the liver, without focal masses or abscess. There was no ductal dilatation or gall bladder wall thickening. Splenomegaly was present without focal lesions within the spleen. Also noted were several enlarged nodes within the porta hepatis and several retroperitoneal nodes in the para-aortic area. The kidneys were normal.

DISCUSSION: CASE 6-1

I. Differential Diagnosis

There were many possible diagnoses to consider in this case. In the general categorization of organic versus nonorganic causes of FTT, the symptoms of diarrhea and later fever were factors supporting an organic cause. Yet, the family history of being noncompliant with getting the nutritional supplements and the fact that this was an overstressed family, with an HIV-positive mother and twin babies, raises some nonorganic factors. The possibility of mixed FTT was very high on the list. As far as organic causes, HIV is a well-known cause of FTT. It is sometimes difficult to distinguish between maternally acquired antibodies and true infection. The positive (times 2) PCR result made true HIV infection one diagnosis. The onset of high spiking fevers then prompted the evaluation for an opportunistic infection.

Diagnostic considerations in an HIV-infected child with fever are diverse. Opportunistic diseases and pathogens to consider include *Pneumocystis carinii* pneumonia, lymphoid interstitial pneumonia (LIP), and cryptococcal infection. Viruses include hepatitis B and C, Epstein-Barr virus, and cytomegalovirus. Other pathogens include *M. avium*, cryptosporidium, *Toxoplasma gondii,* and *Mycobacterium tuberculosis.* Children with HIV are also at risk for focal bacterial infections such as sinusitis, pneumonia, or intraabdominal abscess. A child who is HIV positive and who is febrile requires an exhaustive search to identify an organism.

The initial evaluation should include a search for focal infection and a general assessment of severity of illness. The absence of specific localizing signs presents a greater diagnostic dilemma.

II. Diagnosis

Toxoplasma immunoglobulin M (IgM) was negative, but IgG was positive and the patient was believed to have a clinical picture consistent with disseminated toxoplasmosis. He had hepatitis, pneumonitis, and diffuse lymphadenopathy, with an atypical lymphocytosis on smear. Ophthalmology staff were consulted to check for evidence of retinal changes; none were present. Therapy for toxoplasmosis was started, including pyrimethamine, sulfadiazine, and leucovorin rescue. These medications were to be continued for at least 6 months. **The diagnosis is** *Toxoplasmosis gondii,* **an intracellular parasite.** Infection with this organism is usually asymptomatic in children, but serious infection occurs in immunocompromised hosts and in children with congenitally acquired infections. Infection is lifelong, with acute and chronic stages. Acute illness involves a period of parasitemia after the initial infection. With the chronic infection, the parasite is encysted in the host tissue. The organism may periodically break out of the cells, resulting in local reactivation of the disease. In those patients with immune compromise, the reactivation of disease may result in dissemination and systemic spread.

III. Incidence and Epidemiology

The organism is distributed widely, and it is estimated that between 1 and 3 million people are affected worldwide. Human infection may be asymptomatic to severe, or even fatal in individuals who are immunocompromised. Felines (cats) are the only definitive host.

The routes of transmission in humans include blood transfusion; organ transplantation; transplacental, and ingestion of chicken eggs, meat, milk, or oocysts that contaminate water or vegetables as a result of feline fecal matter. The life cycle of the parasite includes a sexual phase that occurs in cats and an asexual phase that occurs in cats, humans, and other intermediate hosts. The incidence in cats, other animals, and humans varies greatly by location and age of the population studied.

IV. Clinical Presentation

In postnatally acquired toxoplasmosis, 80% of cases are asymptomatic. Among those patients who are immunocompetent, the symptomatic cases involve lymphadenopathy with either tender or nontender nodes. These children have a mononucleosis-like picture. In children who are immunocompromised, multiple organs may be involved. In patients with acquired immunodeficiency syndrome (AIDS), central nervous system involvement is common. Findings include headaches, hemiparesis, and visual disturbances. More severe presentations have included speech abnormalities, seizures, and the syndrome of inappropriate secretion of antidiuretic hormone (SIADH).

Congenital toxoplasmosis is most often asymptomatic and bears no significant signs or symptoms, but 30% to 40% of affected newborns have some findings if evaluated closely. The affected newborns may have hydrocephalus, fevers, hepatosplenomegaly, prolonged hyperbilirubinemia, blindness, deafness, or other manifestations including diarrhea and feeding difficulties. In this case, the main findings were fever and poor feeding leading to FTT.

V. Diagnostic Approach

T. gondii **antibodies.** Serologic tests are most commonly employed and measure the host antibody represented. *T. gondii*-specific IgG serum antibody, at any titer, indicates a risk of active infection in an immunocompromised individual. Testing that shows seroconversion or a four-fold or greater rise in antibody titer in serum samples obtained 3 to 6 weeks apart confirms the diagnosis.

Other studies. The infection can also be confirmed by demonstration of the organism histologically or by identification of nucleic acid (PCR) in a site in which the encysted organism would not be present as part of a latent infection, such as cerebrospinal fluid or bronchoalveolar fluid. When the diagnosis is made in an individual who is thought to be immunocompetent, HIV testing should be considered.

VI.   Treatment

The mainstream of treatment is pyrimethamine, a folic acid antagonist. The combination of pyrimethamine with sulfadiazine acts synergistically. There are also some experimental agents under consideration. Spiramycin is a macrolide that may be effective in treating women during pregnancy. Clindamycin may also be effective when used alone or in combination with pyrimethamine. HIV-infected patients with CD4+ T-lymphocyte counts lower than 100 to 200/mm^3 may require continued suppressive antimicrobial therapy.

VII.   References

1. Freij B, Sever J. Toxoplasmosis. *Pediatr Rev* 1991;12:227–236.
2. Jackson MH, Hutchinson WM. The prevalence and source of toxoplasma infection in the environment. *Adv Parasitol* 1989;28:55–105.
3. Sever JL, Ellenberg JH, Ley AC, et al. Toxoplasmosis: maternal and pediatric findings in 23,000 pregnancies. *Pediatrics* 1988;82:181–192.

Case 6-2: 7-Month-Old Boy

I. History of Present Illness

A 7-month-old white boy was admitted for evaluation of FTT. The patient was a former twin B who was born at 37 weeks' gestation. The mother's pregnancy was uncomplicated, and the patient did well until 3 months of age. At that time, he had bilateral inguinal hernia repair. Since then, he had not been gaining weight. His stools were loose and foul smelling and occurred six to seven times per day. There was no history of fevers or vomiting, and his appetite was described as greater than that of his twin brother, who was thriving.

II. Past Medical History

He was a former 37-week twin B of an uncomplicated pregnancy, labor, and delivery. The mother denied any sexually transmitted diseases. The child took no medications, had no allergies, and was up to date in immunizations. The family history was remarkable for a father with diabetes. The child lived with his mother, father, twin, and 3-year-old sister. Both siblings were healthy. Developmentally, the child was unable to sit unassisted, had not rolled over, and still had some head lag on repeated testing.

III. Physical Examination

T, 37.2°C; RR, 20/min; HR, 110 bpm; BP, 78/50 mm Hg

Height, less than 5th percentile; weight, is much less than 5th percentile

In general, the child was emaciated but interactive. His head was normocephalic, and hi pupils were equal round and reactive to light. The sclerae were anicteric. The tympanic membranes were normal in appearance and mobility. The neck was supple with free range of motion. There were no enlarged lymph nodes or palpable masses. The chest was clear bilaterally. There were no murmurs, gallops, or rubs on cardiovascular examination. The abdomen was soft, nontender, and nondistended with positive bowel sounds. There was no hepatosplenomegaly or masses. The genitalia were normal. There was clinodactyly. Neurologic examination showed global weakness and head lag. The skin had a fine erythematous macular rash over the extremities.

IV. Diagnostic Studies

Complete blood count revealed 1,000 WBCs/mm^3 (2% band forms, 8% segmented neutrophils, 81% lymphocytes, and 9% monocytes); hemoglobin, 2.2 g/dL; platelets, 180,000/mm^3. Serum electrolytes were as follows: sodium, 138 mEq/L; potassium, 3.6 mEq/L; chloride, 103 mEq/L; and bicarbonate, 22 mEq/L. The serum albumin concentration was 4.2 mg/dL. The prothrombin time (PT) and the partial thromboplastin time (PTT) were 12.5 and 31.0 seconds, respectively. A sweat test was normal.

V. Course of Illness

The patient was evaluated for malabsorptive stool pattern. He was shown to have increased fecal fat and evidence of pancreatic insufficiency. This finding in conjunction with findings on physical examination and the complete blood count suggested a diagnosis.

DISCUSSION: CASE 6-2

I. Differential Diagnosis

The differential diagnosis of growth failure due to malabsorption is a long one. Once the type of malabsorption was narrowed down to exocrine pancreatic dysfunction, then the differential narrowed to hereditary and acquired causes. The hereditary causes include cystic fibrosis, Shwachman-Diamond syndrome, Pearson's pancreatitis and bone marrow syndrome, and isolated enzyme deficiency. Acquired causes include chronic pancreatic and surgical conditions.

Other causes of malabsorption are many and include defects in the luminal phase, the mucosal phase, or the transport phase of absorption and digestion. Table 6-4 shows tests that may be used to evaluate the various forms of malabsorption.

II.   Diagnosis

The presence of neutropenia and a skeletal abnormality (clinodactyly) in conjunction with pancreatic insufficiency suggested the diagnosis of Shwachman-Diamond syndrome. **The diagnosis is Shwachman-Diamond syndrome, the second most common cause of hereditary pancreatic insufficiency after cystic fibrosis.** The stool pattern and growth pattern are similar to those of cystic fibrosis, but patients with Shwachman-Diamond syndrome have additional features, which often include short stature with a normal growth pattern. Skeletal deformities have been noted in the thorax and fingers. Some children manifest bone marrow dysfunction, which most often causes neutropenia and frequent infections but may also lead to anemia and thrombocytopenia.

III.   Incidence and Epidemiology

Shwachman-Diamond syndrome appears to be caused by an autosomal recessive gene. The overall incidence is not known.

IV.   Diagnostic Approach

The diagnostic approach is similar to that for a child with cystic fibrosis; the sweat test is normal, but some of the other distinguishing features may be present. There is no single laboratory marker. Shwachman-Diamond syndrome is a clinical phenotype with central features of pancreatitis and bone marrow dysfunction. Other causes of pancreatic dysfunction must be eliminated.

Patients with Shwachman-Diamond syndrome may have a complete blood count with neutropenia, but the platelet count may be low or normal. The PT, PTT, amylase, and lipase values may also be elevated. Bone marrow may show hypoplasia with fibrosis.

TABLE 6-4. *Diagnostic Studies in the Evaluation of Malabsorption*

Initial screening studies
  Stool examination for occult blood, leukocytes, reducing substances, and pH
  Stool examination for *Clostridium difficile* toxin, ova, and parasites
  Stool cultures for infectious and viral pathogens
  Serum electrolytes, albumin, and total protein
  Urinalysis and culture
Quantitative and qualitative tests for malabsorption
  Breath H_2 studies
  D-Xylose absorption for mucosal function
  Fecal fat studies
  Serum iron, vitamin B_{12}, folate
Specific diagnostic studies
  Sweat chloride test
  Biopsy of small intestine for histology and mucosal enzymes
  Contrast radiographic studies: upper gastrointestinal series with small-bowel follow-through and/or
    barium enema
  Provocative pancreatic secretion testing
  Ultrasound studies for biliary tree anomalies
  Endoscopic retrograde cholangiopancreatograph (ERCP) for selective evaluation of biliary or
pancreatic ducts

Adapted from Hill ID. Disorders of digestion and absorption. In: Rudolph CD, Rudolph AM, eds. *Rudolph's pediatrics,* 21st ed. New York: McGraw-Hill, 2003.

V. Treatment

Treatment includes enzyme replacement and nutritional support. Careful attention should be paid to vitamin therapy of the fat-soluble vitamins and treatment for infections and other hematologic manifestations. The response to treatment is good in most cases. Patients may be prone to infections due to the neutropenia. Some patients may also develop acute myelogenous leukemia (AML).

VI. References

1. Mark DR, Forstner GG, Wilchanski M, et al. Shwachman syndrome: exocrine pancreatic dysfunction and variable phenotypic expression. *Gastroenterology* 1996;111: 1593–1602.
2. Baldassano R, Liacouras C. Chronic diarrhea: a practical approach for the pediatrician. *Pediatr Clin North Am* 1991;38:667–674.
3. Rothbaum R, Perrault J, Vlachos A, et al. Shwachman-Diamond syndrome: report from an international conference. *J Pediatr* 2002;14:266–270.

Case 6-3: 20-Day-Old Girl

I. History of Present Illness

This 20-day-old Caucasian female infant was referred to the emergency department by her primary care doctor for FTT. She was born after full-term gestation, weighing 2.53 kg, via spontaneous vaginal delivery with no complications during pregnancy. In the first 36 hours of life, she had poor feeding because of poor suck. She had normal bowel movements and normal urine output in the nursery. After 36 hours of life, she began to feed well and was discharged to home with her mother. Over the ensuing 3 weeks, she was seen several times by her primary physician for weight checks. She failed to regain her birth weight. She was taking 2.5 to 3 ounces of formula every 2 to 3 hours (approximately eight 3-ounce bottles per day). Formula was being made from powder and mixed appropriately. There was no emesis, arching, or irritability with feeds. She had had loose, seedy stools for 2 days before admission. No blood was noted in the stool. There was nasal congestion but no fever. There were no ill contacts, except that the mother had had an illness with fever and headache 1 week before this visit.

II. Past Medical History

The prenatal history was remarkable for maternal tobacco use (one-half pack per day) but no illicit drug use. Peripartum testing for group B *Streptococcus,* hepatitis B, and HIV was negative. The prenatal ultrasound revealed normal fetal movements. The mother took prenatal vitamins but no other medications during pregnancy. The infant was born by vaginal delivery complicated only by the presence of meconium at delivery. The Apgar scores were not known.

There was no family history of stillbirths or miscarriages. There were no known metabolic disorders, congenital heart disease, seizure disorders, or neurologic disease. There was no history of cystic fibrosis.

III. Physical Examination

T, 36.9°C; RR, 40/min; HR, 160 bpm; BP, 96/62 mm Hg

Weight, 2.42 kg (less than 5th percentile); length, 46 cm (less than 5th percentile); head circumference, 35 cm (10th percentile).

In general the patient was cachetic but active. The anterior fontanel was open and flat. The posterior fontanel was approximately 1 cm wide. There were no dysmorphic facial features. The pupils were reactive bilaterally. The oropharynx was clear; specifically, there was no thrush. There was no lymphadenopathy. The heart and lung sounds were normal. The abdomen was soft. The liver edge was palpable 1 cm below the right costal margin. The skin was mottled and pale. A 1-cm hemangioma was located on the left parietal area. The neurologic examination was normal.

IV. Diagnostic Studies

The following laboratory results were obtained: serum sodium, 136 mEq/L; potassium, 5.5 mEq/L; chloride, 100 mEq/L; and bicarbonate, 28 mEq/L. The blood urea nitrogen, creatinine, glucose, calcium, magnesium, and phosphorus values were normal.

V. Course of Illness

This 20-day-old with moderate malnutrition and FTT was admitted for inpatient evaluation, including strict calorie counts and feeding observation. Over the next 2 days, she had adequate caloric intake (as much as 180 to 200 kcal/kg per day) without documented weight gain. She was also noted to have increased stool output, with more output than intake. Her stools were positive for reducing substances. The stool pH was 5.5. All stools were heme negative.

DISCUSSION: CASE 6-3

I. Differential Diagnosis

The differential diagnosis in this case was broad. During feeding, the baby was noted to have a poor suck and swallow. There was a question whether this difficulty with intake was a primary problem (e.g., neuropathy, spinal-muscle atrophy) or secondary due to poor nutrition and weakness. When the child was fed, she gained more strength but still failed to gain weight. When no weight gain was noted despite adequate caloric intake, malabsorption was considered.

II. Diagnosis

Sweat tests were obtained, which showed good sweat volumes over the collection time of 30 minutes. The sweat chloride concentration was 95 and 105 mEq/L at the two sites sampled (normal, less than 40 mEq/L; borderline, 40 to 60 mEq/L; abnormal, greater than 60 mEq/L). The sweat test was repeated and was again abnormal. The patient was diagnosed with cystic fibrosis (CF). A baseline chest radiograph was normal. Supplemental enzymes, vitamin supplementation, and nebulized albuterol and cromolyn were started. She did well with supplemental enzymes, documenting excellent catch-up growth while in the hospital. **The diagnosis of CF was considered when a normal, and eventually a supernormal, calorie intake was achieved but the infant failed to gain weight.** This clinical trial resulted in suspicion of a malabsorption problem, and CF was considered as the most common cause of malabsorption.

III. Incidence and Epidemiology

The incidence of CF varies by population tested. Overall, it is the most common life-shortening inherited disease in North America. CF is inherited as an autosomal recessive disease. Several gene sites have been recognized. The most important is the ΔF508 mutation on the long arm of chromosome 7. In those of northern European extraction, it occurs in 1 in every 2,500 live births. Approximately 4% of whites are carriers of a CF gene. The manifestations of CF are extremely varied. Table 6-5 shows diagnostic criteria for CF.

IV. Clinical Presentation

The clinical presentation and age at presentation are varied. Manifestation may be evident at birth, but in some cases CF does not become apparent until fertility evaluations

TABLE 6-5. *Diagnostic Criteria for Cystic Fibrosis*[a]

Clinical findings and history	Laboratory evidence of abnormal CFTR/CFTR function
One or more characteristic phenotypic features (COPD, exocrine pancreatic insufficiency, sweat salt loss syndrome, male infertility) CF in a sibling or positive newborn screening test	Positive sweat test (sweat chloride concentration >60 meq/L on a sample of at least 100 mg, obtained after maximal stimulation by pilocarpine iontophoresis Identification of two *CFTR* mutations known to cause CF Diagnostic nasal potential difference

CF, cystic fibrosis; CFTR, cystic fibrosis transmembrane conductance regulator (gene); COPD, chronic obstructive pulmonary disease.
[a]Diagnosis requires at least one item from each column.

in young adulthood lead to the diagnosis. All of the following systems may be involved: gastrointestinal, sweat glands, respiratory tract, reproductive, orthopedic, and endocrine/metabolic (hyperglycemia). FTT is one of the most frequent presenting signs. Table 6-6 shows the indications for sweat testing, listing clinical findings in patients with cystic fibrosis.

V. Diagnostic Approach

The diagnostic approach is based on phenotypic presentation together with laboratory confirmation. The laboratory confirmation is usually based on a positive sweat test with a sweat concentration greater than 60 mEq/L on a sweat sample of at least 100 mg. Genetic testing is also available (Table 6-7).

Tissue typing gives the indications for sweat testing and also shows the varied manifestations. Care must be taken, because false-positive and false-negative results may occur, as shown in Table 6-8.

Newborn screening. Earlier diagnosis of CF is possible in some cases, because newborn infants with CF have elevated blood immunoreactive trypsinogen levels caused by obstructed pancreatic ductules. Infants with immunoreactive trypsinogen levels above the 99th percentile typically undergo confirmatory sweat testing and, in some cases, screening for the principal CF gene mutation (ΔF508).

TABLE 6-6. *Indications for Sweat Testing*

Gastrointestinal tract
  Chronic diarrhea
  Steatorrhea
  Meconium ileus
  Meconium plug syndrome
  Rectal prolapse
  Cirrhosis/portal hypertension
  Prolonged neonatal jaundice
  Pancreatitis
  Deficiency of fat-soluble vitamins (especially A, E, K)
Respiratory tract
  Upper
    Nasal polyps
    Pansinusitis on radiographs
  Lower
    Chronic cough
    Recurrent bronchiolitis
    Recurrent wheezing
    Intractable "asthma"
    Recurrent or persistent atelectasis
    Obstructive pulmonary disease
    Staphylococcal pneumoniae
    Pseudomonas aeruginosa (especially mucoid colony types) recovered from throat, sputum, or
      bronchoscopic cultures
Other
  Digital clubbing
  Family history of cystic fibrosis
  Failure to thrive
  Hyponatremic, hypochloremic alkalosis
  Severe dehydration incompatible with clinical history
  Heat prostration
  "Tastes salty"
  Male infertility

Adapted from Orenstein DM. Cystic Fibrosis. In: Rudolph CD, Rudolph AM, eds. *Rudolph's pediatrics,* 21st ed. New York: McGraw-Hill, 2003.

TABLE 6-7. *Characteristics of Various Mutations of the Cystic Fibrosis Transmembrane Conductance Regulator Gene (CFTR)*

Mutation	Geographic/ethnic incidence	Other	Class
ΔF508	70–75% in North America	Pancreatic insufficiency	II
W1282X	50–60% in Ashkenzai Jews; 2% worldwide	Pancreatic insufficiency	I
G42X	3.4% worldwide	Pancreatic insufficiency	I
G551D	2.4% worldwide	Pancreatic insufficiency	III
3905insT	2.1% worldwide	Pancreatic insufficiency	I
N1303K	1.8% worldwide	Pancreatic insufficiency	II
R553X	1.3% worldwide	Pancreatic insufficiency	I
621 + 1G → T	1.3% worldwide	Pancreatic insufficiency	
1717 − 1G → T	1.3% worldwide	Pancreatic insufficiency	
A455E[a]	3–7% in Netherlands; 0–0.2% in North America	Pancreatic insufficiency; mild lung disease	
3849 + 10kb C → T[a]	1.4% worldwide; 4% Israel	Normal sweat chloride; most males not sterile; lung disease varies from mild to severe	I
R1162X	20% of non-ΔF508 CF chromosomes in northeast Italy; rare in rest of world	Pancreatic insufficiency	I
R117H[a]	0.8% worldwide	Pancreatic insufficiency	IV
R334W[a]		Pancreatic insufficiency	IV
P574H[a]		Pancreatic insufficiency	
Y563N[a]		Pancreatic insufficiency	

[a]Compound heterozygotes in most cases have one copy of the mutation noted and one other cystic fibrosis mutation (usually ΔF508).

TABLE 6-8. *Conditions Giving False-Positive and False-Negative Sweat Test Results*

False-positive (>60 mEq/L)
Laboratory error
Adrenal insufficiency syndromes
Anorexia nervosa
Ectodermal dysplasia
Familial cholestasis (Byler syndrome)
Fucosidosis
Glycogen storage disease (type I)
Hypoparathyroidism
Hypothyroidism
Malnutrition
Mauriac syndrome
Mucopolysaccharidoses
Munchausen by proxy syndrome (addition of table salt to sweat sample)
Nephrogenic diabetes insipidus
False-negative (<40 mEq/L)
Laboratory error
Edema, hypoproteinemia
Rare cystic fibrosis mutations

Adapted from Orenstein DM. Cystic fibrosis. In: Rudolph CD, Rudolph AM, eds. *Rudolph's pediatrics,* 21st ed. New York: McGraw-Hill, 2003.

VI. Treatment

Treatment is best accomplished with a multidisciplinary team and involves treatment of the lungs, gastrointestinal nutrition, and psychosocial aspects of the disease, with care being delivered at specialized multidisciplinary center. Although much research has been directed at aggressive treatment of lung disease early in life to improve long-term pulmonary function and survival, recently the nutritional aspects of young children with CF have attracted attention. Konstan et al. demonstrated that nutritional status in children with CF at 3 years of age correlates with pulmonary symptoms later in life. In an observational study of 931 children with CF, they found that children with weight-for-age below the 5th percentile at 3 years of age had lower pulmonary function at age 6 years, compared with those above the 75th percentile. Therefore, poor growth and nutritional status, in addition to lung disease early in life, contribute to pulmonary function later in life.

The median survival rate has steadily increased, from 14 years in 1969 to 32 years in 2000. Gene replacement therapy is under active investigation. Prenatal screening is being attempted and appears to have a high degree of patient satisfaction and understanding. Follow-up in a special CF center is important so that multidisciplinary services may be aimed at nutrition, pulmonary status, and avoidance of bacterial infections.

VII. References

1. Collins F. Cystic fibrosis: molecular biology and therapeutic implications. *Science* 1992;256:774–779.
2. Davis PB, Drumm M, Kontan MW. Cystic fibrosis: state of the art. *Am J Respir Crit Care Med* 1996;154:1229–1256.
3. LeGrys VA. Sweat testing for the diagnosis of cystic fibrosis: practical considerations. *J Pediatr* 1996;129:892–897.
4. Rosenstein BJ, Zeitlin PL. Cystic fibrosis (seminar). *Lancet* 1998;851:277–282.
5. Farrell PM, Fost N. Prenatal screening for cystic fibrosis: where are we now? *J Pediatr* 2002;141:758–763.
6. Konstan MW, Butler SM, Wohl MEB, et al. Growth and nutritional indexes in early life predict pulmonary function in cystic fibrosis. *J Pediatr* 2003;142:624–630.
7. Ratjen F, Doring G. Cystic fibrosis. *Lancet* 2003;361:681–689.

Case 6-4: 5-Day-Old Boy

I. History of Present Illness

A 5-day-old Asian boy was brought to his pediatrician for poor feeding. Compared with his siblings, his parents believed that he had been a poor feeder since birth. He was taking only one-half ounce every 2 to 3 hours. The mother had initially breast-fed the baby, but she had begun supplementing with formula because of jaundice. In the clinic, the child was noted to have respiratory distress and was believed to have a cardiac murmur. He was referred to the emergency department for further evaluation. In the review of symptoms, there were no fevers or vomiting. The urine and stool patterns were normal. There was decreased activity but no diaphoresis with feeds, cyanosis, or abnormal movements. There was no rash. The infant had been in contact with a 2-year-old sibling who had emesis and gastroenteritis.

II. Past Medical History

Prenatal care had been good, and a prenatal ultrasound was normal. The infant was born by spontaneous vaginal delivery at 39 weeks' gestation, with a birth weight of 3,100 g. The mother was positive for group B *Streptococcus* and received intrapartum penicillin. The infant received antibiotics empirically for the first 48 hours of life due to tachypnea but was discharged home with clinical improvement after cultures were negative. The family history was remarkable for leukemia in the maternal grandmother. The infant lived with his mother, father, and a 2-year-old sibling. The maternal grandfather died unexpectedly 2 days before the child's hospital admission.

III. Physical Examination

T, 36.1°C; RR, 44/min; HR, 168 bpm; BP in right arm, 74/44 mm Hg; BP in left arm, 85/53 mm Hg; BP in right leg, 77/57 mm Hg; BP in left leg, 77/53 mm Hg; SpO$_2$, 98% room air

Weight, 2.9 kg

In general, the infant was awake, crying, and vigorous. The anterior fontanel was open and flat. There were no dysmorphic facial features. There were ecchymoses surrounding both eyes. The tympanic membranes were normal in appearance and mobility. There was no rhinorrhea. The mucosa was pink and moist, and the oropharynx was clear. There were mild intercostal retractions, but the lungs were clear to auscultation. A IV//VI systolic murmur was noted at the sternal border and radiated to the back. S1 and S2 were normal, but an S3 gallop was noted. The point of maximal impulse was displaced slightly to the left. The abdomen was soft, and the liver edge was palpable 5 cm below the right costal margin. The spleen was not palpable. There were no palpable abdominal masses. The skin was jaundiced to the waist. Distal pulses were normal and symmetric. The neurologic examination was normal.

IV. Diagnostic Studies

The chest radiograph revealed cardiomegaly and increased interstitial edema but no discrete infiltrates. The complete blood count demonstrated the following: 15,500 WBCs/mm^3 (73% segmented neutrophils, 3% eosinophils, 13% lymphocytes, and 11% monocytes); hemoglobin, 21.5 g/dL; and 140,000 platelets/mm^3. Serum electrolyte findings were as follows: sodium, 140 mEq/L; potassium, 3.9 mEq/L; chloride, 105 mEq/L; and bicarbonate, 15 mEq/L. Tests of liver function were also abnormal: albumin, 3.0 mg/dL; total bilirubin, 17.5 mg/dL, ALT, 54 IU/L; AST, 163 IU/L; and γ-glutamyltransferase (GGT), 700 U/L. The PTT was 28 seconds.

The electrocardiogram showed diffuse T-wave abnormalities but normal voltage. Echocardiography showed a diffusely dilated heart with a particularly large left ventricle. The shortening fraction was 22%. The heart was otherwise structurally normal. Lumbar puncture revealed 17 WBCs and 39 red blood cells per cubic millimeter; the protein and glucose concentrations were normal. No bacteria were seen on Gram staining of the cerebrospinal fluid (CSF). A herpes simplex virus PCR study from the CSF was negative.

V. Course of Illness

On admission, he was believed to have congestive heart failure and was treated with digoxin and furosemide. Initially, cardiomyopathy and myocarditis were considered the most likely causes. Viral infections (coxsackievirus, enteroviruses, TORCH infections), bacterial infections, and metabolic storage diseases were all considered. The infant was initially treated with ampicillin, cefotaxime, and acyclovir until those studies returned negative. A head ultrasound study was normal; specifically, no cerebral arteriovenous malformation was visualized. He continued to have mild elevation in his liver function tests, and an abdominal ultrasound examination was performed on the second hospital day. It was remarkable for several masses of increased echogenicity involving most of the right lobe of the liver.

DISCUSSION: CASE 6-4

I. Differential Diagnosis

This child presented in heart failure as the cause of his growth failure. The cause of heart failure may be cardiac or noncardiac, as shown in Table 6-9. Table 6-10 shows the differential diagnosis of a liver mass in a child.

II. Diagnosis

CT of the abdomen to further evaluate the hepatic lesions revealed large heterogeneous lesions with enhancements in the periphery. The hepatic artery was slightly dilated, which may have been the cause of the significant shunting into the lesion. Magnetic resonance imaging (MRI) of the liver was then performed to obtain better detail of the liver process. On MRI, the patient was believed to have a mass lesion rather than an arteriovenous malformation. He underwent open biopsy of the liver mass and Broviac catheter placement.

TABLE 6-9. *Heart Failure in the Newborn*

Structural heart defects
  At birth—hypoplastic left heart syndrome (HLHS)
    Severe tricuspid regurgitation
    Large systemic arteriovenous fistula
  First week—transposition of great arteries (TGA)
    Premature infant with large patent ductus arterious
    Total anomalous pulmonary venous return
  Weeks 1–4
    Critical aortic stenosis or pulmonic stenosis
    Coarctation of the arteries
Noncardiac causes
  Birth asphyxia resulting in transient myocardial ischemia
  Metabolic (acidosis, hypoglycemia, hypocalcemia)
  Severe anemia (hydrops)
  Overtransfusion or overhydration
  Neonatal sepsis
  Endocardial fibroelastosis (rare primary myocardial disease) causes congestive
    heart failure in infancy. 90% of cases occur in the first 8 months of life.

TABLE 6-10. *Differential Diagnosis of a Liver Mass in a Child*

Diagnosis	Age	Distribution of lesions	α-Fetoprotein level
Benign			
Hemangioendothelioma	<6 mo	Single or multiple	Normal
Mesenchymal hamartoma	<2 yr	Single	Normal
Inflammatory	Any	Single or multiple	Normal
Umbilical venous catheter–related	Infant	Single	Normal
Malignant			
Hepatoblastoma	<3 yr	Single	Elevated
Hepatocellular carcinoma	>3 yr	Single or multiple	Elevated
Undifferentiated sarcoma	6–10 yr	Single	Normal
Metastatic	Any	Single or multiple	Normal

On biopsy and special stains, the mass was believed to be most consistent with a hemangioendothelioma. **The findings in this case resulted from a large hemangioendothelioma or cavernous hemangioma.** These lesions can cause congestive heart failure of the high-output type.

III. Incidence and Epidemiology

Liver tumors are rare in children, and approximately 30% are benign (nonmalignant). Benign liver tumors may be classified into five groups: (a) tumor-like epithelial lesions (e.g., focal nodular hyperplasia); (b) epithelial tumors; (c) cysts and mesenchymal lesions (e.g., cystic mesenchymal hamartomas); (d) benign teratomas; and (e) mesenchymal tumors (e.g., hemangiomas, hemangioendotheliomas). Of these benign lesions, hemangioendothelioma is the most common. Hemangioendotheliomas are soft tissue tumors that demonstrate endothelial proliferation. Like cutaneous hemangiomas, these hepatic tumors increase in size during the first year of life and then undergo involution over a period of several months to years.

IV. Clinical Presentation

Most affected children (85%) present in the first 6 months of life. Before tumor involution, findings may include a palpable liver mass, jaundice, weight loss, anorexia, and fever. Life-threatening complications include rupture with hemorrhage, anemia, obstructive jaundice, and, as in this case, congestive heart failure. Many children have associated cutaneous hemangiomas, particularly if there are multiple hepatic lesions. Similar lesions may be found in the trachea, lungs, gastrointestinal tract, spleen, and pancreas.

V. Diagnostic Approaches

The diagnostic approach is based first on ultrasound examination, followed by CT or MRI with contrast. Measurements of α-fetoproteins (AFP) and liver enzymes are helpful. A young child with multiple lesions and normal AFP most likely has hemangioendothelioma. An older child with elevated AFP most likely has hepatocellular carcinoma.

Complete blood count. Anemia is noted in 50% of patients. Thrombocytopenia, when present, may range from mild to severe.

Liver function tests. AST is frequently elevated. High bilirubin levels are usually caused by obstructive jaundice.

Abdominal ultrasound. Hemangioendotheliomas are usually hypoechoic with well-defined margins. Doppler flow studies reveal high-flow velocity. Differentiation from arteriovenous malformations may be difficult by ultrasonography.

Abdominal computed tomography. On CT, a low-attenuation mass with calcification is seen in approximately 40% of cases. Multifocal lesions are less likely to demonstrate calcification. These lesions usually have peripheral enhancement with central hypoattenuation due to central infarction or hemorrhage in larger lesions.

Abdominal magnetic resonance imaging. On MRI, large lesions are heterogeneous, with occasional high signal on T1-weighted imaging suggesting central hemorrhage.

Other studies. Biopsy is often required to distinguish these tumors from other hepatic masses.

VI. Treatment

A hemangioendothelioma may be resected if it is singular and uncomplicated by thrombocytopenia. Nonoperative treatment with prednisone or interferon-α, or both, is the treatment of choice. Cyclophosphamide has also been used, as has radiotherapy. Liver transplantation may be needed.

VII. References

1. Reis-Filho JS, Paiva ME, Lopes JM. Congenital composite hemangioendothelioma: case report and reappraisal of the hemangioendothelioma spectrum. *J Cutaneous Pathol* 2002;29:226–231.
2. Lu CC, Ko SF, Liang CD, et al. Infantile hepatic hemangioendothelioma presenting as early heart failure: report of two cases. *Chang Gun Med J* 2002;25:405–410.
3. Zenge JP, Fenton L, Lovell MA, et al. Case report: infantile hemangioendothelioma. *Curr Opin Pediatr* 2002;14:99–102.
4. Ayling RM, Davenport M, Hadzic N, et al. Hepatic hemangioendothelioma associated with production of humoral thyrotropin-like factor. *J Pediatr* 2001;138:932–935.
5. Davenport M, Hansen L, Heaton ND, et al. Hemangioendothelioma of the liver in infants. *J Pediatr Surg* 1995;30:44–48.
6. d'Annibale, Piovanello P, Carlini P, et al. Epithelioid hemangioendothelioma of the liver: case report and review of the literature. *Transplant Proc* 2002;34:1248–1251.

Case 6-5: 3-Month-Old Girl

I.   History of Present Illness

A 3-month old girl was referred by her pediatrician to the emergency department because of FTT. She had had problems gaining weight since 1 to 2 months of age and had been monitored weekly for weight checks with poor weight gain. She was initially breast-fed but had poor latching-on and was changed to Enfamil formula with iron, then Enfamil without iron, Lactofree, ProSobee, and now is on Similac with iron. The family had tried thickening feeds with cereal and bananas with no improvement. The child was taking 4 ounces per feeding and was burped after every 2 ounces. Intake was 28 ounces per day. She typically spit and vomited, sometimes forcefully, 1 to 2 ounces per feed. The emesis was nonbloody, nonbilious, and occasionally projectile. The emesis had become worse over the last month. There had been no diarrhea. For the last 3 days, she had been less active than usual and had glassy-appearing eyes. Urine output had decreased; on the day of presentation, she had had only 2 wet diapers, compared with her usual 7 to 10 per day.

II.   Past Medical History

The infant was born to a 16-year-old mother. The mother had prenatal care beginning in the second month of pregnancy. The child was born at term with a weight of 3,440 g. There were no postnatal complications, and she was discharged home at 39 hours of age. Development had been normal. She rolled from front to back at 6 weeks of life. She received no medications. Her immunizations were current. The family history was unremarkable.

III.   Physical Examination

T, 37°C; RR, 18/min; HR, 129 bpm; BP, 68/41 mm Hg

Weight, 3.89 kg (50th percentile for a 1-month-old child)

On examination, the child was crying but consolable. She had markedly decreased subcutaneous fat. The anterior fontanel was sunken. The pupils were reactive to light. There was no nasal discharge. The heart and lungs were normal to auscultation. The abdomen was scaphoid with visible peristaltic waves. The spleen tip was palpable below the left costal margin. The extremities were slightly cool, with capillary refill times of 2 to 3 seconds. The neurologic examination was normal.

IV.   Diagnostic Studies

Complete blood count revealed the following: 8,800 WBCs/mm^3 (1% band forms, 59% segmented neutrophils, 30% lymphocytes, and 10% monocytes); hemoglobin, 12.9 mg/dL; and 195,000 platelets/mm^3. Serum electrolyte analysis revealed the following: sodium, 129 mEq/L; chloride, 65 mEq/L; bicarbonate, 53 mEq/L; blood urea nitrogen, 48 mg/dL; and creatinine, 1.4 mg/dL. Serum transaminases were normal. Other studies included a cholesterol of 206 mg/dL and triglycerides of 313 mg/dL.

V.   Course of Illness

In the emergency department, the patient received approximately 40 mL/kg of normal saline. She was admitted to the intensive care unit due to rapid but periodic breathing. An abdominal radiograph (Fig. 6-1) revealed a markedly distended stomach with a paucity of bowel gas pattern beyond the stomach. Abdominal ultrasound (Fig. 6-2) revealed the diagnosis.

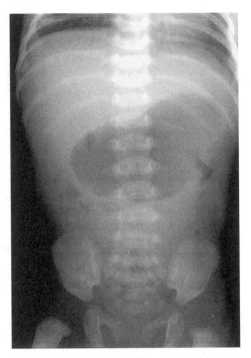

FIG. 6-1. Abdominal radiograph (case 6-5).

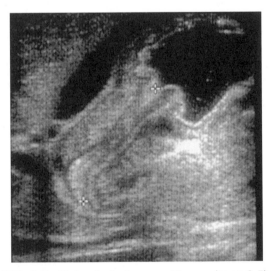

FIG. 6-2. Abdominal ultrasound image (case 6-5).

DISCUSSION: CASE 6-5

I. Differential Diagnosis

The differential diagnosis in this case included some form of upper bowel obstruction. There was a marked hypochloremic alkalosis to support this kind of loss, along with the associated history. Severe gastroesophageal reflux, gastric outlet obstruction, pyloric stenosis, or some kind of duodenal anomaly (e.g., duplication) was possible. The upper gastrointestinal radiograph delineated the lesion of pyloric stenosis. The electrolyte disturbance was characteristic of an upper bowel atresia with loss of sodium, chloride, and hydrogen ion.

II. Diagnosis Pyloric Stenosis

The abdominal ultrasound study showed a thickened and elongated pylorus, with a maximal muscle length measuring 19 mm (Fig. 6-2). The maximal muscle thickness was 5 mm. The gastric antrum was also imaged, and there was evidence of significant fluid and debris from the prior oral feeding. **These findings were consistent with the diagnosis of pyloric stenosis.** Once the patient's metabolic derangement was corrected, she was taken to the operating room for a pyloromyotomy. The postoperative course was uneventful. This case was unusual in terms of the late onset of pyloric stenosis; most cases are identified in the first 3 to 6 weeks of life.

III. Incidence and Epidemiology

Pyloric stenosis occurs in 1 of every 200 male infants and in 1 of every 1,000 females. The mode of inheritance is polygenic and modified by sex. The disorder is associated with smaller family size and higher socioeconomic status. In the United States, it is more common among African-Americans and Asian-Americans than other groups.

IV. Clinical Presentation

The clinical presentation is based on vomiting (often projectile in nature), failure to gain weight, and constipation. There are no other associated symptoms. On examination, the hypertrophied pyloric muscle ("olive") is occasionally palpated in the right upper quadrant.

V. Diagnostic Approach

The palpation of the pyloric olive is often difficult and examiner dependent.

Serum electrolytes. Electrolytes reveal a hypochloremic metabolic alkalosis.

Abdominal ultrasonography. Ultrasound studies typically reveal thickening of the pyloric muscle wall. For a broader differential diagnosis, an upper gastrointestinal barium study should be considered.

VI. Treatment

The treatment is a simple pyloromyotomy, which opens the pyloric channel and allows the passage of food into the small bowel. The symptoms resolve within a few days after surgery. There are no long-term complications, and patients may be discharged postoperatively when they are able to tolerate feeding.

VII. References

1. Garcia VF, Randolph JG. Pyloric stenosis: diagnosis and management. *Pediatr Rev* 1990;11:292–296.
2. Letton RW Jr. Pyloric stenosis. *Pediatr Ann* 2001;30:745–750.
3. Zenn MR, Redo SF. Hypertrophic pyloric stenosis in the newborn. *J Pediatr Surg* 1993;28:1577–1578.
4. Murtagh K, Perry P, Corlett M, et al. Infantile hypertrophic pyloric stenosis. *Dig Dis* 1992;10:190–198.
5. Spicer RD. Infantile hypertrophic pyloric stenosis: a review. *Br J Surg* 1982;69: 128–135.

Case 6-6: 21-Month-Old Boy

I. History of Present Illness
A 21-month-old boy presented with weight loss and crankiness. He had been well until 5 months before admission, when he developed otitis media. This was treated with amoxicillin. The otitis media seemed to recur 1 month later, and he was treated with amoxicillin-clavulanate followed by cefuroxime. At the same time, he began to develop two to four large, mushy, foul-smelling, pale, greasy bowel movements per day. He become a finicky eater with a very variable appetite and also developed intermittent vomiting. He had lost approximately 3 pounds and had not had linear growth in the past 3 months. Vomiting often occurred in the late day or evening and was nonbloody and nonbilious.

II. Past Medical History
This was a full-term infant born to a gravida 1 parity 1 mother. The pregnancy was complicated by preterm labor at 32 weeks' gestation. He was born through meconium-stained fluid with a birth weight of 3,700 g. He had been developing normally but recently began asking to be carried and was not willing to walk for long periods. He tired easily but refused to sleep. His only medication was a multivitamin. The mother was 29 years old and worked as a nurse at a nearby university. The 30-year-old father worked as a materials manager at a pharmaceutical company. The family history was remarkable for a maternal grandmother with ovarian cancer and a maternal grandfather with congestive heart failure and stroke. The family had been to Puerto Rico 5 months before presentation. The diet history revealed that the patient was initially breast-fed, then was changed to Gerber formula with iron at 4.5 months. Cereals were introduced at 6 months of age, followed by vegetables, fruits, and meats. He began to refuse meats at 1 year of age.

III. Physical Examination
Weight, 8.77 kg (less than 5th percentile; 50th percentile for a 7-month-old); height, 80.5 cm (5th percentile; 50th percentile for a 13-month-old). Vital signs are normal.

In general, the child was pale, wasted, and irritable. There were no oral or nasal ulcers. The neck was supple. There was only shotty cervical adenopathy. The lungs were clear to auscultation. The abdomen was distended. There was no hepatosplenomegaly. There was a prominent vascular pattern on the abdomen as well as granular subcutaneous palpable patter. The genitourinary examination was normal. The remainder of the examination was normal.

IV. Diagnostic Studies
Complete blood count revealed the following: 9,300 WBCs/mm^3 (7% band forms, 28% segmented neutrophils, 52% lymphocytes, 4% atypical lymphocytes, and 9% monocytes); hemoglobin, 12.7 g/dL; and 417,000 platelets/mm^3. The mean corpuscular volume was 83 fL, and the reticulocyte count was 1.3%. Other findings were erythrocyte sedimentation rate, 2 mm/hour; PT, 14.2 seconds; PTT, 31.5 seconds; creatinine, 0.5 mg/dL; albumin, 3.8 mg/dL; cholesterol, 142 mg/dL; triglycerides, 172 mg/dL; ALT, 134 IU/L; AST, 98 IU/L; and lactate dehydrogenase, 600 U/L. A sweat test was normal.

V. Course of Illness
In the hospital, upper endoscopy revealed flat villous atrophy of the duodenum and acute inflammation of the lamina propria.

DISCUSSION: CASE 6-6

I. Differential Diagnosis

The differential diagnosis of weight loss is very extensive and potentially involves almost every organ system. For this child, who had grown and developed somewhat normally, one would not expect a psychosocial cause unless there had been some recent change in the child's family constitution or living environment. The loss of weight and linear growth over a short period of time suggest an organic cause. The findings of pallor and abdominal distention also suggest narrowing of the differential diagnosis to a disease-based cause.

II. Diagnosis

The diagnosis made in this case was celiac disease. This is a genetically predisposing disease that manifests in children who eat gluten products or related peptides from other grains. Once the child is exposed to gluten, there is an immunologically triggered reaction to the absorptive surface of the small bowel.

III. Incidence and Epidemiology

With newer diagnostic tests available, the incidence of the disorder has increased. In people of European background, it has been identified in 1 of every 250 individuals in the general population. It has been identified all around the world.

IV. Clinical Presentation

The clinical presentations of celiac disease are many. The classic presentation is that of the case presented: weight loss and growth failure in the second year of life. Table 6-11 identifies other manifestations of the disease.

V. Diagnostic Approaches

The diagnosis has been made by biopsy of the small intestine. Biopsy is the time-proven method and should be performed if there is a clinical suspicion despite enzyme testing. The biopsy shows flat mucosa with villous atrophy and an increased number of lymphocytes. The serologic testing methods for the disease have improved. Antigliaden antibodies of both IgG and IgA are measured. Also measurable are anti-smooth muscle

---

TABLE 6-11. *Clinical Manifestations of Celiac Disease*

"Classic" gastrointestinal form
 Age at onset younger than 2 years; diarrhea, failure to thrive, abdominal distention, proximal muscle
   wasting, irritability
Non-"classic" gastrointestinal form
 Age at onset, childhood to adulthood; diarrhea, intermittent or mild; abdominal pain, bloating, nausea,
   vomiting; change in appetite; constipation
Nongastrointestinal manifestations
 Musculoskeletal system: short stature, rickets, osteoporosis, dental enamel defects, arthritis/arthralgia,
   myopathy
 Skin and mucous membranes: dermatitis herpetiformis, atopic dermatitis, aphthous stomatitis
 Reproductive system: delayed puberty, infertility, recurrent abortions, menstrual irregularities
 Hematologic system: anemia (iron, folate, B_{12}), leukopenia, vitamin K deficiency, thrombocytopenia
 Central nervous system: behavioral changes, epilepsy, dementia, cerebellar degeneration
Associated conditions
 Autoimmune disorders: type I diabetes mellitus, autoimmune thyroid disease, Sjögren syndrome,
   collagen vascular disease, liver disease (PBC), IgA glomerulonephritis
 Miscellaneous associations: selective IgA deficiency, Down syndrome, hyposplenism, colitis
Asymptomatic form
 Patients identified through screening studies

IgA, immunoglobulin A; PBC, primary biliary cirrhosis.

antibodies including anti-endomysium and anti-reticular (IgA). The newest test shows IgA-type antibody to tissue transglutaminase.

VI. Treatment

The therapy involves a life-long removal of gluten from the diet. This is a difficult challenge for children and their parents but is successful.

VII. References

1. Farrell RJ, Kelly CP. Current concepts: celiac sprue. *N Engl J Med* 2002;346:180–188.
2. Kolsteren MMP, Koopman HM, Schalekamp GMA, et al. Health-related quality of life in children with celiac disease. *J Pediatr* 2001;138:593–595.
3. Scoglio R, Sorleti D, Magazzù G, et al. Celiac disease case finding in children in primary care. *J Pediatr* 2002;140:379–380.
4. Walker-Smith JA, Guandalini S, Schmitz J, et al. Revised criteria for diagnosis of coeliac disease. *Arch Dis Child* 1990;65:909–911.

Case 6-7: 18-Month-Old Boy

I. History of Present Illness

An 18-month-old was brought to the emergency department with a chief complaint of draining ear. In the emergency department, it was noted that he was markedly wasted. Vital signs included a body temperature below normal; height, weight, and head circumference were below the 3rd percentile. The heart rate was 40 bpm with a respiratory rate of 26/minute.

The examination of the ears showed bilateral draining otitis media. There was loss of hair that was brittle. There were multiple scabs on the body. The examination was very notable for loss of almost all subcutaneous tissue. Figure 6-3 shows the child at the time of admission. There was no reported weigh loss or diarrhea. The mother reported no other symptoms.

II. Past Medical History

The child had been born in a healthy condition. The mother was married and living in a suburban community. The child had grown normally for several months, but then the mother noted multiple food allergies and placed him on a restrictive diet. She had not sought regular care for the child but frequently sought advice from telephone hotlines and calls to multiple physicians' offices. The child had lost developmental milestones. The mother and father were both college graduates. There was no smoking or drinking in the house. Both parents admitted to using marijuana on a regular basis.

II. Physical Examination

T, 35.9°C; RR, 16/min; HR, 40 bpm; BP, 70/40 mm Hg

Weight and height far below 5th percentile; head circumference, 10th percentile

In general, the child was a weak-appearing and cachectic boy with decreased movement and a weak cry. His hair was stubbled. He had a purulent draining otitis media. There was no adenopathy. The chest was clear. The heart rate was bradycardic with weak pulses. The abdomen was scaphoid with decreased bowel sounds. On the skin, there were

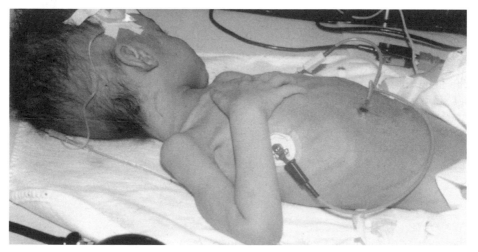

FIG. 6-3. Photograph of patient with marked failure to thrive (case 6-7).

179

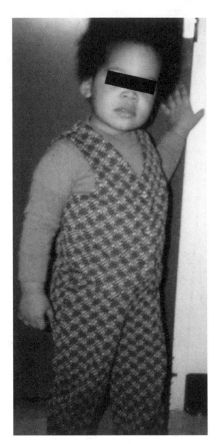

FIG. 6-4. Photograph of same patient as in Figure 6-3, during recovery phase 16 months later (case 6-7).

multiple marks and scars and hyperpigmented macules in the diaper area and diffusely. On neurologic examination, responses were dull, apathetic, and weak. He had decreased muscle mass and muscle tone.

IV. Diagnostic Studies

Laboratory studies were notable for a mild iron deficiency anemia (hemoglobin, 9.6 mg/dL) and mildly decreased serum protein.

V. Course of Illness

The hospital course involved treating the ear infection and starting the child on nutritional support and iron. He responded with weight gain and improvement in development. At the end of 2 weeks in the hospital, he had made tremendous strides in both growth and development. He ate large quantities of food. The parents underwent psychiatric testing and were determined to be unsuitable caretakers. The child recovered completely and was discharged to a foster home (Fig. 6-4).

DISCUSSION: CASE 6-7

I. Differential Diagnosis

The severity of this child's condition prompted the consideration of a wide differential diagnosis. The parent's economic status and educational level at first prompted the medical care team to eliminate psychosocial causes. Yet, the child's response to supportive care and feeding and the normal laboratory pattern that he demonstrated revealed a nonorganic cause for his life-threatening condition.

II. Diagnosis

The final diagnosis was weight loss and developmental repression due to psychosocial causes. The diet that the mother selected for the child was too restrictive in content and calories. Her presenting complaint missed the obvious wasting and was a clue to her lack of perception and parenting ability.

III. Incidence and Epidemiology

The true incidence of psychosocial FTT is not known. Many case series of children with FTT show that 40% to 80% of cases are due to psychosocial causes or a combination of psychosocial and medical causes (so-called mixed FTT). The epidemiology is varied and can result from postpartum depression, lack of knowledge about parenting, or more overt child abuse and willful starvation. It is difficult to sort through the motivation of the parents, yet the results in the child are obvious and disturbing.

IV. Clinical Presentation

Clinical presentations are varied, from children who have minor falling off on their growth parameters to cases of death by starvation. Serial measures of length or height, weight, and head circumference are helpful in sorting through the causes and in differentiating psychosocial and medical causes.

V. Diagnostic Approaches

Diagnostic approach is best directed by the signs and symptoms the child manifests. Without special symptoms, it is best to feed the child in a controlled setting and monitor the weight gain. There is no single battery of laboratory tests to be recommended. Some tests that may be helpful are the complete blood count (iron deficiency anemia), urinalysis (urinary tract infection, renal tubular acidosis), and the purified protein derivative (PPD) test for tuberculosis. HIV infection may also be a cause for FTT. Skeletal survey for trauma may be indicated if there is suspicion of abuse.

VI. Treatment

Treatment for nonorganic FTT requires close follow-up and a multidisciplinary approach to meet the needs of the child and the family. In some cases, the child must be removed from the care of the parents until a system of care and follow-up can be proposed. In this case, a foster home was used initially, and then the child was returned home under close (weekly) supervision. Subsequently, a physical abuse episode resulted in long-term removal of the child. In most cases, the nutritional recovery time equals the duration of the organic deprivation.

VII. References

1. Ludwig S. Failure-to-thrive and starvation. In: Ludwig S, Kornberg A, eds. *Child abuse and neglect: a medical reference,* 2nd ed. New York: Churchill-Livingstone, 1992.
2. Altemeier WA, O'Connor SM, Sherrod KB, et al. Prospective study of antecedents for nonorganic failure-to-thrive. *J Pediatr* 1985;106:360.
3. Sturm L, Drotar D. Prediction of weight for height following intervention in three-year-old children with early histories of nonorganic failure-to-thrive. *Child Abuse* 1989;13:19.
4. Frank DA, Drotar D, Cook J, et al. Failure to thrive. In: Reece R, Ludwig S, eds. *Child abuse: medical diagnosis and management,* 2nd ed. Philadelphia: Lippincott Williams & Wilkins, 2001.

7

Abdominal Pain

Marina Catallozzi

APPROACH TO THE PATIENT WITH ABDOMINAL PAIN

I. Definition of the Complaint

Abdominal pain is a common complaint in pediatrics and has a long list of possible causes, not all of which are gastrointestinal (GI). Abdominal pain is usually stimulated by one of three pathways: visceral pain, somatic pain, or referred pain. Visceral pain is caused by a distended viscus, which activates a local nerve, sending an impulse that travels through autonomic afferent fibers to the spinal tract and central nervous system. Localization of pain is often difficult and frustrating, because there are very few afferent nerves traveling from the viscera, and the nerve fibers overlap. Visceral pain is usually felt in the epigastric region, the periumbilical region, or the suprapubic area. Somatic pain, because it is carried by somatic nerves in the parietal peritoneum, muscle, or skin, is usually well localized and sharp. Referred pain, defined as abdominal pain perceived at a site remote from the actual affected viscera, can be sharp and localized or diffuse. There is a great deal of individual variability with regard to the experience of pain, so that neuroanatomic, neurophysiologic, pathophysiologic, environmental, and psychosocial factors all play a part. The frequency of this chief complaint necessitates categorizing the presentation of abdominal pain as acute, chronic, or recurrent.

With acute abdominal pain, the patient or a parent is usually able to pinpoint the onset of the pain to an event or time of day. Although the pain may be mild initially, it often becomes progressively worse and interferes with sleep and normal activities. Other than intussusception, acute abdominal pain that requires surgical intervention does not recur and is not relieved without intervention. Nausea, vomiting, diarrhea, fever, and anorexia often accompany acute abdominal pain. Patients often appear acutely ill and attempt to protect the abdomen from further examination by their positioning. Chronic abdominal pain is defined as pain that lasts 2 weeks or longer; it usually does not require surgery. Recurrent abdominal pain has several definitions and is frequently referred to as a description rather than a diagnosis. Although formal definitions and guidelines exist, the definition basically includes any recurrent abdominal pain in a child for which the family seeks medical attention. Because of the frustration for the family and child, as well as the extensive differential diagnosis for this problem, a consistent approach is vital. The approach must include a thorough history (arguably the most important component), physical examination, laboratory testing, imaging studies, and empiric interventions.

II. Complaint by Cause and Frequency

Although abdominal pain is a frequent complaint, it is not in itself a diagnosis, and a thorough evaluation of this symptom is required to determine the causative pathology. The causes of abdominal pain in childhood vary by age and can be classified based on whether the abdominal pain is acute, chronic, or recurrent in nature (Table 7-1). They also can be grouped by etiologic category: infectious, toxicologic, metabolic, tumor/oncologic, traumatic, congenital/anatomic, allergic/inflammatory, and functional/other (Table 7-2).

TABLE 7-1. *Causes of Abdominal Pain by Age*

Category	Cause
Acute abdominal pain	
Neonate and infant	
	Colic
	Congential anomalies
	Electrolyte disturbance
	Hypertrophic pyloric stenosis
	Incarcerated hernias
	Infectious gastroenteritis
	Intestinal obstruction
	Intussusception
	Malrotation with or without volvulus
	Necrotizing enterocolitis
	Pyelonephritis/urinary tract infection
	Trauma/child abuse
	Tumors
Toddler and school age	
	Acute appendicitis
	Acute glomerulonephritis
	Cholecystitis
	Cholelithiasis
	Dietary indiscretion
	Diabetic ketoacidosis
	Electrolyte disturbance
	Hemolytic uremic syndrome
	Henoch-Schöenlein purpura
	Hepatitis
	Infectious gastroenteritis
	Infectious mononucleosis
	Intestinal obstruction
	Intussusception
	Meckel diverticulum
	Mesenteric adenitis
	Pancreatitis
	Pneumonia
	Porphyria
	Psoas abscess
	Pyelonephritis/urinary tract infection
	Sickle cell crisis
	Testicular torsion
	Trauma/child abuse
	Tumors
Adolescent	
	Acute appendicitis
	Cholecystitis
	Cholelithiasis
	Diabetic ketoacidosis
	Electrolyte disturbance
	Epididymitis
	Hepatitis
	Herpes zoster
	Infectious gastroenteritis
	Infectious mononucleosis
	Intestinal obstruction
	Meckel diverticulum
	Mesenteric adenitis
	Ovarian cyst
	Pancreatitis
	Pelvic inflammatory disease
	Pneumonia
	Porphyria
	Psoas abscess

TABLE 7-1. *Continued.*

Category	Cause
	Pyelonephritis/urinary tract infection
	Sickle cell crisis
	Testicular torsion
	Trauma/child abuse
	Tumors
Chronic and recurrent abdominal pain	
Neonate and infant	
	Colic
	Disaccharidase deficiency/malabsorbtive syndromes
	Milk protein allergy/eosinophilic gastroenteritis
Toddler and school age	
	Abdominal migraine
	Addison's disease
	Aerophagia
	Carbohydrate malabsorbtion
	Collagen vascular diseaes
	Constipation
	Cystic fibrosis/meconium ileus equivalent
	Functional abdominal pain
	Gastritis
	Gastroesophageal reflux disease
	Heavy metal poisoning
	Hiatal hernia
	Inflammatory bowel disease
	Irritable bowel syndrome
	Parasitic infection
	Peptic ulcer disease
	Recurrent pancreatitis
	Superior mesenteric artery syndrome
	Wilson disease
Adolescent	
	Abdominal migraine
	Addison's disease
	Aerophagia
	Carbohydrate malabsorbtion
	Collagen vascular diseaes
	Constipation
	Cystic fibrosis/meconium ileus equivalent
	Dysmenorrhea
	Endometriosis
	Functional abdominal pain
	Gastritis
	Gastroesophageal reflux disease
	Heavy metal poisoning
	Hematocolpos
	Hiatal hernia
	Inflammatory bowel disease
	Irritable bowel syndrome
	Mittelschmerz
	Parasitic infection
	Peptic ulcer disease
	Recurrent pancreatitis
	Superior mesenteric artery syndrome
	Wilson disease

TABLE 7-2. *Causes of Abdominal Pain in Childhood by Etiology*

Category	Cause
Infectious	
	Cat-scratch disease
	Epididymitis
	Gastroenteritis (viral or bacterial)
	Helicobacter pylori gastritis
	Hepatitis
	Herpes zoster
	Infectious mononucleosis
	Mesenteric adenitis (frequently caused by group A *Streptococcus*)
	Necrotizing enterocolitis
	Parasitic infections (e.g., giardia)
	Pelvic inflammatory disease/Fitz-Hugh–Curtis syndrome/tubo-ovarian abscess
	Pneumonia
	Psoas abscess
	Subdiaphragmatic abscess
	Tuberculosis of the spine
	Urinary tract infection
Toxicologic	
	Black widow spider bite
	Heavy metals (e.g., lead)
	Medications (e.g., anticholinergics, aspirin and nonsteroidal antiinflammatory drugs)
Metabolic	
	Addison's disease
	Diabetic ketoacidosis
	Electrolyte disturbances (especially hypokalemia)
	Hypoglycemia
	Wilson disease
Tumor/Oncologic	
	Any benign or malignant tumor
	Leukemia
	Lymphoma
	Spinal cord tumor
	Testicular neoplasm
	Wilms tumor
Traumatic	
	Child abuse
	Duodenal hematoma
	Splenic rupture
Congenital/anatomic	
	Choledochal cyst
	Cholelithiasis
	Hematocolpos
	Hiatal hernia
	Incarcerated hernia
	Intussusception
	Intestinal obstruction (adhesions)
	Malrotation with or without volvulus
	Meckel diverticulum
	Meconium ileus/meconium ileus equivalent
	Ovarian torsion
	Superior mesenteric artery syndrome
	Renal colic/stones
	Testicular torsion
Allergic/Inflammatory	
	Acute rheumatic fever
	Appendicitis
	Cholecystitis
	Diskitis
	Gastritis
	Glomerulonephritis

TABLE 7-2. *Continued.*

Category	Cause
	Henoch-Schönlein purpura
	Hemolytic-uremic syndrome
	Inflammatory bowel disease
	Milk protein allergy/eosinophilic gastroenteritis
	Pancreatitis
	Peptic ulcer disease
	Serositis associated with collagen vascular disease
	Vasculitis
Functional and other	
	Abdominal migraine
	Aerophagia
	Colic
	Constipation
	Dietary indiscretion
	Disaccharidase deficiency
	Dysmenorrhea
	Ectopic pregnancy
	Endometriosis
	Familial Mediterranean fever
	Functional abdominal pain syndrome
	Gastroesophageal reflux disease
	Hemolytic crisis
	Hypertensive crisis
	Irritable bowel syndrome
	Malabsorptive syndromes
	Mittelschmerz
	Myocarditis
	Nephrotic syndrome with ascites
	Ovarian cyst
	Pericarditis
	Porphyria
	Sickle cell crisis

III. Clarifying Questions

Accurate diagnosis in a child with abdominal pain requires a thorough history and physical examination. There must be consideration of the type and location of pain in order to create a working differential and approach to the individual patient with abdominal pain. The following questions may be helpful in arriving at a diagnosis.

- When did the pain begin, and how long has it lasted?

    — The determination of acute, chronic, or recurrent pain is vital in considering possible causes, in identifying conditions that require surgical intervention and in determining any other life-threatening causes of abdominal pain that do not require surgical intervention. Although gastroenteritis and constipation are considered the most common causes of acute and chronic pain, respectively, other causes must be ruled out.

    Whereas an infant frequently displays pain as a behavior change (e.g., poor oral intake, irritability, inconsolable crying), older children can verbalize the character of the pain. For diagnoses such as irritable bowel syndrome, in which the chronicity of the pain is an important feature of the diagnosis, the duration of pain is vital information. Additionally, with chronic or recurrent pain, the timing of the pain is key. For example, pain that awakens a child from sleep suggests peptic disease, whereas pain that occurs during dinner is often associated with constipation. Paroxysms of pain, in which the child has 20-minute intervals of being well between periods of inconsolability, is classically seen with intussusception.

- What is the location of the pain?

  — Even if abdominal pain seems localized, a thorough examination must be performed to rule out other, non-GI causes of the pain. Certain locations herald specific disease processes. Perhaps the most important of these is the association of appendicitis with acute pain in the right lower quadrant (even more specifically, tenderness over McBurney's point). Although appendicitis is the most common cause for emergency surgery (apart from trauma) in children, the rate of initial misdiagnosis has been found to be between 28% and 57%. (Acute appendicitis often does not result in pain as the first symptom, but other surgical emergencies that are potentially life-threatening and catastrophic do, including malrotation with volvulus, intussusception, and ovarian torsion.) The classic pattern associated with acute appendicitis—periumbilical visceral pain that travels to the right lower quadrant with subsequent nausea, vomiting, and anorexia—is found in only 50% of adults and is far less common in children younger than 12 years of age. For infants, vomiting, pain, diarrhea, fever, irritability, grunting, and refusal to walk or limp are just a few of the nonlocalizing symptoms of acute appendicitis that lead to misdiagnosis and high perforation rates. In children 2 to 5 years of age, the rate of appendicitis is low (less than 5%) but the more classic signs and symptoms are more common. The incidence of appendicitis increases in school-aged children and adolescents, and when the incidence peaks, so do the more common symptoms of vomiting, anorexia, and right lower quadrant pain.

  Right lower quadrant pain can also be associated with Crohn's disease, mesenteric adenitis associated with group A streptococcal pharyngitis, bacterial enterocolitis (particularly *Yersinia enterocolitica* and *Campylobacter jejuni*), Meckel diverticulitis, and intussusception. Right upper quadrant pain should prompt investigation of cholecystitis, cholelithiasis, Fitz-Hugh–Curtis syndrome, and right lower lobe pneumonia. Left upper quadrant pain often indicates splenomegaly, hemolytic crisis, or splenic trauma. Epigastric pain may indicate peptic disease (e.g., peptic ulcer disease, esophagitis secondary to gastroesophageal reflux disease, gastritis), or pancreatitis. Suprapubic pain can suggest a urinary tract infection (UTI), menstrual disorders, or pelvic inflammatory disease. Some disorders commonly cause radiation of pain and should always be investigated: back pain may be observed with pancreatitis or UTI, and gallstones frequently are associated with shoulder pain.

- Has there been a change in stool pattern, has there been blood in the stool, or is the pain relieved with defecation?

  — Questions regarding stool pattern and consistency are important in both acute and chronic abdominal pain. In the acute setting, diarrhea early in the history can point toward an infectious etiology such as viral or bacterial gastroenteritis. Additionally, rectal examination and examination of the stool gives important diagnostic information. Whereas bloody mucoid or currant-jelly stools are seen late in the course of intussusception, hemoccult positivity can be seen earlier. For more chronic etiologies, such as constipation, irritable bowel syndrome, and inflammatory bowel disease, these questions can also clarify the diagnosis.

- Is there associated emesis?

  — Although vomiting can occur with abdominal pain of various causes, vomiting in the absence of abdominal pain often indicates upper intestinal tract disease. Bilious emesis heralds obstruction.

- Can the examination reveal the cause of the abdominal pain?

  — If the diagnosis is unclear and surgical intervention remains a possibility, reassessment and reexamination by the same clinician is an important part of the evaluation. This is particularly important with diagnoses such as appendicitis, for which there is no definitive piece of historical, examination, or laboratory data that will make the diagnosis.

  Certain physical examination findings suggest the diagnosis. These include the Cullen sign (discoloration of the umbilicus) or Grey Turner sign (discoloration of the flank) in hemorrhagic pancreatitis, Murphy's sign (pain with deep palpation of the right upper quadrant) in gallbladder disease, and Rovsing's sign (pain in the right lower quadrant with palpation of the contralateral side) in appendicitis.

- Has there been an ingestion or toxin exposure?

  — Ingestion of certain medications or heavy metals (e.g., lead) can lead to chronic abdominal pain.

- Has there been a preceding illness or recent travel?

  — An upper respiratory tract infection frequently precedes intussusception; a mesenteric lymph node is thought to act as the lead point.

- Is there any significant family history?

  — The family history can be key in diseases such as inflammatory bowel disease and familial Mediterranean fever, as well as genetic disorders such as cystic fibrosis.

- What is the child's weight and height?

  — Failure to thrive indicates a more chronic disease, such as inflammatory bowel disease.

IV. References

1. Ruddy RM. Pain—Abdomen. In: Fleisher GR, Ludwig S, eds. *Textbook of pediatric emergency medicine*, 4th ed. Philadelphia: Lippincott Williams & Wilkins, 2000.
2. Kalloo AN. Overview of differential diagnoses of abdominal pain. *Gastrointes Endosc* 2002:56;255–257.
3. Ashcraft KW. Consultation with the specialist: acute abdominal pain. *Pediatr Rev* 2000:21;363–367.
4. Lake AM. Chronic abdominal pain in childhood: Diagnosis and management. *Am Fam Physician* 1999:59;1823–1830.
5. Thiessen PN. Recurrent abdominal pain. *Pediatr Rev* 2002:23;39–46.
6. Zeiter DK, Hyams JS. Recurrent abdominal pain in children. *Pediatr Clin N Am* 2002:49;53–71.
7. Brown KA. Abdominal Pain. In: Schwartz MW, ed. *The 5-minute pediatric consult*. Philadelphia: Lippincott Williams & Wilkins, 2000.
8. D'Agostino J. Common abdominal emergencies in children. *Emerg Med Clin North Am* 2002:20;139–153.
9. Douglas DA, et al. Irritable bowel syndrome: A technical review for practice guideline development. *Gastroenterol* 1997:112.
10. Okada PJ, Hicks B. Pediatric surgical emergencies: Neonatal surgical emergencies. *Clin Pediatr Emerg Med* 2002:3.
11. Tunnessen WW. Abdominal Pain. In: Tunnessen WW, ed. *Signs and symptoms in pediatrics*, 3rd ed. Philadelphia: Lippincott Williams & Wilkins, 1999.

The following cases represent less common causes of abdominal pain in childhood.

Case 7-1: 13-Year-Old Boy

I. History of Present Illness

A 13-year-old boy presented with recurrent abdominal pain. He reported intermittent right upper quadrant pain for the last year, which occurred two to three times per week and lasted about 1 hour. The pain was sharp and stabbing in nature. It was not associated with eating or defecation and did not radiate. He reported easy bruising, but denied any epistaxis, bloody or tarry stools, headache, nausea, or vomiting. He did report a 2-month history of tea-colored urine and a 5-pound weight loss.

II. Past Medical History

His past medical history was unremarkable. He was a full-term infant with no complications.

III. Physical Examination

T, 37.3°C; RR, 36/min; HR, 80 bpm; BP, 120/77 mm Hg

Height, 75th percentile; weight, 75th percentile

Initial examination revealed an alert and cooperative young man in no acute distress. Physical examination was remarkable for mild scleral icterus. There was good lung aeration bilaterally. On abdominal examination, he had normoactive bowel sounds and tenderness to palpation in the right upper quadrant. Hepatosplenomegaly was present, with the liver 4 cm below the right costal margin (with a span of 10 cm) and the spleen 6 cm below the left costal margin. He was a Tanner stage IV male with normal genitalia and no evidence of trauma. The skin examination was significant for bruises on the lower extremities. His neurologic examination was normal.

IV. Diagnostic Studies

Laboratory analysis revealed 3,400 white blood cells (WBCs)/mm^3, with 2% band forms, 61% segmented neutrophils, 27% lymphocytes, and 3% monocytes. The hemoglobin was 12.8g/dL, and there were 51,000 platelets/mm^3. The erythrocyte sedimentation rate (ESR) was slightly elevated at 12 mm/hour. The hepatic function panel revealed the following: total bilirubin, 2.5 mg/dL; alkaline phosphatase, 450 U/L; albumin, 2.6 g/dL; and elevated transaminases (aspartate aminotransferase, 266 U/L; alanine aminotransferase, 162 U/L; and γ-glutamyltransferase, 500 g/dL). Prothrombin (PT) and partial thromboplastin (PTT) times were 13 and 32 seconds, respectively. Fibrin split products, hepatitis A, hepatitis B, hepatitis C, and monospot testing were all negative. A urinalysis revealed small bilirubin, moderate blood (0 to 2 red blood cells), and a urobilinogen concentration of 2.0 mg.

V. Course of Illness

The patient was hospitalized and an emergency abdominal ultrasound examination was performed, which showed portal venous thrombosis with evidence of portal hypertension, cirrhosis, cholelithiasis, and splenomegaly. There was no evidence of ascites. An enzyme-linked immunosorbent assay (ELISA) test for human immunodeficiency virus (HIV) was negative; an antineutrophil cytoplasm antibody (ANCA) titer was negative; and an antinuclear antibody (ANA) titer was 1:80. Urine copper was elevated at 296 µg/24 hours (normal range, less than 100 µg/24 hours), but ceruloplasmin was within the normal range at 53 mg/dL (normal, 25 to 63 mg/dL). A liver biopsy confirmed the diagnosis (Fig. 7-1).

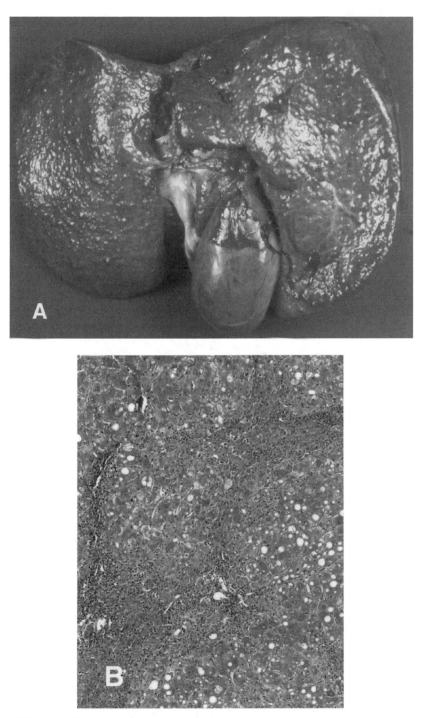

FIG. 7-1. Histopathologic specimens for case 7-1, demonstrating gross appearance of the liver **(A)**, Masson trichrome stain, 100× **(B)**, and Rhodanine stain, 400× **(C)**. (Photomicrographs courtesy of Dr. Bruce Pawel.)

Continued on next page.

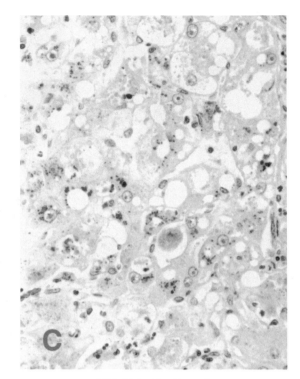

FIG. 7-1. *Continued.*

DISCUSSION: CASE 7-1

I.   Differential Diagnosis

In the pediatric population, the causes of liver disease, in particular hyperbilirubinemia and cirrhosis, are diverse. Common causes include infectious diseases such as viral infections (hepatitis A, B, and C; cytomegalovirus; coxsackievirus; Epstein-Barr virus), bacterial infections, fungal infections, and parasitic infections. Inflammatory causes include ulcerative colitis, ascending cholangitis, and autoimmune hepatitis. Drugs and toxins are another important cause to explore, because common medications such as acetaminophen and acetylsalicylic acid and toxins such as iron can cause liver damage. The differential diagnosis also includes causes of biliary obstruction such as cholecystitis, cholelithiasis, biliary atresia, arteriohepatic dysplasia (Alagille syndrome), primary sclerosing cholangitis, fibrosing pancreatitis, and choledochal cysts. In addition, there is a long and important list of genetic and metabolic diseases that must be ruled out, which includes cystic fibrosis, α_1-antitrypsin deficiency, Wilson disease, and several others.

II.   Diagnosis

Gross appearance of the liver in a patient with a similar condition revealed micronodular cirrhosis (Fig. 7-1A). Histologic examination revealed micronodular cirrhosis with portal–portal bridging, chronic portal inflammation, and fatty change (Fig. 7-1B). Rhodanine stain demonstrated copper (red-brown particulate material) within hepatocytes (Fig. 7-1C). The patient was treated with penicillamine and pyridoxine. Over the next several months, there were improvements in liver function and a stable platelet count of 65,000/mm^3. **The diagnosis is Wilson disease.**

III. Incidence and Pathophysiology

Wilson disease, or hepatolenticular degeneration, was described by Kinnier Wilson in 1912 as a degenerative disease of the central nervous system with asymptomatic cirrhosis, but cases were first recognized as early as the 1880s. Wilson disease is a rare autosomal recessive disorder and is the most common genetic disorder of copper metabolism. Homozygotes for the disease inherit mutations of both alleles of the *ATP7B* gene on chromosome 13. The incidence is 1 in 500,000 to 1,000,000 births. The prevalence of homozygotes with disease is approximately 1 in 30,000. The frequency of heterozygotes (with a single mutation) or carriers is approximately 1 in 90. The disease is found worldwide, but the rate is higher among homogeneous, physically isolated, or culturally isolated populations.

Although copper is a vital trace element and coenzyme for several enzymatic systems, biliary excretion is important to keep the body's copper load in balance. In Wilson disease, the inherited defect in the biliary system's excretion of copper leads to excess copper deposition in the brain, liver, and other organs. Copper's toxic effects include generation of free radicals, lipid peroxidation of membranes and DNA, inhibition of protein synthesis, and altered levels of cellular antioxidants.

IV. Clinical Presentation

The clinical presentation of Wilson disease is variable, with 42% of patients presenting with hepatic manifestations, 34% with neurologic disease, and 10% with psychiatric disease. Although clinical presentation is rare before 5 years of age, symptomatic cases have been reported. Because initial copper accumulation occurs in the liver, in the pediatric population hepatic manifestations usually precede neurologic manifestations. Neurologic symptoms are more common in the second to third decade of life.

Missed or delayed diagnosis of Wilson disease stems from the nonspecific array of clinical manifestations. Very young patients who are diagnosed through family screening or by the incidental finding of Kayser-Fleischer rings on examination are said to be asymptomatic or presymptomatic. There is also wide variability in the spectrum of liver disease seen, ranging from asymptomatic with biochemical abnormalities to acute hepatitis, chronic active hepatitis, cirrhosis, and fulminant hepatic failure. There is a female predominance (2:1) of fulminant hepatic failure in Wilson disease. Central nervous system manifestations include neurologic symptoms (dystonia, tremors, dysarthria, gait disturbance, choreiform movements) and psychiatric symptoms (poor school performance, anxiety, depression, neuroses, psychoses). The ophthalmologic manifestation of the characteristic and diagnostically helpful Kayser-Fleisher rings is a result of accumulation of copper in the cornea and does not affect the function of the eye. Other tissues and systems in which copper deposition does have damaging effects include the endocrine, renal, skeletal, and cardiac systems. Hemolytic anemia of unclear etiology is a common complication of Wilson disease and can be the first manifestation of the disease.

V. Diagnostic Approach

The serious sequelae of a delayed diagnosis indicate that Wilson disease should be seriously considered and investigated in any patient between 3 and 40 years of age who has any unexplained liver or neurologic disease. This is particularly important in children and adolescents with extrapyramidal or cerebellar motor disorders, atypical psychiatric disease, unexplained hemolysis, and elevated transaminases, either with or without a family history of liver or neurologic disease. Additionally, individuals who are asymptomatic but whose family member has confirmed or suspected Wilson disease should be investigated. Because the classic triad of hepatic disease, neurologic involvement, and

Kayser-Fleischer rings usually is not present in the pediatric population, a combination of clinical findings, biochemical tests, and sometimes genetic testing is necessary to establish the diagnosis.

Ophthalmologic examination. Ophthalmic slit-lamp examination of the cornea can demonstrate the characteristic golden-green granular deposits of Kayser-Fleischer rings in patients with concomitant neurologic manifestations. Given the presence of similar corneal rings in other diseases and the frequent absence of Kayser-Fleischer rings in the pediatric population, their presence or absence neither confirms nor negates the presence of Wilson disease. In the presence of neurologic disease, magnetic resonance imaging (MRI) of the brain can delineate the changes commonly seen in the basal ganglia.

Serum ceruloplasmin. Ceruloplasmin is a serum glycoprotein that is synthesized in the liver and contains six copper atoms. The mutation in Wilson disease affects this transport system for copper and leads to decreased incorporation of copper into ceruloplasmin and decreased circulating levels of copper. Therefore, in Wilson disease serum ceruloplasmin is decreased. However, low ceruloplasmin levels can also be seen in other conditions, such as protein-losing enteropathy or nephrotic syndrome, and even in heterozygotes for Wilson disease. Furthermore, ceruloplasmin is an acute phase reactant and can be in the normal range in individuals with Wilson disease. Its production is also induced by hormonal contraceptives.

Urinary copper. Serum copper levels cannot be used in diagnosis of Wilson disease, but their determination is helpful in monitoring adherence and response to therapy. Urinary copper excretion is usually very high (more than 100 μg/24 hours) in symptomatic patients.

Liver biopsy. Currently, liver biopsy with measurement of hepatic copper concentration remains the mainstay of diagnosis. A liver copper concentration of more than 250 μg/g of dry tissue (five times the normal concentration), in combination with characteristic histologic findings on light assay or electron microscopy, is currently considered diagnostic for the disease.

Other studies. In settings in which histologic findings cannot be confirmed, stable copper isotope studies have replaced radioisotope studies for the determination of copper metabolism. The test is helpful only in patients with normal serum ceruloplasmin levels. The genetic heterogeneity of the condition makes the available DNA studies unhelpful diagnostically unless there is a family member in whom Wilson disease has been diagnosed and confirmed.

VI.   Treatment

Therapy should be initiated immediately after confirmation of the disease and continued for the remainder of the patient's life. The goal of therapy is to eliminate symptoms and prevent disease progression. The armamentarium of treatment includes dietary measures, pharmacologic therapy, and liver transplantation.

Although a low-copper diet does not play a large role in the treatment of the disease, it is important for patients to avoid heavy copper-containing foods such as shellfish, nuts, and chocolate.

Penicillamine, an orally administered copper chelator, decreases the body's pool of copper by increasing urinary copper excretion and can effectively reduce or eliminate the effects of copper toxicity. The antipyridoxine effects of penicillamine necessitate concomitant administration of pyridoxine three times a week. The dose can be increased if there is no clinical improvement or decrease in excretion of urinary copper. Adherence to therapy is followed with measurement of either urinary or serum copper and serum ceruloplasmin. Side effects are more common with higher doses. Sensitivity reactions, which include fever, rash, leukopenia, thrombocytopenia, and lymphadenopathy, occur in 10% of patients but can often be overcome with gradual reinstitution of the medication. Penicillamine has consistently shown the successful results, with improvement in liver biopsy findings over time.

Trientine hydrochloride is an alternative chelating agent, particularly for patients with side effects such as nephrotoxicity and lupus-like syndrome from penicillamine. Although there is less urinary copper excretion with this agent, it appears to be equally effective clinically. Iron deficiency or sideroblastic anemia can be seen. Administration of zinc salts three times daily seems to protect hepatocytes by inducing metallothionein in enterocytes, which blocks the intestinal absorption of copper. Sometimes, British antilewisite (dimercaprol) is the only effective agent; it can be particularly helpful in patients with progressive neurologic disease that is unresponsive to treatment with penicillamine, trientine, or zinc.

The indications for liver transplantation in patients with liver disease include acute hepatic failure (especially in association with hemolysis), advanced cirrhosis with decompensation, hepatic insufficiency that progresses in the face of adequate treatment with chelation therapy, and progressive and irreversible neurologic disease (even in the absence of severe hepatic disease). Patients receiving liver transplants display total reversal of the biochemical abnormalities they had previously. Survival rates are variable but have been reported as high as 79% at 1 year.

Future directions of treatment include gene therapy, but presently early detection and chelation therapy are still the most important aspects of treatment.

VII. References

1. Tunnessen WW. Jaundice. In: Tunnessen WW, ed. *Signs and symptoms in pediatrics,* 3rd ed. Philadelphia: Lippincott Williams & Wilkins, 1999:102–112 and 440–447.
2. Chitkara DK, Pleskow RG, Grand RJ. Wilson disease. In: Walker WA, Durie PR, Hamilton JR, et al., eds. *Pediatric gastrointestinal disease,* 3rd ed. Hamilton, Ontario: BC Decker, 2000:1171–1184.
3. Pearce JM. Wilson's disease. *J Neurol Neurosurg Psychiatry* 1997;63:174.
4. Robertson WM. Wilson's disease. *Arch Neurol* 2000;57:276–277.
5. Schilsky ML, Tavill AS. Wilson's disease. In: Schiff ER, Sorell MG, Maddrey WC, eds. *Schiff's diseases of the liver,* 8th ed. Philadelphia: Lippincott–Raven Publishers, 1999:1091–1106.
6. Gaffney D, Fell GS, O'Reilly DS. Wilson's disease: acute and presymptomatic laboratory diagnosis and monitoring. ACP Best Practice No. 163. *J Clin Pathol* 2000;53: 807–812.
7. Sternlieb I. Wilson's disease. *Clin Liver Dis* 2000;4:229–239.
8. Wilson DC, Phillips MJ, Cox DW, et al. Severe hepatic Wilson's disease in preschool-aged children. *J Pediatr* 2000;137:719–722.
9. Balistreri WF. Wilson disease. In: Behrman RE, et al., eds. *Nelson's textbook of pediatrics,* 16th ed. Philadelphia: WB Saunders, 2000.
10. Khanna A, Jain A, Eghtesad B, et al. Liver transplantation for metabolic liver diseases. *Surg Clin North Am* 1999;79:153–162.
11. Durand F, Bernuau J, Giostra E, et al. Wilson's disease with severe hepatic insufficiency: beneficial effects of early administration of D-penicillamine. *Gut* 2001;48: 849–852.

Case 7-2: 5-Year-Old Girl

I. History of Present Illness

A 5-year-old girl was well until 2 days before presentation, when she developed emesis and fever. On the day of presentation, she had two bouts of nonbloody, nonbilious emesis and continued to have fever as high as 39.4°C. The patient pointed to the periumbilical area when describing her pain. Her parents also reported that she had had ear pain and a sore throat for the past 3 days. They denied cough, dysuria, and frequency. She had had a good appetite and no weight loss. The parents reported that about 6 months ago the patient had an episode of abdominal pain. Her primary care physician reportedly felt stool in the abdomen and started her on prune juice. which she had stopped using regularly.

II. Past Medical History

Birth history was normal, with no complications at delivery or birth. She had had mild asthma but no hospitalizations. Three years earlier, she was exposed to tuberculosis and had a positive tuberculin skin test. She was treated with isoniazid for 9 months.

III. Physical Examination

T, 39°C; RR, 24/min; HR, 119 bpm; BP, 106/65 mm Hg

Weight, 22.9 kg (70th percentile); height, 120 cm (70th percentile)

Physical examination revealed an alert, well-nourished, and interactive child. There was no conjunctival pallor. The tonsils were 2+ bilaterally, with mild erythema of the posterior pharynx. Shotty cervical lymphadenopathy was present, with enlarged superior cervical lymph nodes that were mobile and nontender. The lungs were clear, and there was a I/IV systolic ejection murmur at the left lower sternal border. The abdominal examination revealed normal bowel sounds. On palpation, the abdomen was nontender, but a

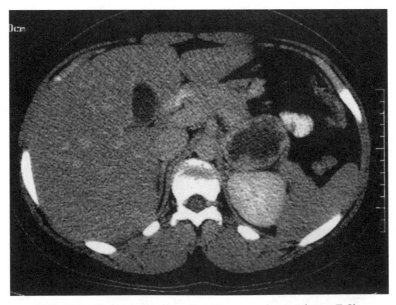

FIG. 7-2. Abdominal magnetic resonance image (case 7-2).

firm mass was felt in the periumbilical region and left upper quadrant. The mass had sharp borders, was approximately 6 × 4 cm, and was slightly mobile. Rectal examination revealed good rectal tone. The rectal vault was full of stool, which was negative for occult blood. She was a Tanner I female with no inguinal lymphadenopathy. Her neurologic examination was normal.

IV. Diagnostic Studies

Laboratory analysis revealed 11,500 WBCs/mm^3, with 2% band forms, 62% segmented neutrophils, 24% lymphocytes, and 9% monocytes. The hemoglobin was 14.3 g/dL, and the platelet count was 251,000/mm^3. Electrolytes, blood urea nitrogen, creatinine, calcium, magnesium, and phosphorus were normal. Liver function tests were normal. The uric acid concentration was 5.3 mg/dL, and the lactate dehydrogenase concentration was 747 U/L. The abdominal radiograph revealed a large amount of stool.

V. Course of Illness

A Fleet enema was given with good results, but the mass was still palpable. Abdominal MRI suggested a diagnostic category (Fig. 7-2). Biopsy of the mass confirmed the diagnosis.

DISCUSSION: CASE 7-2

I. Differential Diagnosis

The finding of an abdominal mass in a child is important and that can be attributed to causes as varied as bladder distention and life-threatening malignancies. The age of the patient, history, physical examination, and specific laboratory and imaging studies are crucial to arriving at the correct diagnosis. Children younger than 5 years of age are the group in which abdominal masses are most commonly identified, and about 60% of abdominal masses that are identified in childhood by physical examination are secondary to organomegaly.

In neonates, retroperitoneal masses that arise from the genitourinary system are the most common type; causes include hydronephrosis, multicystic/polycystic kidneys, mesoblastic nephroma, and renal vein thrombosis, which is seen in infants of diabetic mothers and in those with severe hydration. Other possible causes include pelvic masses such as an ovarian cyst or hydrometrocolpos, which manifests with a suprapubic mass and vomiting as a result of hydronephrosis from obstruction of the ureters. GI causes include intestinal duplication, malrotation, and sacrococcygeal teratoma. Bladder distention, often as a consequence of posterior urethral valves, can also be common in the neonatal period. Hydronephrosis and multicystic/polycystic disease account for as many as 75% of the abdominal masses in neonates.

In infants, the most common malignant solid tumor is neuroblastoma. In childhood, Wilms tumor is the most common childhood abdominal malignancy. The classic presentation is that of an asymptomatic child with an abdominal mass noted by a parent while bathing the child. More than half of Wilms tumors manifest before 5 years of age. Neuroblastomas that arise in the abdomen often cross the midline, and more than half are seen within the first 2 years of life. The tumor can produce catecholamines and therefore can be clinically associated with tachycardia, hypertension, and skin flushing. The variability of the site of the primary tumor makes the clinical presentation variable, but constitutional symptoms such as fever and weight loss often occur. Other retroperitoneal masses seen in infants in children include rhabdomyosarcoma, lymphoma, Ewing's sarcoma, and germ cell neoplasm. There are several liver lesions that can cause abdominal masses in this age group, including benign solid tumors, malignant tumors, vascular lesions, and cystic hepatobiliary disease. In addition, lesions of the stomach (carcinoma, leiomyosarcoma, fibrosarcoma), small bowel (duplication, Meckel diverticulum, lymphoma), colon (fecal mass is also common), and omentum can cause abdominal masses in this age group.

Many of the causes of abdominal masses in infants and children also apply to adolescents, but there are some diagnoses that are more common (pelvic masses in particular). Hematocolpos may not be clinically evident until menarche. Ovarian cystic lesions are common, and more than 85% are benign, with teratomas as the most common lesion of this type. Malignant ovarian lesions include germ cell tumors, dysgerminomas, choriocarcinomas, and gonadoblastomas. In the retroperitoneal region, renal cell carcinoma occurs most commonly at 14 years of age and manifests with flank pain and hematuria.

Physical examination is the most important aspect of early detection of abdominal masses in children. A recent study showed that the majority of malignant abdominal masses in children could be palpated on initial examination.

II.   Diagnosis

MRI of the abdomen (Fig. 7-2) revealed a 6×4.5 cm, multiloculated mass arising from the left adrenal gland. There were no other retroperitoneal masses. During recovery, the biopsy of the tumor revealed ganglioneuroma. A metaiodobenzylguanidine (MIBG) scan was negative, confirming that the tumor was entirely a ganglioneuroma. A chemotherapy protocol was begun to reduce the size of the mass before resection. **The diagnosis is adrenal ganglioneuroma.**

III.   Incidence and Epidemiology

There is a spectrum of neuroblastoma tumors that includes ganglioneuromas, neuroblastomas, and ganglioneuroblastomas that arise from neural crest cells. Unlike neuroblastomas, ganglioneuromas are benign and differentiated tumors. Although the incidence of ganglioneuromas is not known, they are most common in children and young adults. They usually are found in the posterior mediastinum and retroperitoneum, and most often arise from the adrenal medulla. Much like pheochromocytomas, which are tumors of chromaffin cells of the adrenal medulla and adrenergic ganglia, adrenal ganglioneuromas can secrete epinephrine and norepinephrine, giving rise to endocrinologic symptoms. There have been reports of malignant transformation of ganglioneuromas to neuroblastoma and of mixed tumors with pheochromocytoma.

IV.   Clinical Presentation

Apart from the mass effect of any abdominal mass, ganglioneuromas can secrete catecholamines and can cause the paraneoplastic syndrome seen with pheochromocytomas. Hypertension is the most concerning sign, and symptoms can include perspiration, tremor, nausea, vomiting, diarrhea, and other manifestations of Cushing syndrome. Because ganglioneuromas can be associated with neurofibromatosis type I or with von Recklinghausen's disease, clinical manifestations of this disease (e.g., axillary freckling, café-au-lait spots) may be noted.

V.   Diagnostic Approach

Evaluation of an adrenal mass should include studies to detect ganglioneuroma, pheochromocytoma, and neuroblastoma.

Abdominal imaging. The initial study is usually an abdominal radiograph to exclude GI obstruction. Some clinicians next obtain an ultrasound study to determine the organ or origin and identify cysts, hemorrhage, and calcification. Compute tomography (CT) or MRI may be used in lieu of ultrasound. The adrenal gland can be clearly visualized by CT in 95% of patients. In distinguishing pheochromocytoma from other adrenal masses, MRI has a positive predictive value of 83% and a negative predictive value approaching

100%. Additional imaging of the head, spine, or chest may be indicated to exclude metastatic disease.

Complete blood count (CBC). Pancytopenia indicates bone marrow involvement due to malignancy. Isolated anemia suggests either chronic illness or hemorrhage into the mass.

Electrolytes, calcium, phosphorus, uric acid, and lactate dehydrogenase. Abnormalities in these studies are seen with tumor lysis syndrome.

Urine homovanillic acid (HVA) and vanillymandelic acid (VMA). In a patient with an adrenal mass, a spot-check of the urine for HVA and VMA should be obtained to detect neuroblastoma or pheochromocytoma.

Other studies. Plasma concentrations of normetanephrines or metanephrines above the upper reference limits (4 and 2.5 times normal, respectively) indicate a pheochromocytoma with 100% specificity.

VI. Treatment

Treatment of an abdominal ganglioneuroma depends on the patient's clinical manifestations. In general, resection is curative. If the patient has endocrinologic manifestations, they should be stabilized medically before resection.

VII. References

1. Tunnessen WW. Abdominal masses. In: Tunnessen WW, ed. *Signs and symptoms in pediatrics,* 3rd ed. Philadelphia: Lippincott Williams & Wilkins, 1999:484–488.
2. Squires RH. Abdominal masses. In: Walker WA, Durie PR, Hamilton JR, et al., eds. *Pediatric gastrointestinal disease,* 3rd ed. Hamilton, Ontario: BC Decker, 2000: 150–163.
3. Golden CB, Feusner JH. Malignant abdominal masses in children: quick guide to evaluation and diagnosis. *Pediatr Clin North Am* 2002;49:1369–1392.
4. Stratakis CA, Chrousos GP. Endocrine tumors. In: Pizzo PA, Poplack DG, eds. *Principles and practice of pediatric oncology,* 3rd ed. Philadelphia: Lippincott–Raven Publishers, 1997:947–976.
5. Pacak K, Linehan WM, Eisenhoffer G, et al. Recent advances in genetics, diagnosis, localization, and treatment of pheochromocytoma. *Ann Intern Med* 2001;134: 315–329.
6. Celik V, Unal G, Ozgultekin R, et al. Adrenal ganglioneuroma. *Br J Surg* 1996;83:263.

Case 7-3: 11-Year-Old Girl

I. History of Present Illness

The patient, an 11-year-old girl, was well until 1 year before presentation, when she was diagnosed with streptococcal pharyngitis. At that time, she had severe abdominal pain that caused her to double over in pain. Appendicitis was considered, and an abdominal radiograph showed an enlarged loop of bowel. The patient was observed, but neither the clinical picture nor the laboratory results suggested appendicitis, and no surgery was performed. Throat culture revealed a group A *Streptococcus* infection, which was treated. Since that illness, the patient had had multiple illnesses and missed 42 days of school with episodes of headache and abdominal pain. The pain was described as noncrampy but sharp. It consisted of generalized lower abdominal discomfort without radiation. During this time, the patient was diagnosed with three UTIs secondary to pyuria on urinalysis, but all cultures were negative. Her symptoms had been particularly bad since she was diagnosed with mononucleosis 3 months before presentation. She had had a poor appetite and had lost 10 pounds with the mononucleosis and 8 more pounds since then. At presentation, she had decreased intake secondary to a sore throat and difficulty swallowing secondary to pain. She had just completed a full course of antibiotics for pharyngitis, which was diagnosed clinically 3 weeks earlier (cultures were negative). The patient had been missing half-days of school for 2 months and had been sleeping in the afternoons. During the week of presentation, she had had low-grade fevers (37.4 to 37.8°C), neck pain, diffuse abdominal pain, and frontal headache. On the day of admission, the patient was noted to have heme-positive stool at the primary care provider's office after 3 days of diarrhea and loose stools. The primary care provider's workup to date had included a CT scan of the head and sinuses, which was negative; stool for culture, which was also negative; CBC, urinalysis, ESR, Lyme antibody testing, immunoglobulins, ANA, chest radiography, electrolytes, liver function tests, and thyroid testing, all of which were normal.

II. Past Medical History

The patient had had reactive airways disease as a toddler, but it was no longer active. She had had a UTI at 5 years of age, with a negative ultrasound and a vesicoureterogram that could not be completed because of her discomfort. She had sustained a concussion at day camp 2 years earlier. She had no surgical history and was taking no medications except for occasional albuterol with colds. Family history was significant for a maternal grandmother with diverticulitis, a maternal grandfather with ulcers, and a paternal grandmother with irritable bowel syndrome. There was no history of inflammatory bowel disease or childhood illnesses. The patient was in fifth grade and had done very well in school and been very involved in sports before this illness. The patient reported that she missed school and her friends.

III. Physical Examination

T, 38.1°C; RR, 24/min; HR, 124 bpm; BP, 105/71 mm Hg

Weight, 37 kg (75th percentile); height, 155 cm (90th percentile)

Physical examination revealed a thin Caucasian girl who appeared tired and anxious. There was erythema of the pharynx with enlarged tonsils and cobblestoning. There was no exudate and no asymmetry of the tonsillar crypts or soft palate. She had good dentition, halitosis, and cracked red lips. Her neck was supple with no adenopathy. Lungs were clear to auscultation. Cardiac examination revealed no murmurs, rubs, or gallops.

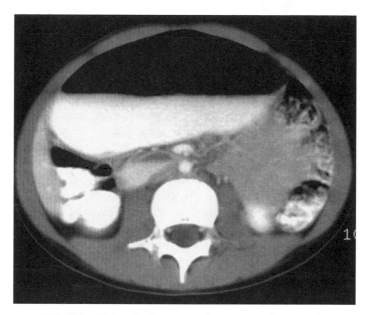

FIG. 7-3. Abdominal computed tomogram (case 7-3).

Abdominal examination revealed good bowel sounds in all four quadrants. There was diffuse tenderness but no guarding, no rebound, and no hepatosplenomegaly. Rectal examination revealed no excoriation, skin tags, fissures, or hemorrhoids. She had good rectal tone without any palpable masses. She was a Tanner II female, and there were no obvious vaginal lesions. The neurologic examination was normal.

IV. Diagnostic Studies

The CBC revealed a 5,800 WBCs/mm^3. Hemoglobin and platelets were normal. ESR was also normal at 14 mm/hour. Electrolytes were as follows: sodium, 144 mEq/L; potassium, 4.2mEq/L; chloride, 101 mEq/L; bicarbonate, 31 mEq/L; blood urea nitrogen, 7 mg/dL, and creatinine, 0.6 mg/dL. Urinalysis showed a high specific gravity of 1.036 as well as 1+ protein, small bacteria, and large mucus. A rapid strep test was positive for group A streptococcal antigen. Amylase was 40 U/L, and lipase was 53 U/L. Stool cultures grew normal flora, and *Clostridium difficile* testing was negative. Abdominal radiographs were normal except for scoliosis of the lumbar spine. There was no obstruction.

V. Course of Illness

An abdominal CT revealed the diagnosis (Fig. 7-3).

DISCUSSION: CASE 7-3

I. Differential Diagnosis

Weight loss in children is a concerning symptom that requires careful thought, especially if it is associated with abdominal pain. Oncologic processes should be considered and are frequently the biggest concern for parents. Acute and chronic infections are probably the most common cause of weight loss in children. With acute infections such as mononucleosis or pharyngitis, the child should regain the weight once the infection clears. The continuing weight loss in this patient is one of the most concerning elements of the history. In such cases, more chronic, insidious infections, such as an abdominal abscess, chronic hepatitis, intestinal parasites, tuberculosis, UTI, or HIV infection, must be considered.

With associated abdominal pain, GI disorders such as chronic constipation, gastroesophageal reflux disease, inflammatory bowel disease (examination of trends in growth parameters is key), pancreatitis, malabsorptive disorders such as celiac disease, and superior mesenteric artery syndrome must be considered.

Endocrinologic disorders associated with weight loss include Addison's disease (abdominal pain and skin discoloration frequently seen), diabetes mellitus (with associated polyphagia, polydipsia, and polyuria), and hyperthyroidism. Cardiopulmonary disorders include asthma, chronic congestive heart failure, cystic fibrosis, and an untreated cardiac disease. Other causes include nutritional deficiencies (iron and zinc), neurologic diseases (increased intracranial disorders that lead to headache and neurodegenerative disorders), connective tissue diseases, and renal failure.

The most common causes of weight loss, particularly in adolescent girls, are dieting, increased physical activity, depression, anorexia nervosa, and bulimia. Although an eating disorder was a possibility in this patient due to her age and preceding illness, it could not explain her associated abdominal pain.

II. Diagnosis

Abdominal CT revealed abnormal dilation of the stomach and proximal duodenum, with tapering of the second part of the duodenum to the level of the space between the superior mesenteric artery and the aorta, consistent with superior mesenteric artery syndrome (Fig. 7-3). **The diagnosis is superior mesenteric artery syndrome.**

III. Incidence and Epidemiology

Superior mesenteric artery syndrome is an uncommon disorder that has also been referred to as cast syndrome, Wilkie's syndrome, duodenal ileus, and arteriomesenteric duodenal compression syndrome. The obstruction is extrinsic and either acute, chronic, or intermittent. It is caused by compression of the transverse portion of the duodenum by the superior mesenteric artery anteriorly and by the aorta and vertebral column posteriorly, which causes classic "megaduodenum" on upper GI series. Although the syndrome was first described in 1861 by Von Rokitansky, many have disputed its existence, believing that it has been confused with other causes of megaduodenum, such as diabetes, collagen vascular diseases, and other causes of chronic intestinal pseudo-obstruction.

The syndrome is most common in older children and adolescents, and it is more common in girls and in those individuals who have risk factors for narrowing the angle between the aorta and the superior mesenteric artery, which results in compression of the duodenum. These risk factors include linear growth during the growth spurt that is not accompanied by weight gain, extreme lumbar lordosis, rapid weight loss that markedly decreases the mesenteric fat pad, severe trauma or surgery that necessitates prolonged bed rest, use of a body cast, and scoliosis surgery. Anatomic predisposition is present in individuals with a short suspensory ligament of Treitz. Recently, there has been a connection with eating disorders, in that the syndrome can appear clinically like an eating disorder and can sometimes precipitate an eating disorder because of the development of food avoidance to avoid pain.

IV. Clinical Presentation

Presenting symptoms can be either acute or chronic (usually with exacerbations) and typically include epigastric and abdominal pain, bilious emesis, and pain after eating. Infrequently, patients present with small-bowel obstruction. Patients with severe cases that have gone undiagnosed may present with signs of malnutrition and dehydration with prostration and electrolyte abnormalities.

V. Diagnostic Approach

Abdominal imaging. Although plain abdominal radiographs are often normal, they can show gastric distention. The diagnosis is usually made by upper GI series, which shows dilatation of the first two portions of the duodenum with a cutoff at the third potion of the duodenum. Hypotonic duodenography can also display the site of obstruction, and CT can provide more detailed information about the aortomesenteric angle and anatomic issues that are creating the obstruction.

VI. Treatment

Treatment should begin with stabilization of the patient. To avoid gastric perforation, nasogastric decompression should be performed and intravenous fluids administered to correct electrolyte imbalances. The patient should be counseled to avoid the supine position, which exacerbates the obstruction, and to remain either upright or in the left lateral decubitus position to open up the aortomesenteric angle. Although some patients cannot tolerate even slow nasogastric feeds, parental nutrition is rarely warranted and nasojejunal feeds are often successful. Metoclopramide may help the patient tolerate feeds. Treatment is conservative until weight gain is achieved. Surgical interventions such as the Ladd procedure or duodenojejunostomy are indicated in cases recalcitrant to other therapies.

VII. References

1. Tunnessen WW. Weight loss. In: Tunnessen WW, ed. *Signs and symptoms in pediatrics,* 3rd ed. Philadelphia: Lippincott Williams & Wilkins, 1999:36–40.
2. Wesson DE, Haddock G. The surgical abdomen. In: Walker WA, Durie PR, Hamilton JR, et al., eds. *Pediatric gastrointestinal disease,* 3rd ed. Hamilton, Ontario: BC Decker, 2000:435–444.
3. Shetty AK, Schmidt-Sommerfeld E, Haymon ML, et al. Radiological case of the month: superior mesenteric artery syndrome. *Arch Pediatr Adolesc Med* 1999;153: 303–304.
4. Jordaan GP, Muller A, Greeff M, et al. Eating disorder and superior mesenteric artery syndrome. *J Am Acad Child Adolesc Psychiatry* 2000;39:1211.
5. Crowther MA, Webb PJ, Eyre-Brock IA. Superior mesenteric artery syndrome following surgery for scoliosis. *Spine* 2002;27:e528–e533.

Case 7-4: 9-Year-Old Girl

I. History of Present Illness

A 9-year-old girl was well until 6 days before admission, when she developed vomiting, abdominal pain, and lethargy. Four days before admission, she was noted to have a fever to 38.9°C and cough. She was seen by her pediatrician 3 days before presentation and was diagnosed with a lower lobe pneumonia with referred abdominal pain. She was treated with amoxicillin. Over the next 2 days, she had worsening of her abdominal pain and increased listlessness. There had been no recent symptoms of upper respiratory tract infection and no diarrhea. Her mother reported that the whites of her eyes had looked yellow for the past 3 weeks.

II. Past Medical History

The patient had had no major illnesses or hospitalizations. She had had four episodes of dizziness over the past 5 months that had been evaluated with an electroencephalogram (EEG) and an electrocardiogram (ECG), both of which were normal. She was not taking medications except amoxicillin for her diagnosis of pneumonia. The family history was significant only for several family members with diabetes mellitus. The mother had required a splenectomy after blunt abdominal trauma.

III. Physical Examination

T, 37.4°C; RR, 30/min; HR, 118 bpm; BP, 91/50 mm Hg; SpO_2, 94% on room air
Weight, 27.9 kg (25th percentile)

The patient was responsive but withdrawn. Physical examination revealed mildly icteric sclera, no oral lesions, and no pharyngeal injection. The neck was supple with shotty lymphadenopathy. The lungs were clear, with equal breath sounds bilaterally. Cardiac examination revealed a normal precordium, mild tachycardia, normal S_1 and S_2 sounds, no gallop, and no murmur. The abdomen was soft and nontender with normal bowel sounds; the liver was palpated 4 cm below the right costal margin, and the spleen tip was palpable. The extremities were warm, but there were diminished pulses in both the upper and lower extremities. The neurologic examination was normal, and the skin revealed no rash.

IV. Diagnostic Studies

A CBC revealed a 9,600 WBCs/mm^3, with 72% segmented neutrophils and 23% lymphocytes. The hemoglobin and platelets were normal. PT, PTT, electrolytes, blood urea nitrogen, and creatinine were all normal. A hepatic function panel revealed a bilirubin concentration of 3.2 mg/dL, with an unconjugated bilirubin concentration of 1.8 mg/dL. Albumin was 3.8 g/dL; alkaline phosphatase, 78 U/L; aspartate transaminase, 54 U/L; lactate dehydrogenase, 237 U/L; and uric acid, 7.3 mg/dL. Lipase was 168 U/L and amylase 63 U/L. An ECG revealed a sinus rhythm at 129 bpm, a PR interval of 0.144 seconds, right axis deviation, normal voltage, and no ST-segment changes. The chest radiograph was abnormal (Fig. 7-4).

V. Course of Illness

The patient had an echocardiogram, which revealed a markedly dilated left ventricle to 5.4 cm, moderate to severe mitral regurgitation, and a markedly decreased shortening fraction of 10% to 18%. Furosemide and milrinone were started. Despite increasing doses, by the fourth hospital day the patient had distended neck veins, increasing dyspnea, cough, and lethargy. Repeat echocardiography showed a decrease in the shortening fraction to less than 10%, with a dilated and thin-walled left ventricle, persistent severe

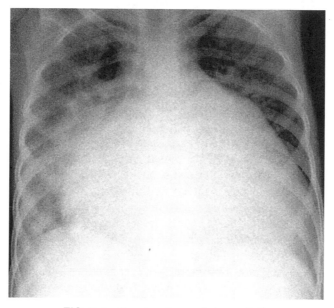

FIG. 7-4. Chest radiograph (case 7-4).

mitral regurgitation, moderate tricuspid regurgitation, and a right ventricular pressure 30 mm greater than that of the right atrium.

DISCUSSION: CASE 7-4

I. Differential Diagnosis

Myocarditis and other forms of heart disease are possible causes for abdominal pain. Cardiomegaly on this patient's chest radiograph gave the first indication of heart disease and heart failure. A possible cause of this heart failure is congenital heart disease, particularly septal lesions, which must be ruled out in the pediatric population at any age. Other possible causes include dilated cardiomyopathy, hypertrophic cardiomyopathy, restrictive cardiomyopathy, arrhythmogenic right ventricular dysplasia, obliterative cardiomyopathy, inflammatory cardiomyopathy (myocarditis), and giant cell myocarditis. In pediatrics, it is most helpful to make the more broad distinction between cardiomyopathy and myocarditis.

II. Diagnosis

Chest radiography revealed dramatic cardiomegaly and prominence of the pulmonary vasculature (Fig. 7-4). Cardiac catheterization with endomyocardial biopsy was done, and the patient was noted to have a decreased cardiac index of 1.47 mm/m^2, a left ventricular end-diastolic pressure of 35 mm Hg, an increased pulmonary capillary wedge pressure of 38 mm Hg, and a right atrial pressure of 18 mm Hg. Biopsy revealed no inflammatory cells. The patient was diagnosed with idiopathic dilated cardiomyopathy and listed for cardiac transplantation. **The diagnosis is idiopathic dilated cardiomyopathy.**

III. Incidence and Epidemiology

Although heart failure represents a major problem in adult medicine, it is far less common in pediatrics and is the cause in fewer than 10% of pediatric heart transplantations.

Excluding infancy, when congenital heart disease is the most common indication for heart transplantation, dilated cardiomyopathy is the primary indication for pediatric heart transplantation throughout the world. Although the majority of cases of dilated cardiomyopathy have no definitive cause, several genetic and molecular lesions have been proposed. These include mutations in the cytoskeleton, troponin, and other sarcomere protein genes. It has long been known that the skeletal muscular dystrophies have cardial involvement, but familial dilated cardiomyopathy, although poorly understood, has been recognized more frequently.

The structural changes that occur in dilated cardiomyopathy include increased left ventricular mass, normal or reduced left ventricular wall thickness, and increased left ventricular cavity size. Histologic samples can show anything from focal myocyte death, to increased interstitial macrophage, to interstitial fibrosis.

Ten percent of cases of new-onset cardiomyopathy can be attributed to myocarditis. Survival rates can be as high as 80% and the infections can be either fulminant (usually with a better prognosis) or insidious. Arguably, insidious cases may be missed and may later contribute to cases of idiopathic cardiomyopathy. Bacterial, spirochetal, fungal, protozoal, parasitic, rickettsial, and viral infectious agents have all been implicated. Worldwide, infections with *Trypanosoma cruzi* (Chagas disease) and with *Corynebacterium diphtheriae* (diphtheria) are the most common causes of myocarditis; in the United States, viral infections are more common. The two major viral etiologies are coxsackievirus B and adenovirus. Other causes of myocarditis include immune-mediated mechanisms and toxins such as medications and heavy metals.

IV. Clinical Presentation

The clinical presentation of dilated cardiomyopathy encompasses that of clinical heart failure, including fatigue, shortness of breath, cough, and abdominal pain. However, the clinical features are varied and can range from asymptomatic patients to those with fulminant cardiac failure. In myocarditis, there is frequently a history of a recent flu-like syndrome and sometimes arrhythmias secondary to the rapid ventricular dilatation.

V. Diagnostic Approach

The distinction between dilated cardiomyopathy and myocarditis is important, because it may alter the management regimen that the child receives. Although clinical symptoms (clinical heart failure, recent flu-like syndrome accompanied by fever) and laboratory findings (leukocytosis, eosinophilia, elevated creatinine kinase or troponin) can be helpful in supporting a diagnosis of myocarditis, they are not sufficient.

Echocardiogram. All patients should have an echocardiogram to rule out structural anomalies.

Myocardial biopsy. Although other noninvasive modalities are important, myocardial biopsy is still the gold standard for diagnosis of myocarditis.

Other studies. Testing for infectious agents (e.g., coxsackievirus, adenovirus, echoviruses, respiratory syncytial virus, cytomegalovirus, Epstein-Barr virus, HIV) and any other possible causes, including autoimmune disease (e.g., lupus) and mitochondrial disease, is warranted in all new cases of pediatric heart failure.

VI. Treatment

Supportive therapy is the mainstay of treatment. Although there is less evidence to support specific treatment of heart disease in the pediatric population, the therapy mirrors that of adult medicine and includes angiotensin-converting enzyme (ACE) inhibitors. Less frequently, β-blockers and digoxin are used. Although there is not a strong literature and controversies persist, the standard is to treat cases of biopsy-proven myocarditis with immunomodulators (ranging from immunoglobulin therapy and steroids to cyclosporine and cytoxan) in an attempt to suppress the inflammation. Patients with progressively worsening heart failure may be candidates for mechanical assist devices (e.g., left ventricular assist device, extracorporeal membrane oxygenation), which may provide stabilization until cardiac transplantation can be achieved.

VII.   References

1. Davies MJ. The cardiomyopathies: an overview. *Heart* 2000;83:469–474.
2. Burch M. Heart failure in the young. *Heart* 2002;88:198–202.
3. Batra AS, Lewis AB. Acute myocarditis. *Curr Opin Pediatr* 2001;13:234–239.
4. Feldman AM, McNamara D. Myocarditis. *N Engl J Med* 2000;343:1388–1398.

Case 7-5: 8-Year-Old Boy

I. History of Present Illness

The patient, an 8-year-old boy, was well until 4 hours before presentation. At that time, he developed crampy periumbilical pain and bilious emesis. His family denied fever, diarrhea, or ill contacts. The pain was described as crampy and intermittent. He had six episodes of emesis before admission. His last bowel movement was 1 day before admission. His mother gave him an enema before presentation, with no relief of symptoms.

II. Past Medical History

The patient was a full-term infant without complications. His first episode of abdominal pain and bilious vomiting occurred about 3 years ago. Over the past few years, the pain and vomiting had been occurring about once every 4 months. The patient would have 2 to 3 days of emesis that was usually bilious and associated with abdominal pain. He had recently been treated with phenobarbital and atropine, without good results. He also had a history of chronic constipation that responded to mineral oil. Three months before presentation, he was admitted with similar symptoms and had a normal abdominal CT. The pain was never associated with eating, and he never missed school. There was no family history of celiac disease, cystic fibrosis, or any GI disorder.

III. Physical Examination

T 36.5°C; RR, 24/min; HR, 110 bpm; BP, 135/85 mm Hg

Weight, 26 kg

Physical examination revealed an alert child who was lying in bed and crying in pain. There were no oral lesions. The neck was supple with no lymphadenopathy. The lungs were clear to auscultation, and the cardiac examination revealed no murmurs, rubs, or gallops. On abdominal examination, there were diminished bowel sounds. Although the

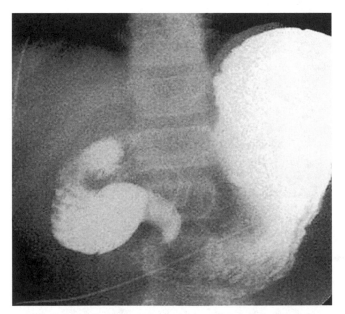

FIG. 7-5. Upper gastrointestinal radiograph (case 7-5).

abdomen was soft, there was intermittent guarding and a question of a mass in the left upper quadrant, with no focal tenderness. There was no hepatosplenomegaly. Rectal examination revealed no fissures or skin tags; hard stool was palpable in the rectal vault on digital examination. He was a Tanner I male. The neurologic examination was normal.

IV. Diagnostic Studies

A CBC showed 14,500 WBCs/mm^3, with 80% segmented neutrophils, 3% band forms, 7% lymphocytes, and 2% eosinophils. The hemoglobin was 12 g/dL, hematocrit 39.4%, and platelet count 314,000/mm^3. Serum bicarbonate was 18 mEq/L, but the electrolytes, blood urea nitrogen, and creatinine were otherwise normal. Liver function tests, amylase, and lipase were also normal. Urinalysis was negative except for the presence of ketones.

V. Course of Illness

The patient had an abdominal radiograph that showed a paucity of bowel gas, stool in the rectum, and no free air. An upper GI series revealed the cause of the patient's cyclic vomiting (Fig. 7-5).

DISCUSSION: CASE 7-5

I. Differential Diagnosis

Although the differential diagnosis of abdominal pain and vomiting is important, the key to the diagnosis in this patient was the cyclic nature of the vomiting. Cyclic vomiting syndrome is an idiopathic disorder characterized by severe episodic vomiting interspersed with periods of normal health. In a study of patients with cyclic vomiting syndrome, 12% were found to have potentially life-threatening disorders such as malrotation with volvulus, obstructive uropathy, or brain tumor. The most common cause of cyclic vomiting, accounting for as many as 50% of cases, is abdominal migraine. The family history is usually significant for migraines. The second most common cause is chronic sinusitis.

Apart from malrotation with intermittent volvulus, other GI causes of cyclic vomiting include chronic idiopathic pseudo-obstruction, intestinal duplication, pancreatitis or pancreatic pseudocyst, peptic ulcer disease, and superior mesenteric artery syndrome. Urinary tract conditions include renal stones and intermittent ureteropelvic junction obstruction. There are also several endocrinologic and metabolic causes for cyclic vomiting, including Addison's disease, porphyria, ornithine transcarbamylase deficiency, methyl malonic acidemia, and hereditary fructose intolerance.

II. Diagnosis

On the upper GI barium study, the ligament of Treitz was located at the midline, in an abnormal position compatible with a midgut malrotation (Fig. 7-5). The intraluminal contrast tapered in the proximal jejunum, in an appearance compatible with the presence of a midgut volvulus. **The diagnosis is malrotation.** The patient underwent a Ladd procedure with appendectomy.

III. Incidence and Epidemiology

It is important to understand the underlying embryology that leads to malrotation. At approximately 10 weeks' gestation, the intestines undergo counterclockwise rotation around the mesenteric artery and finally attach themselves to the posterior abdominal wall. The midgut then rotates 270 degrees around the superior mesenteric artery, with the duodenal-jejunal loop moving posterior to the artery while the cecal-colic loop rotates anterior to it. The duodenum and ascending colon can then attach to the posterior abdominal wall. This process of rotation and attachment helps to support normal GI tract motility and balanced gut-to-mesentery vascular supply.

With malrotation, the normal process is impeded and the cecum is in the right upper quadrant, near the duodenum, while the duodenal-jejunal loop remains to the right of midline. Because there is no mesenteric attachment, volvulus of the midgut is likely to occur with malrotation. The incidence of volvulus in association with malrotation is 44% in all age groups, but in neonates it is more likely to require bowel resection because of more significant damage to the bowel.

IV.   Clinical Presentation

The clinical presentation of malrotation can vary widely. Malrotation is commonly associated with other GI anomalies, namely esophageal atresia, diaphragmatic hernia, jejunal atresia, duodenal atresia, omphalocele, gastroschisis, intussusception, prune-belly syndrome, and Hirschsprung's disease. It can also been in association with heterotaxy and congenital heart disease.

Malrotation with midgut volvulus can occur at any age but is most commonly seen in infancy. Acute volvulus manifests with bilious emesis, abdominal distention, pain (constant, not crampy), and bright red blood per rectum (suggesting ischemia). It is a surgical emergency, and untreated ischemic bowel can lead to shock and sepsis with cardiovascular collapse.

A less commonly seen entity is malrotation with intermittent volvulus. It usually manifests with recurrent abdominal pain and vomiting and signs of failure to thrive.

V.   Diagnostic Approach

Upper gastrointestinal series. Although both the barium enema and the upper GI series can be used, the upper GI series is now preferred because of the possibility of cecal mobility on barium enema and its inability to show volvulus. Findings that are suggestive of malrotation in upper GI series include corkscrew-like deformity of the duodenum, displacement of the duodenum and jejunum in the right upper quadrant, and chronic obstruction of the duodenum.

VI.   Treatment

In neonates, any suggestion of volvulus indicates the possibility of ischemic gut and necessitates immediate surgical intervention. In older patients with rotational abnormalities, definitive surgery is also performed. Timing depends on the presentation. If possible, patients should be prepared for surgery with nasogastric suction, fluid resuscitation, and prophylactic antibiotics to cover the possibility of bowel resection. The Ladd procedure allows definitive treatment with counterclockwise derotation of the midgut volvulus, lysis of bands, appendectomy, and placement of the duodenum in the right side of the abdomen and of the cecum in the left lower quadrant.

VII.   References

1. Tunnessen WW. Cyclic vomiting. In: Tunnessen WW, ed. *Signs and symptoms in pediatrics,* 3rd ed. Philadelphia: Lippincott William & Wilkins, 1999:503–507.
2. Olson AD, Li BU. The diagnostic evaluation of children with cyclic vomiting: a cost-effectiveness assessment. *J Pediatr* 2002;141:724–728.
3. Groff D. Malrotation. In: Ashcraft KW, Holder TM, eds. *Pediatric surgery,* 2nd ed. Philadelphia: WB Saunders, 1993:320–330.
4. Liu PCF, Stringer DA. Radiography: contrast studies. In: Walker WA, Durie PR, Hamilton JR, et al. eds. *Pediatric gastrointestinal disease,* 3rd ed. Hamilton, Ontario: BC Decker, 2000:1555–1591.
5. Shuckett B. Cross-sectional imaging: ultrasonography, computed tomography, magnetic resonance imaging. In: Walker WA, Durie PR, Hamilton JR, et al., eds. *Pediatric gastrointestinal disease,* 3rd ed. Hamilton, Ontario: BC Decker, 2000:1591–1633.

Case 7-6: 2-Year-Old Girl

I. History of Present Illness

The patient, a 2-year-old girl, was well until 1 month before presentation, when she began to experience intermittent periods of abdominal pain. The pain seemed dull, was present throughout the entire abdomen, and did not awaken the patient at night. One week before presentation, she experienced mucousy diarrhea (nonbloody, occurring twice per day). Symptoms of an upper respiratory tract infection developed 2 days before presentation. A sibling had a "cold." She presented to the primary medical doctor with complaints of fever and worsening abdominal pain. A 3-pound weight loss history was elicited. There was a strong history of pica, specifically geophagy. The family had two cats and a new puppy.

II. Past Medical History

The history was significant for breath-holding spells (none recently), with an extensive workup that included a normal EEG, normal Holter monitor results, and a normal EKG. According to her parents, the child's growth was always "a concern." No other information was available with regard to her growth. She had no history of surgery and no drug allergies, her immunizations were up to date, and there was no significant family history.

III. Physical Examination

T, 37.8°C; RR, 20/min; HR, 120 bpm; BP, 92/62 mm Hg

In general, the patient was an alert but pale child. The neck was supple. There was no prominent adenopathy, and the trachea was in the midline. The lung fields were clear. The cardiac examination was unremarkable, with no murmurs, rubs, or gallops. Abdominal examination revealed a soft and nontender abdomen with good bowel sounds, a palpable spleen tip, and a liver edge that was about 2 cm below the right costal margin. The patient was a Tanner I female. The rectal examination revealed good tone, no tenderness on examination, no fissures, no masses, and a small amount of stool in the vault. The neurologic examination was normal.

IV. Diagnostic Studies

A CBC revealed 39,800 WBCs/mm3, with 1% band forms, 18% segmented neutrophils, 53% eosinophils, 17% lymphocytes, and 3% basophils. The hemoglobin was 7.8g/dL. The hematocrit was 29.4%; mean corpuscular volume (MCV), 52.7fL; mean corpuscular hemoglobin content (MCHC), 29.7pg; and red cell distribution width (RDW), 19.5%. The platelet count was 1,000,000/mm3. ESR was 20 mm/hour.

V. Course of Illness

Chest and abdominal radiographs were normal; stool for ova and parasites as well as culture were pending. Serum immunoglobulins were elevated. Anti-A and anti-B isohemagglutinins were markedly elevated (1:16,000 and 1: 512, respectively). ELISA results were pending. The patient was discharged home after a normal ophthalmologic examination and was monitored as an outpatient for resolution of the eosinophilia.

DISCUSSION: CASE 7-6

I. Differential Diagnosis

Diseases that are transmitted from animals to humans are called zoonoses. The presence of pets in more than 50% of homes in the United States and the transmission of zoonoses via fecal-oral or direct contact put children at higher risk for these infections.

Although this patient had a history of abdominal pain and diarrhea, the most important pieces of the history were the family's pets and the patient's history of geophagia. Zoonotic diseases that are transmitted via the fecal-oral route and cause gastroenteritis in children include salmonellosis (Salmonella spp., approximately 5 million cases per year), campylobacteriosis (C. jejuni), cryptosporidiosis (Cryptosporidium parvum), giardiasis (Giardia spp., found in 8% of children in U.S. day care centers), dog tapeworm (Dipylidium caninum), and visceral larval migrans.

II. Diagnosis

The clinical history, together with laboratory abnormalities, supported a diagnosis of visceral larva migrans.

III. Incidence and Epidemiology

Visceral larva migrans, or toxocariasis, is caused by infection with dog ascarid (*Toxocara canis*) or cat ascarid (*Toxocara catis*). The reservoir for latent infection is usually female dogs. The parasite requires 2 to 3 weeks after being shed from feces into soil to be infective. Shedding rates vary from 13% to 75% for dogs and 21% to 55% for cats. Areas that usually harbor infectious ova include playgrounds where children might play. The disease in humans is seen primarily in children, especially those with geophagus pica, who ingest soil that contain the larvae. In the United States, children in kindergarten have been found to have antibody prevalence rates as high as 23%, and disease is diagnosed in 3,000 to 4,000 patients per year.

IV. Clinical Presentation

The clinical manifestations of visceral larva migrans vary from subclinical to primarily visceral to primarily ocular. Apparently, ingestion of infectious eggs leads to penetration of gastric mucosa, followed by incorporation into the portal circulatory system and then into the systemic circulation. Damage from traveling larvae and the marked eosinophilic response cause the clinical manifestations, which can include fever, hepatomegaly, irritability, malaise, and pruritic rash. Pulmonary involvement is observed in up to 86% of infected children and can be severe. Ocular complaints can occur alone, and the subsequent strabismus, failing vision, uveitis, or endophthalmitis can occur secondary to local inflammatory response to the infection. The myocardium and central nervous system are also rarely affected.

V. Diagnostic Approach

Age of the child, history of contact with dogs, and geophagus are all important historical clues to the diagnosis. Definitive diagnosis by biopsy of affected tissue is rarely warranted. With a high index of suspicion and supportive laboratory data, the diagnosis can be made. Elevated serum gammaglobulins, a high WBC count with eosinophilia, and elevated titers of anti-A or anti-B isohemagglutinins (50% of patients) are most common.

VI. Treatment

Although there are reports of success with steroids as well as antiparasitic agents in severe cases, the disease is self-limited. Therapy should focus on avoidance of re-infection.

VII. References

1. Glaser C, Lewis P, Wong S. Pet-, animal-, and vector-borne infections. *Pediatr Rev* 2000;21:219–232.
2. Weller PF. Visceral larva migrans. Available at: https://store.utdol.com/app/index.asp.
3. Despommier D. Toxocariasis: clinical aspects, epidemiology, medical ecology, and molecular aspects. *Clin Microbiol Rev* 2003;16:265–272.
4. Tan JS. Human zoonotic infection transmitted by cats and dogs. *Arch Intern Med* 1997;157:1933–1943.

Case 7-7: 3-Year-Old Girl

I. History of Present Illness

A 3-year-old girl of Sri Lankan descent who was born in the United States presented to the emergency department with a fever of 40.5°C for the past 2 days. She complained of abdominal, knee, and elbow pain while febrile, but she was eating without a change in appetite and was having no problems ambulating. She had no complaint of headache, sore throat, rhinorrhea, cough, diarrhea, or vomiting. Her symptoms had been a recurrent problem for 8 months, since the family took a trip to one of the national parks. After returning from that trip, she had her first episode of fever, with a temperature to 40°C, which lasted 5 days. At that time she complained of a frontal headache, chills, rigors, and abdominal pain. She saw her regular pediatrician, who diagnosed a viral syndrome. At presentation, her mother reported that the episodes occurred at the end of every month. During her second febrile episode, the mother was told that the child's headache and abdominal pain were secondary to sinusitis with postnasal drip, and she was treated for clinical sinusitis with a 3-week course of antibiotics. She continued to have identical episodes every month. She had been treated a total of three times for acute sinusitis based on clinical diagnosis. The mother reported no weight loss, rash, upper respiratory tract symptoms, cough, or joint swelling with these episodes. She has not traveled outside of the country or had any known tick bites. She was seen by her regular doctor on multiple occasions during the episodes, with normal examinations, multiple normal CBCs, and normal Lyme serology. She had had no tuberculosis exposure. She had had normal growth and development and was completely normal between episodes. Her mother stated that the doctor often told her that her daughter's throat was "a little red," but all throat cultures had been negative.

II. Past Medical History

The patient had a normal birth history. She had had no hospitalizations or surgeries and had a diagnosis of allergic rhinitis. Her only medications were acetaminophen and ibuprofen during the febrile episodes. She was appropriately immunized and had had a negative tuberculin skin test within the last 3 months. Her family history was negative for GI disease, autoimmune disease, childhood illnesses, arthritis, cancer, and tuberculosis. She attended day care, and the family had no pets.

III. Physical Examination

T, 39.9°C; RR, 28/min; HR, 112 bpm; BP, 106/73 mm Hg

Weight, 19.8 kg (95th percentile); height, 104 cm (90th percentile)

In general, the patient was talkative, pleasant, and in no acute distress. Her sclerae were anicteric, there was no conjunctival injection, her tympanic membranes were normal, the oropharynx was nonerythematous, and there were no mouth lesions. Neck examination revealed shotty cervical lymphadenopathy. Chest and heart examination were normal. Abdominal examination revealed normoactive bowel sounds, diffuse tenderness without peritoneal signs, and no organomegaly. Neurologic examination was intact, and the skin showed no rashes or discoloration.

IV. Diagnostic Studies

A CBC showed 15,800 WBCs/mm^3, with 64% segmented neutrophils, 22% lymphocytes, and 13% monocytes. The hemoglobin was 11.2g/dL, and the platelet count was 323,000/mm^3. Liver function tests, basic metabolic panel, and immunoglobulins were all normal. Urinalysis, urine culture, blood culture, chest radiograph, sinus films, rapid streptococcal antigen and throat culture, Lyme antibodies, Epstein-Barr virus and cyto-megalovirus serologies, ANA, stool culture, stool for ova and parasites, malaria smear, CT scan of the head and sinuses, and gallium scan with triple-phase bone scan were all negative. ESR was elevated at 66 mm/hour.

V.   Course of Illness

Apart from the mild leukocytosis and elevated ESR, the patient's workup was negative. She became afebrile on hospital day 6 and was discharged home with close follow-up. Her CBC was checked two times a week for 2 months, and her absolute neutrophil count was always normal. During the febrile episodes, she always had an elevated WBC count and ESR, which normalized when she was afebrile. The diagnosis was suggested by the constellation of symptoms including the recurrent fever and pharyngitis.

DISCUSSION: CASE 7-7

I.   Differential Diagnosis

Periodic or recurrent fever has several definitions in the literature. The most common features are that the temperature is at least 38.4°C (some sources require at least 39°C) and continues for 3 to 6 days, occurs at least three times over a 6-month period, has no identifiable cause, is not accompanied by symptoms such as upper respiratory tract infection, and occurs at intervals that are separated by at least 1 week (and usually less than 4 weeks). The intervals without symptoms can be of either variable or predictable duration.

There are several causes that could account for recurrent fevers that occur at irregular intervals. These include infectious diseases such as viral infections (e.g., Epstein-Barr virus, parvovirus B19, herpes simplex virus, repeated viral infections), bacterial infections (e.g., occult bacteremia, recurrent upper respiratory tract infections, relapsing fever caused by Borrelia spp., chronic meningococcemia, dental abscess, brucellosis, Yersinia infections, mycobacterial infection), and parasitic infections (e.g., relapsing malaria with Plasmodium vivax or Plasmodium ovale, reactivation of plasmodium malaria). Other causes of recurrent fevers that occur at irregular intervals include inflammatory diseases (e.g., inflammatory bowel disease, systemic juvenile rheumatoid arthritis, Beçhet's disease), neoplasms such as lymphoma, and drug fevers. Infections and undiagnosed causes are the most common causes of recurrent fevers that occur with irregularity.

There are very few diseases that cause recurrent fevers at predictable and regular intervals. Causes include cyclic neutropenia (which usually recurs at intervals of 21 to 28 days), relapsing fever caused by Borrelia spp. (every 14 to 21 days), and PFAPA (periodic fever, aphthous ulcers, pharyngitis, and adenopathy) syndrome (every 21 to 28 days). There are also a group of hereditary causes of periodic fever that can occur at either regular or irregular intervals and should be considered. These include familial Mediterranean fever, hyperimmunoglobulin D syndrome (HIDS), and tumor necrosis factor receptor-associated periodic syndrome (TRAPS, or familial Hibernian fever). PFAPA and undiagnosed causes are the most common causes of recurrent fevers that occur at predictable intervals.

The clue to this patient's disease was the regularity of her febrile episodes.

II.   Diagnosis

During one of the episodes of fever, the patient was found to have three aphthous mouth ulcers and an erythematous throat. **The diagnosis is PFAPA syndrome.**

III.   Incidence and Epidemiology

PFAPA syndrome is defined by recurrent and periodic episodes of fever (greater than 39°C) that last for 3 to 6 days, occur approximately every 21 to 28 days, and are accompanied by certain clinical findings. There is a slight male predominance, and the disease usually manifests before 5 years of age. There seems to be no pattern of familial inheritance and no seasonal or geographic predilection. Although the etiology of PFAPA is not known, infectious and autoimmune causes have been implicated. PFAPA is considered the most common cause of recurrent fever that occurs at regular and predictable intervals.

IV. Clinical Presentation

Children with PFAPA are generally well in terms of growth and development and present with predictable patterns of fever, as described previously. The three most common clinical findings are aphthous mouth ulcers, pharyngitis, and cervical adenopathy. The aphthous mouth ulcers are frequently missed because these are very small (less 5 mm), few (usually two or three), and painless and resolve very quickly. One case series found reports of associated aphthous mouth ulcers in only 70% of cases of PFAPA. Pharyngitis is found in only 72% of cases and is usually nonexudative. Cervical adenopathy is the most commonly seen sign (88% of cases); it is usually confined to the cervical region and is relatively unremarkable (nodes less than 5 mm). Although symptoms such as abdominal pain, nausea, and headache are sometimes present, upper respiratory tract symptoms are rarely seen and usually indicate a viral upper respiratory tract infection. The most striking features of PFAPA are its predictable recurrence and the overall well-being of the patient, both during the episode and after the episode resolves.

V. Diagnostic Approach

Diagnostic criteria that have been used are clinical in nature and include much of what has already been discussed: (a) regularly recurring fevers with early age at onset (younger than 5 years); (b) constitutional symptoms without upper respiratory tract infection and either aphthous stomatitis, cervical lymphadenitis, or pharyngitis; (c) asymptomatic intervals between episodes; (d) normal growth and development; and (e) exclusion of cyclic neutropenia. Other fever syndromes also have characteristic features (Table 7-3).

Complete blood count. Included in the diagnostic criteria of PFAPA is exclusion of the diagnosis of cyclic neutropenia. This distinction can be difficult because the two disorders have similar features. In cyclic neutropenia, neutropenia recurs approximately every 21 days. Although the fever in cyclic neutropenia usually occurs without accompanying infection, bacterial infection secondary to the neutropenia can occur. The best way to distinguish between the two conditions is with a CBC. In PFAPA, the CBC shows

TABLE 7-3. *Features Associated with Some Fever Syndromes*

Feature	PFAPA	Hyper-Immunoglobin	FMF	TRAPS
Duration of fever (days)	4–5	3–7	1–2	>7
Periodicity (days)	26–30	14–28[a]	7–28[a]	None
Ancestry	None	Dutch, French	Jewish, Turkish, Arab, Armenian	Irish, Scottish
Associated symptoms	Stomatitis, pharyngitis, adenitis	Cervical lymphadenopathy, diarrhea, abdominal pain	Peritonitis, arthritis, splenomegaly	Myalgias Arthralgias Cconjunctivitis Eerythematous macules Edematous plaques

FMF, familial Mediterranean fever; PFAPA, periodic fever, aphthous ulcers, pharyngitis, and adenopathy; TRAPS, tumor necrosis factor receptor-associated periodic fever syndrome.
[a]Often unpredictable.

a mild leukocytosis, and the ESR is also mildly elevated during the episode. These values return to normal in the absence of fever. To diagnose cyclic neutropenia, CBCs with differential must be checked regularly (at least twice per week for two consecutive months), because the neutropenia does not always occur at the time of the fever. In cyclic neutropenia, there is an absolute neutrophil count of less than 500 cells/mm^3 that count recovers on its own.

Other studies. Additional studies may be directed at other diseases in the differential diagnosis. Testing for mutation detection in patients with suspected familial Hibernian fever (TRAPS) is performed by some laboratories. The immunoglobulin D levels are increased in patients with hyperimmunoglobulin D syndrome, although several measurements may be required for confirmation. Genetic testing is also available for familial Mediterranean fever.

VI. Treatment

PFAPA usually persists for several years (more than 4 years) before spontaneous remission occurs. This remission begins with a period during which the episodes occur with decreasing frequency before resolving completely. During the years in which the episodes occur, treatment includes supportive care and planning of family events around the predictable fever. A single dose of corticosteroids at the beginning of an episode has been found to help to shorten the duration and should be the first line of treatment. If this is not effective, prophylaxis with cimetidine can be attempted. Tonsillectomy has been found to effectively stop the episodes in some patients and can be considered if neither corticosteroids nor cimetidine is effective.

VII. References

1. Chandy CJ, Gilsdorf JR. Recurrent fever in children. *Pediatr Infect Dis J* 2002;21: 1071–1080.
2. Thomas KT, Feder HM Jr, Lawton AL, et al. Periodic fever syndrome in children. *J Pediatr* 1999;135:15–21.
3. Long SS. Syndrome of periodic fever, aphthous stomatitis, pharyngitis, and adenitis (PFAPA): what it isn't, what it is. *J Pediatr* 1999;135:1–5.
4. Drenth JPH, van der Meer JWM. Hereditary periodic fever. *N Engl J Med* 2001;345: 1748–1757.
5. Centola M, Aksentijevich I, Kastner DL. The hereditary periodic fever syndromes: molecular analysis of a new family of inflammatory diseases. *Hum Mol Genet* 1998; 7:1581–1588.

8

Altered Mental Status

Nathan L. Timm

APPROACH TO THE PATIENT WITH ALTERED MENTAL STATUS

I. Definition of the Complaint

Altered mental status is a broad, nonspecific term that includes dysfunction of cognition, attention, awareness, or consciousness. Although it is not a defined disease, altered mental status is a symptom of an underlying disease process. The Glasgow Coma Scale provides a structured system for categorizing a child's mental status based on eye opening, verbal response, and motor response. The simpler AVPU (alert, verbal, pain, unresponsive) system provides rapid classification of a child's mental status. The onset of altered mental status may be acute, chronic, or progressive and may be obvious or subtle in its presentation. This chapter focuses on the causes of acute altered mental status in children.

Although all disease processes that manifest themselves as an altered mental status are serious, the life-threatening disorders must be recognized early and treated appropriately. The brain's reticular activating system mediates wakefulness, and disruption of these neurons results in an altered mental status. Infections, toxin-mediated disorders, metabolic conditions, and traumatic injuries are the most common life-threatening disorders affecting the reticulated activating system. Unfortunately, the presentation of even the life-threatening disorders can be subtle, and a high index of suspicion is necessary for the proper diagnosis.

II. Complaint by Cause and Frequency

Altered mental status does not constitute a diagnosis, but it is a symptom of an underlying disease process that requires a thorough investigation. The causes of altered mental status in childhood vary by age (Table 8-1) and may also be grouped based by etiology (Table 8-2).

III. Clarifying Questions

A thorough history is necessary in any child presenting with an altered mental status. Precipitating factors and associated clinical features provide a useful framework for creating a differential diagnosis. The following questions may help provide clues to the diagnosis.

* Was there a preceding illness or fever?

  — Meningitis is a life-threatening cause of altered mental status, and efforts should be made to immediately address this possibility. Toxic appearance, fever, and nuchal rigidity should prompt aggressive use of antibiotics pending cerebrospinal fluid (CSF) cultures. Rashes characteristic of varicella, *Mycoplasma pneumoniae*, and Rocky Mountain spotted fever should be explored as possible causes of encephalitis. Release of Shiga toxin, accompanying *Shigella* gastroenteritis or cerebellitis after varicella or other viral infections, may result in an altered mental status.

TABLE 8-1. *Causes of Altered Mental Status in Childhood by Age*

Disease prevalence	Neonate and infant	Toddler and school age	Adolescent

Common	Infection
	  Meningitis
	  Sepsis
	Hypoxia
	Hypothermia
	Metabolic
	  Acidosis
	  Hypoglycemia
	  Hypernatremia or
	    hyponatremia
	  Hypocalcemia
	Trauma
	  Birth
	  Nonaccidental
		Infection
		  Meningitis
		  Encephalitis
		  Postinfectious
		Accidental ingestion
		Hypoglycemia
		Trauma
		  Accidental
		  Nonaccidental
			Infection
			  Meningitis
			  Encephalitis
			  Postinfectious
			Ingestion
			Hypoglycemia
			Trauma
			  Accidental
			  Nonaccidental
			Psychiatric

Less common	Cardiac anomalies
	  Decreased perfusion
	Seizure
	Metabolic disorders
	  Hyperammonemia
	Hydrocephalus
		Intussusception
		Seizure
		Carbon monoxide
		Hypertension
		Neoplasm
		Heavy metal poisoning
			Carbon monoxide
			Neoplasm
			Hypertension

Uncommon	Stroke
	Kernicterus
		Stroke
		Absence seizure
		Wernicke's syndrome
		  subacute sclerosing
		  panencephalitis
		Central venous thrombosis
			Stroke
			Pseudotumor cerebri
			Wernicke's syndrome

- Is there a history of ingestion or toxin exposure?

  — Drug ingestion of only one tablet can be life-threatening to a toddler. Examples include clonidine, β-blockers, and calcium channel antagonists. Attention should be placed on defining the medications present in the home that the child has the potential to ingest. Furthermore, illness among other family members should prompt concerns of carbon monoxide poisoning. It is also important to remember that toxicologic screens do not test for a number of potentially harmful toxins, including clonidine, organophosphates, and lysergic acid diethylamide (LSD).

- Is there a history of head trauma?

  — Head trauma at any age can result in an altered mental status. Intracranial injury can manifest more than 24 hours after the initial trauma. Evidence of increased intracranial pressure, vomiting, severe headache, or focal neurologic deficits should prompt emergency neuroimaging to rule out intracranial hemorrhage.

TABLE 8-2. *Causes of Altered Mental Status by Etiology*

Category	Cause
Vascular	Cerebral infarction
	Arterial venous malformation
	Central venous thrombosis
	Hypertensive encephalopathy
	Decreased cerebral perfusion
	Congenital heart disease
	Anemia
	Hypovolemia
Infection	Meningitis
	Encephalitis
	Sepsis
	Brain abscess
	Postinfectious
	Gastroenteritis (shigellosis)
Trauma	Intracranial hemorrhage
	Concussion
Toxins	Ethanol
	Carbon monoxide
	Anticonvulsants
	Methemaglobinemia
	Tricyclic antidepressants
	Heavy metals
Metabolic	Hypoglycemia
	Hypernatremia or hyponatremia
	Hypoxia
	Hyperammonemia
	Diabetic ketoacidosis
	Uremia
Gastointestinal	Intussusception
Oncologic	Primary brain tumor
	Metastatic central nervous system disease
Psychiatric	Depression
	Psychosis
	Schizophrenia
	Autism
Neurologic	Seizure
	Postictal
	Temporal lobe epilepsy
	Hydrocephalus
	Shunt malfunction
	Pseudotumor cerebrii

Case 8-1: 6-Year-Old Boy

I. History of Present Illness

A 6-year-old boy was brought to the emergency department because of confusion and "gibberish" talk after waking up that morning. The mother reported that her son was in his usual state of good health when he had two episodes of nonbloody, nonbilious emesis the previous day. Later that day, he complained of headache and neck pain, followed by a fever to 39.7°C, decreased activity, and refusal to move his neck. He awoke the morning of admission and was "not making sense." There were no rashes, trauma, recent travel, or ingestions. A sibling had recently developed severe nonbloody diarrhea.

II. Past Medical History

His past history was remarkable for two hospitalizations for management of asthma; neither required admission to an intensive care unit. He also had had a concussion 2 years earlier that warranted hospitalization for observation. His birth history was significant for a premature birth at 32 weeks' gestation that necessitated ventilatory support for 2 weeks. He did not receive any blood product transfusions.

III. Physical Examination

T, 40.3°C; RR, 20/min; HR, 164 bpm; BP, 110/70 mm Hg

Weight, 50th percentile

Physical examination revealed a sleepy but arousable child in no apparent distress. He was oriented to person but not to place and had slightly slurred speech. Cranial nerves, deep tendon reflexes, motor and sensory examinations were entirely normal. He had no meningismus, joint swelling, or rashes. His abdomen was nontender and nondistended, with active bowel sounds. The remainder of his physical examination was normal.

IV. Diagnostic Studies

Laboratory analysis revealed 5,100 white blood cells (WBCs)/mm^3, with 22% segmented neutrophils, 26% lymphocytes, and 47% band forms. The hemoglobin was 12.1 g/dL, and there were 157,000 platelets/mm^3. Electrolytes, blood urea nitrogen (BUN), and creatinine were normal. Urine and serum toxicology screens were normal. Chest radiography and head computed tomography (CT) results were negative. CSF analysis revealed 0 WBCs, 63 red blood cells (RBCs)/mm^3, a protein concentration of 19 mg/dL, and a glucose concentration of 85 mg/dL. Rapid antigen testing for group A *Streptococcus* was negative. Blood and CSF cultures were subsequently sterile.

V. Course of Illness

The patient remained confused with occasional slurred speech in the emergency department. He was given a normal saline bolus, started on cefotaxime, and admitted with an acute confusional state. Over the next 24 hours, he continued to have persistent mental status changes. Liver function tests and urinalysis were normal. A repeat complete blood count revealed a worsening leukopenia (3,500/mm^3) with more immature forms: 1% myelocytes, 18% metamyelocytes, 32% band, 10% segmented neutrophils, and 16% lymphocytes. His erythrocyte sedimentation rate (ESR) was 38 mm/hour.

The next day he had several large, bloody stools that strongly suggested a diagnosis.

DISCUSSION: CASE 8-1

I. Differential Diagnosis

The most likely diagnosis for the acute onset of confusion with fever and emesis, particularly in the context of an upper respiratory tract infection, is viral encephalitis (enteroviral agents, herpes, Epstein-Barr virus). Other infectious causes to consider include sepsis and meningitis. Ingestion of medications, in particular anticholinergics, should be considered: The classic symptoms are summed up as, "Hot as a hare, mad as a hatter." Other toxic ingestions that result in confusion include sympathomimetics, antihistamines, alcohol, and chronic heavy metal exposures. Central nervous system (CNS) neoplasms should also be considered in the context of fever, emesis, and confusion. Traumatic brain injury resulting in frontal lobe contusion or subdural, epidural, or subarachnoid bleeding may also fit this picture. Metabolic disorders including hypoglycemia, hypernatremia or hyponatremia, and hyperammonemia should also enter into the differential. The feature of this case that made it perplexing was the bloody diarrhea that began almost 48 hours after the child developed fever and began speaking "gibberish."

II. Diagnosis

The stool culture grew *Shigella sonnei*. **The diagnosis is altered mental status secondary to shigellosis.**

III. Incidence and Epidemiology

Shigellosis, a leading cause of diarrhea worldwide, causes almost 650,000 deaths each year. Almost 18,000 cases are reported yearly in the United States, where the gram-negative organism affects mainly children between the ages of 6 months and 5 years. Shigellosis, also known as *bacillary dysentery,* causes a diarrheal stool that contains an inflammatory exudate of polymorphonuclear leukocytes and blood. *S. sonnei* produces the mildest disease and accounts for 60% to 80% of bacillary dysentery cases in the United States. *Shigella dysenteriae* is more common in the developing countries and produces the most severe disease. *Shigella* is unique among diarrhea-inducing culprits in that fewer than 200 organisms can cause disease.

Humans are the only known natural host for *Shigella* species. Close human contact combined with poor sanitation results in the person-to-person transmission of the organisms via the fecal-oral route. *Shigella* species invade the epithelial layer of the large bowel and release Shiga toxin, resulting in a severe local inflammatory response involving polymorphonuclear leukocytes and macrophages. The organism rarely penetrates the intestinal mucosa to invade the bloodstream; however, the host response to the invasion culminates in the characteristic clinical picture of bloody mucopurulent diarrhea.

Shiga toxin is both cytotoxic, resulting in bacillary dysentery, and neurotoxic, participating in the encephalopathy, convulsions, and hallucinations known to occur with *Shigella* infection. These neurologic symptoms are usually benign and do not result in long-term sequelae; however, they often precede the gastrointestinal symptoms by up to 24 hours.

IV. Clinical Presentation

Children with shigellosis typically develop symptoms 12 to 48 hours after exposure to the organism, but symptoms can develop up to 1 week later. Mild infections cause transient watery diarrhea. Children with more severe infections develop fever, crampy abdominal pain, nausea, vomiting, tenesmus, and frequent diarrhea with blood and mucus. Neurologic symptoms such as seizures, hallucinations, and encephalopathy can precede the gastrointestinal symptoms by up to 24 hours. Disseminated intravascular coagulation occurs more often with S. dysenteriae than with other Shigella species.

V. Diagnostic Approach

Shigellosis is suspected clinically by a triad of lower abdominal cramping, rectal burning, and diarrhea. A high index of suspicion is necessary to diagnose shigellosis in a child with altered mental status without gastrointestinal symptoms.

Stool culture. Stool culture provides the definitive diagnosis, distinguishing *Shigella* species from the other microorganisms that cause dysentery (*Campylobacter, Vibrio* *parahaemolyticus, Aeromonas, Plesiomonas, Yersinia,* and *Salmonella* species). Studies to detect *Clostridium difficile* and *Entamoeba histolytica* should also be considered.

Microscopic examination of stool. Fecal leukocytes and RBCs each are present in 70% of cases, although their presence is not specific for *Shigella* infection.

Complete blood count. The peripheral WBC count is frequently normal; however, a left shift is common, with a greater number of band forms than neutrophils.

VI.   Treatment

Therapy for shigellosis should focus on two aspects of care: fluid and electrolyte therapy and antimicrobial therapy. Dysentery, like other diarrheal diseases, can be appropriately managed with oral rehydration. Significant dehydration or persistent emesis may prompt parenteral fluid administration; however, oral hydration should be encouraged as soon as possible. Seizures may develop secondary to fever, electrolyte imbalances, or meningismus and require prompt attention. Antidiarrheal medications such as diphenoxylate (Lomotil) and loperamide provide no benefit and should be avoided.

Unlike the other bacteria that cause gastroenteritis, *Shigella* is effectively eradicated with antibiotic treatment. Treatment with antibiotics both shortens the duration of diarrhea and eliminates the organisms from the feces. Empiric antibiotic therapy depends on local resistance patterns. Ampicillin and trimethoprim-sulfamethoxazole are often effective. Oral or parenteral third-generation cephalosporins (e.g., cefixime, ceftriaxone) or fluoroquinolones are preferred for empiric antibiotic therapy in some areas.

The neurologic symptoms related to shigellosis do not require specific additional therapy. As the bacteria are eradicated, the toxin production diminishes and the neurologic symptoms resolve. The boy in this case was symptom free and had had no further episodes of confusion at his 2-week follow-up appointment with his primary care physician.

VII.   References

1. Diercks DB, Friedland LR, Ernst AA. Hallucinations as the initial presentation of shigellosis. *Pediatr Emerg Care* 2000;16:99–101.
2. Fleisher GR. Infectious diseases emergencies. In: Fleisher GR, Ludwig S, eds. *Textbook of pediatric emergency medicine,* 4th ed. Philadelphia: Lippincott Williams & Wilkins, 2000;757–763.
3. Lopez EL, Prado-Jimenez V, O'Ryan-Gallardo M, et al. *Shigella* and Shiga toxin producing *E. coli* causing bloody diarrhea in Latin America. *Infect Dis Clin North Am* 2000;14:41–65.
4. Procop GW. Gastrointestinal infections. *Infect Dis Clin North Am* 2001;15:1073–1108.
5. Turgeon DK, Fritssche TR. Lab approaches to infectious diarrhea. *Gastroenterol Clin North Am* 2001;30:693–707.

Case 8-2: 3-Year-Old Boy

I. History of Present Illness

A 3-year-old African-American boy, according to his father, became unresponsive soon after he began "acting strange." The father reported that over the course of the afternoon his son complained of a headache and seemed to be sleepier. The boy regained consciousness after his father took him outside into the cold fall air. He was well before that afternoon and did not have any other illness. There was no witnessed ingestion. There were no sick contacts at home; however, that afternoon, both the mother and father developed nausea, headaches, and dizziness. The family had spent the day inside cleaning the attic, starting the furnace, and organizing the kitchen. An 8-month-old sister was taking a nap at home and did not appear to have any symptoms.

II. Past Medical History

The boy had had a febrile seizure at 1 year of age. An inguinal hernia had been repaired at 3 months of age. His past medical history was otherwise unremarkable.

III. Physical Examination

T, 37.5°C; RR, 23/min.; HR, 100 bpm; BP 111/51 mm Hg

Weight, 50th to 75th percentile

Physical examination revealed an alert and playful child in no apparent distress. There were no oral lesions. There was no lymphadenopathy. The lungs were clear, and the heart sounds were normal. His neurologic examination was intact, and the remainder of his examination was also normal.

IV. Diagnostic Studies

During the initial evaluation, the father revealed a key piece of history, prompting a simple blood test that revealed the diagnosis.

DISCUSSION: CASE 8-2

I. Differential Diagnosis

The possible causes of CNS depression in a 3-year-old are diverse. Common causes include accidental toxin exposures, including opiates, carbon monoxide, iron, sedative-hypnotics, clonidine, antihistamines, and alcohol. Metabolic disorders such as hypoglycemia, hypernatremia/hyponatremia, and hypocalcemia should also be considered. Infectious causes such as food poisoning or postviral syndromes may cause multiple family members to experience similar symptoms. Less likely infectious causes are encephalitis and meningitis. Complex partial seizures with a brief postictal period should also be considered. The features of this case that are remarkable are the CNS depression that rapidly resolved when the child was taken outside and the similar symptoms present in other family members.

II. Diagnosis

The father reported that he had turned on the furnace earlier in the day for the first time that fall. The child's carboxyhemoglobin (HbCO) value was 16.9%. **The diagnosis is carbon monoxide poisoning.**

III. Incidence and Physiology

Accidental carbon monoxide poisoning accounts for almost 500 deaths each year in the United States. House fires are responsible for most of these deaths; however, tobacco smoke, automobile exhaust, and faulty heating equipment causing incomplete combustion release carbon monoxide and contribute to accidental exposure. The gas is odorless and colorless and binds to hemoglobin with an affinity 200 to 300 times greater than that of oxygen, leading to tissue hypoxia. Increased minute ventilation and the presence of fetal hemoglobin make young children particularly susceptible to the effects of carbon monoxide.

IV.   Clinical Presentation

A high index of suspicion for carbon monoxide poisoning should be maintained for any child who is a fire victim or has been exposed to other devices that cause incomplete combustion. Clinical symptoms can be categorized as mild, moderate, or severe. Mild symptoms include headache, exercise-induced dyspnea, and confusion. Moderate poisoning causes nausea, vomiting, drowsiness, and incoordination. Severe intoxication leads to coma, convulsions, hypotension, and death. The classic "cherry-red" skin color is rarely seen at any level of exposure.

V.   Diagnostic Approach

Carboxyhemoglobin level. The HbCO level is the diagnostic and often prognostic test for carbon monoxide poisoning. Spectrophotometric detection methods using co-oximetry are most useful clinically because they distinguish between HbCO and oxygenated hemoglobin. HbCO levels may help stratify cases into mild, moderate, or severe intoxication; however, blood HbCO levels fall rapidly over time and may not correlate with persistent cellular dysfunction. Mild symptoms develop with HbCO levels of 20%. HbCO levels of 20% to 60% cause moderate symptoms, and levels higher than 70% are often fatal.

Other studies. Anemia, myoglobinuria, and metabolic acidosis are other significant complications from carbon monoxide poisoning; therefore, a complete blood count, urinalysis, electrolytes, electrocardiogram (ECG), and arterial blood gas analysis should be obtained. Pulse oximetry is likely to be normal, because it does not discriminate between the forms of hemoglobin.

VI.   Treatment

The antidote for carbon monoxide poisoning is oxygen. The half-life of HbCO is approximately 4 hours in a patient breathing room air at sea level. If that same patient is given 100% oxygen, the half-life of HbCO drops to 1 hour. The goal is to administer 100% oxygen until the HbCO level is less that 5%. Hyperbaric oxygen at 2 to 3 atmospheres further reduces the half-life of HbCO to 30 minutes; however, its routine use is still controversial. Risks from hyperbaric oxygen treatment include pneumothorax, oxygen toxicity, tympanic membrane rupture, and decompression sickness. Nevertheless, hyperbaric oxygen is indicated for victims who are neonates, are pregnant, or have history of coma, seizures, or arrhythmias secondary to intoxication, and early consultation with a hyperbaric center should be considered. Other management issues include correcting anemia if the hemoglobin is less than 10 g/dL to maximize oxygen-carrying capacity, decreasing the patient's activity level with bed rest, maintaining urine output at greater than 1 mL/kg per hour if myoglobinuria is present, and monitoring acid-base status and treating metabolic acidosis with sodium bicarbonate if the pH is lower than 7.15.

Neurologic injuries, such as impairment of concentration, attention, memory, and motor function, occur in 25% to 50% of patients who experience loss of consciousness or HbCO levels greater than 25%. These deficits may appear soon after exposure to carbon monoxide or up to 3 weeks later. These symptoms can last 1 month or longer in the most severe cases.

VII.   References

1. Baum CR. Environmental Emergencies. In: Fleisher GR, Ludwig S, eds. *Textbook of pediatric emergency medicine,* 4th ed. Philadelphia: Lippincott Williams & Wilkins, 2000:949–951.
2. Ellenhorn M, ed. *Ellenhorn's medical toxicology,* 2nd ed. Baltimore: William & Wilkins, 1997:1465–1475.
3. Morgan I. In: Bates N, ed. *Paediatric toxicology.* New York: Stockton Press, 1997:321–325.
4. Weaver LK, Hopkins RO, Chan KJ, et al. Hyperbaric oxygen for acute carbon monoxide poisoning. *N Engl J Med<* 2002;347:1057–1067.

Case 8-3: 20-Month-Old Boy

I. History of Present Illness

A 20-month-old African-American boy arrived by flight squad from an outside emergency department. The mother was on her way to the hospital and was not available; however, the squad relayed the history from the previous emergency department. The mother reported that her son had had a week-long upper respiratory tract infection and had developed a fever on the previous day. On the day of presentation, he had four episodes of emesis and was more tired than usual. Several children in his day care center had had bronchiolitis. There was a pet hamster at home.

II. Past Medical History

There was no personal or family history of sickle cell disease. The child was otherwise healthy.

III. Physical Examination

T, 37.5°C; RR, 28/min; HR, 140 bpm; BP, 80/60 mm Hg; SpO_2, 85% in room air
Height, 50th percentile; weight, 50th percentile

Initial examination revealed a pale-appearing, lethargic child who was responsive to painful stimulation. Head and neck examination was significant for pale conjunctivae and scleral icterus. Mucous membranes were moist, and there was no meningismus or lymphadenopathy. Mild subcostal retractions were present, but the lungs were clear to auscultation. The cardiac examination revealed tachycardia and a III/VI systolic ejection murmur at the left upper sternal border. There were no gallops or rubs. Capillary refill was 2 seconds, and peripheral pulses were strong. The abdomen was nondistended and soft. There was no hepatomegaly; however, a mildly tender spleen tip was palpable. The rectal examination was normal. There were no rashes, bruises, or petechiae noted on skin examination.

IV. Diagnostic Studies

Laboratory analysis revealed 30,800 WBCs/mm³, with 77% segmented neutrophils, 14% lymphocytes, 7% monocytes, and 8% nucleated RBCs. The hemoglobin was 3.1 g/dL, and there were 608,000 platelets/mm³. The mean corpuscular volume (MCV) was 90 fL, and the red blood cell distribution width was 21. The reticulocyte count was 10.5%. The blood type was O+ with a negative direct Coombs test. Electrolytes were significant for a BUN of 22 mg/dL; the other electrolytes were normal. The glucose concentration was 117 mg/dL, and liver function tests were significant for a lactic dehydrogenase concentration of 1,250 U/L and a total bilirubin concentration of 5.2 mg/dL (direct fraction, 0.4 mg/dL). A chest radiograph showed no cardiomegaly. The urine was tea colored, and urinalysis revealed hemoglobin. Blood and urine cultures were subsequently negative.

V. Course of Illness

The child was fitted with a 100% nonrebreather face mask, and intravenous access was obtained. The child received 10 mL/kg normal saline. With these interventions, the child's comfort level and vital signs improved: pulse oximeter reading, 96%; HR, 110 bpm; and RR, 22/min. The results of the peripheral blood smear suggested the cause of his severe anemia (Fig. 8-1). The mother arrived and provided an additional piece of information that confirmed the suspected diagnosis.

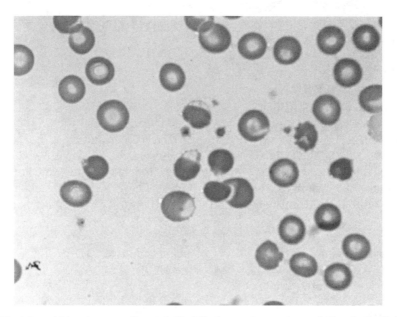

FIG. 8-1. Peripheral blood smear (case 8-3). (Photograph courtesy of Marybeth Helfrich, MT, ASCP.)

DISCUSSION: CASE 8-3

I. Differential Diagnosis

The results of the physical examination (pallor, scleral icterus, splenomegaly) and laboratory tests (anemia, elevated unconjugated bilirubin, elevated reticulocyte count) pointed toward the diagnosis of a hemolytic anemia. Hemolytic anemias can be classified into RBC intrinsic abnormalities and extrinsic forces acting on the RBC. Membrane (spherocytosis) and metabolic deficiencies (glucose-6-phosphatase [G6PD] deficiency, pyruvate kinase deficiency), in addition to the hemoglobinopathies (sickle cell disease and the thalassemias), make up the intrinsic abnormalities of RBCs that lead to hemolysis. The extrinsic causes are autoimmune hemolytic anemia, physical trauma to the RBC (prosthetic valve), infection (malaria), and drug/toxin effects (G6PD deficiency).

II. Diagnosis

The mother provided additional information when she arrived. The child had been seen at an emergency department 4 days earlier when she found a mothball in his mouth. His hemoglobin at that time was 10 g/dL. The peripheral blood smear showed schistocytes, blister cells, bite cells, 3+ anisocytosis, and 4+ poikilocytosis, consistent with RBC hemolysis (Fig. 8-1). **The diagnosis of naphthalene ingestion in a child with glucose-6-phosphatase dehydrogenase deficiency was confirmed.**

III. Incidence and Epidemiology

G6PD deficiency is an X-linked enzyme disorder that affects almost 200 million people worldwide. Kurdish Jews (60%), individuals of Saudi Arabian descent (13%), and African-Americans (11%) are most often affected. The female heterozygote carrier state provides a survival advantage against malaria.

The enzyme G6PD is present in all cells in the body; however, RBCs are most severely affected by its absence. G6PD aids in the biochemical pathway that replenishes glutathione, the chemical responsible for breaking down oxygen free radicals and peroxide. Therefore, the enzyme-deficient patient is at particular risk when confronted with stressors leading to an "oxidative challenge." Fava beans, infection, and drugs such as antimalarial agents, sulfonamides, nitrofurantoin, and naphthalene (mothballs) are the most notorious culprits leading to RBC damage in patients with G6PD deficiency.

IV.   Clinical Presentation

Naphthalene ingestion in a child with G6PD deficiency results in acute hemolytic anemia. Hemolytic anemia can develop as early as 1 day after naphthalene exposure. The oxidative metabolite, α-naphthol, causes a depletion of glutathione. The G6PD-deficient RBC is unable to replenish the glutathione, leading to hemoglobin and protein oxidation. Hemoglobin and proteins are denatured into Heinz bodies, and the RBC membrane is lysed. The spleen removes the Heinz body-containing RBCs, leading to splenomegaly and "bite cells" on the peripheral blood smear. The destruction of the RBCs leads to a normocytic anemia, increased unconjugated bilirubin, increased reticulocyte production, and hemoglobinuria. The clinical features include nausea, emesis, dark urine, icterus, abdominal pain, pallor, and lethargy.

V.   Diagnostic Approach

History and physical examination findings are the mainstay of the diagnosis. Additional laboratory tests to help differentiate the hemolytic anemias include the following.

Complete blood count and peripheral smear. The peripheral blood smear reveals anisocytosis, poikilocytosis, schistocytes, bite cells, and occasional Heinz bodies.

Reticulocyte count. The reticulocyte count is usually elevated after hemolysis to compensate for increased RBC destruction.

Coombs test. Direct and indirect Coombs tests are negative in G6PD but should be performed to exclude autoimmune hemolytic anemia.

Serum haptoglobin. Haptoglobin binds to free hemoglobin and is decreased with hemolysis.

Hepatic function panel. Plasma indirect bilirubin, aspartate aminotransferase, and lactate dehydrogenase are elevated due to the release of intracellular enzymes during hemolysis.

Urinalysis. Increased urine bilirubin is noted. Hemoglobinuria occurs once hemoglobin binding sites in the plasma, such as haptoglobin and hemopexin, are saturated.

Glucose-6-phosphatase assay. A G6PD assay measures the production of reduced nicotinamide adenine dinucleotide phosphate (NADPH) by means of a spectrophotometer. G6PD assay may be normal immediately after a hemolytic episode, despite G6PD deficiency, because younger RBCs (reticulocytes) with normal levels of G6PD will have replaced the older, more deficient population. This screening test should be performed at least 2 weeks after a hemolytic episode. Additional screening tests are also available that utilize dye decolorization techniques that quantify G6PD levels as normal or deficient (less than 30% normal activity). The limitations of these screening tests are that they do not detect heterozygotes and are helpful only for steady-state levels; therefore, they are unreliable during or after active hemolysis.

VI.   Treatment

Supportive care is the mainstay of treatment. Activated charcoal and cathartics are helpful in acute naphthalene ingestions. In addition, patients should avoid milk or fatty meals, which would aid the absorption of the lipophilic naphthalene. The hemolytic anemia is effectively corrected by the bone marrow, and hemoglobin levels return to normal in 3 to 6 weeks. In addition, hemoglobinuria rarely leads to the development of renal failure in children.

VII.   References

1. Cohen AR. Hematologic emergencies. In: Fleisher GR, Luwdig S, eds. *Textbook of pediatric emergency medicine,* 4th ed. Philadelphia: Lippincott Williams & Wilkins, 2000:859–863.
2. Desforges J. Glucose 6 phosphate dehydrogenase deficiency. *N Engl J Med* 1991;324: 169–194.
3. Luzzato L. Hemolytic anemias. In: Nathan D, Orkin S, eds. *Hematology of infancy and childhood,* 5th ed. Philadelphia: WB Saunders, 1988:704–722.
4. Wason S, Siegel E. Mothball toxicity. *Pediatr Clin North Am* 1986;33:369–374.

Case 8-4: 9-Year-Old Boy

I. History of Present Illness

A previously healthy 9-year-old boy presented to his pediatrician 5 days before admission with complaints of headache and malaise. Rales were noted in the right lung, and he was treated with azithromycin for suspected pneumonia. The next day he developed low-grade fevers with decreased oral intake, emesis, lethargy, and weakness. His mother described him as being "out of it." His symptoms worsened over the next 2 days, and he was admitted to an outside hospital with disorientation, slurred speech, weakness, drooling, and bradykinesia. CT of the head was negative, but magnetic resonance imaging (MRI) revealed increased signal intensity in the basal ganglia bilaterally. He was transferred to the regional children's hospital for further management. There was no history of trauma, drug or toxin exposure, ill contacts, or any chronic changes in his behavior or school performance.

II. Past Medical History

The past medical history was remarkable for bronchiolitis requiring hospitalization at 3 months of age. He had a history of enuresis that had improved over the past 6 months. He was a third grader who did well in school. His older half-brother had attention-deficit and hyperactivity disorder, but there was no family history of neurologic or developmental disorders. The boy had been placed in foster care at 5 years of age; however, he had returned to live with his mother, stepfather, stepbrother, and stepsister 2 years ago.

III. Physical Examination

T, 39°C; RR, 18/min; HR, 60 bpm; BP, 114/64 mm Hg; SpO$_2$, 100% in room air
Weight, 50th percentile; height, 50th percentile

General examination revealed a pale boy with masked facies who was occasionally tearful, sitting up in bed. He had minimal spontaneous movement. His general physical examination was unremarkable. He had intact cranial nerves but decreased facial movement. Extraocular movements were intact without nystagmus, and pupils were equally round and reactive. There were no Kaiser-Fleischer rings, and disk margins were sharp. Sensory examination was intact diffusely to light touch, temperature, and proprioception. Motor examination revealed normal tone with diminished strength 3 to 4/5 throughout. He had coordinated but slow movement with finger-nose-finger; however, he had a resting tremor in both hands. Babinski reflexes were downgoing bilaterally without clonus.

IV. Diagnostic Studies

Laboratory results from the outside hospital were as follows. A complete blood count revealed 4,600 WBCs/mm^3, with 57% segmented neutrophils, 33% lymphocytes, 8% monocytes, and 2% eosinophils. Serum electrolytes, BUN, creatinine, and calcium were normal. The serum glucose was 124 mg/dL. Liver function tests were significant for an elevated lactic acid dehydrogenase level, 228 U/L. Ammonia level was 19 µg/dL. Serum ceruloplasmin and lead levels were normal. Carboxyhemoglobin level was normal. Urinalysis and urine tests for heavy metals were negative. Serum and CSF amino acids, pyruvate, and lactate were normal. Lumbar puncture revealed clear CSF with a glucose concentration of 65 mg/dL and a protein concentration of 40 mg/dL, 20 WBCs/mm^3, and no RBCs. Viral and bacterial cultures of blood, urine, and CSF were negative. CSF herpes simplex virus and enteroviral polymerase chain reaction (PCR) assay were also negative.

V. Course of Illness

The child was hospitalized. His medications on arrival included acyclovir, van-comycin, cefotaxime, and erythromycin. He was started on nasogastric feeds due to the profound weakness of his oropharyngeal muscles. He showed no evidence of respiratory or cardiovascular compromise, although the bradykinesia and tremor worsened and his ability to communicate verbally deteriorated during the subsequent 48 hours. The Parkin-sonian-like clinical picture prompted initiation of amantadine. However, the results from a CSF PCR analysis provided the diagnosis.

DISCUSSION: CASE 8-4

I. Differential Diagnosis

The child did not have any change in his level of consciousness; rather, his clinical findings were more consistent with a global cerebral dysfunction, or encephalopathy. Encephalopathy in children is either acute or chronic and can be divided into toxic, meta-bolic, and infectious causes. The most notorious of the toxins are carbon monoxide and lead. Metabolic disorders that involve the basal ganglia should also be considered in the differential diagnosis. Wilson disease (copper accumulation in the brain, liver, and cornea) and Hallervorden-Spatz syndrome (deposition of iron-containing material in the substantia nigra) both affect the basal ganglia and should be considered; however, these are rare disorders that usually manifest as chronic encephalopathy. Encephalitis is inflam-mation of brain matter caused by either direct invasion of the brain by the infectious organism or immune-mediated mechanisms. Viral agents are the common culprits, including herpes simplex virus, human immunodeficiency virus (HIV), and the arthro-pod-borne encephalitides (St. Louis and West Nile). Nonviral pathogens include Lyme disease and rickettsial diseases. Postinfectious encephalitis can also occur after Epstein-Barr virus, influenza, or varicella. Cultures and PCR testing are the most helpful in dis-tinguishing among the various infectious etiologies.

II. Diagnosis

The child's preceding history of clinical pneumonia raised the possibility of a rela-tionship between the two illnesses. *Mycoplasma pneumoniae* PCR assay of the CSF and nasopharyngeal aspirate were positive. **The diagnosis is *M. pneumoniae* encephalitis.**

III. Incidence and Epidemiology

M. pneumoniae, the smallest free-living organism, accounts for one third of all pneu-monias in children 5 to 9 years old and 70% of all pneumonias in children aged 9 to 15 years. In one series, *M. pneumoniae* was implicated as the cause of encephalitis in 11 (7%) of 159 children with encephalitis.

IV. Clinical Presentation

M. pneumoniae pneumonia most commonly manifests with a gradual onset of head-ache, malaise, fever, and rhinorrhea that progresses to cough, dyspnea, and bronchop-neumonia. Other manifestations of infection are maculopapular rashes, erythema multi-forme, and Stevens-Johnson syndrome. Respiratory symptoms usually precede the neurologic symptoms by several days. Nevertheless, encephalitis may occur without res-piratory symptoms. CNS involvement includes Guillain-Barré syndrome, transverse myelitis, meningoencephalitis, cerebellar ataxia, and aseptic meningitis. CNS involve-ment manifests as seizures, altered level of consciousness (disorientation, confusion, coma), and meningeal signs (headache, stiff neck, fever greater than 39°C). The mecha-nism of neurotoxicity is unclear but is hypothesized to be either (a) an autoimmune reac-tion, (b) direct invasion of the CNS, or (c) neurotoxin production.

V. Diagnostic Approach

Detection of *M. pneumoniae*. Diagnosis of *M. pneumoniae* infection is based on four possible findings: (a) a four-fold increase in serum complement-fixing immunoglobulin G (IgG) antibodies to *M. pneumoniae,* (b) a positive test for IgM antibodies in the serum, (c) antibodies to *M. pneumoniae* in the CSF, and (c) detection of *M. pneumoniae* in CSF by PCR analysis.

Lumbar puncture. CSF is normal in 45% to 70% of patients with *M. pneumoniae* encephalitis. Abnormalities, when present, include a mild lymphocytic CSF pleocytosis (fewer than 100 WBCs). The CSF protein may be mildly elevated, but the glucose concentration is normal.

Neuroimaging. CT or MRI of the head is helpful to exclude other conditions. Neuroimaging is abnormal in approximately 45% of cases. Abnormal findings may be similar to those observed in other cases of encephalitis and may include focal edema or ischemia, focal enhancing lesions, or demyelination.

Electroencephalogram (EEG). EEG findings are abnormal in up to 80% of children with *M. pneumoniae* encephalitis. Abnormalities, which are not necessarily specific for *M. pneumoniae,* include generalized slowing, epileptic focus, periodic lateralizing epileptiform discharge, and frontal intermittent rhythmic delta activity.

VI. Treatment

There are no clearcut guidelines for the treatment of *M. pneumoniae* encephalitis. *M. pneumoniae* does not have a cell wall and therefore is resistant to penicillins and cephalosporins. Macrolide antibiotics (erythromycin, clarithromycin, azithromycin), tetracyclines, and fluoroquinolones effectively eradicate the organism; however, there is no evidence that they affect the course of the neurologic illness. There is anecdotal evidence that corticosteroids may be beneficial in treating CNS infection with *M. pneumoniae,* but further investigation is necessary to confirm their effectiveness.

A 10% to 15% mortality rate and a 20% to 30% chance of permanent neurologic damage accompanies *M. pneumoniae* encephalitis. These risks are seven times greater than in children with other forms of encephalitis (excluding herpes simplex viral encephalitis).

VII. References

1. Beskind DL, Keim SM. Choreoathetotic movement disorder in a boy with *Mycoplasma pneumoniae* encephalitis. *Ann Emerg Med J* 1994;23:1375–1378.
2. Bitnun A, Ford-Jones EL, Petric M, et al. Acute childhood encephalitis and *Mycoplasma pneumoniae. Clin Infect Dis* 2001;32:1674–1684.
3. Carpenter TC. Corticosteroids in the treatment of severe mycoplasma encephalitis in children. *Crit Care Med* 2002;30:925–927.
4. Lehtokoski-Lehtiniemi E, Koskiniemi MJ. *Mycoplasma pneumoniae* encephalitis: severe entity in children. *Pediatr Infect Dis J* 1989;8:651–653.
5. Powell DA. Mycoplasmal infections. In: Behrman RE, Kliegman RM, Jenson HB, eds. *Nelson textbook of pediatrics,* 16th ed. Philadelphia: WB Saunders, 2000: 914–917.
6. Rautonen J, Koskiniemi M, Vaheri A. Prognostic factors in childhood acute encephalitis. *Pediatr Infect Dis J* 1991;10:441–446.
7. Thomas NH, Collins JE, Robb SA, et al. *Mycoplasma pneumoniae* infection and neurological disease. *Arch Dis Child* 1993;69:573–576.

Case 8-5: 8-Month-Old Boy

I. History of Present Illness

A previously well 8-month-old boy was brought to the emergency department because of increased sleepiness. The mother reported that her son was well earlier in the day, but over the last few hours had become extremely drowsy. He had had two episodes of non-bloody, nonbilious emesis during this period but no diarrhea. There was no history of fever, cough, or rash. The parents reported that they had been cleaning the house with bleach, and although they did not witness any ingestion, the child's drowsiness seemed to coincide with the cleaning. There were no prescription medications in the house.

II. Past Medical History

He was full-term infant who was delivered via cesarean section for fetal distress but did well and was discharged to home after 48 hours. The pregnancy was complicated by preeclampsia. The remainder of the past history was unremarkable.

III. Physical Examination

T, 36.7°C; RR, 55/min; HR, 133 bpm; BP, 118/57 mm Hg; SpO_2, 99% in room air

Weight, 11.5 kg (greater than 90th percentile); height, 75 cm (75th to 90th percentile)

In general the child was well developed and appeared lethargic. He had moist mucus membranes with no oral ulcers or burns. His pupils were equally round and reactive to light. His neck was supple. Cardiac and lung examination findings were unremarkable. The abdomen was nontender with active bowel sounds. There were no masses. Testes were descended bilaterally, and there were no hernias. Rectal examination revealed normal tone with brown, Hemoccult-positive stool. The neurologic examination was significant for a lethargic-appearing child who moved all four extremities, had symmetric facies, and responded to painful stimulation.

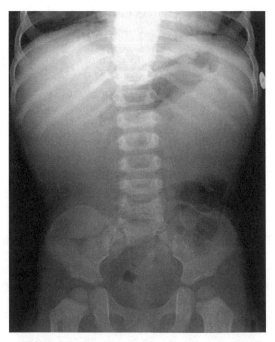

FIG. 8-2. Abdominal radiograph (case 8-5).

IV. Diagnostic Studies

The complete blood count revealed 7,100 WBCs/mm^3, with 70% segmented neutrophils, 1% eosinophils, 23% lymphocytes, and 6% monocytes; hemoglobin, 12.0 g/dL; and platelet count, 274,000/mm^3. Serum electrolytes, calcium, BUN, and creatinine were normal. The serum glucose concentration was 111 mg/dL.

V. Course of Illness

An abdominal radiograph suggested a diagnosis (Fig. 8-2).

DISCUSSION: CASE 8-5

I. Differential Diagnosis

The possible causes of a depressed mental status as described in this patient are diverse; however, clues from the history and physical examination can lead to the diagnosis. Ingestion should be high on the list in this particular age group. The parents were concerned about cleaning products. However, household bleach, soaps, and detergents cause mainly gastrointestinal irritation resulting in vomiting and mild diarrhea. Other possible ingestions resulting in a depressed mental status include alcohol, carbon monoxide, iron, clonidine, opiates, and sedative hypnotics. Closed-head injury with an expanding mass lesion should also be considered in a previously well child who presents with lethargy and vomiting. Although an infectious cause was unlikely given the absence of fever, early shigellosis (described in a previous case) was possible given the vomiting, abdominal pain, and Hemoccult-positive stool. However, shigellosis is an uncommon infection, and there is a much more common diagnosis that occurs in this age group that would explain the vomiting, Hemoccult-positive stool, and depressed mental status.

II. Diagnosis

The history of lethargy and emesis, the finding of Hemoccult-positive stool, and the presence of tachypnea were worrisome. The radiograph showed a paucity of bowel gas in the right abdomen as well as a soft tissue density protruding into a gas-filled loop of transverse colon (Fig. 8-2). These findings were concerning for intussusception. An air contrast enema identified an intussusception in the midtransverse colon that was easily reduced, leading to free retrograde flow of air into the nondilated bowel loops. **The diagnosis is ileocolic intussusception.**

III. Incidence and Epidemiology

Intussusception is the most common cause of intestinal obstruction in children between the ages of 3 months and 2 years. Sixty percent of cases occur in children younger than 1 year of age, and boys are four times more likely to be affected than girls. Ninety percent of the cases are idiopathic, and the most common type occurs when the distal ileum telescopes into the proximal colon. The other 10% of intussusceptions have a lead point such as a Meckel diverticulum, polyp, or lymphoma.

IV. Clinical Presentation

The classic presentation of intussusception is a previously well child who develops intermittent episodes of colicky abdominal pain with "currant-jelly" stools and an abdominal mass. However, almost 15% of children with intussusception present without abdominal pain, only 40% have hematochezia, and only 25% have a palpable mass. Therefore, nonspecific signs and symptoms such as vomiting, irritability, and decreased oral intake may be the only indication that intussusception is present. Lethargy is a well-described presenting complaint of intussusception. Although most cases described were also associated with other findings (e.g., hematochezia, abdominal mass), a high level of suspicion for intussusception must be maintained for any child presenting with altered mental status. Lethargy may be caused by dehydration, shock, or cytokine release by the entrapped bowel wall.

V. Diagnostic Approach

History and physical examination findings raise the clinical suspicion of intussusception.

Abdominal radiograph. Plain radiography is a helpful next step. Free air and obstruction can be identified on abdominal films; however, almost 30% of patients with intussusception have normal abdominal radiographs.

Abdominal ultrasound. Ultrasound, if available, provides a highly sensitive and specific test to diagnose or exclude intussusception. Additional benefits of ultrasound are patient safety and comfort, the ability to characterize lead points, and the ability to make alternative diagnoses. High-risk features such as absence of blood flow and fluid within the intussusception can be detected with the use of ultrasound.

Air or barium contrast enema. If ultrasound is not available, then an air or barium contrast enema should be performed for the diagnosis and treatment of intussusception. Successful reduction rates are 90% for air and 65% to 85% for barium or water-soluble contrast enemas. Contraindications for the use of barium contrast enema include free air on plain films and clinical peritonitis.

VI. Treatment

Barium enema has been the standard diagnostic and therapeutic tool for intussusception for the past three decades. Success rates at reduction approach 80% but drop off when symptoms have persisted for longer than 48 hours. Water-soluble contrast, air, and ultrasound-guided saline enemas have also been described as having equal effectiveness at reduction compared with barium, yet these techniques have the benefits of cleaner methods, less radiation exposure, and reduced risk of chemical peritonitis if perforation occurs. Surgical correction is necessary if enema reduction fails. The recurrence rate of intussusception is greater in children who have definable lead points. Ten percent of intussusceptions recur after enema reduction, whereas surgical correction has a 2% to 5% recurrence rate.

VII. References

1. Birkhahn R, Fiorini M, Gaeta TJ. Painless intussusception and altered mental status. *Am J Emerg Med* 1999;17:345–347.
2. Del-Pozo G, Albillos JL, Tejedor D, et al. Intussusception in children: current concepts in diagnosis and enema reduction. *Radiographics* 1999;19:299–319.
3. Harrington L, Connolly B, Hu X, et al. Ultrasonographic and clinical predictors of intussusception. *J Pediatr* 1998;132:836–839.
4. Kupperman N, O'Dea T, Pinckney L, et al. Predictors of intussusception in young children. *Arch Pediatr Adolesc Med* 2000;15:25000-255.
5. Losek JD. Intussusception: don't miss the diagnosis! *Pediatr Emerg Care* 1993;9:46–51.
6. Lui KW. Air enema for diagnosis and reduction of intussusception in children: clinical experience and fluoroscopy time. *J Pediatr Surg* 2001;36:479–481.
7. Luks FI, Yazbeck S, Perreault G, et al. Changes in the presentation of intussusception. *Am J Emerg Med* 1992;10:574–576.
8. McGuigan MA. Bleach, soaps, detergents and other corrosives. In: Haddad LM, Shannon MW, Winchester JF, eds. *Clinical management of poisoning and drug overdose,* 3rd ed. Philadelphia: WB Saunders, 1998:830–835.
9. Myllyla V. Intussusception in infancy and childhood. *Rontgenblatter* 1990;43:94–98.
10. Sargent MA. Plain abdominal radiography in suspected intussusception: a reassessment. *Pediatr Radiol* 1994;24:17–20.
11. Schnaufer L, Mahboubi S. Abdominal emergencies. In: Fleisher GR, Ludwig S, eds. *Textbook of pediatric emergency care,* 4th ed. Philadelphia: Lippincott Williams & Wilkins, 2000:1519–1521.
12. Wyllie R. Intussusception. In: Behrman RE, Kliegman RM, Jenson HB, eds. *Nelson textbook of pediatrics,* 16th ed. Philadelphia: WB Saunders, 2000:1072–1074.

Case 8-6: 14-Year-Old Girl

I. History of Present Illness

A previously healthy 14-year-old girl was brought to the emergency department after she was found semiconscious on the floor next to an open bottle. Her mother reported that she had been upset lately because her boyfriend was recently diagnosed with HIV. In the ambulance, she was uncooperative en route and refused vital signs. Although she was combative on arrival, within a few minutes she became less and less responsive. Supplemental oxygen was administered. Her initial set of vital signs included HR, 100 bpm and BP, 100/70 mm Hg. Her serum glucose concentration was 110 mg/dL. Naloxone and flumazenil were administered without impact on her deteriorating mental status. She had become responsive only to painful stimulation and required endotracheal intubation. Nasogastric lavage did not reveal pill fragments. Activated charcoal was administered via nasogastric tube. While the results of head CT scanning were awaited, her HR increased to 180 bpm and she became hypotensive. An ECG revealed supraventricular tachycardia. Her blood pressure improved after cardioversion with adenosine.

II. Past Medical History

Her past medical history was unremarkable. She had never attempted suicide. She did not take any prescription medications. Her father had a history of depression.

III. Physical Examination

T, 39.0°C; RR, 16/min; HR, 120 bpm; BP, 110/70 mm Hg

Physical examination revealed an intubated patient who responded only to painful stimulation. Her head and neck examination revealed no evidence of head injury. There was no hemotympanum. The oropharynx was clear. Pupils were 5 mm and reactive to light. Sharp disc margins were present on funduscopic examination. She was mildly tachycardiac without murmurs, rubs, or gallops. The lungs were clear bilaterally. The abdomen was soft with absent bowel sounds and no organomegaly. She was incontinent of stool that was Hemoccult negative. Her skin examination was significant for linear excoriations on her left wrist. Her neurologic examination was significant for a Glasgow Coma Scale score of 4 with response to deep pain only. A gag reflex was present. Babinski reflexes were downgoing bilaterally.

IV. Laboratory Studies

A complete blood count revealed 6,600 WBCs/mm³, with 54% segmented neutrophils and 35% lymphocytes; hemoglobin, 11.4 g/dL; and 180,000 platelets/mm³. Electrolytes were normal. Calcium, magnesium, and phosphorous were normal. BUN was 8 mg/dL with a creatinine of 0.6 mg/dL. Prothrombin time, partial thromboplastin time, and liver enzymes were unremarkable. Urinalysis and a pregnancy test were both negative. A urine toxicology screen was negative for drugs of abuse including phencyclidine, cocaine, amphetamines, cannabinoids, opiates, and barbiturates. Acetaminophen and aspirin levels were undetectable. The head CT was negative. The ECG revealed a QTc of 0.42 seconds with a QRS duration of 0.110 seconds.

V. Course of Illness

The patient remained endotracheally intubated and had two additional episodes of supraventricular tachycardia that responded well to adenosine. Her father arrived soon after her last cardioversion and provided the team with the identity of the bottle's contents.

DISCUSSION: CASE 8-6

I. Differential Diagnosis

An open bottle found next to the patient is an important clue to the diagnosis; however, additional diagnoses beyond overdose need to be considered. Sepsis, meningitis, or encephalitis should always be considered in someone with fever and rapid mental deterioration. Furthermore, an intracranial bleed, either spontaneous or from trauma, should be excluded. Nevertheless, the history directs the differential diagnosis toward an ingestion. The presence of an anticholinergic toxidrome (altered mental status, increased temperature, dilated pupils, absent bowel sounds) leads to a number of possible medications: antihistamines, antipsychotics, and muscle relaxants. Ingestion of jimsonweed and certain species of mushrooms produces similar anticholinergic effects. In addition to the specific anticholinergic toxidrome, a prolonged QRS duration was present on the ECG. Class IA and IC antiarrhythmics, cocaine, propranolol, and digoxin can prolong the QRS duration. However, the father's history of depression provided the final clue to the diagnosis.

II. Diagnosis

The father reported that his bottle of doxepin was missing. He was taking the tricyclic antidepressant (TCA) for his depression. He reported that they were 100-mg tablets and there were approximately 20 pills in the bottle.

III. Incidence and Epidemiology

TCAs are the leading cause of death from a prescription drug overdose in the United States. Despite this propensity for significant mortality after overdose, TCAs continue to be a commonly prescribed medication in the pediatric population for disorders such as enuresis, attention-deficit hyperactivity disorder, and depression. Amitriptyline, imipramine, nortriptyline, clomipramine, and doxepin are the most commonly prescribed TCAs. Although each is unique in clinical effectiveness, the entire group act similarly in overdose. Ingestion of 1 g of TCA can result in life-threatening consequences in adults; in children, only 10 to 20 mg/kg, or just two 50 mg tablets, can be equally devastating.

IV. Clinical Presentation

The clinical picture of TCA toxicity includes the following: hypotension, arrhythmias, seizures, altered level of consciousness, and hyperthermia. α-Adrenergic blockade results in refractory hypotension, the most common cause of death from TCA overdose. Myocardial depression from sodium channel blockade results in PR, QT, and, classically, QRS interval prolongation. Wide-complex tachycardia, either supraventricular or ventricular in origin, is characteristic of the life-threatening arrhythmia from TCA overdose. However, the most common arrhythmia is sinus tachycardia, a result of the anticholinergic properties of TCAs. Altered level of consciousness and hyperthermia constitute the other significant components of the anticholinergic effects. Seizures may occur, usually 1 to 2 hours after ingestion, and are usually generalized and brief. Among patients with seizures, 10% to 20% quickly go on to develop cardiovascular deterioration. The clinical picture can change rapidly with TCA overdose, requiring prompt diagnosis, therapy, and monitoring.

V. Diagnostic Approach

Electrocardiogram. The most helpful diagnostic tool is an ECG. Measurement of the QRS interval is a good prognostic aid. QRS intervals longer than 0.1 second reflect significant risk of seizure, whereas those longer than 0.16 second are associated with increased risk of ventricular arrhythmias. An additional ECG finding associated with increased potential for seizure and arrhythmia is an R wave height of 3 mm or more in aVR.

Other studies. Laboratory testing should be performed, including electrolytes, BUN, creatinine, hemoglobin, prothrombin time, and a screen for additional ingested drugs.

Serum TCA levels are not helpful in the immediate management of a TCA ingestion. TCAs have a large volume of distribution, with tissue concentrations exceeding blood concentrations by 10- to 100-fold; therefore, levels do not correlate well with toxicity.

VI. Treatment

Patients with suspected TCA toxicity are at great risk for rapid clinical deterioration; therefore, evaluation and treatment should be started without delay, and frequent reassessment is a necessity. Attention to airway, breathing, and circulation are the critical components of the initial assessment. Mechanical ventilation may be required to secure the airway, and careful attention to perfusion and temperature is crucial. Cardiac monitoring is mandatory, and a 12-lead ECG should be performed immediately to assess for any evidence of cardiac toxicity, reflected in a prolonged QRS interval, R wave height of 3 mm or more in aVR or ventricular arrhythmias.

If cardiac toxicity is evident as conduction delays, hypotension, or wide-complex tachycardia, serum alkalinization with hypertonic sodium bicarbonate is the treatment of choice. Empiric treatment should not be initiated in the absence of cardiac toxicity, given the potential for arrhythmias, hypocalcemia, and seizures from profound alkalemia. Although the exact mechanism for the effectiveness of alkalinization in treating TCA toxicity is unknown, two theories are correction of acidosis and decrease in the amount of pharmacologically active drug through protein binding. Nevertheless, numerous animal models and anecdotal evidence support the use of alkalinization in reducing QRS prolongation, increasing blood pressure, and reversing ventricular arrhythmias.

The goal for alkalinization is a serum pH of 7.50 to 7.55. This can be accomplished with the use of 1 to 2 mEq/kg boluses of sodium bicarbonate (1 mEq/mL) administered over 1 to 2 minutes, followed by an infusion of sodium bicarbonate (150 mEq $NaHCO_3$ in 1 L of 5% dextrose in water). If arrhythmias are not responding to alkalinization, hypoxia, acidosis, hyperthermia, and hypotension should be corrected and lidocaine may be used as an antiarrhythmic agent. Hypotension is the most common cause of death from TCA overdose and should be managed with normal saline boluses (up to 30 mL/kg) and alkalinization. However, if the hypotension is refractory to fluid administration, norepinephrine and low-dose dopamine may be effective.

Alkalinization should be continued until mental status is back to baseline, hypotension is resolved, and ECG abnormalities are improved. Observation for 24 hours after resolution of toxicity is appropriate. However, patients can be safely discharged to psychiatry services if they have received activated charcoal and show no signs of TCA toxicity after 6 hours of observation.

VII. References

1. Harrigan RA, Brady WJ. ECG abnormalities in tricyclic antidepressant ingestion. *Am J Emerg Med* 1999;17:387–393.
2. Osterhoudt KC, Shannon MD, Henretig FM. Toxicologic emergencies. In: Fleisher GR, Ludwig S, eds. *Textbook of pediatric emergency medicine,* 4th ed. Philadelphia: Lippincott Williams & Wilkins, 2000:925–927.
3. Pentel PR, Keyler DE, Haddad LM. Tricyclic antidepressants and selective serotonin reuptake inhibitors. In: Haddad LM, Shannon MW, Winchester JF, eds. *Clinical management of poisoning and drug overdoses,* 3rd ed. Philadelphia: WB Saunders, 1998: 437–451.
4. Shannon M, Liebelt EL. Toxicology reviews. Targeted management strategies for cardiovascular toxicity from tricyclic antidepressant overdose: the pivotal role for alkalinization and sodium loading. *Pediatr Emerg Care* 1998;14:293–298.

Case 8-7: 4-Year-Old Boy

I. History of Present Illness

A 4-year-old African-American boy presented to the emergency department with a 2-day history of fever. He awoke the day before admission and complained of neck pain and headache in the back of his head. His mother reported that he crawled down the stairs instead of walking and was unable to put food into his mouth. She also reported that he appeared confused. She asked him to bring her a hat and he returned with a book. She stated that he had no history of medication ingestions, vomiting, diarrhea, head injury, or rashes. There were no ill contacts.

II. Past Medical History

He was born at 32 weeks' gestation and had a history of unconjugated hyperbilirubinemia. He had been hospitalized in the neonatal intensive care unit for 2 weeks but did not require endotracheal intubation or antibiotics. He also had a history of plumbism, with a peak lead level of 25 µg/dL; however, a lead level 2 weeks ago was 10 µg/dL. He did not take any medication and had no allergies.

III. Physical Examination

T, 37.5°C; RR, 24/min; HR, 110 bpm; BP, 100/65 mm Hg

Height, 50th percentile; weight, 50th percentile

In general he was a well-appearing boy who was sitting quietly in his mother's arms. He was appropriately interactive during the examination. He had no nuchal rigidity, his tympanic membranes were clear, and his funduscopic examination was normal. Cardiac, pulmonary, and abdominal examinations were normal. The cranial nerves were grossly intact. He had brisk reflexes symmetrically, with downgoing toes. Tone and strength were normal and symmetric throughout. The child displayed truncal ataxia while sitting and was unable to walk without assistance due to ataxia. He also had dysmetria with finger-nose-finger.

IV. Diagnostic Studies

The complete blood count revealed 7,800 WBCs/mm^3 (34% segmented neutrophils, 51% lymphocytes, 10% monocytes, and 5% eosinophils), a hemoglobin of 12.2 g/dL, and a platelet count of 275,000/mm^3. Electrolytes, urinalysis, partial thromboplastin time, prothrombin time, ammonia, and liver function tests were all normal. His serum glucose concentration was 84 mg/dL. Head CT was negative. CSF analysis revealed 3 WBCs/mm^3 and 1 RBC/mm^3, with a glucose concentration of 54 mg/dL and a protein concentration of 15 mg/dL. There were no bacteria on CSF Gram stain. Lead level was 8 µg/dL.

V. Course of Illness

The child was admitted to the hospital and treated empirically with vancomycin, cefotaxime, and acyclovir. The next day he developed a rash that revealed the diagnosis (Fig. 8-3).

DISCUSSION: CASE 8-7

I. Differential Diagnosis

The life-threatening causes of ataxia that must be addressed are acute bacterial meningitis, cerebellar abscess, neoplasm, and metabolic disturbances including hypoglycemia, hyponatremia, and hyperammonemia. Toxin ingestions, particularly alcohol, benzodiazepines, and phenytoin, must also be considered. Posterior fossa tumors and metastatic

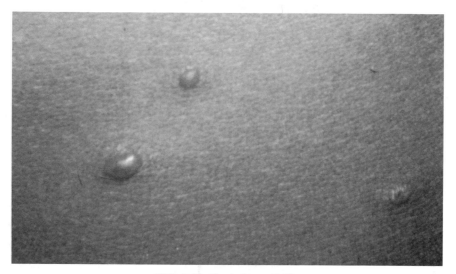

FIG. 8-3. Rash (case 8-7).

malignancies may manifest with ataxia. Guillain-Barré syndrome may also present as ataxia with lower extremity weakness in an otherwise healthy child. Infectious causes include bacterial meningitis and *Listeria* rhombencephalitis. Measles, mumps, and rubella were common precipitants of cerebellar ataxia before the advent of widespread vaccination. However, the vast majority of children with ataxia have postinfectious acute cerebellar ataxia. Common inciting agents are enteroviruses, influenza, Epstein-Barr virus, and varicella.

II. Diagnosis

The next day the boy developed a pruritic vesicular rash on his face and trunk. The rash consisted of clear fluid-filled vesicles with a surrounding irregular margin of erythema resembling "dewdrops on a rose petal" (Fig. 8-3). Several stages of the rash were present in the same area, a finding consistent with varicella. **The diagnosis is acute cerebellar ataxia secondary to varicella infection.**

III. Incidence and Epidemiology

Before the availability of the varicella vaccine, approximately 4 million cases of varicella occurred in the United States annually. Almost 100,000 hospitalizations and 100 deaths occurred each year in the United States from the infection. Ninety-five percent of the cases occurred in people younger than 20 years of age, and almost half of the deaths occurred in children. However, the vaccine licensed in 1995 has resulted in a marked decrease in severe varicella infection in the United States. The vaccine prevents 70% to 85% of cases of mild disease and more than 95% of cases of severe disease.

IV. Clinical Presentation

Varicella is contagious from 24 to 48 hours before the eruption of the rash until all of the vesicles have crusted over. The incubation period is 10 to 21 days, and prodromal symptoms include fever, headache, and malaise. The lesions occur initially on the face and trunk and spread to the extremities. They begin as erythematous macules that evolve to form clear, fluid-filled vesicles with irregular surrounding erythema. These vesicles are classically described as resembling "dewdrops on a rose petal." New lesions erupt as older lesions are crusting. The lesions are typically pruritic.

Varicella is usually a benign and self-limited infection, and complications are rare; however, the two most common complications of varicella are secondary bacterial infections and neurologic disturbances. Group A β-hemolytic *Streptococcus* and *Staphylococcus aureus* are the notorious causes of bacterial superinfection. Neurologic manifestations include cerebellar ataxia and meningoencephalitis. Cerebella ataxia is characterized by gait disturbance, nystagmus, and slurred speech. Signs of meningoencephalitis include seizures, altered level of consciousness, and nuchal rigidity. The neurologic sequelae usually develop 3 to 7 days after eruption of the rash; however, as in this case, they may appear during the incubation phase, making the diagnosis difficult if there is no history of varicella exposure. The mechanism of the neurologic complications is unknown; however, direct invasion by the virus and an autoimmune response are proposed theories.

V. Diagnostic Approach

A thorough history focused on possible ingestions, trauma, and associated symptoms or viral syndromes is necessary with any child presenting with ataxia. Close attention to vital signs, an altered level of consciousness, or weakness helps distinguish life-threatening from more benign causes of ataxia.

Lumbar puncture. CSF examination may be normal or may reveal a mild lymphocytic pleocytosis (fewer than 200 WBCs/mm^3) and elevated protein (50 to 200 mg/dL).

Varicella detection. Varicella may be detected in the CSF by PCR. When lesions are present, direct immunofluorescent staining of epithelial cells from the base of a newly formed vesicle detects viral antigens with great sensitivity and specificity. This rapid test readily differentiates varicella from herpes simplex virus, which can cause similar lesions. Isolation of varicella from tissue culture provides definitive diagnosis, but identification requires 3 to 7 days. Therefore, viral culture serves to confirm a diagnosis already made by clinical examination or rapid antigen testing. Varicella IgM antibody detection should not be used for clinical diagnosis, because the test produces many false-positive and false-negative results.

Neuroimaging. MRI should be considered to exclude posterior fossa tumors. Neuroimaging is necessary if there is a history of trauma, focal neurologic examination, or increased intracranial pressure.

Other studies. Testing of serum and urine for toxic ingestions may help narrow the differential diagnosis. Laboratory studies including glucose and serum electrolytes are also appropriate in the evaluation.

VI. Treatment

Acyclovir is the drug of choice for the treatment of varicella in high-risk patients, including neonates and immunocompromised children. Patients with disseminated varicella disease (pneumonia, encephalitis) also benefit from intravenous acyclovir. However, acyclovir is not recommended in cases of cerebellar ataxia, because it does not alter the course of the illness. Otherwise healthy patients may benefit from acyclovir if the drug is initiated within 24 hours after the appearance of the initial skin lesions; however, this practice remains controversial.

VII. References

1. American Academy of Pediatrics, Committee on Infectious Disease. Varicella vaccine update. *Pediatrics* 2000;105:136–140.
2. Arvin AM. Varicella zoster virus. In: Behrman RE, Kliegman RM, Jenson HB, eds. *Nelson textbook of pediatrics,* 16th ed. Philadelphia: WB Saunders, 2000:973–977.
3. Dangond F, Engle E, Yessayan L, et al. Pre-eruptive varicella cerebellitis confirmed by PCR. *Pediatr Neurol* 1993;9:491–493.

4. DeAngelis C. Ataxia. *Pediatr Rev* 1995;16:114–155.

5. Gieron-Korthals MA, Westberry KR, Emmanuel PJ. Acute childhood ataxia: 10 year experience. *J Child Neurol* 1994;9:381–384.

6. Haslam RHA. In: Behrman RE, Kliegman RM, Jenson HB, eds. *Nelson textbook of pediatrics,* 16th ed. Philadelphia: WB Saunders, 2000:1793–1803.

7. Klassen TP, et al. Acyclovir for treating varicella in otherwise healthy children and adolescents: a systemic review of randomized controlled trials. *BMC Pediatrics* 2002; 2:9(abstract).

8. Skull SA, Wang EL. Varicella vaccination: a critical review of the evidence. *Arch Dis Child* 2001;85:83–90.

9. Ziebold C, von Kries R, Lang R, et al. Severe complications of varicella in previously healthy children in Germany: a 1 year survey. *Pediatrics* 2001;108:E79.

9

Rash

Heather C. Forkey

APPROACH TO THE PATIENT WITH RASH

I. Definition of the Complaint

Rash, a general term applied to any skin eruption, is the presenting problem or secondary complaint for 20% to 30% of visits to pediatricians, emergency departments, and primary care practitioners. Perhaps because rashes are so common and because the skin is the easiest organ of the body to access, patients with skin complaints may receive only cursory examinations and overly hasty diagnoses.

Rashes may be divided into primary and secondary lesions. The primary lesion is the most representative lesion and arises from the disease process itself without alteration by the patient or therapies. Examination of the primary lesion is most helpful in making a specific diagnosis. Secondary lesions result from changes caused by the patient or environment, usually from scratching, medication use, or infection. These change over time. Although they do not usually identify the primary cause, they do give historical clues to the primary lesions.

There are a variety of primary lesions. A *macule* is a flat, nonpalpable area of color change to the skin in any shape. *Papules* are raised lesions less than 0.5 cm in diameter. *Nodules* are raised lesions larger than 0.5 cm in diameter, and *tumors* are larger nodules, usually greater than 2 cm in diameter. *Plaques* are well-circumscribed, wide-based lesions usually created by the convergence of a number of papules. The diameter of a plaque is usually greater than its height. *Wheals* are raised edematous lesions of various sizes that are transient in nature and white, pink, or red in color. *Vesicles* are raised, fluid-filled lesions smaller than 1 cm in diameter, and *bullae* are similar but greater than 1 cm in diameter. *Cysts* are circumscribed tumors that contain fluid or soft contents. *Pustules* are raised, well-demarcated lesions with purulent material inside, and they are usually white or yellow in appearance. *Petechiae* are pinpoint areas of hemorrhage that are caused by leakage of blood into the skin. *Purpura* is the leakage of blood into the skin that results in a flat or elevated lesion. Neither purpura nor petechiae blanch when pressure is applied. *Burrows* are linear lesions caused by the movement of parasites in the skin.

Secondary lesions include *scales,* which are accumulations of dried layers of squamous cells. Scales can appear greasy, yellowish, or silvery. *Crusts* are made by dried exudate overlying damaged skin. *Excoriations* are usually caused by scratching; they are linear lesions of skin that usually indicate pruritus. *Erosions* are lesions of denuded epidermis, and *ulcers* signify a deeper loss of skin into the dermis or subcutaneous tissue. *Fissures* are linear clefts of the epidermis to the dermis. *Lichenification* is an exaggeration of skin markings caused by chronic rubbing or scratching. A *scar* is permanent fibrotic tissue that is found when there has been deep injury to the skin. *Atrophy* is the loss or thinning of the epidermis or dermis.

One of the values of identifying primary lesions and differentiating them from secondary lesions is that doing so allows classification into broad groups of skin disorders that can narrow the differential. These categories are *papulosquamous, vesicobullous, tumor-nodule, vascular reaction, eczematous,* and *pigmentary changes.* Two additional terms define a constellation of findings rather than primary or secondary lesions. *Eczematous* lesions are erythematous inflammatory skin lesions that have poorly defined borders and can acutely become vesiculated. Scale, crust, and lichenification may be seen over time. *Hyperkeratosis* describes lesions with thick and adherent scale.

II.   Complaint by Cause and Frequency
Causes of rashes may be grouped by age and frequency (Table 9-1).

TABLE 9-1. *Causes of Rash in Childhood by Age and Frequency*

Disease prevalence	Newborn and infant	Child and adolescent
Papulosquamous		
Common	Candidiasis	Pityriasis rosea
	Epidermal nevus	Tinea corporis
	Tinea corporis	Scabies
	Chronic dermatitis	Lichen planus
	Scabies	Chronic dermatitis
Uncommon	Ichythyosis	Psoriasis
	Psoriasis	Lupus erythematosus
	Congenital syphilis	Parapsoriasis
	Neonatal lupus	Keratosis pilaris
	Congenital rubella	Secondary syphilis
	Pityriasis rubra pilaris	Dermatomyositis
Vesicobullous		
Common	Miliaria	Impetigo
	Impetigo	Burns
	Herpes simplex	Acute dermatitis
	Burns	Papular urticaria
	Acute dermatitis	Viral blisters
	Sucking blisters	
	Friction blisters	
Uncommon	Varicella	Erythema multiforme
	Scalded skin syndrome	Scalded skin syndrome
	Epidermolysis bullosa	Toxic epidermal necrolysis
	Lymphangioma	Fixed drug eruption
	Aplasia cutis congenita	Dermatitis herpetiformis
		Kerion
		Lupus erythematosus
Tumor nodule		
Common	Epidermal nevus	Warts
	Warts	Corns/callus
	Milia	Microcomedones of acne
	Molluscum contagiosum	Keratosis pilaris
		Molluscum contagiosum
Uncommon	Dermoid cyst	Epidermal nevus
		Epidermal cyst
		Granuloma annulare
		Lipoma
		Mucous cyst
		Rheumoid nodule
		Neurofibroma
		Papular acrodermatitis (Gianotti-Crosti syndrome)
Vascular lesions—blanching		
Common	Mottling	Hemangioma
	Flat hemangioma	Urticaria
	Urticaria	Livedo reticularis
	Erythema toxicum	Scarlet fever
Uncommon	Port wine stain	Erythema multiforme
	Vascular birthmarks	Erythema infectiosum
	Neonatal lupus	Kawasaki disease

TABLE 9-1. *Continued.*

Disease prevalence	Newborn and infant	Child and adolescent
		Morbilliform viral exanthems
		Toxic shock syndrome
		Drug eruptions
		Urticarial lesions of systemic disease
		Erythema chronicum migrans (Lyme disease)
		Syphilis
Vascular lesions— nonblanching (purpuric)		
Common	Trauma	Trauma
Uncommon	Congenital infection	Henoch-Schönlein purpura
	Toxoplasma	Coagulation disorders
	Enteroviruses	ITP
	Rubella	Leukemia
	Cytomegalovirus	Hemophilia
	Herpes simplex	Erythema nodosum
	Syphilis	Meningococcemia
	Coagulation defects	Rocky Mountain spotted fever
	Autoimmune disorders	Atypical measles
	ITP	Herpes simplex purpura
	SLE	Gonococcemia
	Erythroblastosis fetalis	Ecthyma gangrenosum
		Bacterial endocarditis
		Infectious mononucleosis
Eczematous disorders		
Common	Diaper dermatitis	Atopic dermatitis
	Atopic dermatitis	Contact dermatitis
	Seborrheic dermatitis	Nummular eczematous dermatitis
	Contact dermatitis	Drug eruption
	Scabies	Tinea corporis
	Candidiasis	Scabies
Uncommon	Acrodermatitis enteropathica	Candidiasis
	Lenier's disease	HIV infection
	Multiple carboxylase deficiency	Seborrheic dermatitis
	Severe combined immunodeficiency	Histiocytosis X
	Histocytosis X	Lichen planus
	HIV	Dermatitis herpetiformis
Pigmentary changes		
Common	Mongolian spot	Café-au-lait spot
	Café-au-lait spot	Tinea versicolor
	Junctional nevus	Mongolian spot
	Congenital pigmented intradermal nevus	Postinflammatory hypopigmentation or hyperpigmentation
	Piebaldism	Pityriasis alba
	Postinflammatory hypopigmentation or hyperpigmentation	Junctional or intradermal nevus
Uncommon	Ash leaf macules	Halo nevus
	Hypomelanosis of Ito	Scleroderma
	Precursor to strawberry hemangioma	Dermatofibroma
	Lentigo	Urticaria pigmentosa
	Transient neonatal pustular melanosis	Blue nevus
	Linear and whorled hypermelanosis	Lichen sclerosis et atrophicus
		Ash leaf macules
		Piebaldism
		Diffuse endocrine hyperpigmentation
		Melanoma
		Pyogenic granuloma
		Hemangioma
		Incontentia pigmenti
		Nevus of Ota
		Lentigo
		Waardenburg syndrome
		Hypomelanosis of Ito

HIV, human immunodeficiency virus; ITP, idiopathic thrombocytopenia purpura; SLE, systemic lupus erythematosus.

III. Clarifying Questions

The history is vitally important in narrowing the differential diagnosis of skin lesions. Because rash can be the primary manifestation of systemic disease, general questions relating to the child's overall health are important. Determination of age, gender, and racial or ethnic background may be useful, because some skin disorders are found only in particular age groups or are seen more commonly in specific subsets of the population. Specific questions that help narrow the diagnosis include the following.

- What was the progression of the rash over time and the duration of the rash?

  — Viral exanthems can be defined by where they start and where they spread. For example, measles begins at the scalp and hairline and progresses downward, whereas scarlet fever begins on the upper trunk. Duration varies with different types of rashes. Pityriasis rosea may last for weeks, whereas viral exanthems are more limited.

- What is the configuration of the lesion?

  — The shape of the lesion can often be characteristic or provide clues to the etiology. Linear lesions include contact dermatitis and lichen striatus, a self-limited papular dermatitis. Annular lesions, which are ring shaped with central clearing, include tinea corporis, pityriasis rosea, and nummular eczema. Arciform lesions are arc-like or semicircular and are found in erythema multiforme and erythema marginatum.

- Where is the rash distributed on the body?

  — Lesions limited to a particular dermatome may be characteristic of herpes zoster. If contact dermatitis is being considered, the distribution of the rash must be consistent with the area in contact with the suspected irritant. Knowing the typical patterns of disorders in particular types of patients may guide diagnosis. Scabies rarely involves the face, except in infants. Atopic dermatitis is found in the flexural areas of the older child, whereas psoriasis involves extensor surfaces.

- What is the color of the rash?

  — Pigmentation and erythema are clues to the disease process. Pigment changes can include hyperpigmentation and hypopigmentation and usually indicate postinflammatory changes due to increases or decreases in melanin production. Depigmentation is the loss of pigment resulting from an autoimmune effect or congenital disorder.

IV.   References

1. Hurwitz S. *Clinical pediatric dermatology: a textbook of skin disorders of childhood and adolescence,* 2nd ed. Philadelphia: WB Saunders, 1993:1–6.
2. Pomeranz AJ, Fairley JA. The systematic evaluation of the skin in children. *Pediatr Clin North Am* 1998;45:49–63.
3. Shivaram V, Christoph RA, Hayden G. Skin disorders encountered in a pediatric emergency department. *Pediatr Emerg Care* 1994;9:202.
4. Tunnessen WW Jr. A survey of skin disorders seen in pediatric general and dermatology clinics. *Pediatr Dermatol* 1982;1:219.
5. Weston W, Lane AT, Morelli JG. *Color textbook of pediatric dermatology,* 2nd ed. St. Louis: Mosby, 1996:1–16.

Case 9-1: 8-Year-Old Girl

I. History of Present Illness

An 8-year-old girl presented to her primary care physician with a history of bruising of the chest, groin, arms, and legs over a period of several months without any obvious source of trauma. During the months of bruising, the patient had also complained of mild leg pain, which the family had attributed to excessive exercise. A relative noted that she was increasingly pale. She had no history of fever, weight loss, or night sweats.

II. Past Medical History

Three years before this visit, the patient had been neutropenic and thrombocytopenic after a viral illness, but the hematologic abnormalities resolved. The child had congenital conductive hearing loss for which she wore a hearing aid in the left ear; the right ear had been repaired surgically. A maternal grandfather had anemia, but details were not available. The birth history was otherwise unremarkable.

III. Physical Examination

T, 37.3°C; RR, 24/min; HR, 96 bpm; BP, 107/46 mm Hg

Height, 5th to 10th percentile; weight, 5th to 10th percentile

The physical examination was remarkable for mucous membrane pallor. Scattered petechiae were noted on the posterior pharynx and upper chest. There were 1- to 2-cm areas of ecchymoses on the forehead, left hip, left arm, posterior right heel, and right knee. Lung examination revealed decreased breath sounds at the bases. Cardiac examination revealed no murmurs, rubs, or gallops. There was no hepatosplenomegaly and no prominent adenopathy.

IV. Diagnostic Studies

Laboratory analysis revealed 2,300 WBCs/mm^3, with 1% band forms, 14% segmented neutrophils, 84% lymphocytes, 8% eosinophils, and 1% monocytes. The hemoglobin was

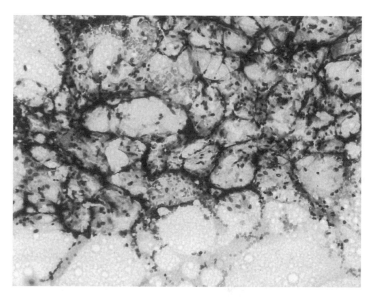

FIG. 9-1. Bone marrow biopsy (case 9-1). (Photograph courtesy of Marybeth Helfrich, MT, ASCP.).

6.2 g/dL, and there were 16, 000 platelets/mm^3. The peripheral blood smear revealed anisocytosis, poikilocytosis, and hypochromia. Electrolytes, blood urea nitrogen (BUN), and creatinine were normal. Alkaline phosphatase was 159 mU/mL. Lactate dehydrogenase was 1,062 IU/L. Serum transaminases, albumin, and bilirubin were normal. Uric acid was normal. Antibodies to Epstein-Barr virus were consistent with past infection. Serologic tests for hepatitis B and C infection were negative.

V. Course of Illness

The patient was admitted to the hospital, where bone marrow biopsy (Fig. 9-1) and a hematologic test were diagnostic for her condition.

DISCUSSION: CASE 9-1

I. Differential Diagnosis

Bruising and petechiae are types of vascular rashes. Given the location of the lesions in areas where accidental trauma is unlikely, first on the differential for a child of this age would be coagulation disorders such as leukemia or immune thrombocytopenic purpura (ITP). Leukemia was possible in this case, given the bone complaints and pancytopenia. ITP is an acute, self-limited illness that manifests with bruising and petechiae 2 to 4 weeks after a minor illness. The timing of this patient's symptoms and the effect on all three cell lines rather than on the platelets alone made this diagnosis unlikely. Because of the slow evolution of her illness and the lack of other systemic symptoms, acute illness causing vasculitis was less likely. Because all three cell lines were affected, clinicians were led to suspect a congenital or acquired aplastic anemia.

II. Diagnosis

Bone marrow biopsy revealed a markedly hypocellular marrow with only rare hematopoietic cells (Fig. 9-1). There also was stromal edema and focal hemosiderosis. Peripheral blood lymphocytes were cultured in the presence of diepoxybutane (DEB), an alkylating agent. The DEB test was considered positive by the presence of consistent chromosomal abnormalities. This indicated the diagnosis of **Fanconi anemia, or congenital aplastic anemia.**

III. Incidence and Epidemiology

Fanconi anemia is transmitted in an autosomal recessive inheritance pattern. More than 600 cases have been reported in many ethnic groups since the disorder was first described by Professor Fanconi in Switzerland in 1927. It now appears that there are at least five separate Fanconi anemia genes, although there seem to be no clinical differences among the Fanconi anemia genotypes.

IV. Clinical Presentation

There are three features of Fanconi anemia: chromosome breakage, pancytopenia, and congenital anomalies. Although chromosomal breakage and pancytopenia are universal features of the disease, congenial anomalies and resultant dysmorphic features are not. More than one half of patients with Fanconi anemia have skeletal abnormalities, including thumb abnormalities or absence of the radii, and one third have renal abnormalities. Other findings in some include short stature and hyperpigmentation. In this case, the absence of obvious congenital anomalies led to delays and difficulties in the diagnosis.

Although pancytopenia is genetically determined, patients do not usually present until after 5 years of age. The onset of progressive bone marrow failure is initially manifested by petechiae and ecchymoses secondary to thrombocytopenia between ages 2 and 22 years (mean age, 7 years). Anemia and neutropenia develop later.

V. Diagnostic Approach

Complete blood count. Disordered erythropoiesis is demonstrated by macrocytosis and increased levels of fetal hemoglobin before marrow failure occurs. Thrombocytopenia is usually noted at presentation, with pancytopenia ultimately developing.

Bone marrow biopsy. Serial bone marrow aspirates show progressive hypocellularity and, finally, frank aplasia.

Chromosomal breakage test. The laboratory diagnosis is made by finding an increased incidence of chromosome breakage induced by alkylating agents such as nitrogen mustards, mitomycin C, and DEB. An increased incidence of spontaneous chromosome breakage is seen in these patients. Prenatal diagnosis is now possible in some experienced laboratories.

VI. Treatment

Supportive therapy, including transfusions of erythrocytes and platelets, is of only temporary benefit. In the past, 75% of these patients died within 2 years after diagnosis. Therapy with pharmacologic doses of androgenic hormones provides hematologic benefit in more than two thirds of the patients and may be maintained for several years. However, complications of androgenic therapy are common, and most patients eventually become refractory to therapy. Bone marrow transplantation has been successful in some patients.

VII. References

1. De Kerviler E, Guermazi A, Zagdanski AM, et al. The clinical and radiological features of Fanconi's anaemia. *Clin Radiol* 2000;55:340–345.
2. Giampietro PF, Davis JG, Auerbach AD. Fanconi's anemia. *N Engl J Med* 1994;330: 720–721.
3. Joenje H, Patel KJ. The emerging genetic and molecular basis of Fanconi's anaemia. *Nat Rev Genet* 2001;2:446–457.
4. Martin PL, Pearson HA. Hypoplastic and aplastic anemias. In: Mc Millan JA, DeAngelis CD, Feigin RD, et al., eds. *Oski's pediatrics: principles and practice,* 3rd ed. Philadelphia: Lippincott Williams & Wilkins, 1999:1459–1460.
5. Woods CG. DNA repair disorders. *Arch Dis Child* 1998;78:178–184.

Case 9-2: 7-Week-Old Girl

I. History of Present Illness

A 7-week-old Caucasian girl had initially presented to a hematologist for evaluation of bruising. Her mother had noted several small purple bruises on her right arm and a linear bruise across her left cheek at age 3 weeks. At 5 weeks of life, she had been noted to have linear and circular bruises along her buttocks and legs. Laboratory evaluation at that time revealed a normal complete blood count and differential, normal prothrombin time (PT) and partial thromboplastin time (PTT), and normal platelet aggregation studies in response to adenosine diphosphate (ADP), collagen, and ristocetin. Epinephrine-induced platelet aggregation studies were mildly low but consistent with testing variability. Factor XIII level was normal.

At 11 weeks of life, she was brought to the emergency department after having had a possible seizure at home. Her father reported that she had an episode of stiffening of her arms and body during her afternoon feeding. Her eyes had rolled back in her head. After stiffening, her body became limp and she had shallow breathing, but no cyanosis. The child had had decreased oral intake during the day before the episode. There was no recent history of fever, vomiting, diarrhea, or trauma. Immunizations, including diphtheria-tetanus-pertussis (DTaP) vaccine, had been given 2 days before the episode.

II. Past Medical History

The child was born at full term, of an uncomplicated pregnancy and delivery, and weighed 3,500 g at birth. She was delivered vaginally without complication. She had previously been evaluated for the bruising at her pediatrician's office at 3 and 5 weeks of age, as noted. Child protective services had been contacted by the pediatrician for the bruising, but the case was determined to be unfounded and was closed. Family history was significant for an uncle with frequent nosebleeds and a first cousin who was born with a "platelet problem" that necessitated platelet transfusion at birth.

III. Physical Examination

T, 37.0°C; RR, 43/min; HR, 180 bpm; BP, 113/53 mm Hg

Height, 50th percentile; weight, 50th percentile

The physical examination was remarkable for a hemangioma of the left occiput, a hematoma of the tip of the tongue, and two ecchymotic areas on the right mandible, each about 1 cm in diameter. She had three 3- to 4-cm ecchymotic areas on the left back. A café-au-lait macule (1 cm) was seen on the left thigh. Lungs were clear. Cardiac examination revealed tachycardia but no murmurs, rubs, or gallops. There was no hepatosplenomegaly and no prominent adenopathy. Neurologically she was alert, crying, and moving all extremities. Funduscopic examination revealed right retinal hemorrhages. The rest of her examination was normal.

VI. Diagnostic Studies

Laboratory analysis revealed 18,800 WBCs/mm^3, with 39% segmented neutrophils, 49% lymphocytes, and 11% monocytes. The hemoglobin was 11.4 g/dL, and there were 406, 000 platelets/mm^3. PT and PTT were normal. Electrolytes, BUN, and creatinine were normal. Alkaline phosphatase was 270 mU/mL. Other liver function studies were as follows: alanine aminotransferase, 100 IU/L; aspartate aminotransferase, 220 IU/L; and γ-glutamyltransferase, 46 IU/L. Examination of the cerebrospinal fluid revealed 8 WBCs/mm^3 and 5,250 red blood cells/mm^3. The glucose concentration was 60 mg/dL, and the protein concentration was 36 mg/dL. There were no organisms on Gram staining of the CSF.

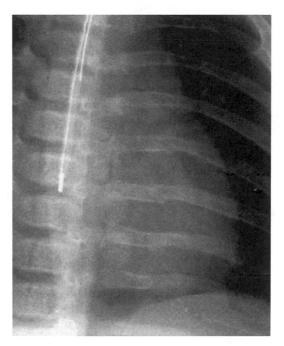

FIG. 9-2. Chest radiograph (case 9-2).

V. Course of Illness

The patient was admitted to the intensive care unit. Electroencephalography revealed no seizure activity but was consistent with diffuse cerebral edema. Examination of the chest radiograph (Fig. 9-2), in conjunction with the clinical examination findings, suggested a diagnosis.

DISCUSSION: CASE 9-2

I. Differential Diagnosis

Bruising caused clinicians to consider hematologic causes primarily. The initial workup was done to evaluate for von Willebrand's disease, which causes decreased platelet adhesiveness, impaired agglutination of platelets in the presence of ristocetin, and prolonged bleeding time. The usual presentation is mild to moderate bleeding involving mucous membranes, including easy bruising, epistaxis, and prolonged bleeding after dental procedures. In boys, hemophilia (factor VIII and IX deficiency) should be considered. These children have bruising with a firm or nodular consistency because of deep soft-tissue bleeding. Vitamin K deficiency can be seen in patients with fat malabsorption syndromes, and hemorrhagic disease of the newborn may be seen in those not given vitamin K at delivery. In these infants, signs and symptoms typically occur within the first few days of life and include diffuse bruising and, rarely, catastrophic central nervous system bleeding. However, the timing in this case was not consistent with vitamin K deficiency. ITP, an acute and self-limited illness that causes bruising and petechiae 2 to 4 weeks after a minor illness, could be considered. This infant did not have any preceding illness, and her platelet count was normal. The peak age for presentation with ITP is 2 to 5 years, and infants who are diagnosed before 1 year of age have a high likelihood of developing chronic symptoms. Leukemia was considered less likely on the basis of a normal complete blood count in the context of significant bruising and bleeding. Anticoagulant ingestions from medications or commercial rat poison have been seen in older children and in cases of Munchausen syndrome by proxy, but this child had normal PT and PTT times, which would not have been the case after ingestion of anticoagulants.

Dermatologic considerations include Mongolian spots, which are rare in Caucasian children and do not progress through the color changes indicative of a healing bruise. These slate-blue patches of skin are commonly seen in pigmented skin. Phytophotodermatitis is a skin reaction to psoralens (a chemical compound in citrus fruits such as limes). After contact with psoralens and on exposure to sunlight, this manifests as red marks that appear as bruises or burns. The locations of the lesions, as well as the child's age and lack of contact with psoralens, made such a diagnosis unlikely. Hemangioma was considered. Unlike this child's lesions, hemangiomas undergo a typical growth pattern of rapid growth for the first 6 months of life, then a slowing of growth until 3 years. This child's lesions resolved and then new ones appeared. Approximately 85% of hemangiomas spontaneously involute or partially regress, but not until later childhood.

Collagen vascular diseases should be considered. Ehlers-Danlos syndrome (EDS) is a congenital defect in collagen synthesis that may lead to easy bruising. Many forms have been identified that involve a variety of basic defects and inheritance patterns. This child did not display the clinical triad seen in these patients: skin hyperextensibility, joint hypermobility, and skin fragility. Osteogenesis imperfecta is a congenital abnormality of quality or quantity of type I collagen synthesis. Of the four subtypes, type I is associated with easy bruising and fractures as seen in this child, but this child did not display other signs, such as blue sclera, hearing impairment, osteopenia, bony deformities, and excessive laxity of joints. Should a question have persisted, a punch biopsy of skin for analysis of collagen synthesis would confirm the diagnosis. Infectious causes were unlikely given the timing of the child's lesions. Child abuse remains the most alarming cause of unexplained bruising in children.

II.   Diagnosis

Chest radiograph revealed fractures of the left sixth and seventh posterior ribs (Fig. 9-2). Computed tomography (CT) of the head revealed right subarachnoid hemorrhage, right subdural hemorrhage in the right interhemispheric fissure, and cerebellar convexity. There was also left intraventricular hemorrhage and left caudothalamic parenchymal hemorrhage. A skeletal survey was obtained, which demonstrated splayed cranial sutures and callused fractures at left tibia. **The diagnosis was child abuse.** The parents continued to deny any knowledge of who could have harmed their child. The child was removed from the home and placed in protective custody with grandparents.

III.   Incidence and Epidemiology

Child abuse is an all too common diagnosis. Soft tissue trauma or skin injuries such as bruising are frequently the earliest and most common manifestation of physical maltreatment. A number of studies have shown that many seriously injured children had been evaluated previously for bruises or burns, just as in this case. Johnson and Showers showed in an epidemiologic study of injury variables that children with evidence of chronic maltreatment, such as these bruises, are at a 50% risk for further abuse and at a 10% risk for fatal injury.

IV.   Clinical Presentation

The diagnosis of child abuse must be considered in all cases in which a child's injuries cannot be explained and there is a discrepancy between the physical findings and the history. In a study of bruises occurring in children 6 to 9 months of age, Carpenter found that all accidentally acquired bruises were on the front of the body and that no bruise was greater than 1 cm. In a larger study of children, Sugar et al. demonstrated that only 2.2% of bruises occurred in infants who did not walk or cruise, and only 0.6% occurred in children younger than 6 months of age. In cases that did not involve abuse, bruises were small, few, and located on bony prominences. Typical accidental bruises involve the skin overlying bony prominences such as the anterior tibia, knees, elbows, forehead, and dorsum of the hands. Parents can usually give explanations for how the bruises occurred, unlike these parents.

The shape of the bruise may also suggest intentional harm. Finger and thumb prints may be found on the arms where a child has been forcefully held. A blunt instrument often leaves a bruise that resembles the shape of the instrument. Loop-shaped marks are caused by a folded extension cord or rope.

V. Diagnostic Approach

The most helpful aid to the diagnosis is a high index of suspicion. The most common reason for missing the diagnosis of abuse is that it was not considered before atypical presentations of medical disorders. Bruises should be evaluated by a history that includes explanation of the injury, with evaluation of that explanation from a developmental perspective. A medical and family history of conditions associated with easy bruisability or those that mimic bruising should be investigated. Any prior maltreatment should also be uncovered. Physical examination should include a detailed description of the injury, identification of patterns associated with abuse, and a search for other injuries. Laboratory studies are indicated only if suggested by the history or physical examination. Unfortunately, it is sometimes difficult to distinguish accidental injury from abuse or to distinguish abuse from diseases or other conditions that produce similar changes. These disorders include bleeding diathesis, connective tissue disorders, dye, paint, folk remedies, and phytophotodermatitis.

Diagnostic studies to consider include the following.

Prothrombin time, partial thromboplastin time, bleeding time. Screening tests for a bleeding diathesis should be obtained if medically indicated.

Roentgenologic bone survey. If physical abuse is suspected in a young child, radiographs of the skull, thorax, and long bones may reveal recent or old fractures. This is important because clinical manifestations of nondisplaced fractures may resolve within 1 week, whereas the radiographic manifestations persist for longer periods. For verbal children (usually older than 4 years of age), radiographs are required only if there is bone tenderness or restricted range of motion on physical examination. Fractures of ribs, scapula, or sternum should arouse suspicion of nonaccidental trauma.

Retinal examination. Retinal hemorrhages should always raise concern for abuse.

VI. Treatment

The injuries suffered by the child should be managed as medically indicated. The state division of child and family services should be notified in all cases of suspected abuse. Removal from the home and placement in foster care may be required. In this case, once the child was removed from the home, no additional lesions were noted.

VII. References

1. Carpenter RF. The prevalence and distribution of bruises in babies. *Arch Dis Child* 1999;80:363–366.
2. Giardino AP, Christian CW, Giardino ER. *A practical guide to the evaluation of child physical abuse and neglect.* Thousand Oaks, CA: Sage Publications, 1997:61–74.
3. Johnson CF, Showers J. Injury variables in child abuse. *Child Abuse Neglect* 1985;9: 207–215.
4. Sugar NF, Taylor JA, Feldman KW. Bruises in infants and toddlers: those who don't cruise rarely bruise. *Arch Pediatr Adolesc Med* 1999;53:399–403.

Case 9-3: 4-Year-Old Girl

I History of Present Illness

A 4-year-old Caucasian girl presented to her primary care physician with a 1-day history of rash on her legs. Four days before admission, she was evaluated by her primary physician for complaints of left knee pain. At that time she had mild swelling and tenderness of the joint without erythema. She had been prescribed ibuprofen, which provided some relief. Three days before admission, she had developed abdominal pain and was evaluated at a nearby hospital. Physical examination and abdominal radiograph and obstructive series were normal. Rectal examination was normal, with Hemoccult-negative stool in the rectal vault. The patient was sent home, but the severe, intermittent abdominal pain persisted. On the day of admission, the child's mother had noted "small red bumps" all over both of her legs while she was giving the child a bath. The mother reported that these lesions became larger and spread on the girl's legs during the day. There was no history of fever, vomiting, or diarrhea. The patient ate well between episodes of abdominal pain. She had had some nasal congestion and rhinorrhea 1 week earlier. There was no history of tick bites or ingestions.

II. Past Medical History

The child was a full-term infant with an uncomplicated birth history. There was no significant family history, travel, or exposures.

III. Physical Examination

T, 37.7°C; RR, 22/min; HR, 124 bpm; BP, 98/65 mm Hg

Height, 50th percentile; weight, 50th percentile

The physical examination was remarkable for 2- to 10-mm, nonblanching, erythematous papules on the lower extremities from the dorsum of her feet to her waist bilaterally. A horizontal 4-cm wide purpuric area on the left leg at the sock line was also noted (Fig. 9-3). The lung examination was normal. Cardiac examination revealed no murmurs, rubs,

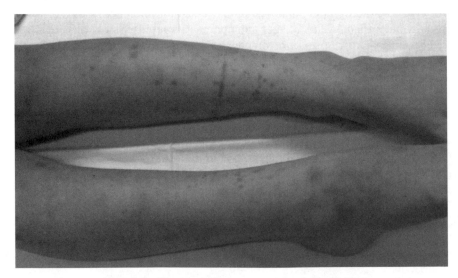

FIG. 9-3. Rash on lower extremities (case 9-3).

or gallops. Active bowel sounds were present, the abdomen was soft and nondistended, and there was no hepatosplenomegaly. Rectal examination was normal with soft, heme-negative stool in the vault. There was no prominent adenopathy. Joint and neurologic examinations were normal.

IV. Diagnostic Studies

Laboratory analysis revealed 10,700 WBCs/mm^3, with 50% segmented neutrophils, 40% lymphocytes, 4% eosinophils, and 6% monocytes. The hemoglobin was 10.9 g/dL, and there were 436,000 platelets/mm^3. Electrolytes, BUN, and creatinine were normal. The erythrocyte sedimentation rate (ESR) was 22 mm/hour. Urinalysis demonstrated a specific gravity of 1.010, with no protein, WBCs, or red blood cells. Blood cultures were obtained.

V. Course of Illness

The patient was admitted to the hospital, where she received medication to manage her abdominal pain. The distribution and character of the rash suggested the diagnosis (Fig. 9-3).

DISCUSSION: CASE 9-3

I. Differential Diagnosis

The nonblanching rash limited to the lower extremities of a well-appearing patient suggested trauma. However, the timing of the rash and the unusual number of lesions on the legs made trauma unlikely. The history of joint and gastrointestinal symptoms suggested leukemia, ITP, hemolytic-uremic syndrome, and septicemia. However, these disorders are less likely with a normal complete blood count, BUN, and creatinine. Purpura due to *Neisseria meningitidis* should also be considered. Juvenile rheumatoid arthritis (JRA) should be considered, but the rash was not typical of the salmon-colored macular rash of JRA, and the timing and joint symptoms were too limited to be consistent with JRA.

II. Diagnosis

The characteristic rash consisting of palpable purpuric lesions on the lower extremities, especially along the sock line of the left leg (Fig. 9-3), along with the constellation of symptoms in this patient led to the clinical diagnosis of **Henoch-Schönlein purpura (HSP), also known as anaphylactoid purpura.** One of the most common vasculitic syndromes affecting children, HSP is characterized by purpuric rash on the buttocks and lower extremities, polyarthritis, colicky abdominal pain, nephritis, or any combination of these symptoms. It is an immunoglobulin A (IgA)–mediated leukocytoclastic vasculitis that involves inflammation of the precapillary, capillary, and postcapillary vessels in the skin, joints, gastrointestinal tract, and kidneys.

III. Incidence and Epidemiology

HSP can occur at any age, but there is a peak at 4 to 5 years of age, and the syndrome is rare before age 1 or after age 10 years. Boys are affected twice as often as girls. The incidence increases in the spring and fall. All races are affected equally.

IV. Clinical Presentation

The clinical picture of HSP is similar to that described in this case, with a previously healthy child who acutely develops a distinctive rash, arthritis or arthralgias, and abdominal pain. The rash is seen in all patients, and half of the patients initially present with the skin rash. Fifty percent of the time the rash occurs on the buttocks, lower extremities, and other areas of dependency. In severe cases, it may include the face, trunk, and arms. The classic lesions are urticarial wheals and erythematous maculopapules that progress to petechiae and purpura. The lesions can occur in crops and can last 3 to 30 days. Nonpitting edema occurs in dependent areas in 35% to 70% of patients and is seen more often in children younger than 3 years of age.

Arthralgia or arthritis is seen in 65% to 85% of patients and precedes the rash in up to 25% of patients. The large joints are most commonly affected. These symptoms usually resolve within a few days.

Gastrointestinal manifestations can be seen in as many as three fourths of patients. Abdominal pain is usually colicky in nature. The abdominal pain may be severe, mimicking appendicitis. Vomiting is common. Abdominal symptoms occasionally precede other manifestations by up to 4 weeks. Although stools often contain occult blood, massive gastrointestinal bleeding occurs rarely. Other gastrointestinal complications include intussusception, bowel infarction, perforation, pancreatitis, and hydrops of the gall bladder. Intussusception, which occurs about 3% of the time, is usually ileoileal (rather than ileocolic) and is seen in the older children.

Renal manifestations range from transient hematuria or proteinuria to nephritis, nephrotic syndrome, and end-stage renal disease. Microscopic hematuria is a constant feature, and up to 40% of patients have gross hematuria. Proteinuria occurs in conjunction with hematuria in two thirds of patients, but proteinuria alone is rarely, if ever, a manifestation of HSP nephritis. Nephritis develops in 20% to 50% of children with HSP. It usually appears days or weeks after the initial symptoms of HSP. It usually resolves, but in 2% of affected patients it progresses to renal failure. The histopathology of HSP renal disease is the same as IgA nephropathy. Those children who present with renal disease with nephritic and nephrotic features are at the highest risk to develop end-stage renal disease.

Neurologic findings, including headaches and behavioral changes, are seen in about one third of the cases. Seizures, focal neurologic deficits, and peripheral neuropathies are rare. They are seen in 2% to 8% of those patients with the disease. Most neurologic findings are transient.

Orchitis develops in up to 10% of boys with HSP. Symptoms may mimic those of testicular torsion.

V.   Diagnostic Approach

The diagnosis is made clinically, because there are no specific laboratory tests to diagnose HSP. Laboratory studies may reveal suggestive features or complications of HSP, but they are more important to help differentiate HSP from other potential causes.

Complete blood count. Leukocytosis is seen in two thirds of the children. Eosinophilia is occasionally present. Anemia is more commonly seen with Crohn's disease and ulcerative colitis than with HSP.

Serum immunoglobulin A level. Serum IgA is elevated during the acute illness in approximately 50% of patients.

Complement levels. C3 and C4 levels are normal in HSP nephritis but may be low in lupus nephritis and poststreptococcal glomerulonephritis.

Urinalysis. Urinalysis should be performed on all the patients to look for findings suggestive of nephritis or nephrotic syndrome, including hematuria and proteinuria. Urinalysis should be repeated every 7 days while the disease is still active to monitor for the development of nephritis.

Radiologic studies. When gastrointestinal signs are present, contrast radiologic studies of the gastrointestinal tract demonstrate small-bowel involvement, with thickened folds, hypomotility, and "thumb-printing," characteristic of submucosal hemorrhages. Ultrasonography can help diagnose intussusception, especially because intussusception proximal to the ileocolic location is often missed by air or liquid contrast enemas.

Other studies. The ESR may be elevated but is rarely helpful in diagnosing HSP. The ESR is always elevated with Crohn's disease and ulcerative colitis. The PT and PTT are normal in children with HSP but frequently are elevated in children with meningococcemia. Blood cultures should be performed for ill-appearing children if HSP cannot be readily distinguished from meningococcemia. Renal biopsy should be considered in children with nephritis complicated by nephrotic syndrome, hypertension, or substantial renal insufficiency, in order to predict prognosis more precisely.

VI. Treatment

Specific treatment is not usually required, and most cases can be managed on an outpatient basis. Hospital admission should be considered for children who develop gastrointestinal hemorrhage, colicky abdominal pain suggestive of intussusception, significant renal disease, or changes in mental status. The duration of illness is typically 3 to 4 weeks. Relapses are uncommon but have occurred in up to 15% of children in some studies.

The use of prednisone (1 to 2 mg/kg per day) has been suggested to hasten improvement of abdominal pain, and it may also reduce the risk of intussusception. Some reports suggest that corticosteroids, alone or in combination with other immunosuppressive agents (e.g., azathioprine, cyclophosphamide), reduce the risk of renal failure in children with HSP nephritis, although prospective trials are still needed.

The prognosis for children who develop HSP is generally good. Approximately 95% of children have complete recovery. However, of those children who require renal biopsy to evaluate persistent renal disease, 18% ultimately develop chronic renal failure. The risk factors for renal failure include age at onset greater than 7 years, severe abdominal symptoms, and persistent purpura.

VII. References

1. Al-Sheyyab M, El-Shanti H, Ajlouni S, et al. The clinical spectrum of Henoch-Schönlein purpura in infants and young children. *Eur J Pediatr* 1995;154:969–972.
2. Hyams JS. Corticosteroids in the treatment of gastrointestinal disease. *Curr Opin Pediatr* 2000;12:451–455.
3. Lanzkowsky S, Lanzkowsky L, Lanzkowsky P. Henoch-Schönlein purpura. *Pediatr Rev* 1992;13:130–137.
4. Saulsbury FT. Henoch-Schönlein purpura in children: report of 100 patients and review of the literature. *Medicine (Baltimore)* 1999;78:395–409.
5. Walker WA, Higuchi L. Henoch-Schönlein syndrome. In: McMillan JA, DeAngelis CD, Feigin RD, et al., eds. *Oski's pediatrics: principles and practice,* 3rd ed. Philadelphia: Lippincott Williams & Wilkins, 1999:2176–2179.

Case 9-4: 14-Year-Old Boy

I. History of Present Illness

A 14-year-old boy presented to the emergency department complaining of a rash on his face. Seven days before admission, he had developed low-grade fevers, sore throat, myalgias, and malaise. His primary pediatrician diagnosed him with the "flu" after antigens of influenza A were detected by immunofluorescence of nasopharyngeal washings. His symptoms gradually improved until the day of admission, when he developed fever to 39.0°C, a rapidly worsening cough, and a rash on his face. In the emergency department, he had an episode of hemoptysis (approximately 250 mL) and subsequently became hypotensive, requiring multiple normal saline boluses and packed red blood cell transfusion. He did not have a history of abdominal or chest pain. The patient recalled striking his head in the shower while coughing, a fact that he had not mentioned to his parents.

II. Past Medical History

This child had a history of recurrent rectal prolapse at 4 years of age that resolved without sequelae. His mother noted that he had a tendency to bruise easily and often had gingival bleeding after brushing his teeth. He had not undergone any surgical procedures. He had no allergies. He had received all of his required immunizations. He was adopted at the age of 4 weeks. His biologic mother died after uterine rupture that complicated the delivery. Details of the family history were not known.

III. Physical Examination

T, 38.5°C; RR, 50/min; HR, 130 bpm; BP, 100/55 mm Hg

Height, 50th percentile; weight, 25th percentile

Physical examination revealed an ill-appearing but alert boy. He had a very thin and narrow face. His sclerae were mildly injected but anicteric. There was no blood in the nares. There was no hemotympanum. His neck was supple. He had mild suprasternal retractions with dullness to percussion approximately half way up the back on the right. There were rales in the region of the right lower and middle lobes. There was no murmur on cardiac examination. Femoral pulses were thready but improved during the fluid resuscitation. He had mild tenderness to palpation at the right costal margin, but the remainder of the abdominal examination was normal. Examination of the skin was remarkable for a large ecchymotic area on the patient's forehead (3 cm), which was tender to palpation. There was a 2-cm wound on his knee. He had numerous thin, atrophic scars on his extremities, especially over his joints.

IV. Diagnostic Studies

Arterial blood gas analysis demonstrated the following: pH, 7.35; carbon dioxide tension (PCO_2), 26 mm Hg; and oxygen tension (PO_2), 60 mm Hg in room air. The WBC count was 1,600/mm^3, with 26% band forms, 26% segmented neutrophils; and 44% lymphocytes. Hemoglobin was 9.8 g/dL and platelets were 270,000/mm^3. The ESR was 35 mm/hour. The PT and PTT were 13.1 and 35.7 seconds, respectively. The fibrinogen was 749 mg/dL, and fibrin split products were 20 μg/mL. The creatinine kinase was 120 U/L. Serum electrolytes were as follows: sodium, 136 mmol/L; potassium, 3.6 mmol/L; chloride, 104 mmol/L; bicarbonate, 18 mmol/L; BUN, 16 mg/dL; creatinine, 1.0 mg/dL; and glucose, 169 mg/dL. Serum aminotransferases and total bilirubin were normal. The urinalysis was normal. A blood culture was obtained. The chest radiograph revealed areas of

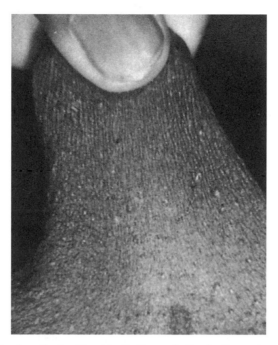

FIG. 9-4. Photograph of patient with skin findings similar to those in case 9-4. (From Tunnessen WW Jr, Krowchuk DP. Pediatric dermatology. In: McMillan JA, DeAngelis CD, Feigin RD, et al., eds. *Oski's pediatrics: principles and practice,* 3rd ed. Lippincott Williams & Wilkins: Philadelphia, 1999:710, with permission).

consolidation in the right lower and right middle lobes, with a moderate right-sided pleural effusion.

V. Course of Illness

The patient received vancomycin and gentamicin empirically. CT of the chest revealed extensive consolidation involving the entire right lower lobe and part of the left lower lobe, with moderate pleural effusions. A chest tube was placed, draining approximately 500 mL of pleural fluid. The pleural fluid contained 7,350 WBCs/mm^3 and 650 red blood cells/mm^3. Initial blood cultures grew *Staphylococcus aureus,* and cultures of the pleural fluid were negative. His chest tube was removed on the third day of hospitalization. After the blood culture results and sensitivities became available, the patient's antibiotics were changed to oxacillin and he recovered uneventfully, completing a 4-week total antibiotic course. Repeat blood cultures were negative. This patient had influenza complicated by bacterial superinfection causing *S. aureus* pneumonia and bacteremia. Close examination of the skin suggested an underlying diagnosis (which predisposed the patient to bruising and hemoptysis) that was confirmed by skin biopsy (Fig. 9-4).

DISCUSSION: CASE 9-4

I. Differential Diagnosis

In this case the bruising, atrophic scars, and bleeding indicated increased vascular permeability or weakness. Use of corticosteroids or Cushing syndrome could have given the patient the atrophic scars as well as the bruising and bleeding, but there was no history of such medications, nor did he demonstrate cushingoid features. Scurvy, secondary to a dietary lack of vitamin C, causes bruising, bleeding, and poor wound healing, but this diagnosis is unlikely in a patient in the United States.

Hematologic causes should be considered. Thrombocytopenia, especially that caused by immune thrombocytopenic purpura or sepsis, occurs in patients with a history of recent illness and fever but can be excluded in this case based on the normal platelet count. Von Willebrand's disease is a relatively common disorder in which there is a deficiency of a circulating plasma protein related to factor VIII. This causes decreased platelet adhesiveness and prolonged bleeding time. As with this patient, there is usually a history of mild to moderate bleeding involving the mucous membranes, including epistaxis and prolonged bleeding after dental procedures. This patient had a history of bleeding with brushing his teeth, nosebleeds, and bruising, but von Willebrand's disease would not explain his atrophic scars.

Collagen vascular disease also needs to be considered. Osteogenesis imperfecta is a congenital abnormality of quality or quantity of type I collagen synthesis. Of the four subtypes, type I is associated with easy bruising. However, this child did not display the other signs of osteogenesis imperfecta, such as frequent fractures, blue sclera, hearing impairment, osteopenia, bony deformities, and excessive laxity of the joints. Ehlers-Danlos syndrome (EDS) is also a congenital defect in collagen synthesis. There are multiple forms of EDS, identified by clinical features (major and minor criteria) and biochemical and molecular findings. Most of the EDS cases are associated with skin hyperflexibility and joint hypermobility.

II.   Diagnosis

Close examination of the patient's skin revealed dramatic hyperextensibility (Fig. 9-4). There were also numerous atrophic, cigarette paper–like scars (papyraceous scarring), most prominently at the joint surfaces. Detailed history revealed that he had always had difficulty with wound healing. He had received sutures once after a laceration, and the wound quickly dehisced. These findings, together with the history of easy bruising, rectal prolapse, and mother's death from uterine rupture, suggested the diagnosis of EDS. The diagnosis was confirmed by skin biopsy with fibroblast cultures, which revealed decreased secretion of type III procollagen, consistent with the diagnosis of **Ehlers-Danlos syndrome type IV (EDS IV)**.

III.   Incidence and Epidemiology

EDS IV is the most severe form of EDS. It occurs because of mutations on the *COL3A1* gene, which encodes type III collagen. EDS IV is inherited as an autosomal dominant condition. This is a very rare condition, with a prevalence of less than 1 per 100,000 individuals worldwide. Possibly as a result of its rarity, the diagnosis is often made only after catastrophic or fatal complication. In fact, the literature suggests that only 16% of patients had symptoms suggesting EDS before a vascular event occurred.

IV.   Clinical Presentation

The clinical diagnosis of EDS IV is made based on the presence of at least two of four clinical criteria: easy bruising, thin skin with visible veins, characteristic facial features (thin facies, pinched nose, large eyes), and rupture of arteries, uterus, or intestines. Because EDS IV is a heterogeneous genetic disorder, various clinical scenarios are seen. Complete expression of the syndrome can involve prematurity, low birth weight, congenital hip dislocation, small joint hyperlaxity, and spontaneous pneumothorax. Type III collagen, the type affected in this syndrome, is found in highly vascular structures such as liver and blood vessels. Therefore, it is these structures that are at risk in patients with EDS IV. These patients usually are not diagnosed until the second or third decade of life.

They often die before 40 years of age, most commonly as a result of an arterial or organ rupture; few survive beyond age 50 years. Although hypermobility of the large joints and hyperextensibility of the skin were present in this patient and are characteristic of the more common forms of EDS, they are seen only occasionally seen with this vascular type.

V. Diagnostic Approach

In addition to the clinical criteria noted, diagnosis is confirmed by the demonstration of abnormal type III procollagen molecules in cultured fibroblasts or by the identification of a mutation in the gene for type III procollagen (*COL3A1*).

VI. Treatment

The prognosis for patients with EDS IV is poor. Approximately 44% die from an arterial or organ rupture before any surgical intervention can be performed, and another 19% die during or immediately after surgeries. Women have a 25% risk of death with each pregnancy. Surviving patients usually succumb to an arterial hemorrhage before middle age.

Genetic evaluation and counseling is crucial for those diagnosed with this disorder. Because it is transmitted in an autosomal dominant pattern, patients and families need to be informed of the 50% risk of transmission to an affected individual's offspring. Although there are no available therapies to delay the onset of complications in patients with EDS IV, knowledge of the diagnosis certainly influences the management of surgery, pregnancy, and reproductive decisions.

VII. References

1. Dame C, Hausser I, Geukens J, et al. Ehlers-Danlos syndrome: classical type. *Arch Pediatr Adolesc Med* 2001;155:1275–1276.
2. Dowton SB, Pincott S, Demmer L. Respiratory complications of Ehlers-Danlos syndrome type IV. *Clin Genet* 1996;50:510–514.
3. Maltz, SB, Fantus RJ, Mellett MM, et al. Surgical complications of Ehlers-Danlos syndrome type IV: case report and review of the literature. *J Trauma Injury Infect Crit Care* 2001;51:387–390.
4. Pepin M, Schwarze U, Superti-Furga A, et al. Clinical and genetic features of Ehlers-Danlos syndrome type IV, the vascular type. *N Engl J Med* 2000;342:673–680.
5. Tunnessen WW. *Signs and symptoms in pediatrics,* 3rd ed. Philadelphia: Lippincott Williams & Wilkins, 1999:790–799.

Case 9-5: 16-Year-Old Girl

I   History of Present Illness

A 16-year-old Caucasian girl presented to the emergency department with an acute onset of epistaxis lasting 3 to 4 hours. Her parents estimated her blood loss to be several cups, and there had been no slowing of the flow with compression. She reported a history of intermittent epistaxis since she was 8 years of age. She reportedly had had at least one nosebleed per year, lasting 20 to 30 minutes each time. The last episode was 1 year earlier, and it lasted approximately 4 hours. She also reported a history of "easy bruising" without any history of prolonged bleeding from prior injuries. There was no history of fever, weight loss, or night sweats. She had no recent trauma. She did note increasing fatigue over the past several months. Her menstrual periods were described as regular with heavy flow during the first 2 days. She also noted an 18-month history of lower extremity pain, primarily in the ankles and knees. The pain usually lasted for minutes, and it occurred twice per week. She had no history of fractures.

II.   Past Medical History

She was born at full term with an uncomplicated birth history. There was no significant history of travel or exposures. Family history was significant for a brother with a deletion of the short arm of chromosome 7, who also had a history of epistaxis. A maternal aunt had systemic lupus erythematosus.

III.   Physical Examination

T, 37.4 C; RR, 36/min; HR, 110 bpm; BP, 151/83 mm Hg

Height, 50th percentile; weight, 50th percentile

Physical examination was remarkable for nonicteric sclerae, a small amount of bleeding from the left nostril, and dried blood in the oropharynx. Lung examination was normal. Cardiac examination revealed no murmurs, rubs, or gallops. The abdomen was soft and nondistended; however, the liver was noted to be 4 cm below the right costal margin, and the spleen was palpable 4 cm below the left costal margin. Rectal examination was normal with soft, heme-positive stool in the vault. There was no prominent adenopathy. An erythematous rash was noted across her cheeks. No petechiae were noted, but there was mild bruising on the lower extremities. The neurologic examination was normal.

IV.   Diagnostic Studies

Laboratory analysis revealed 5,400 WBCs/mm^3, with 4% band forms, 54% segmented neutrophils, and 37% lymphocytes. The hemoglobin was 10.0 g/dL, and there were 46,000 platelets/mm^3. Reticulocyte count was 2.7%. PT and PTT were 12.6 and 34.7 seconds, respectively. Serum electrolytes, BUN, and creatinine were normal. Lactate dehydrogenase was normal, and uric acid was 6.3 mg/dL. The ESR was 35 mm/hour. Antinuclear antibodies, anti–double-stranded DNA antibody, rapid plasma regain test, and Monospot test were all negative.

V.   Course of Illness

Hemostasis was achieved without immediate intervention other than pressure applied to her nares. The patient was admitted to the hospital, where she underwent further evaluation for the bleeding and associated symptoms. Bone marrow biopsy (Fig. 9-5) suggested a diagnosis that was confirmed by a blood test.

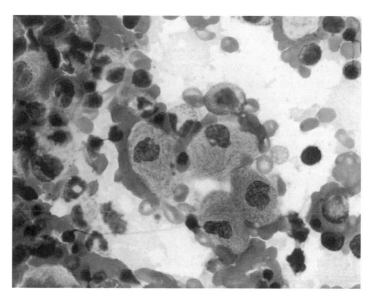

FIG. 9-5. Bone marrow biopsy (case 9-5). (Photograph courtesy of Marybeth Helfrich, MT, ASCP.)

DISCUSSION: CASE 9-5

I. Differential Diagnosis

Bruising and easy bleeding in this older child suggested a vascular disorder. The differential includes immune thrombocytopenic purpura and leukemia. Idiopathic thrombocytopenic purpura (ITP) would have been unlikely given the prolonged duration of the symptoms, because ITP is an acute, self-limited illness. Chronic forms of ITP occur, but it would be rare for the acute phase of the illness to have passed undetected. It was the enlargement of the liver and spleen that caused consideration of autoimmune disorders or a metabolic type of illness. Most of these were eliminated on the basis of the relatively low ESR and negative lupus panel. Finally, infectious causes of thrombocytopenia and enlarged liver and spleen include Epstein-Barr virus–associated or cytomegalovirus-associated infectious mononucleosis or syphilis, but these were eliminated by negative laboratory tests for the conditions.

II. Diagnosis

The bone marrow biopsy showed macrophages with the characteristic "wrinkled tissue paper" appearance of Gaucher cells (Fig. 9-5). The leukocyte glucocerebrosidase activity was 0.85 nmol/hour per milligram of protein (less than 10% of the normal value), consistent with the diagnosis of Gaucher disease. Radiographs of the right femur revealed undertabulation of the distal femoral metaphysis, with marked cortical thinning and sclerosis. Additionally, she had an elevated tartrate-resistant acid phosphatase level of 6.1 U/L (reference range, 2.0 to 4.2 U/L). MRI showed diffuse infiltration of her liver, spleen, and bone marrow. **All of these findings were consistent with Gaucher disease, type I.**

III.   Incidence and Epidemiology

Gaucher disease is an autosomal recessive disorder associated with deficient activity of the lysosomal β-glucosidase, β-glucocerebrosidase. In Gaucher disease, macrophages, the major site of catabolism of glycolipids, accumulate glucocerebroside. There are three forms of the disorder, which vary in severity. This child had type I Gaucher disease, the most common sphingolipid storage disorder. The highest incidence occurs among individuals with Eastern European Jewish ancestry.

IV.   Clinical Presentation

Macrophages are most numerous in the liver, spleen, bone, and lung, so it is not surprising that the manifestations of Gaucher disease are usually related to one of these organs. Patients with Gaucher disease type I can present at any age, although those who are more severely affected present during childhood with splenomegaly and pancytopenia. Patients may complain of easy bruising and chronic fatigue. They may also have hepatomegaly and mild elevation of hepatic transaminases. Cirrhosis and liver failure may develop. As in this patient, infiltration of the bone marrow interferes with bone growth and mineralization and compounds the pancytopenia. Skeletal complications include osteopenia, osteonecrosis, and recurrent bone pain. Pulmonary glycolipid accumulation may lead to lung dysfunction.

The disease is slowly progressive, and many of those affected live well into adulthood. The disease is very stable, with a steady state achieved between lipid accumulation and lipid degradation or loss. Some individuals with the mildest disease are identified only incidentally as adults during evaluation for other conditions. The central nervous system is spared in type I Gaucher disease, so affected children have normal intelligence. Neurologic symptoms develop early in life for infants with type II disease, and death occurs by 2 years of age. In type III disease, children develop visceromegaly early in life and have late-onset neurologic complications.

V.   Diagnostic Approach

The diagnosis of Gaucher disease can now be made by measurement of enzyme levels or by gene mutation analysis.

Glucocerebrosidase levels. Because the glucocerebrosidase gene has been mapped to chromosome 1q21, identification of the underlying enzymatic defect in Gaucher disease is possible from peripheral blood. Decreased glucocerebrosidase activity in peripheral blood leukocytes (usually 10% to 30% of normal levels) is diagnostic of Gaucher disease.

Gene analysis. DNA-based diagnosis can be used if findings from enzymatic testing are equivocal, as is occasionally the case in heterozygotes. The detection of mutations is, however, limited to the previously defined mutations. DNA analysis detects most mutations (greater than 95%) in Ashkenazi Jews but only a few mutations in other populations, in which there is a greater diversity of mutations.

Bone marrow biopsy. Once considered the diagnostic method of choice, bone marrow biopsy has fallen out of favor as a diagnostic tool in Gaucher disease since less invasive and more reliable diagnostic modalities became available. Bone marrow biopsy findings include large, lipid-laden, fusiform macrophages with dense, eccentric nuclei that resemble wrinkled tissue paper or crumpled silk (Gaucher cells). These cells are not pathognomonic of Gaucher disease, because the same type of cell can be found in various leukemias and some infectious disorders. This test is often performed to exclude malignancy in the child presenting with pancytopenia.

Complete blood count. Patients with untreated disease may have anemia, thrombocytopenia, and leukopenia.

Radiologic imaging. Radiography, CT, or MRI of the femur shows the Erlenmeyer-flask deformity, which is caused by expansion of the cortex, as well as cyst-like changes of varying sizes. MRI of various bones shows infiltration of bone marrow.

Other studies. A number of plasma enzyme activities are greatly increased in patients with Gaucher disease. Serum acid phosphatase levels, β-hexosaminidase, and angiotensin-converting enzyme have all been found to be elevated in these patients. Acid phosphatase levels are used to monitor response to therapy; these levels become normal with adequate exogenous enzyme replacement.

VI. Treatment

Treatments used for these patients include symptomatic treatment, exogenous administration of the missing enzyme, and allogeneic bone marrow transplantation. Gene transfer is being explored for future therapy.

Symptomatic measures are used to improve quality of life. Surgical splenectomy can correct the thrombocytopenia, and complete or partial splenectomy is used if the splenomegaly is so massive as to become symptomatic. Patients are advised to avoid activities that put sudden stresses on the skeleton, which can result in fractures. Some patients require joint replacements due to osteonecrosis.

Type I Gaucher disease is particularly responsive to exogenous replacement of the defective enzyme, because the target cell is the macrophage and there is no central nervous system involvement. This enzyme is a macrophage-targeted modified glucocerebrosidase. Patients require enzyme replacement (alglucerase) every 2 weeks. Enzyme replacement therapy has been highly effective in causing regression of the visceral and hematologic manifestations, and to a lesser extent the skeletal manifestations, of Gaucher disease.

Bone marrow stem cell transplantation may be considered in some patients. Because macrophages are derived from the hematopoietic stem cells, stem cell transplantation can be expected to cure Gaucher disease. Indeed, allogeneic bone marrow transplantation has led to correction of the clinical manifestations of the disease. However, marrow transplantation carries substantial risks and is currently reserved for a small subset of patients.

VII. References

1. Balicki D, Beutler E. Gaucher disease. *Medicine (Baltimore)* 1995:74:305–323.
2. Beutler E, Grabowski GA. Gaucher disease. In: Scriver CR, Beaudet AL, Sly WS, et al., eds. *The metabolic and molecular basis of inherited disease,* 8th ed. New York: McGraw-Hill; 2001:3635–3668.
3. Charrow J, Esplin JA, Gribble TJ, et al. Gaucher disease: recommendations on diagnosis, evaluation, and monitoring. *Arch Intern Med* 1998;158:1754–1760.
4. Rosenthal DI, Doppelt SH, Mankin HJ, et al. Enzyme replacement therapy for Gaucher disease: skeletal responses to macrophage-targeted glucocerebrosidase. *Pediatrics* 1995;96:629–637.

10

Pallor

Stephen Ludwig

APPROACH TO THE PATIENT WITH PALLOR

I. Definition of the Complaint

The complaint of pallor indicates a perceived decrease in rubor in the skin and mucous membranes of a child. In general, the finding of pallor indicates color that is associated with decreased blood flow to the skin. The lack of blood flow may be regional (e.g., thrombosis) or systemic (e.g., shock), or there may be normal flow with decreased oxygen-carrying capacity (e.g., anemia).

In most cases, the finding of pallor demands that anemia be ruled out. Some children have a constitutional cause of pallor due to their fair complexion and a lack of sunlight exposure. But most children with pallor should be considered to have low hemoglobin, which should be measured. Ordinarily, a complete blood count with differential count and RBC indices helps the clinician sort through the many causes of anemia and recognize unusual situations in which pallor is not related to anemia.

II. Complaint by Cause and Frequency

Pallor may be separated into those causes involving normal hemoglobin (Table 10-1) and those involving an abnormal hemoglobin level. An abnormal hemoglobin level may be caused by decreased red blood cell (RBC) production, increased destruction, or blood loss. Anemia may also be considered in relation to mechanism, as trauma, toxin, metabolic tumor, congenital, or mixed etiology (Table 10-2), or in relation to RBC morphology (Table 10-3).

III. Clarifying Questions

- What are the child's dietary habits?

    — Because the most common cause of pallor is iron deficiency anemia, an important clarifying question pertains to diet. Diets containing large quantities of cow's milk are suspect for iron deficiency due to lack of iron intake and loss of appetite for food rich in iron. Other related questions for iron deficiencies have to do with sources of loss of iron or blood, such as recent heavy menstruation, black or tarry stools, or multiple blood draws for diagnostic testing.

- Is there a family history of anemia, splenectomy, or gall bladder surgery?

    — A second clarifying question pertains to family history. Many of the membrane disorders and other genetic diseases roots in the family history. Some disorders, such as hereditary spherocytosis and elliptocytosis, frequently necessitate splenectomy due to substantial RBC sequestration. Inherited diseases causing hemolysis, such as sickle cell disease, may be recognized in some families by a history of gall bladder surgery.

TABLE 10-1. *Pallor with Anemia*

Decreased erythrocyte or hemoglobin production
  Nutritional deficiencies
    Iron deficiencies
    Folic acid and vitamin B_{12} deficiency or associated metabolic abnormalities
  Aplastic or hypoplastic anemias
    Diamond-Blackfan syndrome
    Fanconi syndrome
    Aplastic anemia[a]
    Transient erythroblastopenia of childhood
    Malignancy: leukemia, lymphoma, neuroblastoma[a]
  Anemia of chronic disease: renal disease, inflammatory bowel disease, collagen-vascular disease, thyroid deficiency or thyrotoxicosis, malignancy
  Abnormal heme and hemoglobin synthesis
    Lean poisoning[a]
    Sideroblastic anemias
    Thalassemias
Increased erythrocyte destruction
  Erythrocyte membrane defects: hereditary spherocytosis, elliptocytosis, stomatocytosis, pyknocytosis, paroxysmal nocturnal hemoglobinuria
  Erythrocyte enzyme defects
    Defects of hexose monophosphate shunt: glucose-6-phosphate dehydrogenase deficiency most common
    Defects of Embden-Meyerhof pathway: pyruvate kinase deficiency most common
  Hemoglobinopathies
    Sickle cell syndromes[a]
    Unstable hemoglobins
  Immune hemolytic anemia
    Autoimmune hemolytic anemia[a]
    Isoimmune hemolytic anemia
    Infection
      Viral: mononucleosis, influenzas, coxsackie, measles, varicella, cytomegalovirus
      Bacterial: *Escherichia coli, Pneumococcus, Streptococcus,* typhoid fever, *Mycoplasma*
    Drugs: antibiotics, α-methyldopa
    Inflammatory and collagen-vascular disease
    Malignancy[a]
  Microangiopathic anemias
    Disseminated intravascular coagulation[a]
    Hemolytic-uremic syndrome[a]
    Cavernous hemangioma
Blood loss
  Severe trauma[a]
  Anatomic lesions
    Meckel diverticulum
    Peptic ulcer
    Idiopathic pulmonary hemosiderosis[a]

[a]Conditions that are known to manifest with acute, life-threatening anemia or are associated with other serious abnormalities.

TABLE 10-2. *Etiology of Anemia (Common Causes of Pallor) by Mechanism*

Trauma
    Blood loss
    Infection
    Sepsis
Toxin
    Atropine
    Lead poisoning
    Aplastic anemia
Metabolic-inherited
    Iron deficiency
    Thalassemia
    Sideroblastic anemia
    Sickle cell anemia
    Hereditary spherocytosis
    Glucose-6-phosphate dehydrogenase deficiency
    Allergic-immunologic
    Autoimmune hemolytic anemia
    Goodpasture syndrome
    Hemolytic-uremic syndrome
    Systemic lupus erythematosus
Tumor
    Leukemia
    Marrow infiltration
Congenital
    Diamond-Blackfan syndrome
Multiple etiologic
    Acute blood loss
    Anemia of chronic illness
    Recurrent blood loss (e.g., menorrhagia)
    Pulmonary hemosiderosis

Adapted from Poncz M. Pallor In: Schwartz MW, ed. *Pediatric primary care: a problem-oriented approach,* 2nd ed. Chicago: Year Book Medical Publishers, 1987.

- Are there signs of systemic illness, fatigue, growth failure, weight loss, or lymphadenopathy?

    — For children whose anemia is based on an oncologic cause, look to questions that identify other systemic signs of fatigue or of growth or tenderness of lymph nodes.

- Was there exposure to certain medications or toxins?

    — Some questions should be asked about exposure to toxins, which may act directly on blood or bone marrow and may act in conjunction with a genetic defect (e.g., naphthalene exposure in a patient with glucose-6-phosphate dehydrogenase (G6PD) deficiency, leading to anemia).

- Did the pallor develop quickly or gradually?

    — Information about the speed of onset provides clues about the cause. Has there been an insidious onset (e.g., iron deficiency) or an acute onset of pallor with jaundice (e.g., hemolytic disorder)?

TABLE 10-3. *Etiology of Anemia (Low Hemoglobin Level) by Red Blood Cell Morphology*

Microcytic anemia
  Iron deficiency
  Lead poisoning
  Thalassemia
  Sideroblastic anemia
Normocytic anemia
  Low reticulocyte count
    Anemia of chronic disease
    Transient erythroblastopenia of childhood
    Diamond-Blackfan syndrome
    Leukemia
    Marrow infiltration
    Aplastic anemia
  Elevated reticulocyte count
    External blood loss
    Pulmonary hemosiderosis
    Goodpasture syndrome
    Intraerythrocyte defects
    Hemolytic-uremic syndrome
    Sickle cell disease
    Hereditary spherocytosis
    Glucose-6-phosphate dehydrogenase deficiency
Macrocytic anemia
  Low reticulocyte count
    Folate or vitamin B_{12} deficiency
    Preleukemia
    Aplastic anemia
    Diamond-Blackfan syndrome
    Transient erythroblastopenia of childhood
  Elevated reticulocyte count
    Hemolytic anemia and high reticulocyte count
    Autoimmune hemolytic anemia
    Secondary folate deficiency in hemolytic anemia

Adapted from Poncz M. Pallor In: Schwartz MW, ed. *Pediatric primary care: a problem-oriented approach,* 2nd ed. Chicago: Year Book Medical Publishers, 1987.

IV.   References

1. Poncz M. Pallor. In: Schwartz MW, ed. *Pediatric primary care: a problem-oriented approach,* 2nd ed. Chicago: Year Book Medical Publishers, 1987.
2. Segel GB, Hirsh MG, Feig SA. Managing anemia in pediatric office practice: part I. *Pediatr Rev* 2002;23:75–84.

Case 10-1: 3-Week-Old Boy

I. History of Present Illness

A 3-week-old twin B Caucasian male infant presented to an outpatient clinic for evaluation of anemia. He was noted in the nursery to be pale and had a hemoglobin of 12.3 g/dL and a mean corpuscular volume (MCV) of 120 fL. The hemoglobin measurement repeated at 2 weeks of age was 8.1 g/dL with a reticulocyte count of 1.2%. He had initial problems with weight gain that improved after the mother started to pump breast milk and to feed the baby with a bottle. He was described as usually sleepy, including falling asleep during feeds. He had no vomiting, diarrhea, fever, or cough. He had normal gold-colored bowel movements. There had been no change in urine color. There was no rash.

II. Past Medical History

The infant was born at 38 weeks' gestational age after *in vitro* fertilization. The pregnancy was complicated by maternal anemia. The mother's blood type was O-positive. The mother did not receive any medications during pregnancy except for prenatal vitamins. The infant was delivered vaginally. He had a transverse lie and was delivered vertex after external manipulation. The birth weight was 2,470 grams. His twin (twin A) weighed 2,900 g. On the first day of life, the infant was noted to have a swollen right upper leg with significant bruising. The initial radiograph was normal, but a subsequent film showed evidence of a healing fracture that was presumably related to birth trauma. There was no history of jaundice in the newborn nursery.

The family history was remarkable for the mother's anemia which did not require specific treatment. The maternal grandmother also had a history of anemia. Both the maternal grandmother and an aunt had required cholecystectomy for gallstones. The infant received a multivitamin with iron. He did not have any known allergies. He received a diet of breast milk with occasional cow's milk supplementation.

III. Physical Examination

T, 36.7°C; RR, 46 to 66/min; HR, 166 to 230 bpm; BP, 70/37 mm Hg

Weight, 3.1 kg (25th percentile); height, 50 cm (50th percentile); head circumference, 36 cm (approximately 75th percentile)

On examination, the infant awakened easily and cried. He was remarkably pale-appearing. The anterior fontanel was open and flat. The conjunctivae were pale. The sclerae were anicteric. Mucous membranes were moist. The clavicles were intact. The infant was tachypneic, but the lungs were clear to auscultation. On cardiac examination, normal first and second heart sounds (S1 and S2, respectively) were heard. A III/VI systolic murmur was best appreciated at the left upper sternal border. There were no gallops or rubs. No murmurs were heard along the back. The liver edge was just palpable, but the spleen was not palpable. The area of known extremity fracture had minimal edema but no tenderness. There was some widening of the right distal femur compared with the left. The remainder of the examination was normal.

IV. Diagnostic Studies

Complete blood count revealed the following: 11,300 white blood cells (WBCs)/mm^3 (1% metamyelocytes, 43% segmented neutrophils, 34% lymphocytes, and 19% monocytes); hemoglobin, 3.9 g/dL; 430,000 platelets/mm^3; MCV, 117 fL; RBC distribution width (RDW), 17; and reticulocyte count, 0.3%. The peripheral blood smear revealed a few small spherocytes but no schistocytes, burr cells, or target cells.

V. Course of Illness

The child was admitted for evaluation of anemia.

DISCUSSION: CASE 10-1

I. Differential Diagnosis

This male child presented with pallor at a young age. There was no history of jaundice, which lessened the likelihood of a hemolytic anemia. There was no issue of dietary causes because of the baby's young age. No chronic illness was apparent, and there was no history of blood loss. Therefore, the focus shifted to a congenital defect in RBC production. There was a remarkable drop in the hemoglobin and a very poor bone marrow response as far as reticulocyte production. The WBC and platelet concentrations were normal. The anemia was macrocytic. The sum of these findings indicated a defect of RBC production. There was also the physical examination finding of a possible skeletal anomaly at the distal right femur.

RBC aplasia may be congenital or acquired. Most of the acquired forms occur in adults, but some may be seen in adolescent patients. In childhood, the major causes are Diamond-Blackfan anemia, transient erythroblastopenia of childhood, and acquired aplasia of RBCs associated with chronic hemolysis. The aplastic crisis of a sickle cell disease patient is an example of the latter.

In this case, there was no evidence of acute or chronic hemolysis. The patient was too young to be considered for transient erythroblastopenia of childhood. Another possible cause to be considered was Fanconi anemia, an autosomal recessive disorder associated with aplastic anemia, short stature, skeletal defects, pigmentation changes, and other abnormalities. Some cases of Fanconi anemia are diagnosed in the first year of life. The anemia involves all cell lines; bone marrow analysis and genetic studies establish the diagnosis. In this case, there was only RBC involvement, and hence Diamond-Blackfan anemia was the most plausible diagnosis.

II. Diagnosis

The infant was admitted with the diagnosis of anemia secondary to a hypoproductive state. He was believed to have symptomatic anemia with difficulty feeding. He was transfused with a total of 15 mL/kg of packed RBCs administered in three separate aliquots. He underwent bone marrow aspiration, which revealed absence of RBC precursors with normal granulocyte precursors, a finding consistent with Diamond-Blackfan anemia. After the packed RBC transfusion, he had a hemoglobin concentration of 8.7 g/dL. He was more active and was in no respiratory distress. Corticosteroids were started at 2 mg/kg per day, and an additional 5 mL/kg of packed RBCs was given before his discharge home. **The final diagnosis was Diamond-Blackfan anemia.** It is one of the pure RBC aplasias.

III. Incidence and Epidemiology

The precise incidence of Diamond-Blackfan anemia is not known. For all the RBC aplasias, it is estimated that there are 300 to 1,000 new cases annually in the United States. Diamond-Blackfan anemia occurs primarily in infancy. In some studies, 10% of patients are anemic at birth, 25% by 1 month, 50% by 3 months, and 70% by 1 year. This anemia is seen in all ethnic groups, but primarily in Caucasians. There is no gender predominance.

IV. Clinical Presentation

Pallor caused by anemia in the early months of life characterizes this form of anemia. About one third of patients have an associated finding. There are many associated anomalies, including characteristic facies, thumb anomalies, short stature, eye abnormalities including glaucoma, renal anomalies, hypogonads, skeletal anomalies, congenital heart disease, and mental retardation. There is a wide range of involvement. The current median survival rate is 45 years. Some patients progress to full aplastic anemia, and about 5% develop leukemia or myelodysplasia.

V. Diagnostic Approach

Complete blood count and peripheral blood smear. The mean hemoglobin level at diagnosis for all patients with Diamond-Blackfan anemia is 7 g/dL. Infants diagnosed in the first 4 months of life typically have hemoglobin levels of 4 g/dL at presentation. The reticulocyte count is decreased or zero. The peripheral blood smear reveals macrocytes, anisocytosis, and teardrop cells. The WBC count is normal in most patients, but in 20% it is less than 5,000/mm^3.

Bone marrow aspiration. Bone marrow aspirates and biopsies show normal cellularity, myeloid cells, and megakaryocytes. Approximately 90% of patients have erythroid hypoplasia or aplasia. The remaining 10% of patients have either normal erythroblast number and maturation or erythroid hyperplasia with maturation arrest. Despite the variable marrow findings, all patients have reticulocytopenia, indicating some form of ineffective erythropoiesis and delayed precursor maturation.

Other studies. Serum iron, ferritin, folate, vitamin B$_{12}$, and erythropoietin are all elevated. In most cases there is an increase in RBC adenosine deaminase (ADA). Genetic studies have shown one site on chromosome 19, and other gene defects have also been associated.

VI. Treatment

The treatment includes use of corticosteroids. The currently recommended dose is 2 mg/kg per day of prednisone, given in three or four divided doses. Reticulocytes appear within 1 to 2 weeks, but the rise in hemoglobin is delayed for several more weeks. Once the hemoglobin level reaches 10 g/dL, the steroid dose is gradually tapered until the patient is receiving a single daily dose that adequately maintains appropriate hemoglobin levels. Response followed by steroid dependence is seen in 60% of patients. Approximately one fifth of the steroid-responsive patients may ultimately be maintained without steroids.

Approximately 30% to 40% of patients have poor or no response to steroids and require chronic transfusion therapy to maintain normal hemoglobin. These children require leukocyte-depleted packed RBC transfusions every 3 to 6 weeks, with the goal of keeping the hemoglobin level higher than 6 g/dL. Concurrent chelation of iron with subcutaneously administered desferrioxamine may decrease some chronic transfusion-related complications. Complications of chronic transfusion therapy are similar to those seen with other conditions that employ this modality (e.g., thalassemia). Bone marrow transplantation has been successful for some patients.

Median survival time is 43 years, but approximately 13% of patients die within the first 6 years of life. Deaths occur from complications of iron overload, pneumonia, sepsis, and occasionally transplant-related complications, leukemia, and pulmonary emboli.

VII. References

1. Alter BP. Inherited bone marrow failure syndromes. In: Nathan DG, Orkin SH, Ginsburg D, et al., eds. *Nathan and Oski's hematology of infancy and childhood,* 6th ed. Philadelphia: WB Saunders, 2003:280–365.
2. Ball SE, McGuckin CP, Jenkins G, et al. Diamond-Blackfan anaemia in the UK: analysis of 80 cases from a 20 year birth cohort. *Br J Haematol* 1996;94:645–653.
3. Willing TN, Draptchinskaia N, Dianzani I, et al. Mutations in ribosomal protein S19 gene and Diamond-Blackfan anaemia: wide variations in phenotypic expression. *Blood* 1999;94:4294–4306.
4. Willing TN, Gazda H, Sieff CA. Diamond-Blackfan anaemia. *Curr Opin Haematol* 2000;7:85–94.

Case 10-2: 12-Month-Old Girl

I. History of Present Illness

A 12-month-old Caucasian girl presented to the emergency department with pallor. The grandparents had just arrived from Florida. When they were greeted by the child at the airport, they were alarmed at her appearance, prompting a visit to the emergency department. The child had last been seen by her grandparents at Thanksgiving, and at that time she appeared well. The parents conceded that the child did appear more pale than usual. There was no fever, rash, vomiting, or diarrhea. There was no jaundice. Her activity level had been normal. She had not traveled anywhere, but the parents had visited Puerto Rico 2 weeks earlier; their trip was uneventful.

II. Past Medical History

The birth history was unremarkable. She had a febrile illness at 6 months of age. Evaluation at that time included a blood culture that was positive for *Staphylococcus epidermidis*. This was believed to be a contaminant. A complete blood count was also obtained (see later discussion). She had not required hospitalization. Her immunizations were appropriate for age. There were no pets. Her development was normal. She was breastfed until 6 months of age, after which she began drinking whole milk. She was a finicky eater but had been growing well.

III. Physical Examination

T, 36.1°C; RR, 38/min; HR, 145 bpm; BP, 97/53 mm Hg; SpO_2, 99% in room air
Weight, 79th percentile; height, 50th percentile

She was pale but alert and playful. The conjunctivae were pale but without injection or discharge. There was no lymphadenopathy. Her neck was supple. A II/VI systolic murmur was heard at the left upper sternal border without radiation. The lungs were clear to auscultation. There was no splenomegaly or hepatomegaly. There were no rashes or petechiae.

VI. Diagnostic Studies

The complete blood count obtained when the child was 6 months of age revealed the following: 15,200 WBCs/mm^3 (71% segmented neutrophils, 25% lymphocytes, and 4% monocytes); hemoglobin, 11.2 g/dL; and 365,000 platelets/mm^3. At that time, the MCV was 78 fL and the RDW was 17.3.

Her current studies revealed the following: 8,300 WBCs/mm^3 (58% segmented neutrophils, 31% lymphocytes, and 11% monocytes); hemoglobin, 3.4 g/dL; and 410,000 platelets/mm^3. The MCV was 59 fL, and the RDW was 15.1. The reticulocyte count was 1.4%. Stool was Hemoccult negative.

VII. Course of Illness

The history, examination, and laboratory findings suggested a diagnosis that was subsequently confirmed.

DISCUSSION: CASE 10-2

I. Differential Diagnosis

Table 10-4 lists the differential diagnosis of microcytic anemia in children. Causes of iron deficiency include poor bioavailability, decreased iron absorption, disruption of enteric mucosa or loss of functional bowel, blood loss, and insufficient intake. Alkaline gastric pH reduces the solubility of inorganic iron, impeding absorption. Chronic use of acid pump blockers, vagotomy (for severe gastroesophageal reflux), and impaired gastric

TABLE 10-4. *Evaluation of Microcytic Anemia*

	Iron deficiency	Lead	Thalassemia trait	Chronic disease
Hemoglobin	↓	Normal or ↓	↓	↓
MCV	Normal or ↓	Normal or ↓	↓	Normal or ↓
RDW	Normal or ↑	Normal or ↑	Normal	Normal
RBC No.	↓	↓	Normal or ↓	↓
FEP	↑	↑	Normal	↑
Serum iron	↓	Normal	Normal	↓
TIBC	↑	Normal	Normal	Normal or ↓
% Transferrin Saturation	↓	Normal	Normal or ↑	↓
Ferritin	↓	Normal	Normal	Normal or ↑

MCV, mean corpuscular volume; RDW, red cell distribution width; RBC No., red blood cell number; FEP, free erythrocyte protoporphyrin; TIBC, total iron-binding capacity.

parietal cell function in pernicious anemia may compromise iron absorption. Iron absorption may also be disrupted after surgical bowel resection, often performed because of volvulus or intussusception. Iron deficiency in such cases develops slowly and may not become evident for several years. Blood loss is a leading cause of iron deficiency. Common causes of gastrointestinal blood loss in children include Meckel diverticulum, cow's milk protein allergy, and parasitic infestation. Blood loss from hematuria or pulmonary hemorrhage can also occur. In this case, the dietary history suggested a likely cause.

II. Diagnosis

On examination, the child was extremely pale. **The combination of a hypochromic microcytic anemia and paucity of dietary iron implicated iron deficiency as a cause of this child's pallor.** Subsequent tests, including iron level, ferritin, and total iron-binding capacity, supported this diagnosis. The child received a packed RBC transfusion followed by daily iron supplements. Studies performed 1 month later revealed a hemoglobin level of 9.7 g/dL. This case illustrates the importance of the RDW as a marker of iron deficiency that precedes anemia.

III. Incidence and Epidemiology

In developed countries, routine iron fortification of formulas and cereals has led to a significant decrease in early childhood anemia. However, iron deficiency remains a leading cause of anemia. Currently, the prevalence of iron deficiency is approximately 7%. One third of affected children develop anemia. Children living below the poverty level are at greatest risk. More worrisome is the increasing recognition of anemia as only one manifestation of iron deficiency. Even in the absence of anemia, children with iron deficiency may have neurocognitive and behavioral problems. Only some of these problems are reversible with iron supplementation, suggesting the importance of prevention.

IV. Clinical Presentation

The clinical examination in children with mild iron deficiency is usually normal. With moderate or severe iron deficiency, the findings may be similar to those seen with other causes of anemia, including fatigue and pallor. If the anemia develops gradually, as in the child presented here, immediate family members may not notice changes in pigmentation. Other findings may include pica, the compulsive consumption of nonnutritive substances such as soil or ice. Long-standing iron deficiency may lead to angular stomatitis and glossitis. Softening of the fingernails leads to concave deformities descriptively termed "spooning" (koilonychia).

V. Diagnostic Approach

Complete blood count. In children, an elevated RDW is usually the earliest hematologic finding in iron deficiency. As the deficiency progresses, other hematologic parameters are affected (Table 10-4).

Peripheral blood smear. Peripheral blood smear in early disease may reveal anisocytosis. As the iron deficiency progresses, cells become hypochromic and microcytic. With severe iron deficiency, RBCs may be deformed and misshapen and demonstrate poikilocytosis.

Other studies. In the absence of a concurrent inflammatory disease state, the ferritin level decreases, reflecting diminished total tissue iron stores. With continued iron deficiency, reticuloendothelial macrophage iron stores become depleted and serum iron levels decrease. At this point the total iron-binding capacity increases without a change in hemoglobin levels. When the transferrin saturation decreases to approximately 10%, the availability of iron becomes the rate-limiting step for hemoglobin synthesis. This leads to the accumulation of heme precursors called free erythrocyte protoporphyrins. Ultimately, the RBCs become smaller as their hemoglobin content decreases.

VI. Treatment

Treatment of iron deficiency depends on its cause. For children with suspected dietary deficiency, treatment consists of supplemental iron. In children with anemia, an initial therapeutic trial often eliminates the need for expensive laboratory testing in determining the diagnosis. The reticulocyte count usually increases within several days and the hemoglobin concentration within 3 weeks. Patients should be treated until the hemoglobin reaches the normal range and then for at least one additional month to replete the iron stores. Failure of the hemoglobin level to rise within 1 month indicates either poor compliance with iron therapy or incorrect diagnosis.

VII. References

1. Oski FA. Iron deficiency in infancy and childhood. *N Engl J Med* 1993;329:190–193.
2. Segel GB, Hirsh MG, Feig SA. Managing anemia in pediatric office practice: part I. *Pediatr Rev* 2002;23:75–83.
3. Andrews NC. Disorders of iron metabolism and sideroblastic anemia. In: Nathan DG, Orkin SH, Ginsburg D, et al., eds. *Nathan and Oski's hematology of infancy and childhood,* 6th ed. Philadelphia: WB Saunders, 2003:456–497.
4. Lozoff B, Jimenez E, Wolf AW. Long-term developmental outcome of infants with iron deficiency. *N Engl J Med* 1991;325:687–694.
5. Aslan D, Altay C. Incidence of high erythrocyte count in infants and young children with iron deficiency anemia: re-evaluation of an old parameter. *J Pediatr Hematol Oncol* 2003;25:303–306.
6. Centers for Disease Control and Prevention. Iron deficiency—United States, 1999–2000. *MMWR Morb Mortal Wkly Rep* 2002;51:897–899.

Case 10-3: 5-Month-Old Boy

I. History of Present Illness

A 5-month-old African-American boy presented with pallor, difficulty breathing, and lethargy. He had been in his usual state of good health until 4 days before admission, when he developed a fever to 39 to 39.5°C with rhinorrhea. There was no coughing, vomiting, or diarrhea. The patient otherwise seemed well at the time. Over the next few days, he developed increased work of breathing with decreased appetite. One day before admission, the mother noted that he seemed lethargic and irritable. Oral intake was significantly decreased; the infant was taking in only 8 ounces rather than his typical 48 ounces over the day. The patient was brought to the emergency department. In retrospect, the father noted that the child's abdomen seemed to be increasing in size and firmness over the last month, with some tenderness.

II. Past Medical History

The infant was born at term after an uncomplicated pregnancy. He was taken home on the second day of life. He had no known allergies. He did not take any medications. He had received the appropriate immunizations for age, including two doses of the heptavalent pneumococcal conjugate vaccine. The family history was notable for sickle cell disease in a paternal cousin and reactive airways disease, cervical cancer, and ovarian cancer in several maternal relatives. A great uncle died of "jaundice" at 3 years of age and a cousin at 10 years of age.

III. Physical Examination

T, 38.4°C; RR, 58/min; HR, 160 bpm; BP, 83/38 mm Hg

Weight, 5.7 kg

In general, the child was lethargic and responsive only to painful stimuli. He also had severe respiratory distress. The anterior fontanel was sunken. The pupils were equal, round, and reactive to light. The conjunctivae and oral mucosae were pale. The lips were dry and cracked. There were white patches on the buccal mucosa that were easily removed with scraping. There was shotty anterior and posterior cervical adenopathy. The lungs were clear to auscultation, but the child had mild grunting and flaring. There was a II/VI systolic ejection murmur at the left lower sternal border. The abdomen was firm, with a liver edge palpable 5 cm below the right costal margin. The spleen was palpable at the level of the umbilicus. Bowel sounds were present. The extremities were cool with delayed capillary refill (5 seconds). On neurologic examination, the child localized pain but had decreased tone and diminished spontaneous activity.

In the emergency department, the patient had an oxygen saturation of 94% in room air. He received several normal saline boluses as well as sodium bicarbonate and intravenous dextrose. Blood and urine cultures were obtained. Intravenous cefotaxime was given for presumed sepsis.

IV. Diagnostic Studies

The complete blood count revealed the following: 14,100 WBCs/mm³ (2% band forms; 52% segmented neutrophils, 42% lymphocytes, 2% eosinophils, and 2% atypical lymphocytes); hemoglobin, 2.6 g/dL; 184,000 platelets/mm³; MCV, 88 fL; RDW, 17.4. The total bilirubin was 4.6 mg/dL with an unconjugated level of 3.8 mg/dL. Hepatic transaminases, were normal but the lactate dehydrogenase level was 2,984 IU/L (normal range, 934 to 2,150 IU/L). The chest radiograph was normal. There was no cardiomegaly, infiltrates, or mediastinal masses.

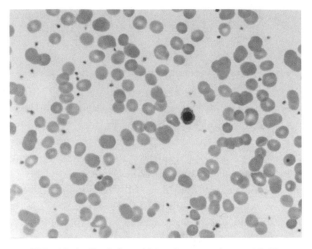

FIG. 10-1. Peripheral blood smear (case 10-3).

V.   Course of Illness

The peripheral blood smear (Fig. 10-1), in conjunction with other laboratory findings, suggested the diagnosis.

DISCUSSION: CASE 10-3

I.   Differential Diagnosis

This child came to the hospital with significant severe pallor of acute onset. The child had had no medications or unusual exposures. It was clear that he was critically ill. Despite the severe illness, the WBC and platelet counts were normal. The most significant finding was the severe anemia. The increased unconjugated bilirubin and lactate dehydrogenase levels suggested a hemolytic process. Other causes of hemolytic anemia were considered, including drug-associated hemolytic anemia, disorders of RBC membrane and cytostructure (e.g., hereditary spherocytosis), abnormalities of RBC metabolism (e.g., G6PD deficiency), as well as sepsis with disseminated intravascular coagulation. The patient was given antibiotics to cover this last possibility. Parvovirus B19 infection can cause severe anemia but usually as a result of bone marrow suppression rather than hemolysis.

Patients with a microangiopathic hemolytic anemia (e.g., hemolytic-uremic syndrome, thrombotic thrombocytopenic purpura) usually have schistocytes rather than spherocytes on peripheral blood smear. Both of these conditions usually present with severe thrombocytopenia. A child of this age should be closely examined for physical abnormalities seen with Diamond- Blackfan syndrome or Fanconi anemia. Laboratory studies allowed differentiation of the diagnostic possibilities.

II.   Diagnosis

The peripheral blood smear revealed a nucleated RBC (erythroid progenitor cell) prematurely released from the bone marrow into the peripheral circulation (Fig. 10-1). There were also many small spherocytes. Polychromasia was also noted, because the bone marrow was releasing large numbers of reticulocytes and nucleated RBCs to compensate for accelerated RBC destruction. A direct antiglobulin (Coombs) test was positive, confirming the presence of antibodies to circulating RBCs. Specifically, this test was positive for immunoglobulin G (IgG) and negative for C3, consistent with the diagnosis of warm agglutinin autoimmune hemolytic anemia (AHA). **The diagnosis is AHA of the warm agglutinin type.**

III.   Incidence and Epidemiology

AHA occurs as the result of binding of antibody, antibody and complement complex, or complement to the RBC. The resulting immunologic reaction destroys RBCs and causes anemia. Infectious agents, drugs, and other agents may stimulate the process. Some autoimmune diseases, such as systemic lupus erythematosus, may also generate anti-RBC antibodies and RBC destruction. The true incidence of AHA is unknown, but is estimated to be 1 to 3 cases per 100,000 population per year. Acute AHA usually manifests in the first 4 years of life.

IV.   Clinical Manifestation

Children usually present with signs and symptoms of severe anemia. In younger children, parents or other family members may note pallor or weakness. Older children may complain of exercise intolerance or dizziness. Jaundice and scleral icterus result from the recycling of unconjugated bilirubin released from hemolyzed RBCs. Dark urine suggests hemoglobinuria. On examination, there is usually mild or moderate splenic enlargement. Some patients present with congestive heart failure related to the rapid development of anemia.

V.   Diagnostic Approach

Complete blood count. The anemia of acute-onset AHA is usually significant. Most children have a hemoglobin level of 4 to 7 g/dL. The MCV may be relatively normal, reflecting the weighted average of small microspherocytes and large reticulocytes. Erythrocyte agglutination within the sample tube may artifactually raise the MCV on an automated counter. An elevated RDW may be a clue that several different RBC populations are present, such as microspherocytes forming after partial splenic ingestion and large reticulocytes. There is an increase in reticulocytes once the bone marrow has a chance to respond. The WBC and platelet counts are typically normal. Concurrent thrombocytopenia indicates Evan's syndrome, aplastic anemia, hemolytic-uremic syndrome, or other conditions, rather than isolated autoimmune hemolytic anemia.

Direct antiglobulin test. A positive Coombs test confirms the suspected diagnosis. To establish a diagnosis, there must be antibody and evidence of hemolysis. The RBC antibodies that react at 37°C (warm antibodies) are usually IgG and do not cause spontaneous agglutination of cells unless Coombs antiserum is added. Cold antibodies are usually IgM and react at 4°C. These are considered complete antibodies, because no antiserum needs to be added to cause the RBC destructive process. There are also cases of mixed-type autoimmune responses.

Other studies. Other tests can provide evidence of an underlying hemolytic process: elevated unconjugated bilirubin, elevated lactate dehydrogenase, decreased serum haptoglobin, and urinalysis revealing blood on dipstick but no RBCs on microscopy (hemoglobinuria). Hepatic transaminases should be normal.

VI.   Treatment

The mainstay of treatment is corticosteroids, given at a dosage of 2 to 10 mg/kg per day. In severely ill patients such as this child, the steroids should be given intravenously. Otherwise, the care is supportive and includes replacement therapy. Compatible cross-matching may not be possible, but if the patient is in extremis blood type group O, Rh-negative blood should be used in aliquots that are given slowly and in amounts sufficient to stabilize the cardiovascular system. The patient should be adequately hydrated to avoid renal involvement. Splenectomy may be necessary if steroid therapy fails.

VII. References
1. Gehrs BC, Friedberg RC. Autoimmune hemolytic anemia. *Am J Hematol* 2002;69: 258–271.
2. Flores G, Cunningham-Rundles C, Newland AC, et al. Efficacy of intravenous immunoglobulin in the treatment of autoimmune hemolytic anemia: results in 73 patients. *Am J Hematol* 1993;44:237–242.
3. Ware RE. Autoimmune hemolytic anemia. In: Nathan DG, Orkin SH, Ginsburg D, et al., eds. *Nathan and Oski's hematology of infancy and childhood,* 6th ed. Philadelphia: WB Saunders, 2003:521–559.

Case 10-4: 6-Year-Old Girl

I. History of Present Illness
A 6-year-old Caucasian girl developed fever, abdominal pain, and pallor 3 days before admission. She had one episode of nonbilious emesis. Two days before admission, the family thought she was more pale and then "yellow." On the day of admission, she had a rash on her buttocks and extremities. She complained of feeling dizzy in the morning. She had decreased oral intake, and her urine appeared slightly dark. She also had several loose stools.

II. Past Medical History
Six years earlier, the patient had been admitted for dehydration and was noted to have anemia at that time. Past surgical history was notable for three surgeries for cleft palate and cleft lip repair. There were no known allergies, and she did not require any medications. Her immunizations were up to date. She had also received the hepatitis A vaccination series before a vacation in Mexico 1 year earlier. There had been no recent travel. She lived with her parents. There were no pets. The mother had had her spleen removed after blunt abdominal trauma sustained in a car accident. The mother had also required supplemental iron therapy for treatment of anemia. A maternal aunt required removal of her gall bladder at 19 years of age. Multiple family members had been diagnosed with diabetes mellitus.

III. Physical Examination
T, 38.5°C; RR, 24/min; HR, 142 bpm; BP, 100/50 mm Hg
Weight, 25 kg (50th percentile).

On general examination, she was very pale but alert and oriented. The sclerae were mildly icteric. The oropharynx had mild erythema but no exudates or vesicles. The lungs were clear to auscultation. A gallop was appreciated on cardiac examination. The abdomen was soft. A tender spleen was palpated 4 cm below the left costal margin. There was no tenderness in the right upper quadrant. Capillary refill was brisk. The remainder of the examination was normal.

IV. Diagnostic Studies
A complete blood count revealed the following: 6,300 WBCs/mm^3 (64% segmented neutrophils, 30% lymphocytes, and 6% monocytes); hemoglobin, 4.5 g/dL; and 179,000 platelets/mm^3. The RDW was elevated at 16.9. The MCV was 78 fL, and the mean corpuscular hemoglobin concentration (MCHC) was 37 mg/dL. The reticulocyte count was 8.4%. Other laboratory findings included the following: total bilirubin, 3.3 mg/dL; unconjugated bilirubin, 2.4 mg/dL; uric acid, 2.3; lactate dehydrogenase, 1,136 U/L. Serum albumin, transaminases, and electrolytes were normal.

V. Course of Illness
This child was admitted for fever and abdominal pain. Significant anemia was noted on complete blood count. The presence of a gallop with severe anemia prompted a gradual transfusion of packed RBCs. She received empiric ceftriaxone after a blood culture was obtained. The peripheral blood smear (Fig. 10-2) suggested a diagnosis.

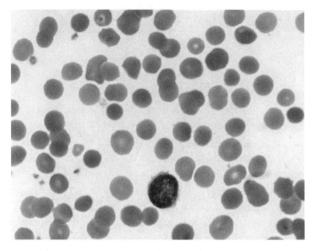

FIG. 10-2. Peripheral blood smear (case 10-4).

DISCUSSION: CASE 10-4

I. Differential Diagnosis

The history of gall bladder surgery in a young aunt certainly raises the possibility of an inherited hemolytic disorder. The mother's history of splenectomy may have been related to splenic laceration due to trauma; however, the history of anemia is intriguing. The differential diagnosis is that of other hemolytic anemias, both congenital and acquired. There are other disorders of the RBC membrane and cytoskeleton, including spherocytosis, elliptocytosis, and stomatocytosis. Also under consideration are disorders of RBC enzymes (e.g., G6PD deficiency), drug-associated hemolytic anemia, and autoimmune hemolytic anemia. The differential diagnostic possibilities are broad, but spherocytosis is the most common of the congenital causes. Basic laboratory testing allows for establishment of the correct diagnosis.

II. Diagnosis

The peripheral blood smear revealed numerous small spherocytes, with a paucity of other abnormal forms and a paucity of normal RBCs (Fig. 10-2). Causes of spherocytosis include conditions that lead to RBC membrane damage, such as immunohemolytic anemias (e.g., autoimmune hemolytic anemia), clostridial toxin, severe burns, Wilson disease, and hereditary spherocytosis. **This child had hereditary spherocytosis,** a congenital hemolytic anemia caused by defects in proteins comprising the RBC skeleton. Subsequent evaluation of other family members revealed mild hereditary spherocytosis in the mother and maternal aunt. The grandparents declined testing.

III. Incidence and Epidemiology

The incidence of spherocytosis in the United States is 1 in 5,000 live births. It is most common in individuals of northern European descent but does occur in other ethnic groups. Inheritance is usually autosomal dominant, but in up to one fourth of the cases family history is negative. In some cases, family members have only minor manifestations. A family history of gall bladder surgery or splenectomy should raise suspicion for underlying hemolytic diseases, including hereditary spherocytosis. In other situations, there may be a new mutation or a recessive pattern of inheritance. The defects for this condition are found on chromosomes 1, 8, 14, 15, and 17.

IV. Clinical Presentation

Presentation depends to some extent on the severity of the spherocytosis. Fatigue due to anemia and episodic jaundice are common complaints. Jaundice may be noted more frequently during viral infections. Most children have splenomegaly (50% of infants and 75% to 90% of older children). During the newborn period, some cases are detected by severe or prolonged hyperbilirubinemia. Some patients present with gallstones.

V. Diagnostic Approach

Complete blood count. Patients with hereditary spherocytosis have varying degrees of anemia, reticulocytosis, elevated MCHC, and hyperbilirubinemia. In mild forms, the hemoglobin may be normal (compensated hemolysis). Those with moderate or moderately severe spherocytosis have a hemoglobin level that ranges from 6 to 10 g/dL and a reticulocyte count of 8% or greater. Those with severe spherocytosis typically have hemoglobin levels lower than 6 g/dL and reticulocyte counts greater than 10%. The MCHC exceeds the normal value in about one third of affected patients. The finding of an MCHC greater than 35 g/dL has a sensitivity of 70% and a specificity of 86% in diagnosing hereditary spherocytosis. The MCV is usually normal, but the RDW is elevated due to the mixed population of small spherocytes and large reticulocytes.

Peripheral blood smear. The finding of spherocytes on peripheral blood smear is characteristic. Spherocytes are round, dense, hyperchromic RBCs that lack the typical central pallor and biconcavity of normal RBCs. They are present in 25% to 35% of patients with mild spherocytosis but in almost all patients with moderate or severe disease. In contrast to some other causes of hemolytic disease, in hereditary spherocytosis spherocytes and microspherocytes are the only abnormal cells visualized on the peripheral blood smear. In severe hereditary spherocytosis, the spherocytes may appear dense, contracted, or budding. Nucleated RBCs are not usually seen. Howell-Jolly bodies are seen in only 4% of patients before splenectomy.

Osmotic fragility test. Normal RBCs have a high surface-to-volume ratio (i.e., more membrane than they need). When normal RBCs are suspended in a hypotonic saline solution, they expand due to the influx of fluid. The extra membrane allows the cells to expand and gradually take the shape of a sphere, a conformation that efficiently minimizes the surface area relative to volume. As the solution becomes progressively hypotonic, the normal RBCs become more spherical and ultimately burst, releasing hemoglobin into the solution. In spherocytes, the RBC surface area is already decreased relative to volume. Cells that start with a low surface-to-volume ratio (e.g., spherocytes) reach the spherical limit at a higher saline (less hypotonic) concentration than normal cells do. Fragility is calculated by measuring the percent lysis at specific saline concentrations.

Other studies. The glycerol lysis test measures the rate rather than the extent of hemolysis. The hypertonic cryohemolysis test is based on the fact that spherocytes are particularly sensitive to cooling in hypertonic solutions. In contrast to the other tests, this determination is independent of the surface-to-volume ratio. Other findings in children with hereditary spherocytosis, such as unconjugated hyperbilirubinemia and increased fecal urobilinogen, reflect chronic hemolysis.

VI. Treatment

Patients with hereditary spherocytosis require folic acid supplementation to keep up with their chronic hemolysis (usually 0.5 to 1 mg/day orally). Patients with spherocytosis may require transfusion in the acute phase. Splenectomy can reduce or eliminate the need for transfusion. Most often splenectomy is delayed until the patient reaches 5 or 6 years of age, a time when the risk of pneumococcal sepsis has decreased considerably. Children evaluated for splenectomy should receive vaccination with both the heptavalent pneumococcal conjugate and the pneumococcal 23-valent polysaccharide vaccines. After splenectomy, penicillin prophylaxis is generally recommended.

Complications related to hereditary spherocytosis include gallstones, hemolytic crises, and aplastic crises. Bilirubinate gallstones may be asymptomatic, or they may cause cholecystitis or biliary obstruction. Ultrasonography detects these pigmented stones, and some specialists recommend routine abdominal ultrasound studies every 5 years. Hemolytic crises occur commonly in children with hereditary spherocytosis, usually in association with viral syndromes. Transient jaundice, emesis, and abdominal pain characterize the hemolytic crisis. Most children do not require specific treatment, but the development of severe anemia may lead to hospitalization and a need for transfusion of packed RBCs. Aplastic crises occur less frequently than hemolytic crises do, but severe anemia may precipitate congestive heart failure. Aplastic crises frequently occur after parvovirus B19 infection.

VII.   References

1. Michaels LA, Cohen AR, Zhao HMA, et al. Screening for hereditary spherocytosis by use of automated erythrocyte indexes. *J Pediatr* 1997;130:957–960.
2. Evans TC, Jehle D. The red cell distribution width. *J Emerg Med* 1991;9:72–74.
3. Gallagher PG, Lux SE. Disorders of the erythrocyte membrane. In: Nathan DG, Orkin SH, Ginsburg D, et al., eds. *Nathan and Oski's hematology of infancy and childhood,* 6th ed. Philadelphia: WB Saunders, 2003:560–684.
4. Tse WT, Lux SE. Red blood cell membrane disorders. *Br J Haematol* 1999;104:2–13.
5. Delhommeau F, Cynober T, Schischmanoff PO, et al. Natural history of hereditary spherocytosis during the first year of life. *Blood* 2000;95:393–397.

Case 10-5: 5-Year-Old Girl

I. History of Present Illness

A 5-year-old African-American girl was brought to the emergency department for complaints of pallor and fatigue. For the past 3 to 4 days she had seemed tired. She had not been eating or drinking as usual and had been relatively inactive. There had been no fevers. She denied nausea, vomiting, and diarrhea. Her urinary pattern has not changed. She had no specific sites of pain or discomfort. The mother stated that the girl's eyes were always somewhat yellow and the color had not changed.

II. Past Medical History

She was the full-term product of a spontaneous vaginal delivery. At 2 years of age, she had developed painful swelling of her hands. Her 5-year-old sibling had witnessed a "bee sting." She was treated with diphenhydramine and corticosteroids for a possible allergic reaction. The swelling resolved over the course of several days. She required emergency department evaluation at 4 years of age for persistent left knee and back pain after falling. Radiographs of her spine, hips, and left femur, tibia, and fibula were normal. She was treated with a combination of ibuprofen and oxycodone. She had not received any medications recently. She was born in Jamaica and moved to the United States at 2 years of age. Her immunizations were reportedly up to date, although written confirmation was not available.

III. Physical Examination

T, 37.3°C; RR, 30/min; HR, 140 bpm; BP, 100/60 mm Hg; SpO$_2$, 95% in room air
Weight, 5th percentile; height, 75th percentile

Physical examination revealed a thin child with obvious scleral icterus. She was in mild respiratory distress. The neck was supple. Several small cervical lymph nodes were palpable. The lungs were clear. There was a I/VI systolic ejection murmur at the lower left sternal border. The abdomen was soft. The liver edge was palpable 1 to 2 cm below the right costal margin. The spleen was massively enlarged and could be felt at the pelvic brim. The remainder of the examination was normal.

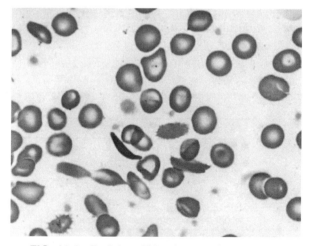

FIG. 10-3. Peripheral blood smear (case 10-5).

IV. Diagnostic Studies

The complete blood count revealed the following: 8,200 WBCs/mm^3 (2% band forms, 23% segmented neutrophils, 61% lymphocytes, 12% monocytes, and 2% eosinophils); hemoglobin, 4.6 g/dL; and 156,000 platelets/mm^3. The reticulocyte count was 16%. The total bilirubin was 2.4 mg/dL. The remainder of the hepatic function panel was normal.

V. Course of Illness

A chest radiograph was normal. The peripheral blood smear revealed the diagnosis (Fig. 10-3).

DISCUSSION: CASE 10-5

I. Differential Diagnosis

The findings on peripheral blood smear were suggestive of sickle cell disease (see later discussion). In patients known to have sickle cell disease who present with the signs of pallor and fatigue, the differential diagnosis consists of four elements: infection, acute RBC aplasia (aplastic crisis), acute hemolytic crisis, and sequestration. Infections until recently were the major cause of mortality in children with sickle cell disease. Infection is usually heralded by fever. Any fever in a patient with sickle cell disease or one of its variants must be taken seriously and treated aggressively. Acute RBC aplasia occurs when RBC production fails to keep up with the need produced by a shortened RBC survival time. Often parvovirus B19 is the cause of his type of acute drop in hemoglobin. Acute hemolysis may also occur and cause a worsening of anemia. Often, the parents detect an increase in jaundice or a darkening of the child's urine. Sequestration can be diagnosed by clinical examination and tends to occur in young children whose spleens have not yet autoinfarcted. Table 10.5 compares the findings in the various manifestations of sickle cell disease.

II. Diagnosis

The peripheral blood smear revealed numerous blunted and boxy sickled cells, a situation most typically seen with SC-type sickle cell disease (Fig. 10-3). This diagnosis was confirmed by hemoglobin electrophoresis. **The clinical picture in light of the peripheral blood smear suggested the diagnosis of sickle cell disease, SC type, with associated splenic sequestration.** In retrospect, the episode of hand swelling at 2 years of age may have been dactylitis, a complication of sickle cell disease in young children. The episode of pain requiring narcotics may have been a vaso-occlusive episode causing pain. Obviously, this would be difficult to prove in retrospect. She promptly received penicillin prophylaxis.

TABLE 10-5. *Comparison of Findings in Sequestration, Aplastic, and Hemolytic Crises in Sickle Cell Disease*

Category	Sequestration crisis	Aplastic crisis	Hemolytic crisis
Onset	Sudden	Gradual	Sudden
Pallor	Present	Present	Present
Jaundice	Normal	Normal	Increased
Abdominal pain	Present	Absent	Absent
Hemoglobin level	Very low	Low or very low	Low
Reticulocytes	Unchanged or increased	Decreased	Increased
Marrow erythroid activity	Unchanged or increased	Decreased	Increased

Cohen A: Hematologic emergencies. In: Fleisher G, Ludwig S, eds. *Textbook of pediatric emergency medicine,* 4th ed. Philadelphia: Lippincott Williams & Wilkins, 2000.

III. Incidence and Epidemiology

The cultural incidence of sequestration is not known. Sickle cell disease affects 1 in every 400 to 500 African-Americans. It also occurs in people of Mediterranean, Arabic, and East Indian origin. There are three major forms of sickle cell disease in the United States population: homozygous sickle cell disease (HbSS, 60%), sickle cell–hemoglobin C disease (HbSC, 30%), and sickle cell–beta-thalassemia (10%). In patients with HbSS, sequestration usually occurs early in life, because the spleen ultimately undergoes autoinfarction. Children with milder forms of disease, typically HbSC, may develop sequestration as late as 10 or 11 years of age.

IV. Clinical Presentation

The manifestations of sequestrations are varied. Patients may have a mild form of sequestration with only a minor drop in hemoglobin, or they may present in full cardiovascular collapse. In all cases, there is splenic enlargement and evidence of a decrease in circulating blood volume. There may be a fatal outcome if therapeutic response is not adequate. Splenic sequestration may recur.

V. Diagnostic Approach

The diagnosis is established by a careful physical examination and a high index of suspicion. Laboratory studies can rule out other conditions in the differential diagnosis, but there is no single laboratory test to confirm sequestration. Part of the high index of suspicion comes in having a well-educated patient and patient population that is capable of recognizing and reporting every sign and symptom.

VI. Treatment

In mild cases with hemodynamic stability, hydration and careful watching in an inpatient setting may be all that is required. In severe cases, prompt transfusion therapy is required. For some patients, a routine transfusion program is begun. If episodes recur frequently, splenectomy may be indicated. Splenic infarct occurs over time, and the splenic function usually is already compromised.

VII. References

1. Ohene-Frempong K. Abnormalities of hemoglobin structure and function. In: Rudolph A, ed. *Rudolph's pediatrics,* 21st ed. New York: McGraw-Hill, 2003.
2. Grover R, Wethers DL. Management of acute splenic sequestration crisis in sickle cell disease. *J Assoc Acad Minor Phys* 1990;1:67–70.
3. Kinney TR, Ware RE, Schultz WH, et al. Long-term management of splenic sequestration in children with sickle cell disease. *J Pediatr* 1990;117:194–199.
4. Mallouh A. Acute splenic sequestration in sickle cell disease. *J Pediatr* 1986;108:1035–1036.
5. Powell RW, Levine GL, Yang YM, et al. Acute splenic sequestration crisis in sickle cell disease; early detection and treatment. *J Pediatr Surg* 1992;27:215–218.

Case 10-6: 2-Year-Old Boy

I. History of Present Illness

A 2-year-old boy was in his usual state of good health until the day of admission, when he visited his grandmother, who felt he was "off his color." She had not seen him for 4 weeks. The mother took his temperature, which was normal. He did not have fever, vomiting, or diarrhea, and his activity level had not changed. At the grandmother's insistence, he was taken to the hospital for evaluation. He had not received any mediations recently. He had had an upper respiratory tract infection approximately 6 weeks earlier, which resolved without intervention.

II. Past Medical History

The infant was born at term by spontaneous vaginal delivery after an uncomplicated pregnancy. The birth weight was 3,400 g. He had not required any hospitalizations or undergone any surgical procedures. He reportedly had had a "rash" with amoxicillin approximately 1 year earlier, during treatment of an otitis media. He had received the appropriate immunizations for his age. He had traveled to Lake George in New York State 2 months before presentation. His developmental history was normal. There were no siblings. The family history was unremarkable.

III. Physical Examination

T, 38.0°C; RR, 25/min; HR, 120 bpm; BP, 113/54 mm Hg; SpO$_2$, 98% in room air

In general the child was alert and in no acute distress. However, he was extremely pale. The conjunctivae were anicteric. The tympanic membranes were normal in appearance. The lungs were clear to auscultation. There were no murmurs on cardiac examination. Distal pulses were strong. The abdomen was soft without hepatomegaly or splenomegaly. The palmar creases were remarkable for loss of pigmentation.

IV. Diagnostic Studies

The complete blood count revealed the following: 8,400 WBCs/mm^3; hemoglobin, 7.2 g/dL; 326,000 platelets/mm^3; MCV, 81 fL; RDW, 12.4. Serum electrolytes, blood urea

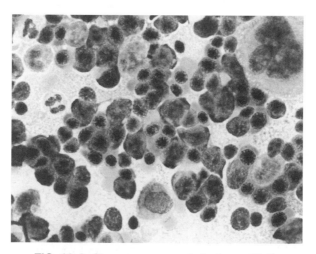

FIG. 10-4. Bone marrow aspirate (case 10-6).

nitrogen, glucose, transaminases, albumin, and lactate dehydrogenase were all normal. The reticulocyte count was 0.2%. A direct Coombs test was negative. Parvovirus IgM and IgG were also negative.

V. Course of Illness

The child was noted to be pale by his grandmother when he went to see her for a visit. This history speaks to the insidious onset of this child's pallor. His mother, who lived with him day by day, had not noticed his pallor. The child had been well except for a mild viral illness. He had no other symptoms. There was no family history of anemia and no previous complete blood counts that suggested any problem. His examination was normal except for the pallor. Laboratory studies indicated a normocytic normochromic anemia and a reticulocyte count of virtually zero. None of the other cell lines was abnormal. The findings indicated a need for a bone marrow aspiration and analysis, which confirmed the diagnosis (Fig. 10-4).

DISCUSSION: CASE 10-6

I. Differential Diagnosis

The differential diagnosis of acquired RBC aplasia includes transient erythroblastopenia of childhood (TEC), anemia associated with parvovirus B19, drug- and chemical-related anemia, and idiopathic anemia. The condition may also be confused with congenital RBC aplasia (Diamond-Blackfan anemia), but the age at onset of TEC is usually older and there are no associated anomalies. Also, TEC is a normocytic anemia, whereas Diamond-Blackfan anemia is usually macrocytic.

II. Diagnosis

The bone marrow aspirate revealed numerous young (nucleated) RBCs, all in the same stage of maturation (Fig. 10-4). **This finding, combined with the normal MCV and low reticulocyte count, suggested the diagnosis of TEC on the verge of recovery.** It is one of the most common acquired RBC aplasias.

III. Incidence and Epidemiology

TEC is a condition that occurs in previously well children. The age at diagnosis is usually about 2 years, with a typical range of 1 to 3 years. There is often a history of a preceding upper respiratory tract infection or other viral illness, but no single agent has been identified. Parvovirus infection usually is not an etiologic agent in this diagnosis.

IV. Clinical Presentation

The presenting signs and symptoms are usually pallor and fatigue. Sometimes tachycardia and feelings of palpitations prompt a visit to the physician's office and subsequent detection. There are no other common significant manifestations, but there have been sporadic cases of TEC associated with neurologic conditions, including papilledema and transient hemiplegia. One recent report has linked TEC and breath-holding.

V. Diagnostic Approaches

TEC should be suspected in a patient of appropriate age who has insidious onset of anemia and no reticulocyte response.

Complete blood count. The median hemoglobin value at presentation is 5 to 6 g/dL but varies significantly depending on whether the diagnosis occurs early or late in the course of disease. Reticulocyte counts are less than 1% except for those children on the cusp of recovery. WBC and platelet counts are typically normal, although exceptions are possible. The MCV in TEC is usually normal, whereas the MCV in Diamond-Blackfan anemia is usually elevated. Other features also help distinguish TEC from Diamond-Blackfan anemia (Table 10-6).

TABLE 10-6. *Features of Transient Erythroblastopenia of Childhood and Diamond-Blackfan Anemia*

Feature	TEC (%)	DBA (%)
Age >1 year at diagnosis	80	10
Physical anomalies	0	30
Adenosine deaminase	Normal	Elevated
Elevated mean corpuscular volume at diagnosis	5	80
Elevated fetal hemoglobin (HbF) at diagnosis	20	100
Elevated i antigen at diagnosis	20	100

DBA, Diamond-Blackfan anemia; TEC, transient erythroblastopenia of childhood.
Adapted from Alter BP. Inherited bone marrow failure syndromes. In: Nathan DG, Orkin SH, Ginsburg D, et al., eds. Nathan and Oski's hematology of infancy and childhood, 6th ed. Philadelphia: WB Saunders, 2003:280–365.

Bone marrow aspiration. During the illness, the bone marrow reveals significant erythroblastopenia with maturation arrest. During the recovery phase, patients with TEC produce a cohort of "fetal-like" erythrocytes that evolve into normal RBCs. All marrow RBCs are at the same stage of maturation.

Other studies. Interpretation of MCV, fetal hemoglobin, and i antigen depends on stage of illness. During the recovery phase the MCV, fetal hemoglobin, and i antigen may all be elevated. Ultimately, the distinction is often made when the patient with TEC begins recovery.

VI. Treatment

Treatment is supportive. A blood transfusion may be needed for hemodynamic instability. Resolution typically occurs within 1 to 3 months after diagnosis. Approximately 5% to 10% of children have begun to recover by the time medical care is sought. There are no other associated hematologic problems. The prognosis is excellent.

VII. References

1. Skeppner G, Kreuger A., Elinder G. Transient erythroblastopenia of childhood: prospective study of 10 patients with special reference to viral infections. *J Pediatr Hematol Oncol* 2002;24:294–298.
2. Chan GC, Kanwar VS, Williams J. Transient erythroblastopenia of childhood associated with transient neurologic deficit: report of a case and review of the literature. *J Paediatr Child Health* 1998;34:299–301.
3. Cherrick I, Karayalcin G, Lanzkowsky P. Transient erythroblastopenia of childhood: prospective study of fifty patients. *Am J Pediatr Hematol Oncol* 1994;16:320–324.
4. Hays T, Lane PA Jr, Shafer F. Transient erythroblastopenia of childhood: a review of 26 cases and reassessment of indications for bone marrow aspiration. *Am J Dis Child* 1989;143:605–607.
5. Tam DA, Rash FC. Breath-holding spells in a patient with transient erythroblastopenia of childhood. *J Pediatr* 1997;130:651–653.

11

Fever

Samir S. Shah

APPROACH TO THE PATIENT WITH FEVER

I. Definition of the Complaint

The complaint of fever accounts for a large portion of ambulatory pediatric visits. Although fever is classically defined as a temperature greater than 38.0°C for neonates or 38.5°C for older children, the term is subject to significant interpretation. An isolated temperature measurement of 38.0°C in a toddler may not be meaningful, but repeated daily temperatures of 38.0°C over a period of several weeks may indicate underlying pathology.

Practitioners must also recognize that body temperature normally fluctuates throughout the day, tending to be lower in the early morning and peaking in the evening. Certain conditions or activities (e.g., exercise, warm baths, hot drinks) also affect the measured temperature. Additionally, axillary measurements of temperature may be 0.5 to 1.0°C lower than oral, rectal, or tympanic measurements. To compensate for such discrepancies, parents are sometimes instructed to add 0.5° or 1.0°C to axillary measurements to approximate the "real" temperature. Such "corrections" may further cloud evaluation of the febrile child.

II. Complaint by Cause and Frequency

Fever may develop in response to injury, infection, autoimmune disease, or malignancy. The release of endogenous pyrogens triggers a cascade of reactions that ultimately raise the hypothalamic set-point. Fever may also be caused when the body's heat production or environmental heat overwhelms heat loss mechanisms or when heat loss mechanisms are deficient. Viruses are the most common cause of fever in children. Specific common causes of fever are too numerous to list here, but less common causes are listed in Table 11-1.

III. Clarifying Questions

Certain clarifying questions may help provide clues to the diagnosis.

• What temperature value is the parent using to define a fever?

— Although 37°C (98.6°F) is commonly considered to be the normal body temperature, normal temperature exhibits significant daily variation, with a nadir in the early morning and a peak in the early evening.

• Are there symptoms of specific illness?

— The presence of certain complaints, such as bloody diarrhea, cough, and stiff neck, suggests specific diagnostic categories.

• Has there been exposure to animals?

— In addition to pets in the home, inquiry should be made about contact with rodents or farm animals and consumption of unpasteurized dairy products. For example,

TABLE 11-1. *Less Common Causes of Fever*

Diagnostic category	Examples
Infection	Endemic fungi (histoplasmosis, blastomycosis)
	Enteric diseases (*Salmonella* spp., *Shigella* spp.)
	Human immunodeficiency virus
	Infectious mononucleosis (Epstein-Barr virus, cytomegalovirus)
	Protozoa (malaria, toxoplasma)
	Tickborne diseases (Lyme disease, Rocky Mountain spotted fever)
	Tuberculosis
	Zoonoses (cat-scratch, tularemia, brucellosis)
Collagen vascular disease	Systemic juvenile rheumatoid arthritis
	Systemic lupus erythematosus
	Dermatomyositis
	Scleroderma
	Sarcoidosis
	Vasculitis (e.g., Kawasaki, Behçet, Wegener granulomatosis)
Malignancy	Leukemia
	Lymphoma
Inflammatory bowel disease	Crohn's disease
	Ulcerative colitis
Drug fever	Penicillins
	Cephalosporins
	Sulfonamides
	Phenytoin
	Methylphenidate
	Cimetidine
	Acetaminophen
Factitious fever	Pseudofever
	Munchausen syndrome by proxy
Recurrent fever syndromes	Familial Mediterranean fever
	Hyperimmunoglobulin D syndrome
	PFAPA syndrome
	Tumor necrosis factor receptor-associated periodic fever
Centrally mediated fever	

PFAPA, periodic fever, aphthous ulcers, pharyngitis, and adenopathy syndrome.

exposure to house mice may suggest lymphocytic choriomeningitis virus, and exposure to farm animals suggests brucellosis as a potential cause. Household contacts with occupational exposure to potentially infectious animals should also be sought.

- Have there been recent tick or flea bites?

 — Tularemia, ehrlichiosis, Rocky Mountain spotted fever, and Lyme disease may be acquired in this manner.

- Has there been any recent travel?

 — Travel to regions where certain diseases are endemic may shift the differential diagnosis. For example, travel to the Indian subcontinent raises the suspicion for typhoid fever and malaria. Coccidioidomycosis would be included in the differential diagnosis of a child with atypical pneumonia who has traveled to the southwestern United States.

- What medications is the child receiving?

 — Medications, including penicillins, cephalosporins, acetaminophen, anticonvulsants, and methylphenidate, can cause fever.

- What is the pattern of fever?

  — The evaluation of acute, prolonged, and recurrent fevers differs dramatically. If differentiating between prolonged and recurrent fevers is difficult, documenting the fevers in a "fever diary" may help clarify the pattern.

- Are there family members with recurrent episodes of fever?

  — Familial dysautonomia, familial Mediterranean fever, and cyclic neutropenia are some of the hereditary disorders that cause recurrent fever.

IV. References

1. Calello DP, Shah SS. The child with fever of unknown origin. *Pediatr Case Rev* 2002; 2:226–239.
2. Nizet V, Vinci RJ, Lovejoy FH Jr. Fever in children. *Pediatr Rev* 1994;15:127–135.
3. Saper BC, Breder CD. The neurologic basis of fever. *N Engl J Med* 1994;330: 1880–1886.
4. Tunnessen WW Jr. Fever. In: Tunnessen WW Jr, ed. *Signs and symptoms in pediatrics,* 3rd ed. Philadelphia: Lippincott Williams & Wilkins, 1999:3–7.

Case 11-1: 18-Month-Old Girl

I. History of Present Illness

An 18-month-old girl presented with a 1-day history of fever to 38.0°C and cough. While in the examination room, she had tonic flexion of her upper extremities and eye deviation to the left. This episode lasted 10 minutes and resolved spontaneously. Mild perioral cyanosis developed just before the end of the seizure. Afterward, the child was tired and irritable. There was no history of rash, eye pain, neck pain, or emesis. There were no alterations in gait or balance. There was no antecedent witnessed trauma. The only pet was a recently acquired goldfish. Several children at her daycare center had had symptoms of upper respiratory tract infection. The remainder of the review of systems was unremarkable.

II. Past Medical History

She was born at term after an uncomplicated pregnancy. She had not previously required hospitalization. Her immunizations were up to date and included the pneumococcal conjugate vaccine. She had received supplemental iron starting at 12 months of age for treatment of "anemia." The maternal grandmother had type 2 diabetes treated with glyburide, a sulfonylurea oral hypoglycemic agent. There was no family history of febrile seizures, but one relative supposedly had a seizure and drowned while swimming. The family was not able to provide further details.

III. Physical Examination

T, 39.1°C; RR, 26/min; HR, 132 bpm; BP, 97/53 mm Hg; SpO_2, 98% in room air
Weight, 25th percentile

The child was crying and seemed mildly disoriented. There were no bruises or abrasions on her face or scalp. Her tympanic membranes were mildly erythematous but mobile. There was copious purulent nasal discharge. The neck was difficult to assess due to the child's lack of cooperation. While yelling and screaming, she was able to arch her back and neck without apparent limitation. There was no cervical lymphadenopathy. The

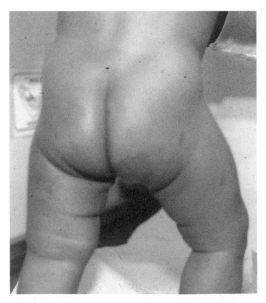

FIG. 11-1. Photograph of patient's skin findings (case 11-1).

heart and lung sounds were normal. The abdomen was soft without organomegaly. There were no focal neurologic deficits, but the child appeared groggy and irritable and was slow to respond to her mother's voice. Several hyperpigmented macules were noted on her skin as her clothes were removed for the lumbar puncture (Fig. 11-1).

IV. Diagnostic Studies

A complete blood count revealed the following: 15,500 white blood cells (WBCs)/mm^3 (61% segmented neutrophils, 22% lymphocytes, 15% monocytes, and 2% eosinophils); hemoglobin, 12.1 g/dL; and 282,000 platelets/mm^3. Serum electrolytes, calcium, and glucose were normal. Urinalysis revealed no WBCs or nitrites. Lumbar puncture revealed 2 WBCs and 19 red blood cells per cubic millimeter. No bacteria were visualized on Gram staining. The cerebrospinal fluid (CSF) protein and glucose concentrations were normal. Blood and CSF cultures were subsequently negative.

V. Course of Illness

The skin findings (Fig. 11-1) suggested a diagnosis that was subsequently confirmed with further evaluation.

DISCUSSION: CASE 11-1

I. Differential Diagnosis

This child presented with fever and seizures. Given her age and the difficult examination, a lumbar puncture was performed to exclude meningitis as a cause of seizures. The reassuring CSF findings led to other diagnostic considerations. The maternal grandmother used an oral hypoglycemic agent, making an ingestion-induced hypoglycemic seizure possible. However, the child's serum glucose concentration was normal. The history of a cousin drowning during a reported seizure raised the possibility of a cardiac condition such as prolonged QT syndrome, Wolff-Parkinson-White syndrome, or hypertrophic cardiomyopathy as a possible cause of hypoxic seizures. The electrocardiogram, performed in light of this history, was normal.

In an 18-month-old girl who presents with a brief (less than 10-minute) seizure in the context of fever, typical febrile seizure is the most likely diagnosis. However, it is possible that the fever lowered the seizure threshold in a child with an underlying seizure disorder. Potentially important clues in this case were the hyperpigmented macules on this child's skin. Café-au-lait spots are characteristic for neurofibromatosis type 1 (NF1) but may also be noted in unaffected children and in children with other disorders. The critical factor in this case was the number of spots seen; fewer than 0.1% of normal individuals have more than six café-au-lait spots. Inherited disorders associated with café-au-lait spots are summarized in Table 11-2.

II. Diagnosis

Examination of the skin revealed approximately 15 hyperpigmented macules substantially greater than 5 mm in diameter (Fig. 11-1). Axillary freckling was also noted on physical examination. An ophthalmology examination revealed findings suspicious for an optic glioma. **These findings confirmed the diagnosis of neurofibromatosis type 1.** As is common in children with NF1, this child's seizures were not related to a structural lesion in the brain. This child's febrile seizures were likely related to her NF1, but the relationship among seizure type, presence or absence of brain lesions, and evolution of epilepsy in children with NF1 is not clear.

III. Epidemiology and Incidence

NF1 and NF2 are genetic disorders in which affected patients develop both benign and malignant tumors at increased frequency. NF1 is associated with cutaneous lesions, vision loss, and skeletal problems; cataract formation and hearing loss are more typically associ-

TABLE 11-2. *Inherited Multisystem Diseases Associated with Café-au-lait Spots*

Disease	Key features
Ataxia telangiectasia	Bulbar telangiectasia, progressive ataxia, oculomotor apraxia, recurrent sinopulmonary infection
Bannayan-Riley-Ruvalcaba syndrome (formerly Riley-Smith, Ruvalcaba-Myhre, and Bannayan syndromes)	Macrocephaly, subcutaneous lipomas, pigmentary changes of penis, polyposis of colon, hypotonia, joint hyperextensibility, seizures
Bloom syndrome	Short stature, malar hypoplasia, facial telangiectatic erythema, propensity to develop malignancy
Fanconi syndrome	Pancyotpenia, mental retardation, hypoplastic radii and thumbs, microcephaly, microphthalmia, genitourinary tract anomalies, generalized hyperpigmentation
McCune-Albright syndrome	Polyostotic fibrous dysplasia, precocious puberty, nevi with irregular ("coast of Maine") borders
Multiple lentigines syndrome (LEOPARD syndrome)	*L*entigines, *E*CG abnormalities, *O*cular hypertelorism, *P*ulmonic stenosis, *A*bnormal genitalia, *R*etardation of growth, *D*eafness
Multiple endocrine neoplasia type 2b	Medullary thyroid carcinoma, pheochromocytoma, parathyroid adenoma, marfanoid habitus, mucosal neuromas
Neurofibormatosis type one	See text
Russell-Silver syndrome	Intrauterine growth retardation, congenital hemihypertrophy, precocious puberty, small/triangular face
Tuberous sclerosis	Abnormal hair pigmentation, adenoma sebaceum, shagreen patches, seizures

ated with NF2. NF1, also known as von Recklinghausen's neurofibromatosis or peripheral neurofibromatosis, is an autosomal dominant condition. Half of the cases occur in patients with a family history of NF1, and the other half occur as spontaneous mutations. The incidence is approximately 1 in 3,000. The clinical manifestations of NF1 result from alterations of the NF1 gene located on chromosome 17. The gene product, termed neurofibromin, is thought to function as a tumor suppressor, but research is still ongoing.

IV.   Clinical Presentation

Despite advances in our understanding of the molecular basis for NF1, the diagnosis remains one that is largely based on clinical criteria. Clinical diagnosis of NF1 requires the presence of at least two of the seven consensus criteria stipulated by the National Institutes of Health (NIH) (Table 11-3). Children with sporadic rather than inherited cases may not meet the NIH diagnostic criteria until later in life. At 1 year of age, approximately 50% of individuals with sporadic disease lack two or more of the cardinal clinical features permitting diagnosis, but by age 8 years, 95% meet NIH criteria.

The most visible features of NF1 are flat, evenly pigmented macules known as café-au-lait spots. These macules, often present at birth, increase in both number and size over the first few years of life. One or two café-au-lait macules are present in up to 25% of the normal population, but the presence of six or more macules should raise suspicion for NF1. These macules are easier to visualize with the use of a Wood's lamp. Skinfold freckling, another pigmentary change associated with NF1, usually occurs in the axillae, groin, nape of the neck, or under the chin. By 6 years of age, approximately 80% of children with NF1 demonstrate axillary or inguinal freckling.

Lisch nodules are benign pigmented hamartomas of the iris that occur in patients with NF1. These nodules do not interfere with vision. Lisch nodules may not be apparent in young children, but they are present in more than 95% of adolescent and adult patients. Detection of Lisch nodules on bedside examination is challenging, and diagnosis frequently requires a slit-lamp examination by an experienced ophthalmologist. In contrast to Lisch nodules, optic nerve tumors, such as optic nerve gliomas, occur primarily in

TABLE 11-3. *Diagnostic Criteria for Neurofibromatosis Type 1*[a]

Six or more café-au-lait spots
>1.5 cm in postpubertal children
>0.5 cm in prepubertal children
Two or more neurofibromas or any type of plexiform neurofibroma
Freckling in the axillary or inguinal regions (Crowe sign)
Optic glioma
Two or more Lisch nodules
Benign iris hamartomas
Distinctive bony lesions
Dysplasia of sphenoid bone or long bone cortex
First-degree relative with neurofibromatosis type 1
Includes parent, sibling, or offspring

[a]Two or more criteria must be present to make the diagnosis.

younger children. They are often associated with asymmetric, noncorrectable vision loss, diminished peripheral vision and color discrimination, and proptosis.

Subcutaneous or cutaneous (dermal) neurofibromas are rarely seen in young children but appear during or just before adolescence. Neurofibromas are present in 48% of 10-year-old patients and 84% of 20-year-old patients. Cutaneous lesions frequently begin as small papules on the face, scalp, trunk, and extremities. Deep lesions may be detected only through palpation. These lesions represent a major cosmetic problem but do not transform into malignant tumors. In contrast, plexiform neurofibromas surround soft tissue and bone, causing aberrant growth. Plexiform neurofibromas, present in 30% of patients, are locally invasive and may undergo malignant transformation. They may be accompanied by overlying hypcrpigmcntation or hypertrichosis. Other tumors that occur with higher frequency in patients with NF1 include pheochromocytomas, juvenile chronic myeloid leukemia, and rhabdomyosarcomas.

Seizures occur in approximately 4% to 5% of patients with NF1. Seizures may be generalized or partial. In a study by Korf et al., 22 of 359 NF1 patients developed seizures. The seizures were most often characterized as complex-partial (9 patients), febrile (6 patients), or generalized epilepsy (3 patients). Other manifestations of NF1 include learning disabilities, pain, scoliosis, headaches, stroke, and bowel or bladder complications (secondary to pelvic plexiform neurofibromas).

V. Diagnostic Approach

NF1 is diagnosed by the presence of the clinical features mentioned previously. Evaluation should focus on symptoms associated with NF1, such as neurocognitive deficits, visual complaints, progressive neurologic deficits, altered bowel or bladder function, weakness, seizures, and headaches. Other medical complications associated with NF1 include hypertension, short stature, and precocious puberty. Once the diagnosis is made, the following strategies may be used.

Orthopedic referral. Tibial dysplasia appears at birth with anterolateral bowing of the lower leg. The presence of tibial bowing should prompt referral to an orthopedic surgeon who is familiar with the management of orthopedic problems in children with NF1.

Ophthalmologic referral. Symptomatic optic gliomas are diagnosed during the first year of life in 1% of NF1 patients, although they typically develop between 4 and 6 years of age. They are ultimately present in 15% of patients with NF1 and cause symptoms in 2% to 5% of cases. An annual vision evaluation by an experienced ophthalmologist is part of the routine follow-up for children with NF1.

Head magnetic resonance imaging (MRI). Routine presymptomatic screening for central nervous system tumors is *not* necessary. However, any evidence of optic nerve dysfunction, seizures, or neurologic abnormalities warrants neuroimaging with special attention to the orbits.

Other radiology studies. Plain radiographs may detect a variety of bony abnormalities. They should be ordered if the clinical findings suggest bony erosion secondary to an adjacent plexiform neurofibroma, scoliosis, or bone pain.

Genetic evaluation. Families who have a child with NF1 may benefit from genetic counseling. A protein truncation assay is available in some settings to genetically confirm the diagnosis. However, this test detects the abnormality in at most 65% of patients with a clear clinical diagnosis of NF1, making it less useful diagnostically. Linkage analysis may be used to track the NF1 gene through generations of affected family members, allowing prenatal diagnosis in some situations.

Other studies. Children with NF1 should be monitored for blood pressure elevations associated with renal artery stenosis or pheochromocytomas. Approximately 6% of patients with NF1 develop hypertension, and a secondary cause (e.g., renal artery stenosis) is identified in one third of cases. Learning disabilities are seen in 40% to 60% of children with NF1. Children should undergo evaluation for cognitive and motor function, with prompt referral or intervention as required. Plexiform neurofibromas grow in early childhood, are difficult to remove, and tend to regrow. A multidisciplinary team that includes the primary pediatrician as well as surgeons, radiologists, and oncologists should manage these neurofibromas.

VI. Treatment

No specific therapy is currently available. In the future, targeted therapies for NF1-associated tumors may be designed to inhibit growth-promoting pathways activated in the absence of neurofibromin. Other potential therapies focus on blockade of angiogenic factors that could potentially decrease tumor growth.

Routine office visits should focus on detection and management of complications, as discussed previously. Annual ophthalmologic examinations are important to detect optic nerve lesions. Interval history should focus on subtle sensory or motor symptoms such as paresthesia or muscle atrophy. Pediatricians should also inquire about incontinence, given the risk of spinal cord neurofibromas. Consultation with specific surgical specialists is warranted based on the location of neurofibromas. Laser treatment has not yet proved successful in permanently removing café-au-lait spots.

VII. References

1. Gutmann DH, Aylsworth A, Carey J, et al. The diagnostic evaluation and multidisciplinary management of neurofibromatosis 1 and neurofibromatosis 2. *JAMA* 1997;278:51–57.
2. DeBella K, Szudek J, Friedman JM. Use of the National Institutes of Health criteria for diagnosis of neurofibromatosis 1 in children. *Pediatrics* 2000;105:608–614.
3. Jones KL. *Smith's recognizable patterns of human malformation,* 5th ed. Philadelphia: WB Saunders, 1997.
4. Korf BR, Carrazana E, Holmes GL. Patterns of seizures observed in association with neurofibromatosis 1. *Epilepsia* 1993;34:616–620.
5. Listernick R, Darling C, Greenwald M, et al. Optic pathway tumors in children: the effect of neurofibromatosis 1 on clinical manifestations and natural history. *J Pediatr* 1995;127:718–722.
6. Lynch TM, Gutmann DH. Neurofibromatosis 1. *Neurol Clin* 2002;20:841–865.
7. Reynolds RM, Browning GGP, Nawroz I, et al. Von Recklinghausen's neurofibromatosis: neurofibromatosis type 1. *Lancet* 2003;361:1552–1554.
8. Riccardi VM, Eichner JE. Neurofibromatosis: past, present, and future. *N Engl J Med* 1991;324:1283–1285.
9. Tekin M, Bodurtha JN, Riccardi VM. Café au lait spots: the pediatrician's perspective. *Pediatr Rev* 2001;22:82–90.

Case 11-2: 10-Year-Old Boy

I. History of Present Illness

A 10-year-old boy presented with a 4-day history of worsening cough. Three days before presentation, he developed chills and fever to 38.9°C. Two days before presentation, he had increasingly frequent posttussive emesis. He also had occasional episodes of hemoptysis. He complained of abdominal pain with coughing. He also complained of "not having any energy." There was no weight loss or night sweats. There were no known contacts with a chronic cough or history of tuberculosis. No family members lived or worked in nursing homes. He had not traveled outside of the state of Pennsylvania. Before this illness, he was actively participating in soccer at school. He had also assisted with household chores that included washing dishes, mowing the lawn, and sweeping the chimney.

II. Past Medical History

His birth history was unremarkable. He required hospitalization at 1 year of age for *Salmonella* gastroenteritis leading to dehydration. Epidemiologic investigation attributed a local *Salmonella* outbreak occurring during that time to a pet store that engaged in improper import of reptiles. The family turtle, purchased from that store, was held culpable for this child's illness and was removed from the home at the family's request. The only other pet was a healthy cat acquired 2 years ago. The patient did not require any medications. He had received the appropriate childhood immunizations. A paternal uncle had been diagnosed with adult-onset diabetes.

III. Physical Examination

T, 38.3°C; RR, 24 to 28/min; HR, 108 bpm; BP, 111/72 mm Hg; SpO$_2$, 97% in room air

Weight, 95th percentile

On examination, the patient was alert and cooperative. His oropharynx was clear. There was no cervical lymphadenopathy. There were no rales or wheezing on lung examination. Heart sounds were normal. There was no hepatomegaly or splenomegaly. There were two mildly tender erythematous nodules on the anterior aspect of his left tibia. There were no other rashes.

IV. Diagnostic Studies

A complete blood count revealed the following: 20,400 WBCs/mm^3 (83% segmented neutrophils, 5% eosinophils, and 11% lymphocytes); hemoglobin, 12.2 g/dL; and 372,000 platelets/mm^3.

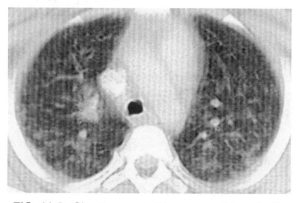

FIG. 11-2. Chest computed tomogram (case 11-2).

V. Course of Illness

Chest radiograph revealed ill-defined pulmonary nodules. Chest computed tomography (CT) was performed to better delineate the radiographic findings (Fig. 11-2). Skin testing for tuberculosis was negative.

DISCUSSION: CASE 11-2

I. Differential Diagnosis

The differential diagnosis of reticulonodular infiltrates on chest radiograph or chest CT includes tuberculosis, blastomycosis, coccidioidomycosis, and histoplasmosis. Tuberculosis is possible, particularly given the hemoptysis, but is less likely with a negative tuberculin skin test. Knowledge of this patient's travel history virtually excludes blastomycosis and coccidioidomycosis. In an adolescent, *Mycoplasma pneumoniae* can cause hilar adenopathy as well as diffuse lung infiltrates.

Hypersensitivity pneumonitis, sarcoidosis, and vasculitis (particularly Wegener granulomatosis) can cause similar findings. Sarcoidosis, a multisystem granulomatous disease, usually manifests with generalized lymphadenopathy and prominent cervical involvement. Associated findings include erythema nodosum and uveitis. Granuloma formation occurs in the eyes, skin, liver, spleen, and parotid glands. Blacks are more commonly affected than whites. Wegener granulomatosis is relatively uncommon in children.

II. Diagnosis

The chest CT revealed bilateral hilar lymphadenopathy (Fig. 11-2). The largest hilar lymph node on the right measured 1.7×2.2 cm. The CT also revealed numerous pulmonary nodules, ranging in size from a few millimeters to 1 cm. No acid-fast bacilli were detected in serial sputum samples. *M. pneumoniae* polymerase chain reaction (PCR) analysis of a nasopharyngeal aspirate was negative. Antigens to influenza A and B; parainfluenza types 1, 2, and 3; adenovirus; and respiratory syncytial virus were not detected by immunofluorescence of nasopharyngeal washings. **The diagnosis of pulmonary histoplasmosis was confirmed by detection of *Histoplasma capsulatum* antigen in the urine and a four-fold increase in *H. capsulatum* antibody between acute and convalescent serum samples.** The chimney cleaning most likely contributed to the development of pulmonary histoplasmosis. The child improved clinically over the next 3 days without specific treatment. A repeat chest radiograph was normal 2 weeks later.

III. Epidemiology and Incidence

H. capsulatum is a dimorphic fungus that grows as a yeast-like organism at temperatures greater than 37°C and as a spore-forming mold at lower temperatures. It is endemic in certain areas of the United States and Latin America. Between 1958 and 1965, a total of 275,558 military recruits raised in different areas of the United States underwent *Histoplasma* skin testing. Recruits from states bordering the Ohio and Mississippi River valleys, along with Maryland and Virginia, had the highest rates of reaction. *Histoplasma* was also prevalent in portions of Pennsylvania and Texas. This study by Edwards et al. remains the largest study of histoplasmosis endemicity in the United States.

H. capsulatum resides in the soil in endemic areas. Excretions of birds and bats facilitate growth of the organism. As a consequence, *H. capsulatum* infections are associated with aerosolization of debris from sites where birds or bats roost, as may occur by cutting firewood, sweeping chimneys, playing in hollow trees, barns, or caves, or other activities. Infection occurs after inhalation of spores, which transform to the yeast phase in the lung. Hematogenous dissemination may occur after primary pulmonary infection. Rarely, the skin or intestinal mucosa serves as the portal of entry.

IV. Clinical Presentation

Severity of illness depends on the exposure intensity and the host's immune status. Low-intensity exposure usually results in asymptomatic infection in immunocompetent hosts. Higher-intensity exposures lead to pulmonary infection, manifested as fever, cough, malaise, and poor appetite. Some patients experience pleuritic chest pain. Rales and wheezing may also occur. Erythema nodosum and other hypersensitivity reactions to infection occasionally develop. Symptoms are self-limited and last 2 or 3 days. In a small number of children, symptoms persist for longer than 2 weeks. Symptoms persisting for longer than 3 weeks after acute histoplasmosis suggests progressive disease or dissemination. In the immunocompetent host, extrapulmomary dissemination is rare. Infants younger than 2 years of age are at higher risk for disseminated disease than are older children. Features of disseminated histoplasmosis include prolonged fever, failure to thrive, and hepatosplenomegaly. Pericardial and pleural effusions occur rarely.

In the immunocompromised host, the illness begins with fever and cough, followed by worsening respiratory distress. Disseminated histoplasmosis is more likely to occur in immunocompromised patients. These patients usually have diarrhea, weight loss, hepatomegaly, splenomegaly, and skin lesions. Less commonly, dissemination leads to bone marrow involvement, meningitis, pericarditis, or chorioretinitis.

V. Diagnostic Approach

H. capsulatum does not comprise the normal flora of humans, so its isolation from mucous membranes, skin lesions, deep organs, or body fluids usually indicates infection.

Chest radiograph. In those with respiratory symptoms, abnormalities seen on chest radiography include hilar adenopathy and localized or diffuse reticulonodular lung infiltrates. In patients with previous pulmonary infection (symptomatic or subclinical), single or multiple calcified nodules may be detected in the lungs, hilar lymph nodes, spleen, or liver. Cavitary lesions resembling those of tuberculosis may be seen in patients with chronic pulmonary histoplasmosis (rare in children).

Histologic examination of tissue. Ovoid yeast forms are frequently visible on microscopic examination of bone marrow and biopsy specimens.

Culture. Culture of the organism on standard mycologic media, including brain-heart infusion agar or broth, requires a 2- to 6-week incubation period, making culture methods less useful in the acute setting (but important for confirmation of the organism in certain cases). Specimens appropriate for culture depend on the site of infection (pulmonary, cutaneous, or disseminated) and include sputum (for pulmonary disease), skin lesion biopsy specimens, blood, bone marrow, and organ biopsy specimens.

Histoplasmin skin test. In endemic areas, the prevalence of skin test positivity due to previous asymptomatic infection approaches 60% in young adults. This high prevalence limits the usefulness of histoplasmin skin testing in diagnosing adults. However, fewer than 5% of asymptomatic children younger than 5 years of age had positive skin tests in one study, suggesting that skin testing might be useful in immunocompetent young children. Patients with disseminated rather than isolated pulmonary disease are less likely to have a positive skin test. This may be related to the fact that disseminated disease typically develops in immunocompromised patients. The inability of skin test positivity to clearly distinguish asymptomatic past infection from symptomatic current infection makes it less useful as a diagnostic tool. Currently its use is limited to epidemiologic investigations.

Serum *H. capsulatum* antibody. This test is recommended for routine detection of infection in otherwise healthy children. Antibodies are detectable 2 to 4 weeks after infection. Antibody titers greater than 1:8 or a four-fold increase between acute and convalescent titers suggests acute infection. Titers revert to negative 12 to 18 months after infection. Cross-reaction from *Blastomyces* or *Coccidioides* antibodies can occur, but the travel history usually differentiates these from *H. capsulatum.*

H. capsulatum urinary antigen detection. This test is most useful in diagnosing disseminated disease in young children or infection at any site in immunocompromised patients, in whom antibody titers can be falsely negative. In a study by Fojtasek et al., *H. capsulatum* antigenuria was detected in all 22 children with disseminated histoplasmosis. Declining antigenuria levels correlate with clinical improvement.

Other studies. Any child with hilar adenopathy requires evaluation, including tuberculin skin testing, to exclude tuberculosis. Findings in disseminated infection may include pancytopenia, anemia, and coagulopathy.

VI. Treatment

Antifungal treatment clearly benefits those with progressive forms of histoplasmosis (e.g., disseminated infection). Other manifestations for which antifungal therapy should be considered include pulmonary infection with protracted symptoms (greater than 4 weeks), severe acute pulmonary infection (e.g., hypoxia), and granulomatous adenitis obstructing critical structures such as blood vessels and bronchi. Whether antifungal therapy shortens the course of illness in those patients with self-limited acute pulmonary disease remains unknown.

Options for treatment include ketoconazole, itraconazole, and amphotericin B (deoxycholate or lipid preparations). Fluconazole is less effective than either itraconazole or amphotericin B. Ketoconazole, although effective, is poorly tolerated compared with the other antifungal agents and is associated with a higher rate of hepatotoxicity. Voriconazole, a new triazole antifungal agent, demonstrates comparable or better *in vitro* activity than either itraconazole or amphotericin against *H. capsulatum* but requires additional clinical evaluation. In general, patients who are well enough to require outpatient therapy may receive itraconazole, whereas those requiring hospitalization should receive amphotericin B.

Duration of therapy depends on the type of histoplasmosis and the underlying immunocompetence of the host. Those with acute pulmonary disease who require treatment usually receive 3 months of therapy. Those with chronic pulmonary disease require 12 to 24 months of treatment. Disseminated infection requires 6 to 18 months of therapy in otherwise healthy patients, but those with the acquired immunodeficiency syndrome (AIDS) require lifelong treatment. Duration of therapy for serious *H. capsulatum* infections is usually determined in conjunction with an infectious diseases specialist.

VII. References

1. Edwards LB, Acquaviva FA, Livesay VT. An atlas of sensitivity to tuberculin, PPD-B, and histoplasmin in the United States. *Am Rev Respir Dis* 99;1:1969.
2. Flynn PM, Hughes WT. Histoplasmosis. In: Chernick V, Boat TF, eds. *Kendig's disorders of the respiratory tract in children,* 6th ed. Philadelphia: WB Saunders, 1998: 946–953.
3. Fojtasek MF, Kleiman MB, Connolly-Stringfield P, et al. The *Histoplasma capsulatum* antigen assay in disseminated histoplasmosis in children. *Pediatr Infect Dis J* 1994; 13:801–805.
4. Kleiman MB. *Histoplasma capsulatum* (histoplasmosis). In: Long SS, Pickering LK, Prober CG, eds. *Principles and practice of pediatric infectious diseases,* 2nd ed. New York: Churchill-Livingstone, 2003:1233–1238.
5. Leggiardo RJ, Barrett RD, Hughes WT. Disseminated histoplasmosis of infancy. *Pediatr Infect Dis J* 1986;7:799–805.
6. Wheat J, Sarosi G, McKinsey D, et al. Practice guidelines for the management of patients with histoplasmosis. *Clin Infect Dis* 2000;30:688–695.

Case 11-3: 14-Year-Old Boy

I. History of Present Illness

A 14-year-old boy was brought to the emergency department for evaluation of prolonged fever and new seizures. Eight days before admission, he developed fever to 38.3°C. Two days before admission, he complained of headache and continued fevers. On the day before admission, he was standing in the kitchen talking to his aunt when he fell to the floor and had tonic flexion of his arms associated with eye deviation. This event lasted approximately 2 minutes. He was evaluated at a nearby hospital. His temperature was 38.6°C, but his physical examination was normal. He was discharged after a normal noncontrast head CT study was obtained. On the day of admission, he was taken to his pediatrician's office for evaluation of continued fever. Shortly after arriving at the office, he had a similar event with arm flexion and eye deviation. It did not resolve spontaneously, and the boy was rushed to the hospital by ambulance. He received several doses of lorazepam without termination of apparent seizure activity. He required endotracheal intubation due to respiratory failure. Seizures were ultimately controlled with the combination of fosphenytoin and valproic acid.

His aunt, the primary caretaker, related that over the past month he had several episodes of fecal soiling. Additionally, he had a documented 8-pound weight loss. The most striking information, however, was the marked deterioration in handwriting that had occurred over the same time period. Furthermore, in the past month he had frequently neglected his household chores, a change from his baseline demeanor that was attributed to "teenage hormones." Aside from the two recent events, she did not recall any seizure activity. There were no rashes, emesis, or diarrhea. He had performed well in school except during the past month, during which he had failed several tests. This change in school performance was attributed to poor vision, and an ophthalmology appointment had been scheduled for later in the month.

II. Past Medical History

He had not previously required hospitalization. He was adopted by his aunt in infancy while his birth mother struggled with drug addiction. The mother had recently died, but the aunt did not know the cause of death. The patient lived in an urban area and had no pets.

III. Physical Examination

T, 38.4°C; RR, 18/min; HR, 93 bpm; BP, 193/98 mm Hg

Before endotracheal intubation, his Glasgow Coma Score was 8. After stabilization, corneal reflexes were present. The gag reflex was intact. The tongue was midline. However, there was no spontaneous eye opening. Though he did not respond to voice or blink with direct visual confrontation, he localized painful stimuli. His tone was increased in the lower extremities. His Babinski sign was negative bilaterally. His neck was supple. Heart and lung sounds were normal. The liver was palpable 3 cm below the right costal margin, with a total span of 11 cm.

IV. Diagnostic Studies

Serum electrolytes were normal. The serum glucose concentration was 119 mg/dL. The serum ammonia level was normal. A complete blood count revealed the following: 11,500 WBCs/mm^3 (73% segmented neutrophils and 22% lymphocytes); hemoglobin, 11.7 g/dL; and 785,000 platelets/mm^3. Prothrombin and partial thromboplastin times, fibrinogen, and fibrin split products were normal. Noncontrast head CT, obtained before lumbar puncture, revealed normal-sized ventricles and no masses. CSF analysis revealed

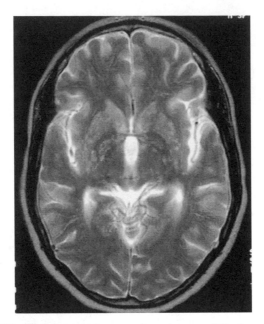

FIG. 11-3. Magnetic resonance image of the head (case 11-3).

1 WBC and 630 red blood cells per cubic millimeter. The protein and glucose concentrations were 53 and 52 mg/dL, respectively.

V.   Course of Illness

Gram staining of the CSF revealed some yeast forms. MRI of the head was significantly abnormal (Fig. 11-3).

DISCUSSION: CASE 11-3

I.   Differential Diagnosis

The boy's initial complaint of prolonged fever precipitated medical evaluation. However, the history of behavioral changes, worsening school performance, and seizures was even more alarming. The development of status epilepticus at the pediatrician's office ultimately prompted a more thorough investigation of his symptoms. It was not clear at this point whether the patient had an encephalitis or encephalopathy. Although bacterial meningitis causes fever and seizures, the absence of CSF pleocytosis and the chronicity of symptoms made typical bacterial meningitis unlikely. Bacterial causes of encephalitis include *Borrelia burgdorferi, Bartonella henselae* (cat-scratch disease), and *Rickettsia rickettsii*. Residence in an urban area made *B. burgdorferi,* the causative agent of Lyme disease, unlikely. Patients critically ill with *R. rickettsii* (Rocky Mountain spotted fever) infection typically have hyponatremia, hypoalbuminemia, anemia, and mild thrombocytopenia, findings not present in this case. Most but not all patients with cat-scratch disease have a clear history of contact with a cat or, more likely, a kitten. Again, the chronic symptoms in this child, if related to the fever and seizures, are not typically seen with any of the illnesses already described.

Viral causes of encephalitis include enteroviruses, arthropod-borne viruses (e.g., West Nile virus, St. Louis encephalitis virus, Eastern equine encephalitis virus), herpes simplex virus, Epstein-Barr virus, adenovirus, influenza, and human immunodeficiency virus (HIV). In adolescents, herpes simplex virus usually causes focal seizures and radiologic changes localized to the temporal lobe. There were no clear risk factors for HIV based on the initial history. The other viruses do not usually cause the progressive neurologic symptoms seen in this child.

Though this child did not have history worrisome for immunodeficiency, several infectious conditions can manifest with subacute symptoms in immunocompromised patients. Patients with humoral deficiencies may develop a chronic enteroviral meningoencephalitis. Those with cell-mediated immune deficiencies are at risk for subacute herpes simplex virus encephalitis, varicella-zoster virus encephalitis, and progressive multifocal leukoencephalopathy. Patients with AIDS can develop central nervous system infection with *Toxoplasma gondii* or *Cryptococcus neoformans*, an encapsulated yeast. These patients can also develop HIV-related encephalopathy.

The finding of yeast forms on Gram staining of the CSF is helpful. Occasionally degenerating WBCs are mistaken for yeast forms, but additional investigation of this finding is clearly warranted. Meningitis due to *Candida* species typically occurs in patients with indwelling venous catheters, sustained neutropenia, or hyperglycemia due to diabetes, glucocorticoids, or hyperalimentation; none of which was present in this patient. In this case, the finding of yeast forms on Gram staining of the CSF strongly suggested the diagnosis of cryptococcal meningitis.

Noninfectious causes include acute drug or medication ingestions as well as lead intoxication. Central nervous system vasculitis caused by either systemic lupus erythematous or polyarteritis nodosa should be strongly considered in the differential diagnosis.

II. Diagnosis

Head MRI revealed dilatation of the Virchow-Robin spaces in the white matter, especially in the basal ganglion and thalamus, a finding seen with cryptococcal meningitis (Fig. 11-3). The MRI also showed dilatation of the lateral and third ventricles and sulci, which is seen with HIV encephalitis. There was also abnormally increased signal in the periventricular white matter bilaterally, a finding consistent with HIV-related encephalitis. *C. neoformans,* the yeast identified on Gram staining of the CSF, was isolated from cultures of blood and CSF. Serum cryptococcal antigen was positive at 1:1024. The CSF cryptococcal antigen was also elevated at 1:512. HIV antibody testing was positive. Additional data-gathering by the family revealed that the patient's birth mother had died from HIV-related complications. The family did not previously know the birth mother's HIV status, and as a consequence the patient had never undergone HIV testing. **The diagnosis was perinatally acquired HIV infection manifesting as cryptococcal meningitis and HIV encephalitis.** The patient died on the third day of hospitalization.

III. Epidemiology and Incidence

C. neoformans, a ubiquitous encapsulated yeast, causes diseases ranging from asymptomatic pulmonary colonization to life-threatening meningitis. Cryptococcal infection may occur in healthy persons, but most infected patients have some immunocompromising factor such as immune suppression related to organ transplantation or HIV infection. Primary infection occurs through inhalation of aerosolized soil particles containing *C. neoformans.* Central nervous system involvement results from hematogenous dissemination.

Cryptococcal infection has been documented in up to 2.8% of organ transplant recipients, most often in those receiving renal transplants (80% of infections) but occasionally after liver (10% of infections) or heart (5% of infections) transplantation. Cryptococcal infection occurs in up to 15% of HIV-infected adults, typically when the CD4-positive T-lymphocyte count declines to less than 50 cells/mm^3. In contrast, this infection occurs in fewer than 2% of HIV-infected children, probably reflecting their lower exposure to sources of *C. neoformans* in the environment. *C. neoformans* antibodies are detectable in only 4% of school age children but in two thirds of adults. Sources of *Cryptococcus* include pigeon droppings and soil.

IV.   Clinical Presentation

Cryptococcal infection may manifest with acute or chronic symptoms. In children, findings in acute primary pulmonary infection have not been adequately characterized, because most cases are disseminated at the time of diagnosis. One half of adults with primary pulmonary cryptococcal infection develop cough and chest pain. Less often, they present with fever, hemoptysis, and weight loss. In immunocompromised patients, the risk of dissemination is high enough that patients presenting with findings of pulmonary cryptococcal infection are presumed to have extrapulmonary disease. In severely immunocompromised patients, pulmonary involvement may be minimal if dissemination occurs shortly after exposure. On examination, signs of respiratory involvement include tachypnea, accessory muscle use, and decreased breath sounds.

Symptoms of cryptococcal meningitis include low-grade fever, malaise, and headache. Nausea, vomiting, altered mentation, and photophobia are less common. Stiff neck, focal neurologic deficits, and seizures are rare. Physical examination findings of cryptococcal meningitis are not sufficiently characteristic to distinguish it from other causes of meningitis, but findings include nuchal rigidity and photophobia. These findings are not always present, particularly in immunocompromised patients.

Cutaneous manifestations of cryptococcal infection include erythematous or verrucous papules, nodules, or pustules. Occasionally acneiform lesions or granulomas are noted. The lesions are usually located on the face and neck but may occur anywhere on the body.

V.   Diagnostic Approach

Sputum culture. Sputum fungal culture can be used to diagnose cryptococcal pneumonia.

Blood culture. *C. neoformans* may grow in 3 days but occasionally takes up to 3 weeks.

Cryptococcal polysaccharide antigen by latex agglutination. The cryptococcal antigen test can be performed on serum and CSF specimens. This test should be performed on the serum of any HIV-infected patient who develops pneumonia and has a CD4+ count lower than 200 cells/mm^3. This test should also be performed in any patient with suspected cryptococcal pneumonia. A positive serum test indicates disseminated infection.

Lumbar puncture. CSF should be examined in all immunocompromised patients with suspected cryptococcal infection, even if signs and symptoms of meningitis are absent. CSF specimens should be sent for cell count; protein; glucose; cultures for bacterial, fungal, and viral pathogens; and cryptococcal polysaccharide antigen by latex agglutination. There are typically fewer than 100 WBCs/mm^3 (mostly lymphocytes and monocytes), although some patients may not demonstrate a pleocytosis. The glucose concentration is less than 50 mg/dL in 65% of patients, and there may be a mild elevation of the CSF protein. CSF cultures are positive in 90% of patients with cryptococcal meningitis. CSF cryptococcal antigen titers of 1:4 or higher also confirm the diagnosis. Budding yeast are visualized by India ink stain in 50% of cases, but this test is not required if cryptococcal antigen testing is performed.

Serum electrolytes. Hyponatremia complicates cryptococcal meningitis, and its development portends a poor prognosis.

Radiologic studies. Chest radiography reveals diffuse nodular infiltrates and, occasionally, small bilateral pleural effusions. CT or MRI of the head may demonstrate granulomatous lesions (cryptococcomas), white matter changes, and increased intracranial pressure.

Human immunodeficiency virus testing. All patients diagnosed with cryptococcal meningitis or disseminated cryptococcal infection should undergo evaluation for immune deficiency, particularly HIV infection.

VI.   Treatment

Clinical management varies depending on the extent of disease and the immune status of the host. An asymptomatic normal host with isolated pulmonary nodules does not require treatment if the serum cryptococcal antigen test is negative. Patients with extensive pulmonary disease or evidence of extrapulmonary infection require treatment with fluconazole or itraconazole for 6 to 12 months or intravenous amphotericin B for 3 to 6 months. HIV-negative immunocompromised patients with either pulmonary or extrapulmonary disease are treated in the same fashion as patients with central nervous system disease (see later discussion). After primary therapy is complete, there is no consensus on how long HIV-negative immunocompromised patients require fluconazole prophylaxis. Most experts suggest providing prophylaxis for 1 year after the completion of acute antifungal treatment and then reassessing its ongoing need based on the level of immunosuppression at that time. Treatment may be discontinued if the immune function has returned to normal (e.g., after completion of chemotherapy).

HIV-negative patients with meningitis are treated with intravenous amphotericin plus flucytosine for 2 weeks; if the CSF culture is negative on repeat lumbar puncture, they may receive fluconazole for an additional 10 weeks.

HIV-infected patients with pulmonary or disseminated cryptococcal infection require treatment with fluconazole that continues indefinitely. HIV-infected patients with cryptococcal meningitis require intravenous amphotericin B plus flucytosine for at least 2 weeks, followed by lifelong fluconazole therapy once the CSF culture is negative. The rate of relapse in HIV-infected patients is 100% without maintenance antifungal therapy. The relapse rate decreases to 18% to 25% with itraconazole prophylaxis and 2% to 3% with fluconazole prophylaxis. Due to advances in antiretroviral therapy, some authors propose discontinuation of secondary prophylaxis for cryptococcal meningitis in HIV-infected patients if the CD4+ count has increased to more than 100 cells/mm^3 and the HIV RNA level has been undetectable for longer than 3 months. This proposal remains controversial.

Untreated cryptococcal infection in HIV-infected patients is uniformly fatal. Survival rates are high with early diagnosis and treatment, but relapse rates are high without lifelong antifungal prophylaxis. Factors associated with poor prognosis include hyponatremia and alteration in mental status at the time of diagnosis.

VII. References

1. Buchanan KL, Murphy JW. What makes *Cryptococcus neoformans* a pathogen? *Emerg Infect Dis* 1998;4:71–83.
2. Chuck SL, Sande MA. Infections with *Cryptococcus neoformans* in the acquired immunodeficiency syndrome. *N Engl J Med* 1989;321:794–799.
3. Gonzalez CE, Shetty D, Lewis LL, et al. Cryptococcosis in human immunodeficiency virus-infected children. *Pediatr Infect Dis J* 1996;15:796–800.
4. Husain S, Wagener MM, Singh N. *Cryptococcus neoformans* infection in organ transplant recipients: variables influencing clinical characteristics and outcome. *Emerg Infect Dis* 2001;7:375–381.
5. Mirza SA, Phelan M, Rimland D, et al. The changing epidemiology of cryptococcosis: an update from population-based active surveillance in 2 large metropolitan areas, 1992–2000. *Clin Infect Dis* 2003;36:789–794.
6. Pappas PG, Perfect JR, Cloud GA, et al. Cryptococcosis in human immunodeficiency virus-negative patients in the era of effective azole therapy. *Clin Infect Dis* 2001;33:690–699.
7. Powderly WG. Current approach to the acute management of cryptococcal infections. *J Infect Dis* 2000;41:18–22.
8. Saag MS, Graybill RJ, Larsen RA, et al. Practice guidelines for the management of cryptococcal disease. *Clin Infect Dis* 2000;30:710–718.
9. Saag MS, Powderly WG, Cloud GA, et al. Comparison of amphotericin B with fluconazole in the treatment of acute AIDS-associated cryptococcal meningitis. *N Engl J Med* 1992;326:83–89.

Case 11-4: 7-Month-Old Girl

I. History of Present Illness

A 7-month-old Japanese girl developed fever to 38.9°C associated with cough, rhinorrhea, and loose stools. Over the next few days, the respiratory symptoms and diarrhea resolved, but her fever persisted. Six days before admission, she was evaluated by her primary pediatrician and diagnosed with cellulitis involving the labia majora. She was treated with cephalexin, an oral first-generation cephalosporin. She presented to the emergency department because of continued fevers and worsening cellulitis and was admitted for intravenous antibiotic therapy and additional evaluation.

II. Past Medical History

Her birth history was remarkable for unconjugated hyperbilirubinemia. Her bilirubin level peaked at 16 mg/dL and returned to normal without phototherapy. Two months before admission, she developed otitis media that resolved after treatment with a 10-day course of amoxicillin. Cephalexin was her only medication at the time of admission. She had received all of the appropriate immunizations, including three doses of the heptavalent pneumococcal conjugate vaccine. The family history was remarkable for hepatitis A in the maternal grandmother approximately 2 months earlier.

III. Physical Examination

T, 40.3°C; RR, 50/min; HR, 160 bpm; BP, 104/60 mm Hg; SpO$_2$, 98% in room air
Weight, 75th percentile

Examination revealed an ill but not toxic-appearing infant. The anterior fontanel was open and flat. Tympanic membranes were mildly erythematous but had normal mobility bilaterally. There were no oropharyngeal lesions. Capillary refill was brisk. The heart and lung sounds were normal. The spleen was palpable just below the left costal margin. Examination of the genitalia revealed significant erythema and induration of the left labia majora with mild fluctuance. There was no crepitus. There were no other skin lesions.

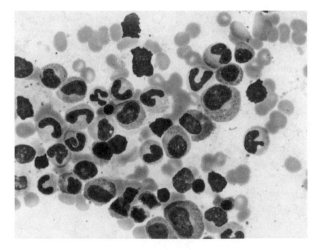

FIG. 11-4. Bone marrow aspirate (case 11-4).

IV. Diagnostic Studies

The WBC count was 3,100/mm^3, with 2% segmented neutrophils, 28% monocytes, and 70% lymphocytes. The absolute neutrophil count (ANC) was 62 cells/mm^3. Hemoglobin was 12.3 mg/dL, and platelets were 337,000/mm^3. A repeat complete blood count produced similar results. Lactate dehydrogenase and uric acid concentrations were normal. Urinalysis did not reveal pyuria or hematuria. Blood and urine cultures were obtained.

V. Course of Illness

Gram staining after percutaneous drainage of the labial abscess demonstrated many gram-negative rods. She received ticarcillin-clavulanate to provide adequate coverage for *Staphylococcus aureus* and gram-negative organisms, including *Pseudomonas aeruginosa*. Gentamicin was added to provide additional coverage against gram-negative organisms. A bone marrow aspirate suggested the underlying diagnosis (Fig. 11-4).

DISCUSSION: CASE 11-4

I. Differential Diagnosis

Neutropenia, defined as an absolute decrease in the number of circulating neutrophils in the blood, can be caused by decreased production, increased peripheral utilization, or increased destruction. The ANC is calculated by multiplying the total WBC count by the total percentage of band forms and segmented neutrophils: ANC = total WBC × (percent bands + percent segmented neutrophils). In general, patients may be characterized as having mild (1,000 to 1,500 cells/mm^3), moderate (500 to 1,000 cells/mm^3), or severe (fewer than 500 cells/mm^3) neutropenia. Blacks tend to have lower neutrophils counts; therefore, in some patients an ANC of 900 cells/mm^3 may be considered normal.

The differential diagnosis of neutropenia in infancy includes a wide range of conditions (Table 11-4). In a child who was previously healthy, the most likely causes are alloimmune neonatal neutropenia, cyclic neutropenia, autoimmune neutropenia (AIN) in infancy, and Kostmann syndrome. Alloimmune neutropenia, a condition occurring in neonates, is analogous to Rh hemolytic disease. Maternal sensitization to fetal neutrophils results in maternal immunoglobulin G (IgG) antibodies' crossing the placenta and causing an immune-mediated destruction of fetal neutrophils. The neutropenia lasts several weeks but rarely persists beyond 6 months of age, making it an unlikely diagnosis in this 7-month-old patient. Cyclic neutropenia can be diagnosed by serial WBC counts.

Less likely causes include neutropenia related to infection. Neutropenia associated with increased peripheral utilization is possible in the context of a serious cellulitis. Infections such as Epstein-Barr virus and parvovirus B19 can also cause neutropenia, but the normal hemoglobin and platelet count in this case make these infections less likely. The mother does not have AIN, a finding that sometimes leads to transient secondary neutropenia in newborn infants.

II. Diagnosis

Bone marrow aspiration revealed a hypercellular marrow (Fig. 11-4). There was an increased number of granulocytes with maturation to the band stage, but there were no mature neutrophils. Quantitative serum immunoglobulins (IgA, IgE, IgG, and IgM) were normal. **These findings combined with the neutropenia suggest the diagnosis of autoimmune neutropenia of infancy.** Antibodies to the neutrophil-specific cell surface antigen NA1 were detected, confirming the diagnosis of AIN of childhood. Culture of the labial cellulitis revealed *P. aeruginosa*. The patient's infection resolved with a 10-day

TABLE 11-4. *Differential Diagnosis of Neutropenia in Infancy*

Category	Examples
Congenital	Kostmann syndrome
	Cyclic neutropenia
	Faconi syndrome
Metabolic	Shwachman-Diamond syndrome
	Propionic academia
	Glycogen storage disease type Ib
	Methylmalonic acidemia
Immune-mediated	Alloimmune neonatal neutropenia
	Autoimmune neutropenia in infancy
	Secondary autoimmune neutropenia
	Felty syndrome
Nutritional	Vitamin B_{12} deficiency
	Folate deficiency
	Copper deficiency
Primary immunodeficiency	X-linked agammaglobulinemia
	Hyper-immunoglobulin M syndrome
	Common variable immune deficiency
	Reticular dysgenesis
	Cartilage-hair hypoplasia
Hematologic	Aplastic anemia
	Myelodysplastic syndromes
Drug-induced	Antibiotics (sulfonamides, penicillin)
	Baribiturates
	Propylthiouracil
	Penicillamine
	Others
Infection	Epstein-Barr virus
	Rickettsiae
	Human immunodeficiency virus
	Malaria
	Others

course of ticarcillin-clavulanate. Serial absolute neutrophil counts over the next 6 weeks revealed persistent neutropenia, effectively excluding the diagnosis of cyclic neutropenia. She experienced no additional infections. Her neutropenia resolved by 20 months of age. The episode of otitis media did not appear to be related to her neutropenia.

III. Epidemiology and Incidence

AIN can occur as an isolated phenomenon (primary AIN) or in association with a known precipitating factor (secondary AIN), such as other autoimmune disorders, infections, medications, and malignancies. In infants and young children, the term *primary AIN* usually refers to AIN in infancy (formerly known as chronic benign neutropenia). The average age at diagnosis of AIN in infancy is 8 months (range, 1 to 38 months). Two thirds of patients are diagnosed between 5 and 15 months of age. The estimated frequency is 1 per 100,000 children, making it more common than the severe chronic neutropenias such as cyclic neutropenia.

IV. Clinical Presentation

Most patients with AIN in infancy suffer from mild infections such as otitis media, gastroenteritis, lymphadenitis, superficial skin infections, or upper respiratory tract infections. In one series, 6 (23%) of 26 girls developed cellulitis of the labia majora, and 3 of these 6 infections were caused by *P. aeruginosa.* Approximately 10% to 15% of patients have serious infections, including pneumonia, sepsis, or meningitis. In approximately

10% of children, the diagnosis is suspected only after a routine complete blood count reveals neutropenia.

V. Diagnostic Approach

Complete blood count. At presentation, the ANC is less than 500 cells/mm^3 in 70% of children (mean, 200/mm^3). Most of the remaining children have an ANC between 500 and 1,000 cells/mm^3. The hemoglobin level and platelet count are usually normal. The complete blood count is repeated two or three times per week for a period of 1 month to exclude the diagnosis of cyclic neutropenia.

Neutrophil-specific antibodies. Neutrophil-specific antibodies (usually to the NA1 antigen) are initially detected in 70% of children with AIN in infancy. In the remaining 30%, antibody titers are so low that antibody screening is negative initially; repeated antibody testing on up to three additional blood samples at intervals of 2 to 4 weeks is sometimes necessary to make the diagnosis. The testing is hampered in part by the need for a sufficient number of isolated neutrophils. Occasionally, administering hydrocortisone before the test increases the peripheral neutrophil count and facilitates antibody detection. Patients receiving granulocyte colony-stimulating factor (G-CSF) may show a false-positive antibody test result. Patients diagnosed shortly before spontaneous remission may not have detectable antibodies.

Coombs test. A Coombs test should be considered to evaluate for the presence of a concomitant red blood cell autoantibody.

Bone marrow aspiration. This test is not routinely required, particularly if the patient appears well and has a normal hemoglobin level and normal platelet count. When the test is performed, the bone marrow aspirate is usually normocellular to hypercellular. The marrow contains a reduced number of mature neutrophils, and occasionally there is maturation arrest at earlier stages. Bone marrow examination is normal in 30% of cases and hypocellular in 3% of cases.

Other studies. Serum immunoglobulin determinations (IgA, IgG, IgE, and IgM) should be requested if an underlying primary immunodeficiency associated with neutropenia is suspected. Examples include X-linked agammaglobulinemia, hyper-IgM syndrome, and common variable immunodeficiency. Serum vitamin B$_{12}$ and red blood cell folate levels are indicated in patients with suspected nutritional deficiency. Other tests to consider in the patient with neutropenia include antinuclear antibody (ANA) for collagen vascular disease, serum copper level, and evaluation for metabolic diseases (e.g., glycogen storage disease type Ib, Shwachman-Diamond syndrome).

VI. Treatment

Most patients require only appropriate antibiotic therapy to treat bacterial infections as they occur. Prophylactic antibiotics are not routinely used, because the efficacy of such prophylaxis is unclear. Some patients benefit from antibacterial mouthwashes for occasional mouth sores and gingivitis. G-CSF, corticosteroids, and intravenous gammaglobulin administration are not routinely required but have been used to increase neutrophil counts in patients with *serious* or *recurrent* infections (15% of patients with AIN in infancy). In such cases, approximately 50% of children respond to corticosteroids and 75% respond to gammaglobulin. G-CSF is effective in almost all patients. The neutropenia resolves spontaneously in 95% of patients, usually within 7 to 24 months. Disappearance of autoantibodies precedes spontaneous normalization of the neutrophil count.

VII. References

1. Bux J, Behrens G, Jaeger G, et al. Diagnosis and clinical course of autoimmune neutropenia in infancy: analysis of 240 cases. *Blood* 1998;91:181–186.
2. Taniuchi S, Masuda M, Hasui M, et al. Differential diagnosis and clinical course of

autoimmune neutropenia: comparison with congenital neutropenia. *Acta Paediatr* 2002;91:1179–1182.

3. Boxer LA. Neutrophil abnormalities. *Pediatr Rev* 2003;24:52–61.
4. Jonsson OG, Buchanan GR. Chronic neutropenia during childhood: a 13-year experience in a single institution. *Am J Dis Child* 1991;145:232–235.
5. Alario AJ, O'Shea JS. Risk of infectious complications in well-appearing children with transient neutropenia. *Am J Dis Child* 1989;143:973–976.
6. Dinauer MC. The phagocyte system and disorders of granulopoiesis and granulocyte function. In: Nathan DG, Orkin SH, Ginsburg D, et al., eds. *Nathan and Oski's hematology of infancy and childhood,* 6th ed. Philadelphia: WB Saunders, 2003:923–1010.

Case 11-5: 6-Year-Old Boy

I. History of Present Illness

A 6-year-old boy presented with a 2-week history of low-grade fevers. One week before admission, he had had an episode of nonbilious emesis and subsequently began complaining of neck pain. There was no cough, diarrhea, rash, abdominal pain, or joint pain. Although he never complained that light bothered his eyes, he did not play outside with his friends during the day. His mother initially attributed this to the summer heat. He received several doses of ibuprofen for complaints of a headache. He was brought for evaluation after the mother learned of a meningococcal meningitis outbreak at a local school from the evening news broadcast. She became concerned about the possibility of meningitis and, after speaking with her pediatrician, rushed the child to the emergency department. There were no ill contacts. Neither the child nor his two siblings attended the school where several children had developed meningitis.

II. Past Medical History

The child had an unremarkable birth history. At the age of 8 months, he required hospitalization for management of rotavirus gastroenteritis-induced dehydration. Two months before admission, he was bitten on the hand while feeding deer during a hiking trip in the Pocono Mountains in Pennsylvania. Three weeks before admission, he developed a severe contact dermatitis on his arms and face that was attributed to poison ivy. He recovered uneventfully after treatment with oral antihistamines and cool compresses. He had developed a rash while being treated with amoxicillin-clavulanate after the deer bite and had completed his prophylactic antibiotic course with clindamycin. The family history was unremarkable. The child lived with his parents and two brothers in southern New Jersey.

III. Physical Examination

T, 38.1°C; RR, 28/min; HR, 100 bpm; BP, 101/53 mm Hg; SpO$_2$, 100% in room air
Weight, 50th percentile for age

In general the child was a thin but healthy-appearing boy. He had mild photophobia. There was no Kernig or Brudzinski sign, but there was difficulty with terminal neck flexion. There was no cervical lymphadenopathy. The heart and lung sounds were normal. There was no hepatomegaly or splenomegaly. The cranial nerve examination was normal. The skin examination revealed a rash that had appeared recently. The rash suggested the diagnosis (Fig. 11-5).

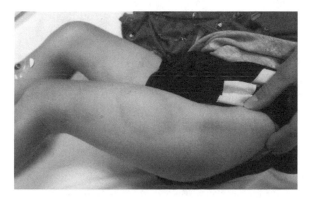

FIG. 11-5. Photograph of patient's rash (case 11-5).

IV. Diagnostic Studies

A complete blood count revealed the following: 8,600 WBCs/mm^3 (71% segmented neutrophils, 22% lymphocytes, and 7% monocytes); hemoglobin, 11.1 g/dL; and 461,000 platelets/mm^3. Serum glucose was 96 mg/dL. Lumbar puncture revealed 21 WBCs (3% segmented neutrophils, 77% lymphocytes, and 20% monocytes) and 1 red blood cell per cubic millimeter. The CSF protein and glucose concentrations were 23 and 63 mg/dL, respectively. No bacteria were noted on the CSF Gram stain. The CSF and blood cultures were subsequently negative.

V. Course of Illness

The diagnosis suggested by the rash was confirmed by additional testing.

DISCUSSION: CASE 11-5

I. Differential Diagnosis

Aseptic meningitis refers to a syndrome of meningeal inflammation without evidence of pathogens by traditional bacterial culture methods. A specific cause is identified in fewer than 60% of cases. Enteroviruses, including echoviruses, coxsackieviruses, and numbered enteroviruses, are the most common causes of aseptic meningitis. They account for up to 95% of cases when a specific pathogen is implicated. In the summer, other infectious causes of aseptic meningitis include Lyme disease (*B. burgdorferi*), Rocky Mountain spotted fever (*R. rickettsii*), ehrlichiosis, and arboviruses such as West Nile virus, St. Louis encephalitis virus, and Eastern and Western equine encephalitis viruses. Some parainfluenza viruses occur throughout the year, including summer. Other viruses include herpes simplex virus, varicella zoster virus, Epstein-Barr virus, and human herpesvirus 6. Less common causes of aseptic meningitis include tuberculosis, syphilis, various fungi (e.g., *C. neoformans*), and parasites. Noninfectious causes include Kawasaki disease, systemic lupus erythematosus, and polyarteritis nodosum.

This relatively well-appearing child presented with subacute symptoms and a CSF pleocytosis. The CSF WBC count does not point to a particular etiology. Although tuberculous meningitis is important to consider in any patient with aseptic meningitis, it usually manifests with characteristic CSF findings, including a dramatically elevated protein level and a low glucose concentration—findings not present in this case. Although a rash is associated with several of the mentioned conditions, children with Rocky Mountain spotted fever, ehrlichiosis, herpes simplex virus, varicella, or syphilis are often quite ill. Additionally, children with Rocky Mountain spotted fever and ehrlichiosis typically result in leukopenia and thrombocytopenia. The rash of herpes simplex virus or varicella, when present, is characteristic and does not resemble the rash on this patient. The rash shown in Figure 11-5 was characteristic of early disseminated Lyme disease.

II. Diagnosis

Examination of the skin revealed multiple annular lesions on the chest, back, and legs, ranging from 5 to 15 cm in diameter (Fig. 11-5). These macular erythematous lesions with partial to complete central clearing were characteristic of erythema migrans (EM). **This finding of multiple EM lesions, combined with headache, photophobia, and CSF pleocytosis, suggested the diagnosis of Lyme meningitis.** Serum antibodies revealed an IgM titer of 27.3 (reference, 0 to 0.8) and an IgG titer of 0.4 (reference, 0 to 0.8). This positive IgM test was also confirmed by Western blotting. CSF enterovirus PCR and bacterial culture were negative. An electrocardiogram did not reveal evidence of heart block, a feature associated with early disseminated Lyme disease. The child was treated with intravenous ceftriaxone for 3 weeks and recovered completely.

III. Epidemiology and Incidence

Lyme disease, caused by the tick-borne spirochete, *B. burgdorferi,*was initially identified during investigation of a cluster of children with arthritis in Lyme, Connecticut. Features of the disease had previously been described in Europe under various names, including erythema chronicum migrans, acrodermatitis chronica atrophicans, and Bannwarth syndrome. Lyme disease is now endemic in the United States in more than 15 states. The infection is also common in middle Europe, Scandinavia, and parts of Russia, China, and Japan. Several closely related ticks that are part of the *Ixodes ricinus* complex (*Ixodes scapularis, Ixodes pacificus, Ixodes ricinus,* and *Ixodes persulcatus*) comprise the vectors of Lyme disease. They vary in their geographic distribution. In the United States, *I. scapularis* is the vector in the northeast and midwest, whereas *I. pacificus* predominates on the west coast.

Most infections occur between May and July. After injection of *B. burgdorferi* into the skin by the *Ixodes* tick, the spirochete multiplies locally at the site of the bite and within days to weeks may disseminate to other sites. The risk of Lyme disease after a tick bite is discussed later.

IV. Clinical Presentation

Lyme disease typically manifests in three stages: localized infection, early (disseminated) infection, and late infection. Localized infection usually occurs 7 to 14 days (range, 3 to 32 days) after the tick bite. Early infection occurs 2 to 6 weeks after the tick bite, and late infection occurs 6 to 12 weeks (range, up to 12 months) after the tick bite. Localized infection refers to development of EM lesions at the site of the tick bite. It usually begins as an erythematous macule or papule and expands to a median diameter of 15 cm, with intensely erythematous macular borders and central clearing or induration. Occasionally, the central area becomes vesicular or necrotic. Complaints such as malaise, headache, arthralgias, myalgias, fever, and regional lymphadenopathy may accompany the lesion. Most children (60% to 70%) present with the localized form of Lyme disease.

Features of early disseminated infection include multiple EM lesions (23% of all Lyme disease cases), carditis (0.5%), cranial nerve palsy (3%), meningitis (2%), and acute radiculopathy (less than 0.5%). The most common cranial nerve palsy involves the seventh (facial) nerve, but palsy of cranial nerves III, IV, or VI may develop. Most children with Lyme meningitis have symptoms for 2 to 3 weeks before the diagnosis is made. They initially develop low-grade fevers, followed by mild neck pain or stiffness with extreme flexion. In some patients with Lyme meningitis, EM rash or concomitant cranial nerve palsy, rather than neck pain, brings the child to medical attention. Cardiac manifestations include fluctuating degrees of atrioventricular block (first degree, Wenckebach, or complete) and, less commonly, myocarditis, pericarditis, or cardiomegaly. Carditis is thought to occur in 5% of patients with untreated Lyme disease.

Arthritis, the most common late manifestation of Lyme disease, involves the knee in 90% of cases. The spirochete occasionally affects the hip, ankle, wrist, or elbow. The joint is swollen and warm but, in contrast to bacterial septic arthritis, only mildly tender. Signs and symptoms of systemic illness are rare.

V. Diagnostic Approach

The diagnosis is usually suspected based on characteristic clinical findings, history of exposure in an endemic area, and antibody testing. Diagnosis of Lyme meningitis requires a high level of suspicion, careful history and examination, serum antibody studies, and lumbar puncture. Diagnosis of other manifestations of Lyme disease is discussed later.

Serologic diagnosis. For serologic testing, the U. S. Centers for Disease Control and Prevention recommends a two-tiered approach to testing. An enzyme-linked immunoassay (EIA) is performed initially. The EIA test is very sensitive, but false-positive results occur due to cross-reactive antibodies in patients with other spirochetal infections or certain viral infections or autoimmune diseases. Those with equivocal or positive results by EIA should undergo confirmatory testing by Western blot analysis of the initial sample. An IgM determination is considered positive if two of three specific bands (23, 39, or 41 kd) are detected by Western blotting. An IgG Western blot is considered positive if at least 5 of 10 specific bands are present.

Only 40% of children with localized EM have detectable antibodies. On repeat testing 4 weeks after detection of the EM lesion, 70% have detectable antibodies; suggesting that early antibiotic treatment of the EM lesion may blunt antibody response. In children with early disseminated infection (e.g., Lyme meningitis), IgM antibodies are present in more than 95% of cases and IgG antibodies in 70%. Children with late infection should have detectable IgG and may have detectable IgM.

Peripheral blood smear. Patients with Lyme disease frequently are coinfected with another tickborne pathogen. In a study by Krause et al., 22% of patients with Lyme disease were coinfected with babesiosis, and 4% were coinfected with human granulocytic ehrlichiosis. The diagnosis of babesiosis depends on microscopic identification of intraerythrocytic parasites in Giemsa- or Wright-stained thick and thin blood smears. In approximately 50% of patients with ehrlichiosis, morulae are detected in peripheral blood neutrophils. Peripheral blood smears should be examined in any patient with Lyme disease who has continued symptoms despite amoxicillin therapy. These coinfecting pathogens should also be considered in any patient with leukopenia, thrombocytopenia, hemolysis, or jaundice—findings that are more typical of other tickborne diseases rather than Lyme disease.

Lumbar puncture. In children with Lyme meningitis, CSF analysis reveals a mild mononuclear (lymphocytes and monocytes) pleocytosis (mean, 100 WBCs/mm^3; range, 10 to 500/mm^3). In a study by Turnquist et al., 23 of 24 children with Lyme meningitis had less than 10% segmented neutrophils in the CSF. The CSF glucose is normal and the protein may be normal or mildly elevated. CSF antibody studies may provide supporting evidence of Lyme meningitis. CSF Lyme PCR analysis has not been useful in diagnosing Lyme meningitis due to its poor sensitivity.

Joint aspiration. In cases of Lyme arthritis, joint aspiration typically reveals between 30,000 and 50,000 WBCs/mm^3. Results of Lyme PCR testing of joint fluid are positive in approximately 85% of patients with suspected Lyme arthritis. False-positive PCR results from joint fluid are uncommon.

Other studies. There does *not* appear to be a role for Lyme PCR testing of urine or blood samples. Because clinically it may be difficult to distinguish Lyme meningitis from other causes of aseptic meningitis, studies to detect other causes (e.g., enteroviral CSF PCR, serum antibodies and CSF PCR for arboviruses) should be considered. Results of additional studies such as peripheral WBC count and erythrocyte sedimentation rate are relatively nonspecific for Lyme disease, but certain findings (e.g., leukopenia) can suggest an alternative or concomitant infection.

VI. Treatment

Treatment of Lyme disease depends on the clinical manifestation. Localized disease may be treated with amoxicillin for 14 to 21 days. Other reasonable agents include doxycycline (if the patient is 8 years of age or older), cefuroxime, erythromycin, or azithromycin. Some controversy exists as to the appropriate management of children with facial nerve palsy. Although some experts recommend CSF evaluation for all patients with a Lyme-associated cranial palsy, others reserve lumbar puncture for those with clinical evidence of CNS infection (e.g., headache, neck stiffness, photophobia). An oral regimen, as discussed previously, is reasonable to treat isolated cranial nerve palsy caused by Lyme disease.

Children with carditis may be treated either orally or parenterally (ceftriaxone, cefotaxime, or penicillin) depending on the severity of cardiac involvement. Children with third-degree atrioventricular heart block are at risk for life-threatening complications and require parenteral therapy and initial hospitalization for monitoring. Children with first- or second-degree heart block may be treated with an oral antibiotic for part of the recommended 14- to 28-day course. This decision is frequently made in conjunction with an infectious diseases specialist.

Children with evidence of Lyme meningitis or radiculopathy usually require parenteral therapy for 21 to 28 days. Children with Lyme arthritis often respond well to 28 days of oral therapy. For those with poor initial response to oral therapy, parenteral ceftriaxone should be considered. Children with Lyme arthritis may have recurrence of the arthritis. Recurrences of arthritis after successful initial treatment can be managed with nonsteroidal anti-inflammatory agents.

Although early studies of the efficacy of prophylaxis after tick bites failed to show a protective effect, a recent study of adults showed that a single 200-mg dose of doxycycline administered within 72 hours after a recognized *I. scapularis* bite had an efficacy of 87% in preventing EM. The rate of EM was 3.2% in the placebo group, compared to 0.4% in the doxycycline prophylaxis group. However, adverse events, including nausea and vomiting, occurred in approximately 30% of those who received doxycycline. Because transmission is unlikely if the tick in not engorged (which usually requires at least 36 hours of attachment), many experts consider prophylaxis only if the tick is engorged and known to be an *Ixodes* tick. The benefit of such prophylaxis in children and with other antibiotics is not known.

VII. References

1. Gerber MA, Zemel LS, Shapiro ED. Lyme arthritis in children: clinical epidemiology and long-term outcomes. *Pediatrics* 1998;102:905–908.
2. Gerber MA, Shapiro ED, Burke GS, et al. Lyme disease in children in southeastern Connecticut. *N Engl J Med* 1996;335:1270–1274.
3. Hayes EB, Piesman J. How can we prevent Lyme disease? *N Engl J Med* 2003;348: 2424–2430.
4. Krause PJ, McKay K, Thompson CA, et al. Disease-specific diagnosis of coinfecting tickborne zoonoses: babesiosis, human granulocytic ehrlichiosis, and Lyme disease. *Clin Infect Dis* 2002;34:1184–1191.
5. Nadelman RB, Nowakowski J, Fish D, et al. Prophylaxis with single-dose doxycycline for the prevention of Lyme disease after an *Ixodes scapularis* tick bite. *N Engl J Med* 2001;345:79–84.
6. Newland JG, Zaoutis TE, Shah SS. The child with aseptic meningitis. *Pediatr Case Rev* 2003;3;179–182.
7. Steere AC. Lyme disease. *N Engl J Med* 2001;345:115–125.
8. Turnquist JL, Shah SS, Zaoutis TE, et al. Clinical and laboratory features allowing early differentiation of Lyme and enteroviral meningitis in children. *Pediatr Res* 2003;53:106A.
9. Wormser GP, Nadelman, Dattwyler RJ, et al. Practice guidelines for the treatment of Lyme disease. *Clin Infect Dis* 2000;31:S1–S14.

12

Constipation

Robert A. Nordgren

APPROACH TO THE PATIENT WITH CONSTIPATION

I. Definition of the Complaint

Constipation, a common problem in childhood, accounts for 10% to 25% of all referrals to pediatric gastroenterologists. Although constipation is usually characterized by the painful passage of hard stool, the term refers to both the consistency and the frequency of stools. The precise definition of constipation is difficult because the normal stooling pattern differs among individuals and varies by age. The frequency of stools in most children decreases from a mean of four per day in the first week of life, to two per day by 16 weeks of age, and one stool per day at 4 years of age.

All cases of constipation involve a failure to evacuate the lower colon completely with a bowel movement. A child who has two small stools per day may not have evacuated the colon, whereas a child who has two large stools weekly may not be constipated. The child who has experienced pain with defecation may aggressively contract the external sphincter to prevent expulsion of stool when the urge to defecate arises. In such cases, increased amounts of stool collect in the rectum, and over a period of weeks to months the rectum gradually dilates, becoming less capable of peristaltic activity.

II. Complaint by Cause and Frequency

Although functional fecal retention is the most common cause of childhood constipation, a number of other causes must be considered in the differential diagnosis (Table 12-1).

III. Clarifying Questions

A diagnosis of constipation can readily be made by the history and physical examination findings. However, attention needs to be paid to certain historical details. The following questions may provide clues to the diagnosis:

- What is the stool consistency, caliber, and volume?

  — Small, pellet-like stools indicate incomplete evacuation. Intermittent, massive stools are characteristic of functional fecal retention.

- Did the child have a bowel movement in the first 24 hours of life?

  — In a child with constipation, failure to pass melonium in the first 24 to 48 hours of life increases the likelihood of Hirschsprung's disease.

- Were there any neonatal complications or prior surgeries?

  — Neonatal gastrointestinal complications such as necrotizing enterocolitis or prior surgery can lead to strictures or adhesions and predispose a child to constipation and small-bowel obstruction.

- Is the child going through any transitions such as changes from breast- to bottle-feeding, diapers to toilet training, or home care to childcare center or school?

TABLE 12-1. *Differential Diagnosis of Constipation*

Category	Cause
Functional	
	Functional fecal retention
	Protracted vomiting
	Lack of bulk in diet
	Irritable bowel syndrome
Neurologic	
	Aganglionosis (Hirschsprung's disease)
	Neuronal dysplasia (hyperganglionosis)
	Hypoganglionosis (Chagas disease)
	Familial dysautonomia
	Hypotonia syndromes
	Spina bifida occulta
	Myelomeningocele
	Paraplegia
	Cauda equina tumor
	Tethered cord syndrome
Obstructive	
	Anterior ectopic anus
	Congenital or acquired anal ring stenosis
	Small left colon
	Meconium ileus (cystic fibrosis)
	Rectal or sigmoid stricture (postoperative, postnecrotizing enterocolitis)
	Adenocarcinoma
	Pelvic tumor, mass or pregnancy
Endocrine and metabolic	
	Congenital pseudo-obstruction
	Visceral myopathy, neuropathy
	Amyloidosis
	Collagen-vascular (scleroderma, lupus, dermatomyositis)
	Diabetes
	Renal tubular acidosis
	Vitamin D intoxication
	Idiopathic hypercalcemia
	Hypokalemia
	Hypothyroidism
	Hyperparathyroidism
	Multiple endocrine adenoma
	Pheochromocytoma
	Porphyria
	Graft versus host disease
Medicinal	
	Laxative abuse
	Diuretics
	Tricyclic antidepressants
	Narcotics
	Aluminum antacids
	Vincristine
	Calcium channel blockers
	Iron overload
	Lead poisoning

— Developmental and social transition periods are the most common times for functional constipation to begin. Asking about transitions such as a move into childcare can help identify a possible cause of constipation and can also give parents insight into the diagnosis.

• Is there a history of sexual abuse?

— The emotional trauma of sexual abuse can predispose a child to constipation.

- Is the child taking any medications?

    — Several medications can cause constipation (Table 12-1).

- Are there any other symptoms (e.g., fever, blood in stool)?

    — Symptoms associated with constipation point to an organic cause.

- Has the family kept a journal of the child's stooling patterns and diet?

    — A 5- to 7-day journal of stooling patterns and diet can help both the clinician and the family objectively assess the true extent of constipation. A diet history can help identify a cause of constipation and also can serve as a starting point for therapy for functional constipation.

Case 12-1: 11-Month-Old Girl

I. History of Present Illness

An 11-month-old girl with a history of chronic constipation presented to the emergency department with her last bowel movement having been 3 weeks ago. Her regular bowel pattern was been two stools per month, which were accompanied by significant straining. No blood or mucus was noted with any of these stools. Two days before presentation she had fever, decreased oral intake, and decreased urine output. She also seemed to be having increased abdominal distention. These symptoms did not improve with several phosphate enemas at home. Before this episode, she had normal weight gain without vomiting or diarrhea.

II. Past Medical History

The patient was delivered at term gestation, and there were no complications during the pregnancy. She was evaluated at 4 days of life because she had not passed meconium. Over the next few months there were several interventions for constipation, including prune juice, increased water intake, and changes in formula. Each intervention seemed to produce more frequent bowel movements initially, and then the pattern would worsen again. Bowel movements tended to be loose, watery, and small in volume. Otherwise, her review of systems was negative. The patient had been taking docusate since 9 months of age. She had had two episodes of otitis media. Thyroid function tests, including thyroid-stimulating hormone, were normal.

III. Physical Examination

T, 38.2°C; RR, 36/min.; HR, 140 bpm; BP 90/60 mm Hg

Weight, 8.7 kg (25th to 50th percentile); height, 74.5 cm (50th percentile); head circumference, 45.5 cm (75th percentile)

Initial examination revealed a quiet but uncomfortable infant. The physical examination was remarkable for mild erythema of the posterior oropharynx and erythematous tympanic membranes with decreased mobility. The abdomen was distended and bowel sounds were distant. The abdominal examination also revealed palpable stool in the left quadrant. On the rectal examination, there were no fissures, the anus was patent, and there was no stool in the ampulla.

IV. Diagnostic studies

Serum chemistry studies revealed the following: sodium, 130 mEq/L; potassium, 5.0 mEq/L; chloride, 107 mEq/L; bicarbonate,14 mEq/L; blood urea nitrogen, 66 mg/dL; and creatinine, 0.3 mg/dL. An abdominal obstruction series showed increased stool with dilated loops of bowel but no air–fluid levels (Fig. 12-1).

V. Course of Illness

In the emergency department, she was treated for dehydration with intravenous normal saline fluid boluses. She was treated with amoxicillin for otitis media. She also received two pediatric phosphate enemas that produced small amounts of liquid stool. She subsequently had three episodes of bile-tinged emesis. Later, on the first day of admission, she became more irritable and had an increasing abdominal girth. Cultures of the blood and urine were negative.

Serial abdominal obstruction series did not show any changes during the first two days of admission. However, with continuing enemas the patient's abdominal girth decreased (from 48 cm to 41cm) as her stool output increased. On the third day of hospitalization, a radiographic barium enema was performed (Fig. 12-2) and suggested the diagnosis.

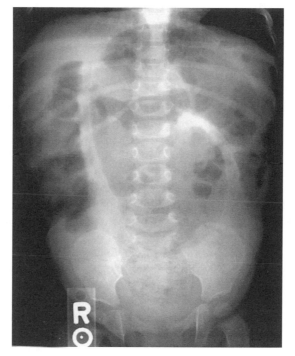

FIG. 12-1. Abdominal radiograph (case 12-1).

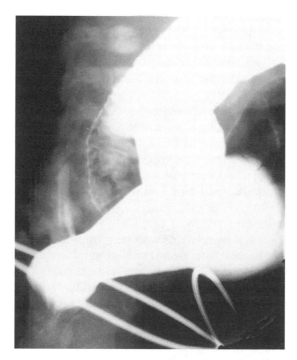

FIG. 12-2. Radiographic enema from a patient with a diagnosis similar to that in case 12-1.

DISCUSSION: CASE 12-1

I. Differential Diagnosis

Based on the history, the patient had been constipated for her entire life. She also failed to pass meconium during the first 48 hours of life. Therefore, Hirschsprung's disease should be at the top of a differential list. However, other diagnoses should also be considered. Hypothyroidism can cause constipation in the infant. Thyroid studies on this patient were reported to be normal. Some obstructive conditions present in infancy, such as anterior ectopic anus and congenital anal ring stenosis. Infants of diabetic mothers may have a small left colon that predisposes them to constipation and obstruction. Neuronal dysplasia is associated with increased numbers of ganglion cells (hyperganglionosis) in the lower colon. It may manifest throughout childhood with variable constipation or features of pseudo-obstruction. Sacral nerve abnormalities, which usually are associated with spina bifida occulta or a tethered cord, can also cause constipation.

II. Diagnosis

The barium enema (Fig. 12-2) revealed a funnel-shaped transition zone that suggested the diagnosis of Hirschsprung's disease. The transition zone probably would have been more obvious had the patient not received several phosphate enemas before the study was performed. Endoscopic rectal suction biopsy was inconclusive. **A full-thickness surgical biopsy showed no ganglion cells in 100 sections and was diagnostic for Hirschsprung's disease.** The patient underwent a successful Duhamel pull-through procedure.

III. Incidence and Epidemiology

Hirschsprung's disease, or aganglionosis of the bowel, is the most common cause of lower intestinal obstruction in neonates. It occurs in 1 of every 5,000 live births. The overall male/female ratio is 3.8:1. In 80% of patients, the aganglionic segment does not extend above the sigmoid; however, the entire colon and some small bowel may be involved in 3%. Recurrent abdominal distention, emesis, failure to thrive, and acute enterocolitis allow diagnosis of 60% of patients by 3 months of age. Approximately 3% of patients have Hirschsprung's disease associated with Down syndrome, cardiac anomalies, or coexistent neuroblastoma.

Hirschsprung's disease is characterized by abnormal innervation of the distal bowel, beginning at the anus and extending proximally for a variable distance. The defect results from a failure of neural crest cell caudal migration. The primary histologic finding is the absence of Meissner and Auerbach plexuses, which are hypertrophied nerve bundles located between the circular and longitudinal muscles and in the submucosa. This abnormal innervation leads to abnormal tone and motility of the bowel and predisposes to obstruction.

IV. Clinical Presentation

Approximately 95% of full-term infants with Hirschsprung's disease fail to pass meconium during the first 24 hours of life. Normal full-term infants pass meconium within 24 hours (90%) to 48 hours (99%) of life. Therefore, Hirschsprung's disease should be suspected in any neonate who fails to pass meconium within 48 hours. These infants may also develop vomiting and abdominal distention during the first week of life. Enterocolitis, a consequence of delayed diagnosis in a neonate with significant bowel involvement, is characterized by fever, abdominal distention, and explosive, foul-smelling, bloody diarrheal stools.

Findings in the older child include a history of severe constipation from birth, failure to thrive, and abdominal distention. Older children may come to attention by presenting with either complete intestinal obstruction or enterocolitis. The rectal ampulla is usually empty on digital rectal examination.

V. Diagnostic Approach

Abdominal radiographs. In children with Hirschsprung's disease, a plain film of the abdomen may show distended loops of colon; air is usually present in the small bowel proximal to the obstruction.

Barium enema. Barium enema is suggestive in approximately 80% of cases. A barium enema should be performed without bowel preparation, so that the large rectum dilated with stool can be appreciated. The characteristic appearance of the barium enema occurs because aganglionosis of the distal colon results in hypertonic contraction of the affected bowel. The normal proximal bowel becomes dilated. Between the two segments, a transition zone of bowel develops. This transition zone lacks innervation but partially distends under the influence of the peristaltic activity of the normal bowel, which pushes the bowel contents into the contracted distal segment. This transition zone is generally funnel-shaped. Variations of this appearance include an abrupt transition from dilated to narrowed bowel and, in some cases, funneling of the bowel incrementally over a long segment of bowel, making the change barely perceptible. Dilation of the rectum to the anal verge is diagnostic of functional constipation and rules out Hirschsprung's disease.

Anal manometry. Anal manometry is also useful in the diagnosis of Hirschsprung's disease, with a reported sensitivity of 95%. This study demonstrates the failure of the internal sphincter to relax in Hirschsprung's disease.

Rectal biopsy. The absence of ganglion cells in the myenteric (Auerbach) and submucous (Meissner) plexuses by rectal suction biopsy is diagnostic for Hirschsprung's disease. Staining for the presence of acetylcholinesterase may be more reliable than visual recognition of the absence of ganglion cells. If the suction biopsy is not conclusive, a full-thickness biopsy is mandatory. Complications of mucosal suction biopsy are rare. In a review of 1,340 mucosal biopsies, there were 3 cases of hemorrhage that required packed red blood cell transfusion and 3 clinical perforations.

Other studies. In children with enterocolitis, the complete blood count frequently reveals anemia and leukocytosis.

VI. Treatment

Operative intervention is necessary to treat Hirschsprung's disease. The original operation (Swenson procedure) consists of removal of the defective distal colon, with an end-to-end anastomosis 2 cm above the anal canal. With this procedure, the defective aganglionic tissue is completely resected and the proximal ganglionated colon and anal canal are left in the normal anatomic position.

For total colonic aganglionosis, some surgeons prefer to perform an initial defunctionalizing colostomy or ileostomy to avoid the hazards of enterocolitis. Definitive surgery is usually performed 6 to 12 months after the initial colostomy. The endorectal pull-through procedure is widely used. This procedure involves stripping the aganglionic rectum of its mucosa and then bringing the normally innervated colon through the rectal muscular cuff, bypassing the abnormal bowel from within. The advantage to this procedure is the preservation of rectal function with minimal risk of injury to the pelvis.

The other commonly used procedure is the retrorectal transanal pull-through (Duhamel procedure). In the Duhamel procedure, the normally innervated bowel is brought behind the abnormally innervated rectum approximately 1-2 cm above the pectinate line, and an end-to-side anastomosis is performed. A neorectum is created, with the anterior half having normal sensory receptors and the posterior half having normal propulsion. The advantages to the Duhamel procedure are that it reduces pelvic dissection to a minimum and retains the sensory pathway of rectal reflexes.

The overall mortality rate for surgical repair is low (approximately 1%). The most common immediate postoperative complications are stricture and leakage at the anastomosis site. Some patients experience recurrent enterocolitis. Repeat operations are required in up to one fourth of cases, although the long-term outcome is quite good. In a study by Rescorla et al., the majority of patients considered their bowel habits normal; 27% ultimately required stool softeners or occasional enemas, and 8% reported soiling.

VII. References

1. Baillie CT, Kenny SE, Rintala RJ, et al. Long-term outcome and colonic motility after the Duhamel procedure for Hirschsprung's disease. *J Pediatr Surg* 1999;34:325–329.

2. Bees BI, Azmy A, Nigam M, et al. Complications of rectal suction biopsy. *J Pediatr Surg* 1983;18:273–275.

3. Fortuna RS, Weber TR, Tracy TF Jr, et al. Critical analysis of the operative treatment of Hirschsprung's disease. *Arch Surg* 1996;131:520–525.

4. Klish WJ. Functional constipation and encopresis. In: McMillan JA, DeAngelis CD, Feigin RD, et al., eds. *Oski's pediatrics: principles and practice.* Philadelphia: Lippincott Williams & Wilkins, 1999:1637–1639.

5. Rescorla FJ, Morrison AM, Engles D, et al. Hirschsprung's disease: evaluation of mortality and long-term function in 260 cases. *Arch Surg* 1992;127:934–941.

6. Rudolph CD, Benaroch L. Hirschsprung disease. *Pediatr Rev* 1995;16:5–11.

7. Swenson O. Hirschsprung's disease: a review. *Pediatrics* 2002;109:914–918.

Case 12-2: 3-Year-Old Boy

I. History of Present Illness

A 3-year-old boy was well until approximately 9 months before admission. At that time, he developed discomfort and difficulty with passage of large stools, which led to further stool withholding, all during the time when he was starting to toilet-train. The patient had bowel movements in his pull-ups but would refuse to sit on the toilet. When stools were passed they were of normal texture, but he would complain of pain. The patient received several enemas followed by mineral oil orally and since then had had passage of stool on a daily basis. However, 6 weeks earlier, he developed perianal irritation. This started as a small pustule around the anus and evolved to a larger lesion. He was admitted to an outlying hospital 1 month before this, admission at which time the anus was described as having a 3- to 4-cm, raised, red excoriating lesion concentrically around the anus. He was diagnosed with perianal cellulitis and was treated for cellulitis with intravenous oxacillin followed by an oral first-generation cephalosporin. After a medical and social evaluation, sexual abuse was excluded. The patient continued to have constipation. His review of systems was negative aside from the symptoms already described.

II. Past Medical History

His birth history was unremarkable. He had had no other hospitalizations or significant illnesses other than those mentioned previously.

III. Physical Examination

T, 37.0°C; RR, 22/min.; HR, 122 bpm; BP, 94/61 mm Hg

Weight, 16.2 kg (50th percentile); height, 98 cm (25th percentile)

The patient was alert and in no acute distress. The examination was remarkable for a 2-cm circumferential lesion around the anus. The lesion was erythematous, and there was purulent exudate soiling in the underpants. A digital rectal examination could not be performed due to the lack of patient cooperation with the examination.

IV. Diagnostic Studies

Laboratory studies showed 9,000 white blood cells (WBCs)/mm^3, with 45% segmented neutrophils, 49% lymphocytes, and 6% monocytes. Hemoglobin was 11.0 g/dL, and platelets were 400,000/mm^3. The mean corpuscular volume was 73 fL, and the red cell distribution width was elevated at 19.1%. The erythrocyte sedimentation rate was 55 mm/hour. Electrolytes, blood urea nitrogen, creatinine, and liver function tests were all normal. The cholesterol concentration was 265 mg/dL.

V. Course of Illness

Two weeks later, the patient underwent an endoscopy and colonoscopy for suspected Crohn's disease. On colonoscopy, a verrucous mass was visualized, which was circumferential to the anus up to the anal verge. Multiple biopsies were taken. The patient was noted to have a normal-appearing descending colon, sigmoid, and rectum. The esophagus, stomach, and duodenum were normal.

During the week after the biopsy, he developed a rash on his back that, in the clinical context, suggested a diagnosis (Fig. 12-3). He was also noted to have increased "swelling" around the eye. On examination, he had left eye proptosis with mild ptosis. Red reflexes were noted, but a full funduscopic examination could not be obtained. Magnetic resonance imaging (MRI) of the head demonstrated multiple lytic lesions around the skull in the frontal and parietal areas, with a left retro-orbital sphenoid mass. The

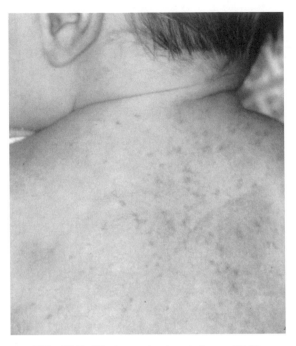

FIG. 12-3. Photograph of rash (case 12-2).

biopsy results became available that same day, confirming the diagnosis suggested by the rash.

DISCUSSION: CASE 12-2

I. Differential Diagnosis

In any 3-year-old boy presenting with difficulty stooling, functional constipation will be first on a differential diagnosis. However, this patient had complicating factors that forced the provider to widen the differential. The perianal lesion should lead to consideration of sexual abuse. Inflammatory bowel disease can also manifest with perianal lesions, but there were no other symptoms, such as diarrhea or bloody stools, to support that diagnosis. A child with inflammatory bowel disease would also most likely present with other symptoms such as fevers or poor weight gain. The symptoms of proptosis and ptosis were worrisome and required additional evaluation. The differential diagnosis of an orbital mass includes leukemia, neuroblastoma, and orbital abscess.

II. Diagnosis

The rash consisted of infiltrated, crusted papules and petechiae (Fig. 12-3). **The biopsy results revealed cells consistent with Langerhans cell histiocytosis (LCH, formerly called histiocytosis X).** The findings of exophthalmos and lytic bone lesions strongly suggested the diagnosis.

III. Incidence and Epidemiology

Since the Langerhans cell was discovered to be the proliferative cell responsible for the various syndromes in the "histiocytosis X" category, the term *Langerhans cell histiocytosis* has replaced the previously used terminology. LCH, or the class I histiocytoses, include the clinical entities *eosinophilic granuloma, Hand-Schüller-Christian disease,* and *Letterer-Siwe disease,* Normally the Langerhans cell is an antigen-presenting cell of the skin. The hallmark of LCH is the presence of a clonal proliferation of cells of the monocyte lineage containing the characteristic electron microscopic findings of Langerhans cells. LCH is not a malignancy, but rather a manifestation of complex immune dysregulation. The proliferation of these "normal" cells causes destruction or impairment of other organ systems.

LCH affects approximately 4 per million persons worldwide, with a male/female ratio of 2:1. Only 2% of cases are known to be familial, but many researchers suspect a genetic basis for the disease. Features that implicate a genetic cause include (a) a greater than expected incidence of malignant disease preceding the onset of LCH, (b) a younger age at onset for identical twins with LCH than for other family pairs, and (c) the finding of monoclonality of the pathologic Langerhans cell in LCH. There is no seasonal or geographic distribution.

IV. Clinical Presentation

LCH has an extremely variable presentation. The skeleton is affected in 80% of patients and may be the only affected site. Lytic bone lesions may be singular or numerous, and they are seen most commonly in the skull. These lesions may be asymptomatic, or they may be associated with pain and local swelling. Lesions can involve weight-bearing long bones and may result in fractures. Exophthalmos, when present, is often bilateral and is caused by retroorbital accumulation of granulomatous disease. Hypertrophic gingivitis and loose teeth signify underlying mandibular LCH.

About 50% of patients have skin involvement, usually a seborrheic dermatitis of the scalp or diaper region, which can spread to involve the back, palms, and soles. The rash frequently consists of infiltrated, crusted papules with areas of hemorrhage. Lymphadenopathy may be part of disseminated disease or associated with local disease affecting adjacent skin or bone. Fewer than 10% of children present with lymphadenopathy. Various degrees of hepatic malfunction can occur, including jaundice and ascites. In severe cases, liver fibrosis and failure occur. Five percent of patients have splenomegaly at presentation. Lung involvement is common in multisystem disease. Children with uncontrolled LCH can develop pulmonary cysts, pneumothorax, and chronic respiratory failure. Central nervous system (CNS) involvement may also occur. Approximately 15% of children develop diabetes insipidus as a consequence of hypothalamic and pituitary histiocytic involvement. Subtle neurologic defects such as hyporeflexia, ataxia, vertigo, nystagmus, and tremor may develop later during the course of illness. Early treatment may prevent the development of some of these features.

The most severely affected patients may have systemic manifestations such as fever, weight loss, malaise, irritability, and failure to thrive. Bone marrow involvement causes anemia and thrombocytopenia.

V. Diagnostic Approach

Plain radiography. Plain radiography remains the first-line approach for detecting bone lesions. Lesions consist of irregularly marginated lytic lesions, usually with adjacent soft tissue swelling.

Bone marrow biopsy. Bone marrow infiltration occurs in 18% of patients with multisystem disease and in 33% of patients with hematologic system involvement.

Tissue biopsy. Diagnostic tissue biopsy is easiest to perform on skin or bone lesions.

Other studies. Once the diagnosis has been made, a thorough clinical and laboratory evaluation should be undertaken. This should include a series of laboratory tests (complete blood count, liver function tests, coagulation studies, chest radiography, urine osmolality, and skeletal survey) and a detailed evaluation of any organ system that has been shown to be involved by physical examination, history, or the laboratory studies.

VI. Treatment

Single-system disease carries a high chance of spontaneous remission and is generally benign. Treatment in such cases should be minimal and should focus on arresting the progression of a lesion that could result in permanent damage. Local radiation therapy is the treatment of choice for single-system disease.

For multisystem or systemic disease, chemotherapy is the treatment of choice. The intensity of the regimen is modified after risk stratification. Children with no organ dysfunction have a better prognosis than do those with one or more involved organs. The initial response rate of children without pulmonary, hepatosplenic, or hematopoietic involvement is 90%, with a survival rate of 100%. In those with an unfavorable prognosis, the mortality rate ranges from 20% to 50%. The mortality rate is greater than 90% in children with multisystem LCH who had a poor response to initial therapy with prednisolone, vincristine, and etoposide. Other chemotherapeutic agents with activity against LCH include glucocorticoids, vinblastine, and methotrexate.

VII. References

1. Arceci RJ, Brenner MK, Pritchard J. Controversies and new approaches to treatment of Langerhans cell histiocytosis. *Hematol Oncol Clin North Am* 1998;12:339–357.
2. Arico M, Egeler RM. Clinical aspects of Langerhans cell histiocytosis. *Hematol Oncol Clin North Am* 1998;12:247–258.
3. Gadner H, Heitger A, Grois N, et al. A treatment strategy for disseminated Langerhans cell histiocytosis. *Med Pediatr Oncol* 1994;23:72–80.
4. Grois N, Tsunematsu Y, Barkovich AJ, et al. Central nervous system disease in Langerhans cell histiocytosis. *Br J Cancer* 1994;70:s24–s28.
5. Ladisch S, Jaffe ES. The histiocytoses. In: Pizzo PA, Poplack DG, eds. *Principles and practice of pediatric oncology,* 3rd ed. Philadelphia: Lippincott–Raven, 1997: 615–631.
6. Minkov M, Grois N, Heitger A, et al. Response to initial treatment of multisystem Langerhans cell histiocytosis: a prognostic indicator. *Med Pediatr Oncol* 2002;39: 581–585.
7. Willman, CL, Busque L, Griffith BB, et al. Langerhans cell histiocytosis (histiocytosis X): a clonal proliferative disease. *N Engl J Med* 1994;331:154–160.

Case 12-3: 3-Month-Old Boy

I. History of Present Illness

A 3-month-old boy was referred from his pediatrician to the emergency department for evaluation. The parents reported that 5 days earlier they had noticed a change in his stooling pattern. Instead of the usual four stools per day, he began passing only one stool per day, and by the time of presentation he had not stooled in 2 days. He was taken to the pediatrician for evaluation of his constipation. The parents noted that the child's feeding intake had decreased from vigorous breast-feeding every 3 hours to relatively poor feeding attempts, and he often had to be wakened for feeds. On the day of admission, they commented that he was not holding onto his pacifier well and that he has been drooling more during the past week. He also was not holding his head up as well as he had 2 weeks earlier. He had had no fevers, and his review of systems was otherwise negative.

II. Past Medical History

The patient weighed 4,100 g at birth, and the pregnancy was uncomplicated. Nasolacrimal duct obstruction that was noted shortly after birth and resolved by 2 months of age. His development had been progressing normally.

III. Physical Examination

T, 36.5°C; RR, 47/min.; HR, 175 bpm; BP, 87/39 mm Hg; SpO_2, 96% on room air
Weight, 6.3 kg

The initial examination revealed an infant in no acute distress. He was awake and alert but was not making any vigorous movements. He had a weak cry and a moderately weak gag. His heart sounds were normal. Femoral pulses were strong, and capillary refill was brisk. His abdomen was soft without organomegaly. He had poor truncal tone. The remainder of the physical examination was normal.

IV. Diagnostic Studies

Electrolytes, blood urea nitrogen, creatinine, and glucose were normal except for a bicarbonate level of 16 mEq/L. Serum aminotransferases and bilirubin were normal. The WBC count was 11,400 cells/mm^3, with 71% segmented neutrophils, 25% lymphocytes, and 3% monocytes. Hemoglobin was 9.5 g/dL, and platelets were 425,000/mm^3. Examination of the cerebrospinal fluid (CSF) revealed 3 WBCs/m^3 and 10 red blood cells/mm^3. CSF protein was 24 mg/dL, and CSF glucose was 67 mg/dL. There were no organisms on CSF gram stain. Blood, CSF, and urine cultures were obtained.

V. Course of Illness

The infant was treated with intravenous cefotaxime for a presumed bacterial infection while culture results were pending. On the third day of hospitalization, his respiratory effort worsened, he had difficulty handling oral secretions, his gag reflex diminished, and he required endotracheal intubation.

DISCUSSION: CASE 12-3

I. Differential Diagnosis

Infectious diseases such as meningitis and encephalitis must be considered in any child who presents with lethargy. Dehydration can cause lethargy and altered stooling patterns. Children with viral or bacterial gastroenteritis usually have vomiting or diarrhea, although constipation may be present in the severely dehydrated child. Neonatal myasthenia gravis may cause neurologic abnormalities including lethargy and ptosis, but it does not usually result in constipation or changes in stooling pattern. Several inborn errors of metabolism may manifest with lethargy, but usually there are other symptoms such as vomiting or irritability. Congenital myopathies (e.g., myotubular myopathy, central core disease, nemaline rod disease) can cause muscular weakness and hypotonia. Focusing on the change in stooling pattern in this patient, hypothyroidism must also be considered as a cause. Other possible diagnoses include Guillain-Barré syndrome, poliomyelitis, anticholinergic poisoning, and cerebrovascular accident. However, the constellation of neurologic changes associated with the change in stooling pattern most strongly suggest infant botulism.

II. Diagnosis

On examination, the infant had marked hypotonia. Because of the rather rapid progression of symptoms, infant botulism was suspected. Electromyography revealed a modest decremental response, consistent with infant botulism. **A stool sample was positive for *Clostridium botulinum* toxin, confirming the diagnosis of infant botulism.** He received botulism immune globulin on the 7th day of hospitalization. He was extubated on the 10th day of hospitalization and required nasogastric feeds for a total of 3 weeks.

III. Incidence and Epidemiology

Infant botulism results from an intestinal infection by *C. botulinum,* an anaerobic, gram-positive, spore-forming bacillus. *C. botulinum* spores are ubiquitous in the environment and can be cultured from soil and many agricultural products. Honey is one dietary source that has been linked to infant botulism by laboratory testing and epidemiologic studies. Corn syrup does not appear to be a risk factor for infant botulism. In the 1980s, a U. S. Food and Drug Administration study found botulism spores in commercially prepared corn syrup. Since changes in corn syrup production were made, spores have not been identified in corn syrup.

C. botulinum spores from various sources are ingested by infants. These spores colonize the colon and release the organism. The organism produces a toxin that causes disease. In contrast, the adult form of botulism occurs after ingestion of the preformed toxin. Botulinum toxin is divided into types A through G, with types A, B, E, and F producing human disease. Cases occur in infants younger than 1 year of age, with 95% of cases occurring during the first 6 months of life. Affected infants are most commonly breast-fed, Caucasian, and residents of rural or suburban areas. The intestinal microflora of breast-fed infants, as compared with bottle-fed infants, may make them more susceptible to colonization with *C. botulinum.* Once the neurotoxin is produced by the organism, it is taken up by nerve endings and irreversibly blocks acetylcholine release in peripheral cholinergic synapses. Cranial nerves are usually affected first, leading to difficulty swallowing and loss of protective airway reflexes. The recovery phase begins when terminal motor neurons regenerate and new motor end-plates develop.

IV. Clinical Presentation

Clinical signs and symptoms usually develop between 2 weeks and 6 months of age. The patients are afebrile. Constipation is the classic initial complaint. Additional presenting complaints include poor feeding, weak suck, weak cry, and hypotonia. Although often described as lethargic, the infant is typically alert but unable to move or smile. Within 1 week after the initial presentation, additional neurologic symptoms are seen, including ptosis, facial diplegia, dysconjugate gaze, weak suck, impaired swallowing or gag reflex, and worsening hypotonia. Paralysis develops in a descending manner, and all cranial nerves are eventually involved. A normal initial response of the pupillary light reflex fatigues with repeated stimulation over 1 to 2 minutes. This sign can be helpful in distinguishing infant botulism from congenital myasthenic syndromes. Deep tendon reflexes are initially normal despite profound hypotonia, but hyporeflexia develops later in the course. Autonomic dysfunction is common. Decreased tearing and salivation gradually develop. Blood pressure and heart rate may fluctuate dramatically.

There are several complications that lead to the morbidity and mortality associated with infant botulism. Most infants have progressive weakness over a 1- to 2-week period, culminating in respiratory failure. Inability to swallow or protect the airway from oral secretions leads to nasogastric tube feeding and endotracheal intubation. The symptoms remain at a nadir for 1 to 2 weeks before improving. Most infants require hospitalization for 4 to 5 weeks. The syndrome of inappropriate secretion of antidiuretic hormone (SIADH) occurs due to venous pooling, diminished left atrial filling, and subsequent stimulus for antidiuretic hormone production. SIADH complicates approximately 17% of cases. Secondary infections such as urinary tract infection and aspiration pneumonia also occur.

V. Diagnostic Approach

The clinical presentation usually suggests infant botulism, but the definitive diagnosis is made by testing stool samples.

Detection of organism. A small enema with nonbacteriostatic water (not saline solution) may be used judiciously to obtain stool for diagnostic testing. The most reliable confirmatory test is detection of *C. botulinum* toxin in the infant's stool by means of the mouse inoculation toxin neutralization assay. Specimens for toxin assay are transported at 4°C to either the state health department or the Centers for Disease Control and Prevention laboratories for testing. *C. botulinum* can be cultured from stool after anaerobic incubation on selective egg yolk agar; however, this is rarely required given the reliability of the toxin assay. Serum testing reveals the diagnosis in fewer than 10% of cases.

Electromyography. Electromyography reveals (a) motor unit action potentials of brief duration, small amplitude, and abundant motor-unit potentials (BSAP), (b) incremental response in the muscle action potential produced by high-frequency stimulation, (c) normal nerve conduction velocity, and (d) no significant response to injection of edrophonium chloride or neostigmine (to distinguish this condition from myasthenia gravis).

Other studies. Lumbar puncture, often performed because of concern for meninigitis, reveals normal CSF cell count, protein, and glucose. Once the diagnosis is made, serum electrolytes should be checked periodically to detect SIADH.

VI. Treatment

The main emphasis of treatment has been on supportive care. Attention should be directed at protecting the airway, providing adequate ventilation and nutrition, and preventing nosocomial complications.

Endotracheal intubation, required by approximately 70% of children with infant botulism, should be performed if impairment of the infant's ability to cough, gag, or swallow occurs. In the past, tracheostomies were performed in up to 50% of patients in anticipation of prolonged requirement for mechanical ventilation. Before the use of antitoxin, the mean duration of mechanical ventilation was 21 days. Currently, the duration of mechanical ventilation is shorter, and late sequelae of airway trauma induced by prolonged endotracheal intubation (e.g., subglottic stenosis) are rare. Prophylactic tracheostomy is not routinely required.

Nasogastric tube feedings are usually required during the course of illness to prevent aspiration of formula. Small-volume, continuous enteral feeding stimulates gut motility and obviates the need for central venous catheterization. Oral feeding may be resumed after the gag, swallow, and suck reflexes have returned. Intake, output, weight, and serum electrolytes must be carefully monitored during this period due to the risk of SIADH.

Antibiotic therapy is often stared empirically while meningoencephalitis and sepsis are being excluded. Specific antibiotic therapy is not required for treatment of infant botulism but may be required to treat nosocomially acquired infections. Aminoglycoside antibiotics may precipitate rapid deterioration; they contribute to neuromuscular blockade and should be avoided in children in whom the diagnosis of infant botulism is suspected.

Human-derived botulism immune globulin (HBIG) has been under investigation. In a randomized study, HBIG was given to infants with infant botulism within 3 days after their initial hospital admission. HBIG decreased the mean duration of hospitalization from 5.5 to 2.5 weeks and decreased intensive care unit stay from 3.5 to 1.5 weeks. The study also showed a decrease in the rate and duration of endotracheal intubation. The illness usually lasts from 1 to 2 months, and the prognosis is excellent. Case-fatality rates are less than 1%.

VII.   References

1. Arnon SS. Infant botulism. In: Feigin RD, Cherry JD, eds. *Textbook of pediatric infectious diseases,* 4th ed. Philadelphia: WB Saunders, 1998:1570–1577.
2. Graf WD, Hays RM, Astley SJ, et al. Electrodiagnosis reliability in diagnosis of infant botulism. *J Pediatr* 1992;120:747–749.
3. Hatheway CL, McCroskey LM. Examination of feces and serum for diagnosis of infant botulism in 336 patients. *J Clin Microbiol* 1987;25:2334–2338.
4. Long SS. *Clostridium botulinum* (botulism). In: Long SS, Pickering LK, Prober CG, eds. *Principles and practice of pediatric infectious diseases,* 2nd ed. New York: Churchill Livingstone, 2003:984–991.
5. Long SS. Epidemiologic study of infant botulism in Pennsylvania: report of the infant botulism study group. *Pediatrics* 1985;75:928–934.
6. Olsen SJ, Swerdlow DL. Risk of infant botulism from corn syrup. *Pediatr Infect Dis J* 2000;19:584–585.
7. Schreiner MS, Field E, Ruddy R. Infant botulism: a review of 12 years' experience at The Children's Hospital of Philadelphia. *Pediatrics* 1991;87:159–165.

Case 12-4: 12-Month-Old Girl

I. History of Present Illness

A 12-month-old girl was brought to her pediatrician for evaluation of constipation. She usually stooled once per day but recently had been stooling only once per week. There had been no apparent change in appetite or activity level. She had had no fevers or emesis, and otherwise her review of systems was negative. She had had normal growth and development.

II. Past Medical History

The patient had a normal birth history. Her birth weight was 3,600 g. She passed meconium during the first 24 hours of life. She had not required previous hospitalization. She was not receiving any medications.

III. Physical Examination

T, 36.2°C; RR 17/min; HR, 90 bpm; BP, 90/50 mm Hg

Height, 25th percentile; weight, 50th percentile

On examination, the patient was a well-appearing girl. Her examination was significant for the presence of a 1×1 cm fleshy mass at the base of her tongue that did not appear to cause her any discomfort. The heart and lung sounds were normal. Her abdomen had an easily reducible umbilical hernia with a 1 cm fascial defect. There was a 2×2 cm macular area of hypopigmentation on her lower abdomen. Her tone was slightly decreased symmetrically, but she was able to sit without support. The neurologic exam was otherwise normal.

IV. Diagnostic Studies

A nuclear medicine test confirmed the diagnosis (Fig. 12-4).

DISCUSSION: CASE 12-4

I. Differential Diagnosis

As with any child who goes from a normal to a constipated stooling pattern, functional constipation must first be considered. In this case, the findings on physical examination,

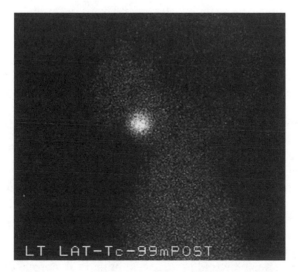

FIG 12-4. Radionuclide scan (case 12-4). (Photograph courtesy of Dr. Martin Charron.)

mass at the base of the tongue, umbilical hernia, and hypotonia led to the diagnosis. In a 1-year-old with constipation, other causes can be considered. The patient was taking no medication, but this must be explored in the history. Although this child is old for infant botulism, this diagnosis must be considered in any infant presenting with new constipation.

II.   Diagnosis

Laboratory studies revealed the following: thyroid-stimulating hormone (TSH), 24.0 μIU/mL (normal range, 0.6 to 6.2 μIU/mL); free thyroxine (T4), 5.4 μg/dL (normal range, 6.8 to 13.5 μg/dL); total T4, 6.2 μg/dL (normal range, 5.3 to 10.8 μg/dL); resin triiodothyronine (T3) uptake, 36.9% (normal range, 28.0% to 47.0%); resin T3 uptake ratio, 0.92 (normal range, 0.70 to 1.18). The patient had an ectopic thyroid gland leading to hypothyroidism. **Thyroid scintigraphy (Fig. 12-4) revealed increased uptake at the base of the tongue, confirming the diagnosis of hypothyroidism due to an ectopic thyroid gland.**

III.   Pathology and Epidemiology

Causes of congenital hypothyroidism include dyshormonogenesis (deficiency of an enzyme involved in the formation of thyroid hormones), transient congenital hypothyroidism, disorders of thyroxine synthesis, thyroid hormone resistance, and thyroid dysgenesis. Iodide transport defects and iodine organification defects are included among the 15 known disorders of thyroxine synthesis. Thyroid dysgenesis is the most frequent cause of hypothyroidism in infancy. Common types of thyroid dysgenesis include aplasia, hypoplasia, and ectopia (ectopic thyroid). The thyroid gland can be totally absent or, as in this case, ectopic. In some cases, the deficiency of thyroid hormone are severe and symptoms develop during the first weeks of life. As in this case, lesser degrees of deficiency can occur, with manifestations delayed for months. In North America, the incidence of congenital hypothyroidism is 1 in every 3,500 to 5,000 live births. The male/female ratio ranges from 1:2 to 1:3.

IV.   Clinical Presentation

Most infants with congenital hypothyroidism are asymptomatic at birth, even if there is complete agenesis of the thyroid gland. This is attributed to the transplacental passage of moderate amounts of maternal T4, which accounts for 33% of the infant's T4 levels at birth.

Soon after birth, children with congenital hypothyroidism often develop poor feeding, prolonged hyperbilirubinemia (longer than 7 days), hypotonia, large posterior fontanelle (larger than 1 cm), and macroglossia. Within the first 2 months of life, children who are hypothyroid usually develop constipation and are seen as sedate or placid infants. They also have abdominal distention and an umbilical hernia. There are several other common clinical manifestations, including subnormal temperature, edema of the genitals and extremities, slow pulse, cardiac murmurs, cardiomegaly, and goiter. By 3 to 6, months these symptoms have progressed. Development is delayed; children with hypothyroidism often appear lethargic and are late in learning to sit or stand. Growth retardation is one of the main manifestations in childhood, and it is accompanied by delayed skeletal maturation.

Children with an ectopic thyroid gland usually have some viable thyroid tissue, so symptoms of hypothyroidism are mitigated. These children represent a spectrum of severity of thyroid deficiency.

V.   Diagnostic Approach

Although neonatal screening programs vary from state to state, most in North America measure levels of T4 and run TSH levels on the lowest 10th percentile for a given day. The rate of false-negative results is 5% to 10%. Abnormal tests on a state-established screen should prompt immediate evaluation of T4 and TSH levels to confirm the diagnosis of hypothyroidism.

Thyroid function tests. Initial evaluation includes determinations of TSH and T4. T3 may be measured if ectopic thyroid is suspected initially. A normal or near-normal level of circulating T3 in the presence of a low T4 suggests the presence of residual thyroid tissue.

Thyroid scintigraphy. All children with proven congenital hypothyroidism should undergo radionuclide scanning if possible. The thyroid gland is the only organ in the body that stores iodine to any significant extent, making radioactive isotopes of iodine (e.g., sodium iodide 123) and ions with charge and radius similar to iodine (e.g., technetium Tc 99m pertechnetate) useful for thyroid imaging. No uptake of ^{123}I or ^{99m}Tc occurs if the thyroid gland is absent. Ectopic thyroid glands are usually characterized by areas of increased uptake at the base of the tongue, but other potential locations include the larynx, mediastinum, and lateral neck. Therefore, images must be obtained from the oropharynx to the upper mediastinum to exclude an ectopic gland. Ectopic thyroid glands are usually hypofunctioning; for this reason, ^{123}I, which produces less background activity than ^{99m}Tc does, is the preferred isotope. The demonstration of ectopic thyroid is diagnostic for thyroid dysgenesis and establishes the need for evaluation and treatment of hypothyroidism. A normally placed thyroid with a normal or active uptake of radioisotope in the context of hypothyroidism suggests a defect in thyroid hormone biosynthesis.

VI. Treatment

The treatment of choice for children with hypothyroidism is L-thyroxine given orally. The goal of therapy is to normalize T4 levels as quickly as possible. Levels of T3 and T4 rapidly return to normal in treated infants. TSH levels may not come into the normal range for several weeks, even with good T4 values. Treatment is lifelong. If the child was even mildly symptomatic at the time of diagnosis, the parents may notice an increase in activity, improvement in feeding, and increased urination and bowel movements soon after treatment begins. If bone maturation was delayed at the time of diagnosis, it will normalize within approximately 1 year. Early diagnosis and treatment usually results in normal IQ and motor development. Delayed diagnosis may result in variable deficits in intelligence that amount to several IQ points for every week of delayed treatment.

To guarantee adequate hormone replacement, T4 levels should be maintained in the upper half of the normal range during therapy. Low T4, high TSH, and poor growth suggest poor compliance or undertreatment. Excessive L-thyroxine over a prolonged period (3 to 6 months) can cause osteoporosis, premature synostosis of cranial sutures, and advancement of bone age. Prognosis is excellent if treatment is begun during the first 4 weeks of life.

VII. References

1. Bongers-Schokking JJ, Koot HM, Wiersma D, et al. Influence of timing and dose of thyroid hormone replacement on development in infants with congenital hypothyroidism. *J Pediatr* 2000;136:292–297.
2. Fisher DA. Disorders of the thyroid in the newborn and infant. In: Sperling MA, ed. *Pediatric endocrinology,* 2nd ed. Philadelphia: WB Saunders, 2002:161–185.
3. Germak JA, Foley TP. Longitudinal assessment of L-thyroxine therapy for congenital hypothyroidism. *J Pediatr* 1990;117:211–219.
4. Grant DB, Smith I, Fuggle PW, et al. Congenital hypothyroidism detected by neonatal screening: relationship between biochemical severity and early clinical features. *Arch Dis Child* 1992;67:87–90.
5. Gruters A. Congenital hypothyroidism. *Pediatr Ann* 1992;21:15–28.
6. Pollock AN, Towbin RB, Charron M, et al. Imaging in pediatric endocrine disorders. In: Sperling MA, ed. *Pediatric endocrinology,* 2nd ed. Philadelphia: WB Saunders, 2002:725–756.

Case 12-5: 9-Year-Old Girl

I. History of Present Illness

A 9-year-old girl who was previously healthy presented with a complaint of constipation. She had developed lower back pain approximately 3 months earlier and at that time complained of some difficulty stooling. She tried various therapies. including mineral oil, senna, and phosphate-supplemented enemas, with an improvement in stooling pattern. However, her back pain did not remit. Initially the pain was intermittent and was controlled to some extent with ibuprofen. It began in the lower back and flank area and then radiated down the buttocks to both lower legs. It was worse with standing and walking. Over the past 2 weeks, the pain had increased in intensity and become more constant; it now interfered with her daily activities. The mother initially believed that the child was about to start menstruating.

She had been evaluated in the emergency department of a nearby hospital about 2 weeks before admission and was diagnosed with pyelonephritis. She was treated with ciprofloxacin without improvement. She was reevaluated 1 week before admission, and at that time computed tomography of the abdomen was normal; specifically, there were no renal stones. At the time of the presentation, she had severe low back pain and had not stooled in 4 days. There had been no recent dysuria, urgency, or frequency. There was no headache, fatigue, weight loss, night sweats, or abdominal pain. Menarche has not occurred. She denied recent trauma or infection.

II. Past Medical History

She had had problems with constipation as an infant and received mineral oil periodically until 3 years of age. She had not previously required hospitalization. She was taking no medications. There was no family history of thyroid disorders or autoimmune diseases.

III. Physical Examination

T, 37.4°C; RR, 16/min; HR, 90 bpm; BP 110/65 mm Hg

Weight, 25th percentile

On examination, she was alert and cooperative but in obvious distress. She was lying on the examination table moaning and holding her back. Her conjunctivae were pink and anicteric. Her neck was supple. There were no murmurs on cardiac examination. Her abdomen was soft without heptaosplenomegaly. The back was tender along the lumbar spine and flanks bilaterally, with significant muscle spasm. Range of motion was limited due to pain. Straight-leg raising produced pain in the posterior thighs at approximately 45 degrees bilaterally. The sensation in the lower extremities was intact at all levels. Motor tone was normal. Deep tendon reflexes at the patellar tendon and ankles were normal bilaterally.

IV. Laboratory Studies

Laboratory evaluation included a WBC count, which revealed 4,100 cells/mm^3, with 35% segmented neutrophils, 55% lymphocytes, 8% monocytes, and 2% eosinophils. Hemoglobin was 12.0 g/dL, and platelets were 204,000/mm^3. Mean corpuscular volume was 87 fL, and red cell distribution width was normal at 12.4. Serum chemistry findings included the following: sodium, 141 mmol/L; potassium, 3.9 mmol/L; chloride, 105 mmol/L; bicarbonate, 25 mmol/L; blood urea nitrogen, 11 mg/dL; creatinine, 0.5 mg/dL; and glucose, 97 mg/dL. The total bilirubin was 0.2 mg/dL. Serum albumin, alkaline phosphatase, and transaminases were normal. Urinalysis revealed a specific gravity of 1.011, pH 6.5, and no WBCs, red blood cells, or protein. Fibrinogen was 411 mg/dL. Pro-thrombin and partial thromboplastin times were 13.7 and 31.5 seconds, respectively.

V. Course of Action

Radiographs of the lumbar spine showed no fracture, dislocation, or degenerative changes of the vertebral bodies. MRI of the spine revealed an intradural, intramedullary lesion measuring 5.2 × 2.0 cm at the level of T12–L1. There was displacement of the nerve roots and the distal tip of the cauda equina ventrally.

DISCUSSION: CASE 12-5

I. Differential Diagnosis

Although this patient's most consistent symptom was back pain, functional constipa-tion must be considered. Constipation can also lead to difficulty urinating, but this patient had not complained of urinary symptoms despite her earlier diagnosis of pyelonephritis.

Back pain and tenderness along the spine are abnormal and potentially serious find-ings in a child. Once this history and physical findings have been elicited, spinal cord processes must be considered. Several disease processes can affect the spinal cord and cause the symptoms described. Trauma must also be considered in any child with severe back pain. Trauma can lead to hematomas, vertebral fractures, and dislocations in the spine. Bacterial infections can cause epidural abscesses, and viral infections can cause transverse myelitis. Intravertebral disc herniation and spinal tumors also cause back pain in children. Guillain-Barré syndrome is occasionally considered in the evaluation of back pain. In this child's presentation there was neither a history of trauma nor signs of infec-tion. Imaging studies and biopsy were warranted to make the final diagnosis.

II. Diagnosis

Diagnosis by frozen section was intramedullary spinal ependymoma.

III. Incidence and Epidemiology

Tumors of the spinal cord can be extramedullary or intramedullary. Extramedullary tumors erode the bony vertebral column and compress sensory and motor tracts located laterally within the spinal cord. Extramedullary lesions are usually metastases from pri-mary tumors such as neuroblastoma, sarcoma, or lymphoma. Dysembryoblastic extramedullary tumors are associated with teeth, bones, or calcification; there may be a sinus tract that leads from the surface and extends intraspinally. Intramedullary tumors are usually either astrocytomas or ependymomas, though oligodendrogliomas also occur.

Ependymomas are CNS tumors that arise within or adjacent to the ependymal lining of the ventricular system or the central canal of the spinal cord. They account for 5% to 10% of primary childhood CNS tumors. Most ependymomas are located in the posterior fossa, but approximately 10% occur in the spinal cord. Ependymomas vary from well-differentiated tumors with no anaplasia and little polymorphism to highly cellular lesions with significant mitotic activity and necrosis.

IV. Clinical Presentation

Signs and symptoms of spinal cord tumors can be insidious and misleading. Com-plaints may be vague, and few specific signs occur early in the disease. Most children with a spinal cord tumor ultimately present with a combination of extremity weakness, gait disturbance, scoliosis, and back pain, depending on the location of the tumor. Incon-tinence as a presenting sign may be overlooked in very young children who may not be fully toilet-trained. A clue to the presence of neurogenic bladder is incontinence of urine associated with crying or straining at stool.

Changes in posture, nonspecific complaints of back pain, or even unexplained abdominal pain can be associated with disease of the spinal cord. The child may have difficulty sleeping because of pain. Any pain that is exacerbated by Valsalva maneuvers, such as straining at stool or coughing, should be evaluated. Tumor attached to nerve roots can cause segmental pain, paresthesias, and weakness. The presence of hyperreflexia, clonus, and upgoing toes suggest corticospinal tract disease. Defects in proprioception, vibration sense, or sensory level should also raise suspicion for an intraspinal process.

V.   Diagnostic Approach

Spine radiographs. Anterior-posterior and lateral projections are obtained, as well as oblique projections for the cervical spine. Destructive bone lesions are associated with metastatic disease. Increased interpedicular distance suggests a long-standing intramedullary process. Slow-growing spinal tumors may cause scoliosis.

Spinal magnetic resonance imaging with gadolinium. MRI allows for differentiation of intramedullary from extramedullary masses.

Cystourethrogram. This study can evaluate bladder function and can confirm the diagnosis of neurogenic bladder.

Ophthalmologic examination. Spinal cord tumors are occasionally associated with increased intracranial pressure and papilledema, probably related to decreased CSF absorption due to hemorrhage within the tumor or dramatically elevated CSF protein.

VI.   Treatment

After confirmation by neurodiagnostic procedures, surgical laminectomy and exploration with removal of the tumor should be considered. Ependymomas expand symmetrically in a rostral-caudal fashion. A tissue plane can be readily identified, facilitating surgical excision. Irradiation is recommended for most spinal cord tumors, but adjuvant chemotherapy is not generally effective. Five-year survival rates for spinal cord ependymomas range from 95% to 100%.

Children with spinal cord tumors often face long-term deficits ranging from partial paralysis of one limb to quadriplegia. Physical therapy, serial casting, and tone-reducing medication may be required for moderate spasticity. Neurogenic bladder problems also require appropriate prophylactic antibiotics, intermittent catheterization, and cystometric evaluation. Multidisciplinary postoperative care includes input from pediatrics, oncology, orthopedics, urology, neurosurgery, and physical therapy.

VII.   References

1. Cohen ME, Duffner PK. Tumors of the brain and spinal cord including leukemic involvement. In: Swaiman KF, Ashwal S, eds. *Pediatric neurology: principles and practice,* 3rd ed. St. Louis: Mosby, 1999:1049–1098.
2. McCormick PC, Torres R, Post KD, et al. Intramedullary ependymoma of the spinal cord. *J Neurosurg* 1990;72:523—532.
3. Chesney RW. Brain tumors in children. In: Behrman RE, Kliegman RM, Jenson HB, eds. *Nelson textbook of pediatrics,* 16th ed. Philadelphia: WB Saunders, 2000: 1858–1862.

13

Neck Swelling

Stephen Ludwig

APPROACH TO THE PATIENT WITH NECK SWELLING

I. Definition of the Complaint

Neck swelling in children is a finding that elicits immediate parental concern and often a prompt visit to the physician. The finding of a neck mass provokes response because it is often associated with malignancy. Although malignancy is part of an extensive differential diagnosis, it is not the most common cause by far. More primary considerations include reactive adenopathy, infections (either acute or subacute), and congenital anomalies. There are oncologic causes as well. Because children often have palpable lymph nodes that are normal, a significant neck mass must be defined as a swelling that exceeds 2 cm in diameter. In only rare cases, smaller nodes may have characteristics that deserve diagnostic attention. Congenital lesions, although present at birth, may not become apparent until the child is school age or older. Neck masses may be categorized by their location in the neck. Location may help to limit the diagnostic possibilities. Another defining characteristic is the feel of the swelling: hard or spongy, painful or nonpainful to palpation. Hospitalization is required if neck masses are present in conjunction with systemic symptoms such as fever, fatigue or pallor; if the nodes are large enough to compromise the airway; or if the masses have not responded to outpatient therapy.

II. Complaints by Cause and Frequency

A differential diagnosis list for neck masses is shown in Table 13-1. This list of potential diagnoses is extensive and often requires a thorough diagnostic evaluation. Table 13-2 indicates the conditions that require immediate diagnosis and treatment. Table 13-3 shows the most common causes of neck swelling. Table 13.4 indicates the type of mass by location.

III. Clarifying Questions

- Is the airway compromised?

  — The first and most important question to be asked relates to the presence of airway compromise. If present, airway compromise demands immediate attention. Airway compromise may result from an intrinsic occlusion or from extrinsic compression of the airway. Airway edema may result from swelling caused by trauma or allergic reaction. Neck masses may also be associated with intrathoracic masses that cause respiratory distress.

- Is the swelling adenitis or adenopathy?

  — With this question one should determine whether there ae signs of active infection or adenitis. Signs of adenitis include swelling, redness, warmth, and tenderness. Adenopathy is more indicative of a reaction of the nodes. With adenopathy, swelling may be present, and possibly mild tenderness, but not redness, warmth, or exquisite pain.

TABLE 13-1. *Differential Diagnosis of Neck Mass by Etiology*

Category	Cause
Congenital	
	Thyroglossal duct cyst
	Brachial cleft cyst
	Cystic hygroma (lymphangioma)
	Squamous epithelial cyst (congenital or posttraumatic)
	Pilomatrixoma (Malherbe's calcifying epithelioma)
	Hemangioma
	Dermoid cyst
	Cervical rib
Inflammatory	
Infection	
	Adenopathy—secondary to local head and neck infection
	Cervical adenitis—streptococcal, staphylococcal, fungal, mycobacterial; cat-scratch disease, tularemia
	Secondary to systemic "infection"—infectious mononucleosis, cytomegalovirus, toxoplasmosis, others
	Focal myositis—inflammatory muscular pseudotumor
"Antigen"-mediated	
	Local hypersensitivity reaction (sting/bite)
	Serum sickness, autoimmune disease
	Pseudolymphoma (secondary to phenytoin)
	Mucocutaneous lymph node syndrome (? infectious)
	Sarcoidosis
	Caffey-Silverman syndrome
Trauma	
	Hematoma
	Sternocleidomastoid tumor of infancy (fibromatosis coli)
	Subcutaneous emphysema
	Acute bleeding
	Arteriovenous fistula
	Foreign body
	Cervical spine fracture
Neoplasms	
Benign	
	Epidermoid
	Lipoma, fibroma, neurofibroma
	Keloid
	Goiter (with or without thyroid hormone disturbance)
	Osteochondroma
	Teratoma (may be malignant)
	"Normal" anatomy or variant
Malignant	
	Lymphoma—Hodgkin's disease, non-Hodgkin's lymphoma
	Leukemia
	Rhabdomyosarcoma
	Neuroblastoma
	Histiocytosis X
	Nasopharyngeal squamous cell carcinoma
	Thyroid or salivary gland tumor

- Is the swelling acute, subacute, or chronic?

  — This question also gives insight to possible etiologies. Bacterial infections are usually acute and progressive. Other infections are more subacute, including Epstein-Barr virus (EBV) infection, cat-scratch disease, or tuberculosis. Congenital defects may be more chronic, perhaps with an acute flare that draws attention. Tumors may progressively increase in size over a variable time course, depending on the histologic characteristics of the tumor.

TABLE 13-2. *Life-Threatening Causes of Neck Mass*

Hematoma secondary to trauma
  Cervical spine injury
  Vascular compromise or acute bleeding
  Late arteriovenous fistula
Subcutaneous emphysema with associated airway or pulmonary injury
Local hypersensitivity reaction (sting/bite) with airway edema
Airway compromise with epiglottitis, tonsillar abscess, or infection of floor of mouth or retropharyngeal
  space (with adenopathy)
Bacteremia/sepsis associated with local infection of a cyst (cystic hygroma, thyroglossal, or brachial cleft
  cyst)
Non-Hodgkin's lymphoma with mediastinal mass and airway compromise
Thyroid storm
Mucocutaneous lymph node syndrome with coronary vasculitis
Tumor—leukemia, rhabdomyosarcoma, histiocytosis X

From McAneney CM, Ruddy R. Neck mass. In: Fleisher G, Ludwig S, ed. *Textbook of pediatric emergency medicine,* 4th ed. Philadelphia: Lippincott Williams & Wilkins, 2000.

TABLE 13-3. *Common Causes of Neck Mass*

Benign reactive adenopathy
Cervical adenitis (bacterial)
Hematoma
Congenital—thyroglossal duct cyst, branchial cleft cyst, cystic hygroma
Benign tumors—lipoma, keloid

TABLE 13-4. *Differential Diagnosis of Neck Mass by Location*

Area	Causes
1. Parotid	Cystic hygroma, hemangioma, lymphadenitis, parotitis, Sjögren's and Caffey-Silverman syndrome, lymphoma
2. Postauricular	Lymphadenitis, brachial cleft cyst (1st), squamous epithelial cyst
3. Submental	Lymphadenitis, cystic hygroma, thyroglossal duct cyst, dermoid, sialadenitis
4. Submandibular	Lymphadenitis, cystic hygroma, sialadenitis, tumor, cystic fibrosis
5. Jugulodiagastic	Lymphadenitis, squamous epithelial cyst, brachial cleft cyst (1st), parotid tumor; *normal:* transverse process C2, styloid process
6. Midline neck	Lymphadenitis, thyroglossal duct cyst, dermoid, laryngocele; *normal:* hyoid, thyroid
7. Sternomastoid (anterior)	Lymphadenitis, brachial cleft cyst (2nd, 3rd) pilomatrixoma, rare tumors
8. Spinal accessory	Lymphadenitis, lymphoma, metastasis (from nasopharynx)
9. Paratracheal	Thyroid, parathyroid, esophageal diverticulum
10. Supraclavicular	Cystic hygroma, lipoma, lymphoma, metastasis; *normal:* fat pad, pneumatocele of upper lobe
11. Suprasternal	Thyroid, lipoma, dermoid, thymus, mediastinal mass

Modified from May M. Neck masses in children: diagnosis and treatment. *Clin Pediatr* 1976;5:17.

- Are there systemic signs of illness?

  — Also helpful in the differential diagnosis process is a determination of the presence or absence of systemic signs such as fever, weight loss, anorexia, night sweats, lethargy, or fatigue. Some elements of the differential diagnosis are associated with these systemic markers, and others are clearly more local.

Case 13-1: 6-Year-Old Girl

I. History of Present Illness

A 6-year-old girl was well until 2 weeks before presentation, when she began to complain of tenderness on the right side of her neck. This continued for 1 week, and then the parents began to notice swelling on the right side of her neck. Swelling and tenderness increased, and the patient developed decreased range of motion. There was no dysphagia and no symptoms of upper respiratory tract infection. She had no history of trauma and no known exposure to cats. A purified protein derivative (PPD) test obtained 3 months earlier was negative; no anergy was panel placed at that time.

II. Past Medical History

She had had chickenpox 1 month earlier. There were no known allergies. She was taking no medications, and her immunizations were up to date. There had been no recent travel and no exposure to rabbits or cats.

III. Physical Examination

T, 37.8°C; RR, 20/min; HR, 96 bpm; BP, 106/69 mm kg

Weight, 23 kg (75th to 90th percentile); height, 44.5 cm (25th to 50th percentile)

On general examination, she was alert and in no acute distress. The optic discs were sharp, and the pupils were equal, round, and reactive to light. The tympanic membranes were gray bilaterally with normal mobility. There was no rhinorrhea. There were no oral lesions, but the mucous membranes were notable for pallor. A few petechiae were noted in the posterior pharynx. On the right side, the neck was supple with no prominent adenopathy. On the left side, a swollen, erythematous area was noted just to the right of midline and approximately 4 to 5 cm cephalad from the clavicle (Fig. 13-1). The mass

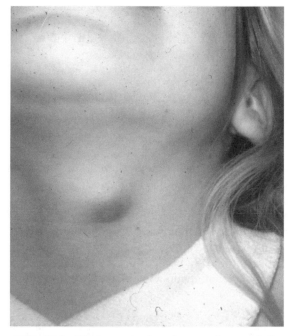

FIG. 13-1. Photograph of neck mass (case 13-1).

itself was 3×4 cm in size and tender to palpation, with well-defined borders. It moved with swallowing but not with tongue movement. The lungs were clear. The heart sounds were normal. There was no hepatosplenomegaly or intraabdominal masses.

IV.   Diagnostic Studies

A complete blood count (CBC) revealed 9,100 white blood cells (WBCs)/mm³, with 54% segmented neutrophils, 34% lymphocytes, 5% eosinophils, and 5% monocytes. The hemoglobin was 11.2 g/dL, and platelets were 565,000/mm³. The erythrocyte sedimentation rate (ESR) was 45 mm/hour. *Bartonella henselae* antibody titers were 1:32 (negative). Thyroid-stimulating hormone and triiodothyronine (T3) levels were normal. Computed tomography (CT) of the neck revealed a 5×6 cm solid right-sided mass, consistent with a thyroid nodule, with minimal tracheal deviation. Also noted were several 3-mm apical lung nodules.

V.   Course of Illness

The child had evidence of an acute infection. There was tenderness, swelling, and limitation of range of motion. Because of the acute nature of this illness, the size of the mass, and the progression of neck swelling, hospitalization was indicated. Biopsy of the mass revealed the diagnosis that was suggested by the clinical examination, along with a slightly surprising result.

DISCUSSION: CASE 13-1

I.   Differential Diagnosis

The location of the mass on the midline raised a moderately broad differential diagnosis. It was known that the child had had no cat exposure and that her PPD test had been negative just 3 months earlier. There had been no trauma. The mass did not feel like a routine infected lymph node, nor was it in the position of one. The differential diagnosis in this case included an infected thyroglossal duct cyst. Adenitis was possible, although the location unusual. If adenitis was consistent with the standard organisms, then *Staphylococcus aureus* or group A β-hemolytic streptococcus would be most likely. Cat-scratch disease and tuberculosis were ruled out by specific tests, and the CBC did not yield any clues to a specific cause.

In the location of this neck swelling, one must also consider thyroid-related masses such as tumors arising from the thyroid or from an aberrant thyroid gland. Thyroid function studies were normal. The CT scan showed a mass that was larger than clinically appreciated. There was also minimal tracheal deviation that was suggestive of a thyroid nodule. Therefore, it was determined that a tissue diagnosis was required without delay.

II.   Diagnosis

Culture of the mass revealed *Eikenella corrodens*. The diagnosis was that of a thyroglossal duct cyst secondarily infected with *Eikenella*, probably as a consequence of occult dental infection.

III.   Incidence and Epidemiology

Thyroglossal duct cysts are congenital remnants that occur when the thyroid migrates from the base of the tongue to its position in the neck. They can occur anywhere from the base of the tongue through the hyoid bone to just above the thyroid cartilage. Although thyroglossal duct cysts are asymptomatic while dormant, they may become symptomatic when infected.

IV.   Clinical Presentation

Thyroglossal duct cysts may be evident at birth, or they may be dormant for many years until they become infected, producing redness, swelling, and pain. The mass of a thyroglossal duct cyst may enlarge to the point of respiratory compromise. *E. corrodens* is a slow-growing organism that has been reported to cause a variety of clinical infections, from infected neck masses to brain abscesses, lung infections, bite wound infections, and bone and joint space infections.

V.   Diagnostic Approach

The diagnosis is suspected clinically by position of the mass and movement with swallowing or protrusion of the tongue.

Radiologic imaging. CT scanning may further delineate the size and location of the mass. Ultrasound may also be helpful in distinguishing a solid from a cystic mass. The possibility of an aberrant thyroid must be ruled out. The cyst may contain elements of thyroid tissue; therefore, if the cyst shows solid elements, they should be identified with a nuclear scan before surgery, lest they be inadvertently removed. Thyroglossal duct cysts are the most common midline lesions.

E. corrodens was isolated in this case. It is an unusual organism but one that should be considered if the patient has active periodontal disease or deteriorated oral health. It is also more common in individuals who are immunocompromised, although that was not the circumstance in this patient. Ultimately, excisional biopsy is the usual method to confirm the diagnosis. Frequently, infection is treated before surgery is performed.

VI.   Treatment

The ultimate treatment is surgical. Removal of the cyst and the other remnants of the migration tract is important. This is difficult and detailed surgery in a field with many other important vital structures. Before surgery, antibiotic therapy may be helpful in lessening the inflammation and aiding the postoperative healing process. Antibiotics to cover gram-positive organisms are customary. *E. corrodens* is a common gram-negative organism that probably derives from active periodontal disease. Treatment may be effective with a wide range of antibiotics; however, in most cases the combination of antimicrobial therapy and surgical drainage is required to effect complete recovery.

VII.   References

1. Paul K, Patel SS. *Eikenella corrodens* infections in children and adolescents: case reports and review of the literature. *Clin Infect Dis* 2001;33:545–561.
2. Knudsen TD, Simko EJ. *Eikenella corrodens*: an unexpected pathogen causing a persistent peritonsillar abscess. *Ear Nose Throat J* 1995;74:114–117.
3. Drake AF, Wolf GT, Fischer JJ. *Eikenella corrodens* as a cause of recurrent and persistent infections of the head and neck. *Am J Otolaryngol* 1986;7:426–430.
4. Marra S, Hotaling AJ. Deep neck infections. *Am J Otolaryngol* 1996;17:287–298.
5. Sheng WS, Hsueh PR, Hung CC, et al. Clinical features of patients with invasive *Eikenella corrodens* infections and microbiological characteristics of the causative isolates. *Eur J Clin Microbiol Infect Dis* 2001;20:231–236.
6. Cheng AF, Man DW, French GL. Thyroid abscess caused by *Eikenella corrodens*. *J Infect* 1988;16:181–185.

Case 13-2: 2-Year-Old Girl

I. History of Present Illness

A 2-year-old Vietnamese girl had been well until a few days before presentation, when her mother noticed a bump under her jaw. She had not had any fever, symptoms of upper respiratory tract infection (e.g., cough, rhinorrhea), or sore throat. She had been acting well. The bump did not hurt and was not red, but over the last 2 to 3 days it had increased from pea-sized to 4 to 5 cm and turned purple. She had normal oral intake and urine output. There was no vomiting, diarrhea, or rash. The patient had sweats at night, but this was not new. There had been no weight loss or change in appetite. Sleep pattern was normal. There was no history of animal bites. There was no dyspnea or wheezing.

II. Past Medical History

She was born by spontaneous vaginal delivery after an uncomplicated pregnancy. She required hospitalization at 14 months and again at 16 months due to pyelonephritis. She was diagnosed with grade 3 vesicoureteral reflux and received prophylactic amoxicillin until 2 weeks before presentation. She had not had pneumonia or any skin or soft tissue infections. Her immunizations were up to date. There was no family history of immune deficiency or other medical problems. The patient lived in suburban New York state. Her maternal grandmother served as her baby-sitter. She did not attend daycare. An aunt had a cat that was declawed. There was no known exposure to tuberculosis or other ill contacts. The child was known to put dirt in her mouth frequently, and there had been a significant amount of landscaping going on in their neighborhood.

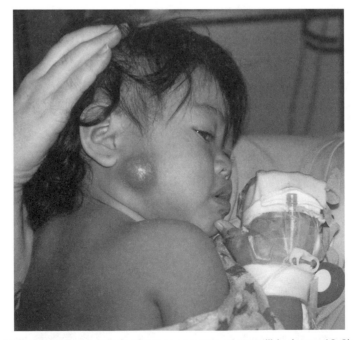

FIG. 13-2. Photograph of mass at angle of mandible (case 13-2).

III. Physical Examination

T, 36.0°C axillary; RR, 22/min; HR 108 bpm; BP, 121/60 mm Hg
 Weight, 25th percentile; height, 50th percentile; head circumference, 25th percentile
 On general examination, the patient was alert and cooperative. There was a 5-cm firm nodule with superficial fluctuance at the angle of the right mandible (Fig. 13-2). Despite the purplish hue, the mass had only trivial tenderness. The lungs were clear. There was no hepatosplenomegaly. The remainder of the examination was normal.

IV. Diagnostic Studies

Serum electrolytes, lactate dehydrogenase, and uric acid values were normal.

V. Course of Illness

She was initially treated with amoxicillin-clavulanate, and the mass increased in size over the next 2 weeks. Because of the lack of response, a fine-needle aspiration was performed, which was inconclusive. She was switched to clarithromycin for 2 weeks, with some mild decrease in size of the mass. A PPD was placed, and she had a reaction of 10 mm. A chest radiograph was obtained, which revealed bilateral paratracheal and mediastinal adenopathy. A chest CT revealed right paratracheal adenopathy (5 × 4 cm mass in right paratracheal area consistent with lymphadenopathy) but no focal lung abnormalities. She was referred to surgery and admitted for excisional biopsy of the mediastinal mass and the left mandibular mass; a bronchoscopy was also performed simultaneously. Examination of the biopsy material suggested the diagnosis.

DISCUSSION: CASE 13-2

I. Differential Diagnosis

The patient was characterized by having an increased neck mass. The mass in this case did not hurt, nor was it red or warm. This differential is from an acute adenitis with a usual bacterial organism. The location of the mass was over the mandible, in a position typical for a lymph node. The patient was treated with antibiotics without response. In addition, there were two other findings of importance, a positive PPD and positive chest radiograph. These findings required that a tissue diagnosis be made, so the patient was sent for biopsy and bronchoscopy after less invasive diagnostic studies failed to reveal a cause. The pathology results showed a pattern consistent with atypical mycobacterial infection. This was consistent with the child's course of an acute enlargement of a lymph node but not with the signs of an acute bacterial infection. The next set of diagnoses to consider was infection with subacute agents such as cat-scratch disease, tuberculosis, or atypical mycobacterial infection. There were no issues of altered immunology and only questionable presence of systemic signs. There was no history of trauma. The location of the mass was not usual for a congenital lesion.

II. Diagnosis

The pathology results revealed necrotizing granulomas consistent with atypical mycobacterial infection. Patient was discharged after 4 days on no antibiotic therapy. Culture of the material grew *Mycobacterium avium* complex. **The diagnosis was atypical mycobacterial infection adenitis in neck and mediastinum.** Given the extent of infection, an evaluation for cellular immune deficiency and macrophage and neutrophil defects was undertaken. No underlying immune deficiency was found in this patient.

III. Incidence and Epidemiology

Most cases of mycobacterial adenitis in children are caused by atypical mycobacteria (now called nontuberculous mycobacteria). In a study by White et al., 19 children with nontuberculous adenitis were reported. Their median age was 5.2 years. Most did not have underlying immunologic problems. Nodes were enlarged 1 to 2 months before diagnosis. Most patients had no systemic symptoms, and most had a negative chest radiograph.

IV. Clinical Manifestations

Atypical mycobacteria can produce both intrathoracic and extrathoracic manifestations. In the chest, the findings are relatively silent and relate primarily to enlargement of paratracheal lymph nodes. Extrathoracic major findings are adenitis that has a subacute quality, with enlargement of the nodes without findings of a suppurative infection.

V. Diagnostic Approach

In this case, the diagnosis was strengthened by findings of enlarged mediastinal nodes and the notation of a positive PPD test. The PPD may be positive in tuberculosis and in atypical mycobacterial infections. Although there was strong suspicion for atypical mycobacterial infection, there was a need to confirm the diagnosis with biopsy and bronchoscopy findings. Skin testing is of inconsistent value. PPD testing may be positive in some cases but cannot be relied upon. Skin testing with specific antigens is the best **method overall.**

VI. Treatment

The treatment in cases of atypical mycobacteria is excision. Many nodes regress on their own if left alone, but the need to establish a diagnosis usually prompts excision. Although these organisms are often susceptible to clarithromycin, antibiotic treatment alone is rarely successful. Once the infected lymph node has been excised, no antibiotic therapy is required.

VII. References

1. Altman RP, Margileth AM. Cervical lymphadenopathy from atypical mycobacteria: diagnosis and surgical treatment. *J Pediatr Surg* 1975;10:419–422.
2. Lai KK, Stottmeier KD, Sherman IH, et al. Mycobacterial cervical lymphadenopathy: relation of etiologic agents to age. *JAMA* 1984;251:1286–1288.
3. White MP, Bangash H, Goel KM, et al. Non-tuberculous mycobacterial lymphadenitis. *Arch Dis Child* 1986;61:368–371.
4. Dhooge I, Dhooge C, DeBaets F, et al. Diagnostic and therapeutic management of atypical mycobacterial infections in children. *Eur Arch Otorhinolaryngol* 1993;250: 387–391.
5. Benson-Mitchell R, Buchanan G. Cervical lymphadenopathy secondary to atypical mycobacterial in children. *J Laryngol Otol* 1996;110:48–51.
6. Danielides V, Patrikakos G, Moerman M, et al. Diagnosis, management and surgical treatment of non-tuberculous mycobacterial head and neck infection in children. *J Otorhinolaryngol* 2002;64:284–289.

Case 13-3: 2-Month-Old Boy

I. History of Present Illness

A 2-month-old boy presented with a 3-day history of neck swelling. The parents did not think that there had been any swelling before the past 3 days. He had had fevers at home for the past day. His oral intake had been adequate. There was no emesis, diarrhea, respiratory symptoms, or rash. There was no exposure to cats or to persons with tuberculosis. The parents noted small lesion on the boy's right neck and a question of an abrasion.

II. Past Medical History

There had been no hospitalizations. The patient was born at term during an uncomplicated delivery. He had not yet received any immunizations. There were no known allergies. The patient had not received any medications. Family history was notable for no significant illnesses. The mother and father had arrived from West Africa 6 months earlier.

III. Physical Examination

T, 38.5°C; RR, 44/min; HR, 176 bpm; BP, 112/76 mm Hg; SpO_2, 97% in room air

Weight, 6.2 kg (75th to 90th percentile); length, 60 cm (90th percentile); head circumference, 41cm (90th percentile).

On examination, the infant was not in any distress. The head was normocephalic, and the anterior fontanelle was open and flat. The oropharynx was clear. The right side of the neck was indurated. An erythematous mass arose from the angle of the jaw and extended to the chin. There was no fluctuance. The lung and heart sounds were normal. There was no hepatomegaly.

IV. Diagnostic Studies

The CBC revealed 15,300 WBCs/mm³, with 9% band forms, 65% segmented neutrophils, and 26% lymphocytes. The hemoglobin was 11.7 g/dL, and the platelets were 296,000/mm³. Serum electrolyte values were as follows: sodium, 135 mEq/L; potassium, 5.3 mEq/L; chloride, 103 mEq/L; bicarbonate, 24 mEq/L; blood urea nitrogen, 4 mg/dL; creatine, 0.2 mg/dL; and glucose, 113 mg/dL. Cerebrospinal fluid examination revealed 1 WBC, no red blood cells, and a glucose concentration of 68 mg/dL. There were no bacteria on Gram staining. Blood, cerebrospinal fluid, and urine culture were obtained. CT scan revealed an abscess in the right neck.

V. Course of Illness

On day 2 of hospitalization, there was significant drainage from the lesion on the neck. The patient underwent operative drainage of the mass.

DISCUSSION: CASE 13-3

I. Differential Diagnosis

This mass was obviously congenital in origin, because it was manifested at age 2 months. Its location was adjacent to the angle of the jaw, again pointing to a branchial cleft cyst that had become infected. The mass was warm, erythematous, and increasing in size, indicating that an infection had complicated the anomaly. The child was febrile, another likely marker of infection. Other possible lesions besides a branchial cleft cyst are cystic lymphoma and hemangioma. Congenital injury to the sternocleidomastoid muscle is usually present at birth and does not expand over time. Congenital torticollis lesions also have a firm, almost calcified, feel to them. A tumor is possible but less likely in this age range. Also, a tumor would not have the inflammatory signs that were evident in this child.

II.   Diagnosis

The diagnosis is branchial cleft cyst with secondary infection.

III.   Incidence and Epidemiology

Branchial cleft cysts are the most common congenital lesions on the midline structure. Most thyroglossal duct cysts occur above the level of the thyroid bed, but the location of branchial cleft cysts depends on which branchial arch is the source of the congenital defect. The first arch is located in the parotid region. The second is located off the angle of the mandible. The third branchial cleft is located in the middle to lower part of the neck. The fourth branchial cleft occurs in the lower neck area.

IV.   Clinical Presentation

The clinical presentation depends on the location and on the state of infection of the cyst. Most do not cause any symptoms other than the local effects.

V.   Diagnostic Approach

The diagnosis may be aided by ultrasound examination but is primarily made by CT scan of the neck. There are no supportive studies to lead to the diagnosis.

VI.   Treatment

The therapy is excision. Removal of the entire cyst is often difficult, and recurrences do occur if remnants are left *in situ*. Antibiotic treatment is used to decrease the acute inflammatory response before surgery. Broad-spectrum antibiotics aimed at gram-positive organisms are typically used.

VII.   References

1. Nusbaum AO, Som PM, Rothschild MA, et al. Recurrence of a deep neck infection: a clinical indication of an underlying congenital lesion. *Arch Otolaryngol Head Neck Surg* 1999;125:1379–1382.
2. Ungkanont K, Yellon RF, Weissman JL, et al. Head and neck space infections in infants and children. *Otolaryngol Head Neck Surg* 1995;112:375–382.
3. Mouri N, Muraji T, Nishijima E, et al. Reappraisal of lateral cervical cysts in neonates: pyriform sinus cysts as an anatomy-based nomenclature. *J Pediatr Surg* 1998;33: 1141–1144.
4. Palacios E, Valvassori G. Branchial cleft cyst. *Ear Nose Throat J* 2001;80:302.

Case 13-4: 2-Year-Old Boy

I. History of Present Illness

A 2-year-old African-American boy was brought to the emergency department by his mother because of swelling under his chin. The swelling had never been noticed before this visit, but the child had developed complaints of difficulty swallowing before coming to the emergency department. He had no history of fever. He had no rash, sweats, or weight loss.

II. Past Medical History

The patient was born at 32 weeks' gestation with a birth weight of 1,300 g. He was hospitalized for 2 to 3 months after birth. The mother could not provide detailed information regarding his perinatal course. However, he was discharged home on an apnea monitor for 4 to 5 months. He had an inguinal hernia repaired before he was discharged from the hospital. The mother had been treated with rifampin due to a positive PPD test. Her chest radiograph was reportedly normal. The child had never received a tuberculin skin test.

III. Physical Examination

T, 38.1°C; RR, 24/min; HR, 113 bpm; BP, 103/73 mm Hg

Weight, 12.9 kg

In general, the child was alert and watchful and in no acute distress. The tympanic membranes were normal in appearance and mobility. There was no nasal discharge. The neck was supple with a full range of motion. There was a 2×2 cm mobile lymph node in the right submandibular area. It was not erythematous or tender. There was also a 2×4 cm mobile, nontender postcervical and postauricular node. There was shotty axillary, anterior cervical, and inguinal adenopathy. The chest was clear to auscultation. There were two small (subcentimeter) hyperpigmented macules on the upper back. There were no other skin lesions.

IV. Diagnostic Studies

There were 7,600 WBCs/mm^3, with 22% segmented neutrophils, 2% eosinophils, 66% lymphocytes, and 10% monocytes. The hemoglobin and platelet counts were normal. The total bilirubin was 0.4 mg/dL. Aspartate aminotransferase (AST) and alanine aminotransferase (ALT) were 40 and 21 U/L, respectively. ESR was 1 mm/hour. EBV titers revealed undetectable levels of viral capsid antigen (VCA) immunoglobulin M (IgM), VCA IgG, and EBV nuclear antigen antibody, consistent with no previous or current evidence of EBV infection. A PPD and anergy panel were placed.

V. Course of Illness

The patient was discharged to home with a diagnosis of rule out mycobacterial disease. He received follow-up care in the clinic with his primary care doctor. He continued to have remarkable right-sided cervical adenopathy. The week after his emergency department visit, his ESR had increased to 67 mm/hour and further studies were sent. Over the course of his evaluation, the patient had negative titers for toxoplasmosis, repeat negative EBV, cat-scratch titers of less than 1:32, and negative cytomegalovirus (CMV) serology. He was taken for excisional lymph node biopsy; Gram staining showed many WBCs but no bacteria. A culture grew coagulase-negative staphylococci, and a culture and smear for acid-fast bacilli was negative. Histologic examination of the biopsy specimen revealed an infiltration of histiocytes filling the sinuses of the lymph nodes.

DISCUSSION: CASE 13-4

I. Differential Diagnosis

Early in the course of this disorder, the lymph node enlargement may be similar to that seen in many other causes of lymphadenopathy, including bacterial infections or viral infections like mononucleosis, adenovirus, or CMV. As the nodes become more and more enlarged with few signs or symptoms, oncologic diagnoses become more likely. Rosai-Dorfman disease is a unique entity that is characterized by self-limited proliferation of the histiocytes.

II. Diagnosis

The progression of this child's neck mass and the elimination of the other causes of massive neck swelling prompted biopsy of the lymph nodes. **The biopsy confirmed the diagnosis of sinus histiocytosis with massive lymph adenopathy (SHML), or Rosai-Dorfman disease.** In this disease, which was first described in 1969, there is a most likely viral trigger, followed by a massive overresponse of the immune system to produce histocytes. The lymph nodes become greatly enlarged and then regress spontaneously.

III. Incidence and Epidemiology

The incidence of this condition is unknown, and it is presumed to be rare. No single etiologic agent has been determined. There is a male predominance in both Caucasian and African-American children. Most cases have been described in children, although there are reports across the age spectrum.

IV. Clinical Presentation

The clinical presentation is usually that of bilateral cervical adenopathy that continues to increase in size despite attempted therapies (87% of cases). Any lymph nodes may be involved, and there are reports of extranodal involvement in nasal cavities, salivary glands, sinuses, tonsils, trachea, eyes, and orbits. It is characteristic that the enlargement of the nodes is relatively painless. There may be a concomitant increase in total WBC count, and particularly the neutrophils. There is also an increase in the ESR.

V. Diagnostic Approach

Lymph node histology. The diagnosis is based on histologic findings on biopsy. Histiocytes with benign cytologic characteristics fill the sinuses of the affected lymph nodes. The histiocytes contain normal-appearing lymphocytes within their cytoplasm. This finding is termed lymphophagocytosis or emperipolesis. CT scan of the involved areas may offer diagnostic clues.

VI. Treatment

Treatment is primarily supportive. Adenopathy may increase to the point of producing airway compromise, and artifical means of airway stabilization may be needed. Surgery may be needed for certain life-threatening circumstances. Treatment with corticosteroids and vinca alkaloids has sometimes appeared to be successful.

VII. References

1. Rosai J, Dorfman FR. Sinus histiocytosis with massive lymphadenopathy: a pseudolymphomatous benign disorder. *Cancer* 1972;30:1174–1188.
2. Faucar E, Rosai J, Dorfman RF. Sinus histiocytosis with massive lymphadenopathy (Rosai-Dorfman disease): review of the entity. *Semin Diagn Pathol* 1990;7:19–73.
3. Ünal ÖF, Köyba S, Kaya S. Sinus histiocytosis with massive lymphadenopathy (Rosai-Dorfman disease). *Int J Pediatr Otorhinolaryngol* 1998;44:173–176.
4. Ahsan SF, Madgy DN, Poulik J. Otolaryngologic manifestations of Rosai-Dorfman Disease. *Int J Pediatr Otorhinolaryngol* 2001;59:221–227.
5. McGill TJI, Wu CL. Weekly Clinicopathological Exercises: case 19-2002. A 13-year-old girl with a mass in the left parotid gland and regional lymph nodes. *N Engl J Med* 2002:346:1989–1996.

Case 13-5: 2-Year-Old Girl

I. History of Present Illness

A 2-year-old white girl presented to the emergency department with a 6-day history of fever. Three days before presentation, according to the girl's mother, she awoke with her head twisted to the left and an estimated 3-cm swollen lymph node in the right cervical region. She was brought to her primary physician, who prescribed amoxicillin-clavulanate, but her fevers continued. She had recently visited a friend's house where there were several cats, but no cat scratch had been noted. She had vacationed in Texas 2 weeks earlier. While in Texas, she developed an erythematous "goosebump-like" rash on her trunk and back. The rash resolved spontaneously and was not associated with any other symptoms: no fever, malaise, or pruritus. Over the past 2 days, the parents had noticed increased irritability, fevers, chills, and night sweats. She had had decreased oral intake over the past 3 days, but had no emesis or diarrhea, and she had had no bowel movement in 3 days. There was no joint swelling.

II. Past Medical History

She was a full-term infant, born of a spontaneous vaginal delivery with no complications. Her past medical history was notable for β-thalassemia minor, diagnosed at 9 months of age on a screening CBC. She had not required hospitalizations. She had no known allergies, and her immunizations were up to date. Her only medication was the amoxicillin-clavulanate prescribed by her pediatrician. The family history was notable for β-thalassemia minor. Her father had juvenile polyps, and her paternal grandmother had systemic lupus erythematosus.

III. Physical Examination

T, 40.0°C; RR, 26/min; HR, 153 bpm; BP, 135/77 mm Hg

Weight, 10th percentile

The patient was fussy and difficult to console. The tympanic membranes were slightly erythematous, but there was no middle ear fluid. The sclerae were injected. The lips were dry and cracked (Fig. 13-3A). The oropharynx was mildly erythematous. A 1.5 × 3 cm lymph node was palpable on the right side of the neck. The chest was clear to auscultation. The heart sounds were normal. There was mild right upper quadrant tenderness but no rebound or guarding. The extremities were erythematous and swollen (Fig. 13-3B).

IV. Diagnostic Studies

The WBC count was 16,700/mm^3. The hemoglobin was 8.8 g/dL, and the platelet count was 410,000/mm^3. The ESR was 65 mm/hour. The ALT and AST were 205 and 136 U/L, respectively. The albumin concentration was 3.1 mg/dL. Amylase and lipase were normal. Urinanalysis revealed 30 WBCs per high-power field. The urine culture was negative.

V. Course of Illness

EBV antibodies were negative. Viral antigens to influenza and adenovirus were not detected by immunofluorescence. Throat culture was negative. The clinical presentation strongly suggested a likely diagnosis.

DISCUSSION: CASE 13-5

I. Differential Diagnosis

The patient had adenopathy that was not increasing or becoming suppurative, but she did have prolonged fever. The fever persisted despite antibiotic therapy. There was also a history of rash, and on presentation she had red cracked lips and injected sclerae. This

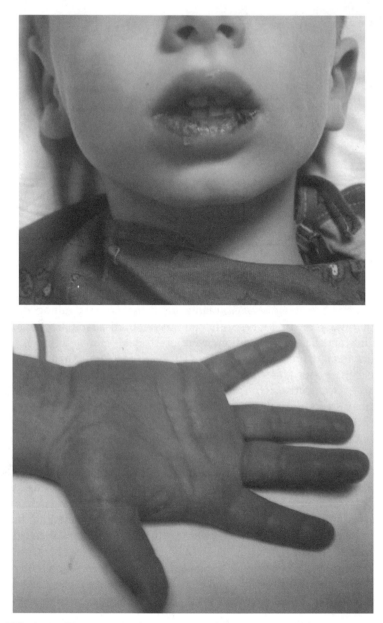

FIG. 13-3. Photograph of patient's lips **(A)** and hands **(B)** (case 13-5).

constellation of findings and the absence of any other diagnosis led to the possibility of Kawasaki disease. Kawasaki disease is the leading cause of acquired heart disease in the United States. Cervical adenopathy is one of the key features. The findings on echocardiography further strengthened the diagnosis. The pathophysiology of Kawasaki disease includes a superantigen response to a microorganism that results in a vasculitis of small and medium arteries. This child was evaluated for a number of causes of acute lymph node enlargement, including group A β-hemolytic *Streptococcus* infection, mononucleosis, cat-scratch disease, hepatitis, CMV, adenovirus, and other infectious causes. All of those infections are in the differential diagnosis. The adenopathy was not progressive to a suppurative state but was more subacute in its course. Other considerations would be tuberculosis and atypical mycobacterial infection.

II. Diagnosis

The final constellation of symptoms and clinical course best fit the diagnosis of Kawasaki disease. The child was treated with intravenous gammaglobulin and had an excellent response.

III. Incidence and Epidemiology

The peak incidence of Kawasaki disease is in early childhood. Fifty percent of patients are younger than 2 years of age, and 80% are younger than 4 years. It is extremely rare beyond 8 years of age. Children of Japanese and Korean descent are at highest risk, including those living in the United States. The incidence in Japan and Korea is 50 to 100 cases per 100,000 children younger than 5 years old. In the United States, the rates are 5 per 100,000 among Asian-Americans, 1.5 per 100,000 among African Americans, and fewer than 1 per 100,000 among European- and Hispanic-Americans. Kawasaki disease is more prevalent in the winter and spring.

IV. Clinical Presentation

The criterion for the diagnosis is to identify the common clinical presentations. This includes fever higher than 38.2°C for longer than 5 days, and the presence of at least four of five clinical criteria: (a) nonpurulent conjunctivus; (b) polymorphous mass; (c) mucous membrane changes, particularly cracked red lips; (d) adenopathy greater than 1.5 to 2 cm; and (e) extremity changes, usually swelling of the hands and feet. Despite this set of clinical criteria, there are many other potential manifestations, including cardiac disease, vasculitis symptoms, aseptic meningitis, hydrops of the gall bladder, hepatic dysfunction, pyuria, and arthritis/arthralgia, among others. Young children with this disease are often extremely irritable, and the irritability and fever often abruptly resolve with treatment. Children younger than 1 year of age often do not meet all of the diagnostic criteria and are often considered to have "atypical Kawasaki disease." Many authors have described the clinical manifestations in terms of three phases: acute, subacute, and convalescent.

V. Diagnostic Approach

The diagnosis is not based on any single laboratory test but on a confluence of the clinical findings. Beyond documentation of the findings, there may be suggestive laboratory evidence, including elevation of the ESR, increased WBC count, increased platelets, and sterile pyuria. Electrocardiography and echocardiography may show cardiac findings, in particular coarctation of the coronary arteries, mitral or tricuspid regurgitation, or left ventricular dysfunction, as in the case described here. Treatment response is considered by some to be another aspect of the diagnostic approach.

Complete blood count. The WBC count is greater than 10,000 cells/mm^3 in 95% of patients and greater than 15,000/mm^3 in 50%. Thrombocytosis develops during the second week of illness, and peak platelet counts (at approximately 3 weeks) are often greater than 750,000/mm^3.

Urinanalysis. Many children with Kawasaki disease have a sterile pyuria due to urethritis. This is more effectively detected on a freshly voided urine specimen than on one obtained by catheterization.

Other studies. Hepatic transaminases are elevated in 30% of cases. The alkaline phosphatase is elevated in the presence of gall bladder hydrops. Hypoalbuminemia is common.

VI. Treatment

Initial treatment is with intravenous immune globulin (IVIG), 2 g/kg infused over 12 hours. Often aspirin is prescribed for its antiplatelet adherence effects. The role of corticosteroids remains controversial. Patients also need supportive care, depending on their symptom complex. Regular follow-up care with a pediatric cardiologist is indicated.

VII. References

1. Shulman ST, Inocencio J, Hirsh R. Kawasaki's disease. *Pediatr Clin North Am* 1995; 42:1205–1222.
2. Newburger JW, Takahashi M, Beiser AS, et al. A single intravenous infusion of gamma globulin as compared with four infusions in the treatment of acute Kawasaki syndrome. *N Engl J Med* 1991;324:1633–1639.
3. Mori M, Imagawa T, Yasui K, et al. Predictors of coronary artery lesions after intravenous [gamma]-globulin treatment in Kawasaki disease. *J Pediatr* 2000;137; 177–180.
4. Shinohara T, Tanihira Y. A patient with Kawasaki disease showing severe tricuspid regurgitation and left ventricular dysfunction in the acute phase. *Pediatr Cardiol* 2003;24:60–63.

Case 13-6: 16-Year-Old Boy

I. History of Present Illness

A 16-year-old boy was transferred from a referral hospital for management of evolving respiratory failure. He had been in his usual state of good health until 1 week before admission. He had been helping friends renovate a house and developed sore throat, swollen glands in his neck, malaise, occasional vomiting, and fever to 38.9°C. His mother noted changes in his voice that this time. He went to his primary physician, who noted "kissing tonsils" and a pharyngeal exudate and diagnosed mononucleosis. He was started on oral prednisone and sent home with follow-up the next day. The next day, his voice had improved, and the regimen was continued.

He was seen in the emergency department at a community hospital 1 day before admission because of ongoing swelling of his glands and the development of chest pains and trouble sleeping (increased pain while lying down). A chest radiograph was initially reported as negative, but the family was called the next day because the reviewing radiologist believed that cardiomegaly was present. The patient returned to his primary physician and was referred for evaluation of chest pain, shortness of breath, orthopnea, fever, chills, and diaphoresis. In the emergency department, his respiratory rate was 40/min and his SpO_2 was 83% in room air. He had scattered petechiae on his trunk, face, and extremities. Chest radiography showed bilateral pneumothoraces and effusions. A chest tube was emergently placed, followed by resolution of the pneumothorax. An echocardiogram showed a mildly enlarged heart, small pericardial effusion, and no vegetations. Blood, urine and pleural fluid samples were sent for culture, and he was started on levofloxacin, ceftriaxone, vancomycin, and doxycycline. The patient continued to deteriorate from a respiratory point of view and required endotracheal intubation.

II. Past Medical History

Immunizations were not up to date. He had not received his tetanus booster or the hepatitis B vaccine series. There were no pets in the home, but he had exposure to friends' cats and dogs. There were no known tick exposures. The patient lived with his mother and three brothers. The only ill contact was his mother, who had a sore throat.

III. Physical Examination

T, 39°C; RR, 20/min (ventilator rate); HR, 110 bpm; BP, 110/70 mm Hg

On examination, the patient was intubated and sedated. There were multiple 1- to 2-cm submandibular lymph nodes and generalized swelling of the neck and face. There was no hepatosplenomegaly. The scrotum and extremities were very edematous. A Foley catheter was in place. There were no splinter hemorrhages or subcutaneous nodules on the extremities. There were a few scattered petechiae on the trunk.

IV. Diagnostic Studies

The WBC count was 25,600 cells/mm³, with 31% band forms, 50% segmented neutrophils, and 16% lymphocytes. The hemoglobin was normal, but the platelet count was 33,000/mm³. Serum electrolyte values were consistent with mild acute renal failure. ALT and AST were 99 and 81 U/L, respectively. The prothrombin time and partial thromboplastin time were mildly prolonged.

V.   Course of Illness

The constellation of pharyngitis, neck pain, and clinical deterioration accompanied by face and neck swelling suggested a likely cause.

DISCUSSION: CASE 13-6

I. Differential Diagnosis

This case was remarkable in that what started as a simple febrile illness with generalized adenopathy and neck swelling rapidly advanced to pneumonia, pneumothoracic pleural effusion, and respiratory failure. One of the initial questions in the evaluation of any neck mass should be, "Is there evidence for airway compromise?" In this case, the pursuit of the answer to that question and the rapid deterioration of the patient led to the appropriate diagnosis. In assessing neck swelling, it may be important to assess other sites in the pulmonary system, including airways and lungs. At the beginning of the course in this patient, the differential diagnosis included streptococcal pharyngitis, mononucleosis, adenovirus, CMV, and other mononucleosis-like virus illnesses. As the process advanced and as a pulmonary component was identified, infection with other organisms, both viral and bacterial (aerobic and anaerobic), were considered. The presence of pleural fluid prompted its analysis to identify the organism. *Fusobacterium varium* was eventually isolated.

II. Diagnosis

A *Fusobacterium* species was isolated from the pleural fluid, suggesting the diagnosis of septic thrombophlebitis of the internal jugular vein (Lemierre's syndrome). *Fusobacterium* species are generally susceptible to penicillin. However, given the severity of this patient's disease and the inability to obtain good visualization of the posterior pharynx or axial imaging at the time, coverage for polymicrobial infection was started. In addition, progressive Lemierre's disease can involve both the mediastinum and the carotid artery, possibly leading to septic emboli, including septic brain emboli. Metronidazole was continued to provide central nervous system and anaerobic coverage.

The diagnosis is Lemierre's syndrome. This syndrome includes acute tonsillopharyngeal adenopathy, neck pain, fever, and the development of supportive thrombophlebitis of the internal jugular vein. Neck swelling may be moderate to more severe and may be accompanied by severe neck pain. The organism that causes this syndrome is *Fusobacterium,* a gram-negative anaerobic organism that normally inhabits the oral cavity. Lemierre's syndrome is also called postanginal septicemia.

III. Incidence and Epidemiology

This is a rare condition that appears in only isolated case reports in the literature. The condition occurs in adolescents and young adults.

IV. Clinical Manifestations

The infection begins as a simple tonsillopharyngeal infection and then advances. Neck swelling and pain are localized to enlarged submandibular nodes at first and then become more generalized. The course often evolves to pulmonary involvement. Septic emboli may develop and may be showered to other body sites, causing symptoms in the central nervous system and elsewhere. In the past, the syndrome was uniformly fatal. However, with early detection by CT scanning and aggressive antibiotic therapy, good results have been reported.

V. Diagnostic Approach

If the specific origin of neck swelling cannot be determined, CT scanning or magnetic resonance imaging of the neck is indicated to determine the location and nature of the swelling. In Lemierre's syndrome, the finding of suppurative thrombophlebitis is central to the diagnosis. Recovery of the *Fusobacterium* isolate from abscess drainage or from pleural fluid confirms the diagnosis.

VI. Treatment

Treatment includes the use of broad-spectrum antibiotics and at times surgical drainage of the phlebitis. Treatment may need to be prolonged over several weeks. Anticoagulation therapy has also been used in some cases. There have not been any large case series or clinical trials to determine the best course of therapy.

VII. References

1. Alvarez A, Schreiber JR. Lemierre's syndrome in adolescent children: anaerobic sepsis with internal jugular vein thrombophlebitis following pharyngitis. *Pediatrics* 1995; 96:354–359.
2. Weesner CL, Cisek JE. Lemierre syndrome: the forgotten disease. *Ann Emerg Med* 1993;22:256–258.
3. Moreno S, Garcia AJ, Pinilla B, et al. Lemierre's disease: postanginal bacteremia and pulmonary involvement caused by *Fusobacterium necrophorum. Rev Infect Dis* 1989; 11:319–324.
4. DeSena S, Rosenfeld DL, Santos S, et al. Jugular thrombophlebitis complicating bacterial pharyngitis (Lemierre's syndrome). *Pediatr Radiol* 1996;26:141–144.
5. Sinave CP, Hardy GJ, Fardy PW. The Lemierre syndrome: suppurative thrombophlebitis of the internal jugular vein secondary to oropharyngeal infection. *Medicine (Baltimore)* 1989;68:85–94.

14

Chest Pain

Debra Boyer

APPROACH TO THE PATIENT WITH CHEST PAIN

I. Definition of the Complaint

Chest pain is a relatively common complaint in children, with a frequency of 6 per 1,000 outpatient visits. It occurs equally in boys and girls, with a median age at presentation of 12 years. Traumatic causes occur more often in boys, and costochondritis and psychogenic causes are diagnosed more frequently in girls. The most common causes of chest pain in children are generally benign, but this complaint causes much anxiety among parents and patients due to concern for a cardiac etiology (Table 14-1).

In understanding the multiple causes for chest pain, one must consider the various innervation patterns that occur throughout the chest. As an example, musculoskeletal pain is transmitted via intercostal nerves, whereas the vagus nerve innervates the large bronchi and trachea. Pain fibers from the parietal pleura travel via intercostal nerves, and the visceral pleura lacks pain fibers. Diaphragmatic disease also is transmitted through intercostal fibers and therefore can cause referred pain in the chest wall. The pericardium has multiple innervations, including the phrenic, vagal, and recurrent laryngeal nerves, as well as the esophageal plexus. Therefore, pericardial disease can manifest with diverse sensations and can be difficult to diagnose. Finally, cardiac pain itself transmits via the thoracic sympathetic chain and other cardiac nerves. In summary, "chest pain" is a very general term that can describe a variety of symptoms and causes. Only by a very careful history and physical examination can one accurately determine the cause of the patient's discomfort.

II. Complaint by Cause and Frequency

Causes of chest pain in children can be separated on the basis of patient age (Table 14-2) or etiology (Table 14-3). Chest pain is classified as idiopathic in 23% to 45% of cases. Children younger than 12 years of age are more likely to have a cardiac or respiratory etiology, whereas children older than 12 years of age more often have psychogenic causes for their chest pain. Furthermore, this is often a chronic complaint, with 20% of patients having chest pain for longer than 3 years.

III. Clarifying Questions

A complete history and physical examination will often reveal the diagnosis in a patient with chest pain. It is essential to have the patient describe the pain in detail: time

TABLE 14-1. *Common Causes of Chest Pain in Children*

Musculoskeletal	Asthma
Cough	Psychogenic
Pneumonia	Costochondritis
Idiopathic	Gastroesophageal reflux

TABLE 14-2. *Causes of Chest Pain in Childhood by Age*

Disease prevalence	School age	Adolescent

Common	Idiopathic
	Cough
	Asthma
	Pneumonia
	Musculoskeletal causes
	   Muscle strain
	   Trauma
	   Costochondritis
		Idiopathic
		Psychogenic
		Cough
		Asthma
		Musculoskeletal causes
		   Muscle strain
		   Trauma
		   Costochondritis
		Pneumonia

Less common	Gastroesophageal reflux Pneumothorax Pneumomediastinum Pleural effusion	Trauma Cocaine/tobacco use Methamphetamine use Gastroesophageal reflux Pleural effusion Pneumothorax Pneumomediastinum Gynecomastia Pubertal breast development Fibrocystic breast disease

Rare	Cardiovascular
	   Structural (aortic/pulmonic stenosis, hypertrophic cardiomyopathy, mitral valve prolapse)
	   Coronary artery disease (anomalous coronary artery, Kawasaki disease, long-standing diabetes mellitus)
	   Congenital heart disease
	   Myocarditis
	   Pericarditis
	   Arrhythmias
	Sickle cell disease
	Pulmonary embolism
	Esophageal foreign body
	Pleurodynia (coxsackievirus)
	Tietze's syndrome
	Slipping rib syndrome
	Precordial catch syndrome
	Peptic ulcer disease
		Cardiovascular
		   Structural (aortic/pulmonic stenosis, hypertrophic cardiomyopathy, mitral valve prolapse)
		   Coronary artery disease (anomalous coronary artery, Kawasaki disease, long-standing diabetes mellitus)
		   Congenital heart disease
		   Myocarditis
		   Pericarditis
		   Arrhythmias
		Sickle cell disease
		Pulmonary embolism
		Esophageal foreign body
		Pleurodynia (coxsackievirus)
		Tietze's syndrome
		Slipping rib syndrome
		Precordial catch syndrome
		Fitz-Hugh–Curtis syndrome
		Shingles
		Chest wall tumors
		Cholecystitis
		Pancreatitis
		Abdominal aortic aneurysm
		Peptic ulcer disease

of onset, duration, frequency, intensity, location, radiation, and precipitating and relieving factors. The patient's activity at the time of diagnosis can often provide valuable information. The following questions may provide clues to the diagnosis.

• Is the chest pain associated with exertion, syncope, or palpitations?

— Chest pain that is associated with exertion, syncope, or palpitations is more concerning for cardiopulmonary disease and warrants further investigation. With exercise, coronary artery blood flow is decreased; therefore, disease states with abnor-

TABLE 14-3. *Causes of Chest Pain in Childhood by Etiology*

Category	Causes
Musculoskeletal	Muscle strain
	Costochondritis
	Cough
	Tietze's syndrome
	Slipping rib syndrome
	Precordial catch syndrome
	Pleurodynia
	Trauma
Pulmonary	Asthma
	Pneumothorax/pneumomediastinum
	Pneumonia
	Pleural effusion
	Pulmonary embolism
Gastrointestinal	Gastroesophageal reflux
	Esophageal foreign body
	Peptic ulcer disease
	Cholecystitis
	Pancreatitis
	Fitz-Hugh–Curtis syndrome
Cardiac	Structural
	Aortic/pulmonic stenosis
	Hypertrophic cardiomyopathy
	Mitral valve prolapse
	Coronary artery disease
	Anomalous coronary artery
	Kawasaki disease
	Long-standing diabetes mellitus
	Myocarditis
	Pericarditis
	Arrhythmias
	Supraventricular tachycardia
	Ventricular tachycardia
Psychiatric	Hyperventilation
	Conversion reaction
Miscellaneous	Sickle cell disease
	Abdominal aortic aneurysm (Marfan syndrome/Ehlers-Danlos syndrome)
	Cocaine, tobacco, methamphetamine use
	Breast
	Gynecomastia
	Fibrocystic disease
	Adolescent breast development
Idiopathic	

mal coronary arteries often manifest symptoms at this time. In some cases, syncope may also occur. Palpitations may indicate an underlying arrhythmia such as supraventricular tachycardia or ventricular tachycardia.

- What is the duration of the pain?

  — Pain caused by myocardial ischemia usually lasts for less than 1 hour. In contrast, chest pain from a noncardiac origin may last for hours.

- Is there a family history of sudden death?

  — Hypertrophic cardiomyopathy is inherited in an autosomal dominant fashion, so there may be a family history of sudden death. These patients may have a murmur that is augmented with standing or with Valsalva maneuver. Furthermore, chest pain in these patients may be most severe with exercise. Similarly, in congenital hyperlipidemia, patients may present at a young age with myocardial infarction and may have a family history of sudden death.

- Is the pain relieved with changes in position?

  — Patients with pericarditis often have precordial pain with radiation to the left shoulder. The pain is worse while lying down and is improved with sitting and leaning forward.

- Is there a history of precipitating trauma?

  — In the trauma patient, tachycardia and hypotension may be secondary to a hemothorax or other vascular injury. In patients with poor perfusion and decreased cardiac output, myocardial contusion, tension pneumothorax, and cardiac tamponade should be considered.

- Is there a prior history of cardiorespiratory disease?

  — Patients with a history of asthma, cystic fibrosis, or a connective tissue disorder have an increased risk of pneumothorax and pneumomediastinum.

- Can the pain be reproduced on physical examination?

  — Musculoskeletal pain usually can be elicited by palpation of the chest wall. Costochondritis, most commonly seen in teenage girls, is associated with palpable pain over the rib cartilage. Muscle strain usually results in palpable pain over the affected muscle.

- Is the child taking any medications?

  — Oral contraceptives increase the risk of pulmonary embolism. Steroids and nonsteroidal antiinflammatory medications (NSAIDs) increase the risk for gastritis.

- Does the pain relate to meals?

  — Chest pain caused by gastroesophageal reflux commonly occurs after meals. Medication trials may be helpful to confirm the diagnosis.

- Have there been any recent stressors in the patient's life?

  — Psychogenic chest pain may occur in patients with recent major stressful events in their lives. These patients often have multiple somatic complaints in addition to chest pain. A family history of depression or a somatization disorder increases the likelihood that a child will develop psychogenic pain.

- Does the pain wake the child from sleep?

  — Children who awake from sleep secondary to chest pain are more likely to have an organic cause of their pain.

- Is there a history of substance use or abuse?

  — Tobacco use may be associated with a chronic cough and chest pain. Cocaine and methamphetamine abuse may lead to coronary artery vasospasm and ischemic chest pain.

IV. References

1. Chest pain. In: Tunnessen WW, ed. *Signs and symptoms in pediatrics.* Philadelphia: Lippincott Williams & Wilkins, 1999:361–369.
2. Kocis KC. Chest pain in pediatrics. *Pediatr Clin North Am* 1999;46:189–203.
3. Leung AKC, Robson WLM, Cho H. Chest pain in children. *Can Fam Physician* 1996; 42:1156–1164.
4. Patterson MD, Ruddy RM. Pain—chest. In: Fleisher GR, Ludwig S, eds. *Textbook of pediatric emergency medicine.* Philadelphia: Lippincott Williams & Wilkins, 2000: 435–440.
5. Rosenstein BJ. Chest. In: Hoekelman RA, Friedman SB, Nelson NM, et al., eds. *Primary pediatric care.* St. Louis: Mosby, 1997:888–890.
6. Selbst SM. Chest pain in children. *Pediatr Rev* 1997;18:169–173.

The following cases represent less common causes of chest pain in childhood.

Case 14-1: 17-Year-Old Boy

I. History of Present Illness

A 17-year-old boy was in good health until 3 days before his admission. At that time, he fell playing basketball and noted some pain in his right thigh. He also began to complain of shortness of breath and chest discomfort when lying flat. He denied fever, rash, joint pains, and cough.

II. Past Medical History

Bilateral inguinal hernia repairs were performed in infancy, but he had had no other hospitalizations. He was not taking any medications. A paternal uncle required renal transplantation at 43 years of age for an unknown diagnosis. A maternal grandmother had systemic lupus erythematosus (SLE).

III. Physical Examination

T, 37.2°C; RR, 20/min; HR, 92 bpm; BP 151/66 mm Hg; SpO$_2$, 100% in room air
Weight, 50th percentile; height, 75th percentile

Initial examination revealed a teenage boy who was awake and alert and in no respiratory distress. His chest examination demonstrated decreased breath sounds at the right base. No wheezes or rales were noted. His cardiac examination was significant for slightly diminished heart sounds but no murmurs or rubs. His right thigh was swollen, with a circumference 6 cm greater than the left thigh. He also had swelling of his right calf, which was 2 cm greater in circumference than the left calf. Flexion of the right knee was limited, and there was mild calf pain with dorsiflexion of the right foot. The remainder of his physical examination was normal.

IV. Diagnostic Studies

Laboratory analysis revealed a peripheral blood count with 6,000 white blood cells (WBCs)/mm^3, including 79% segmented neutrophils and 14% lymphocytes. The hemoglobin was 12.9 g/dL, and the platelet count was 156,000/mm^3. The erythrocyte sedimentation rate was elevated at 101 mm/hour. Prothrombin and partial thromboplastin times were 13.6 and 31.9 seconds, respectively. Urinalysis revealed large blood and 3+ protein. A Doppler ultrasound study of the right lower extremity revealed a thrombus extending from the superficial femoral vein to the calf vein.

V. Course of Illness

The patient was admitted and treated with intravenous heparin at 20 units/kg per hour for his deep vein thrombosis (DVT) and with furosemide for his hypertension. A chest roentgenogram in conjunction with further laboratory work suggested an underlying condition that predisposed to this presentation (Fig. 14-1).

DISCUSSION: CASE 14-1

I. Differential Diagnosis

As mentioned previously, chest pain in children and adolescents is rarely life-threatening. The majority of cases of chest pain in these age groups are classified as idiopathic. Among adolescents, the most common nonidiopathic causes are psychogenic origin, cough, asthma, pneumonia, and musculoskeletal pain. Less common causes include trauma, drug use or abuse, gastroesophageal reflux, and pneumothorax. Cardiac causes are exceedingly uncommon but should be considered in certain clinical situations, such as a patient with syncope and exertional or positional symptoms.

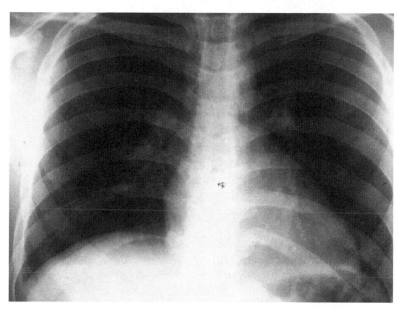

FIG. 14-1. Chest radiograph (case 14-1).

This patient had many physical and laboratory findings that warranted further evaluation. The two most worrisome findings were his chest pain when supine and his DVT. Shortness of breath and chest pain that worsen with supine lying suggest possible pericardial disease. The development of DVT in an otherwise healthy adolescent is extremely uncommon. In this situation, one should suspect underlying hypercoagulation disorders. Finally, this DVT in conjunction with shortness of breath and chest pain suggested pulmonary embolus as a possible diagnosis.

II. Diagnosis

The chest roentgenogram revealed blunting of the right costophrenic angle, suggesting a small right pleural effusion, and cardiomegaly (Fig. 14-1). An echocardiogram demonstrated a small to moderate-sized pericardial effusion that accounted for the finding of cardiomegaly on the chest radiograph. A ventilation-perfusion (VQ) scan suggested a low probability of pulmonary embolus.

As his hospitalization progressed, his hemoglobin dropped acutely to 10.3 g/dL and Coombs positive warm antibodies were demonstrated. A 24-hour urine collection demonstrated 8.5g protein per day. The antinuclear antibody (ANA) titer was elevated at 1:1,280, and complement C3 and C4 concentrations were decreased. Autoantibody studies were positive including anti-Smith, anti-RNP, anti-SSA, anti-SSB, anti-SCL 70 and anti-JO 30. As part of his hypercoagulation workup, he was found to have anti-cardiolipin antibodies and anti-phospholipid antibodies.

These laboratory values along with his clinical picture suggested the underlying diagnosis of SLE. He was treated with prednisone for his nephritis. After a period of time, his anticoagulation regimen was changed to low-molecular-weight heparin, and he was discharged home on the 10th day of hospitalization.

III. Incidence and epidemiology

SLE is a multisystemic autoimmune disorder that can manifest in children and adolescents. Determining the incidence of SLE in children is difficult with minimal data.

However, national registries in Canada and Finland have suggested a mean annual incidence of 0.36 per 100,000 and 0.37 per 100,000 population, respectively. Studies in the United States have suggested an annual incidence of 0.53 to 0.60 per 100,000 population.

SLE rarely develops before the age of 5 years and most often has its onset during adolescence. Girls are more commonly affected than boys, with a ratio of approximately 5:1. There is a suggestion of a higher incidence in African-Americans, followed by Hispanic children and adolescents.

IV.   Clinical Presentation

SLE has a quite variable presentation, and children often have more severe presentations than adults do. The most common presenting signs and symptoms are fever, arthralgias or arthritis, rashes, lymphadenopathy, hepatosplenomegaly, malaise, and weight loss. However, almost all organ systems have the potential for involvement.

Constitutional symptoms are common at diagnosis and with disease flares. Cutaneous findings may include the classic butterfly rash, discoid rash, or even mucosal ulcerations. Arthralgias and arthritis, as well as aseptic necrosis of the femoral head, may occur. Classic cardiac findings can include pericarditis, pericardial effusions, myocarditis, and Libman-Sacks endocarditis. Pulmonary manifestations occur in approximately 50% of patients. Both pleural and parenchymal involvement can occur, with pleuritis and pneumonitis most often seen. Neurologic findings include seizures, psychosis, cerebrovascular accidents, peripheral neuropathies, and pseudotumor cerebri. Ocular findings includes papilledema and retinopathy. From a hematologic standpoint, patients with SLE are at a higher risk for development of the anti-phospholipid syndrome, placing them at high risk for thromboembolic events. Finally, renal disease is also common, with the development of glomerulonephritis, nephrotic syndrome, and hypertension. These renal manifestations are probably the major prognostic factor in patients with SLE.

V.   Diagnostic Approach

With such a variable presentation, attempts have been made to provide criteria for the diagnosis of SLE. The most recent revision by the American College of Rheumatology (1997) included the following criteria for SLE:

- Malar (butterfly) rash
- Discoid-lupus rash
- Photosensitivity
- Oral or nasal mucocutaneous ulcerations
- Nonerosive arthritis
- Nephritis
  - Proteinuria >0.5 g/24 hr
  - Cellular casts
- Encephalopathy
  - Seizures
  - Psychosis
- Pleuritis or pericarditis
- Cytopenia
- Positive immunoserology
  - Antibodies to dsDNA
  - Antibodies to Sm nuclear antigen
  - Positive finding of antiphospholipid antibodies based on:
    (a) Immunoglobulin G (IgG) or IgM anti-cardiolipin antibodies, or
    (b) Lupus anticoagulant, or

(c) False-positive serologic test for syphilis for at least 6 months, confirmed by *Treponema pallidum* immobilization or fluorescent treponemal antibody absorption test
- Positive ANA test

In general, patients with a minimum of 4 of the 11 are diagnosed with SLE. In childhood, these criteria have a sensitivity of 96% and a specificity of 100% for diagnosis of SLE.

Acute phase reactants. Most acute phase reactants, including erythrocyte sedimentation rate and serum ferritin levels, are elevated in lupus exacerbations. There is also a hypergammaglobulinemia.

Hematologic studies. Approximately 50% of children with SLE have anemia of chronic disease. Other findings include an acute hemolytic anemia, leukopenia, and thrombocytopenia. As mentioned previously, a high proportion of SLE patients have a hypercoagulable state, with the presence of anti-phospholipid antibodies.

Autoantibodies. The majority of SLE patients have detectable ANAs. The ANAs that can be seen in SLE include anti-dsDNA, anti-DNP, anti-Ro (SS/A), anti-La (SS/B), anti-Sm and anti-histone antibodies. Various other autoantibodies include anti-erythrocyte, anti-lymphocytotoxic, anti-tissue-specific, and anti-phospholipid antibodies, as well as rheumatoid factors. In terms of diagnosis, antibodies against dsDNA are considered pathognomonic of SLE.

Complement levels. Decreased complement levels are particular indicators of active disease in SLE. One can measure either complement components C3 and C4 or total hemolytic complement, as measured by the ability of a test sample to hemolyze 50% of antibody-coated erythrocytes (CH_{50}).

Urinalysis. The most common abnormality on urinalysis in SLE is proteinuria. Hematuria and red blood cell casts also occur. Further tests to evaluate for lupus nephritis include creatinine clearance, glomerular filtration rate studies, renal ultrasonography, and biopsy.

VI.   Treatment

There is no standard protocol to treat patients with SLE, because each child has a unique presentation. The primary goal is to prevent exacerbations, rather than to treat each flare episodically. Certain recommendations are universal, including the need to avoid exposure to excessive sunlight.

A variety of pharmacologic agents are available to treat symptoms of SLE. NSAIDs are typically used for the treatment of musculoskeletal complaints. Patients with anti-cardiolipin antibodies often receive low-dose aspirin to decrease the risk of thromboembolism. Hydroxychloroquine can be very effective in conjunction with glucocorticoids to minimize disease exacerbations. However, these agents may not always be effective in controlling the disease, and other immunosuppressive agents, such as azathioprine, cyclophosphamide, and methotrexate, may be needed.

VII.   References

1. Lawrence EC. Systemic lupus erythematosus and the lung. In: Lahita RG, ed. *Systemic lupus erythematosus.* New York: John Wiley and Sons, 1987:691–708.
2. Petty RE, Cassidy JT. Systemic lupus erythematosus. In: Cassidy JT, Petty RE, eds. *Textbook of pediatric rheumatology,* 4th ed. Philadelphia: WB Saunders, 2001: 396–438.
3. Tucker LB. Caring for the adolescent with systemic lupus erythematosus. *Adolesc Med* 1998;9:59–67.

Case 14-2: 15-Year-Old Boy

I. History of Present Illness

A 15-year-old boy was well until 1 week before presentation. At that time, he developed the acute onset of chest pain accompanied by fever and chills. He described the pain as sharp and intermittent. It was midsternal and did not radiate. The pain did not increase with exertion but was worse while lying supine or with subtle movement. He denied any syncope, shortness of breath, or diaphoresis. He did not have night sweats, cough, or weight loss.

II. Past Medical History

He had no significant past medical history. He had emigrated from Liberia 6 weeks before his presentation. He had received bacille Calmette-Guérin immunization 5 years earlier and was noted to have a 12-mm induration after tuberculin PPD (purified protein derivative) skin testing on arrival in the United States.

III. Physical Examination

T, 36.8°C; RR, 24/min; HR, 80 bpm; BP, 111/64 mm Hg

Weight, 25th to 50th percentile

In general, he was a thin adolescent boy in no acute distress. His cardiac examination revealed normal first and second heart sounds (S1 and S2, respectively), with a regular rate and rhythm. No cardiac murmur was appreciated. His chest examination demonstrated clear breath sounds bilaterally. The liver edge was minimally palpated just below the right costal margin. The remainder of his physical examination was within normal limits.

IV. Diagnostic Studies

The complete blood count revealed 6,800 WBCs/mm^3. The hemoglobin was 12.8 g/dL, and the platelet count was 426,000/mm^3. Serum electrolytes, blood urea nitrogen, and creatinine were normal. Calcium, albumin, AST, alkaline phosphatase, total bilirubin, and prothrombin and partial thromboplastin times were also normal. Lactate dehydrogenase was elevated at 904 U/L. A chest roentgenogram was initially interpreted as normal.

V. Course of Illness

The patient was discharged home with ibuprofen for his chest pain. The chest roentgenogram was reviewed the following day, and the revised interpretation indicated cardiomegaly, suggesting a diagnostic category for his chest pain. Computed tomography (CT) of the chest and abdomen also revealed bilateral nodular pulmonary infiltrates and splenomegaly. The specific cause of his chest pain was determined by pericardial biopsy.

DISCUSSION: CASE 14-2

I. Differential Diagnosis

Chest pain in an adolescent boy is rarely life-threatening. However, a careful history and physical examination must be undertaken to determine which cases require further investigations.

The majority of cases of chest pain in childhood are classified as idiopathic. Adolescents are more likely to have psychogenic causes for their chest pain than younger children, with this diagnosis being more common in girls. Musculoskeletal causes are quite common, including muscle strain, trauma, and costochondritis. Other common causes are cough, asthma, and pneumonia. Less commonly, chest pain in adolescents is caused by gastroesophageal reflux, pneumothorax, pneumomediastinum, or pleural effusion. In an adolescent with chest pain, it is important to inquire about tobacco, cocaine, and methamphetamine use, all of which can be associated with chest pain. In adolescent girls, one should consider pubertal breast development or fibrocystic breast disease, and in boys, gynecomastia. Rarely, but importantly, one should consider cardiovascular causes of chest pain, including structural diseases (e.g., idiopathic hypertrophic cardiomyopathy), coronary artery disease, myocarditis, pericarditis, and arrhythmias.

The features of this case that warrant further evaluation include the acute onset of the chest pain and the variability with positional changes.

II. Diagnosis

The chest roentgenogram revealed cardiomegaly. An echocardiogram demonstrated a 10-mm circumferential pericardial effusion with nodular areas noted alongside the myocardial surface. Electrocardiography (ECG) revealed ST elevation. A repeat PPD test demonstrated a 19-mm area of induration. The patient underwent pericardial window placement with pericardial biopsy. Stains of pericardial fluid were negative for acid-fast bacilli, but microscopic examination of the pericardial tissue revealed numerous granulomas, and acid-fast smear of the tissue demonstrated organisms. *Mycobacterium tuberculosis* was detected from culture of the pericardial tissue 12 days after inoculation. **The diagnosis is tuberculous pericarditis.** He was treated with isoniazid, rifampin, pyrazinamide, and ethambutol.

Sputum was acid-fast stain and acid-fast culture negative. His family refused human immunodeficiency virus (HIV) testing. He was ultimately discharged home to complete his treatment under directly observed therapy.

III. Incidence and Epidemiology

M. tuberculosis infections are the most frequent cause of deaths worldwide from a single infectious organism. Approximately one third of the world's population has been infected with *M. tuberculosis*. Usually, infection occurs through inhalation of droplet nuclei and causes pulmonary infections. The HIV epidemic has significantly increased the infection rate worldwide.

Pericarditis may result from infectious or noninfectious causes (Table 14-4). Pericarditis, an uncommon complication of tuberculosis infection, can be fatal even with

TABLE 14-4. *Most Common Causes of Pericarditis*

Category	Causes	Category	Causes
Infectious		Noninfectious	
Bacteria	Streptococcus pneumoniae	Cardiac injury	Acute myocardial infarction
	Staphylococcus aureus		Blunt or penetrating trauma
	Neisseria meningitidis		Irradiation
	Haemophilus influenzae	Malignancy	Primary
	Mycobacterium tuberculosis		Metastatic
	Peptostreptococcus species	Collagen	Systemic lupus erythematosus
	Prevotella species	vascular	Rheumatic fever
Viruses	Coxsackieviruses	disease	
	Echoviruses	Drug-induced	
	Adenovirus	Idiopathic	
	Influenza		
	Epstein-Barr virus		
Fungi	Histoplasma capsulatum		
	Cryptococcus neoformans		
	Candida albicans		
Parasites	Toxoplasma gondii		
	Entamoeba histolytica		

proper diagnosis and treatment. Tuberculous pericarditis occurs by extension of an adjacent focus of infection, such as mediastinal or hilar nodes, lung, spine, or sternum. It occurs less commonly in association with miliary tuberculosis.

Tuberculous pericarditis is believed to occur in 0.4% to 4% of children with tuberculosis. The prevalence of tuberculosis varies by geographic region. Its relationship to HIV disease is well known. In many African countries where tuberculosis and HIV are endemic, pericarditis in an HIV-positive patient is considered to be tuberculosis until proved otherwise.

IV.　Clinical Presentation

The presentation of pericarditis varies depending on the cause. The pain associated with pericarditis is often retrosternal, radiating to the shoulder and neck. The pain is typically worsened by deep breathing, swallowing, and supine positioning. Tuberculous pericarditis can have both acute and insidious presentations. The most common symptoms are cough, dyspnea, and chest pain. Other associated symptoms include night sweats, orthopnea, weight loss, and edema. Physical examination may reveal fever, tachycardia, and pericardial rub. Pulsus paradoxus, hepatomegaly, pleural effusions, and muffled heart sounds are often associated with the condition.

V.　Diagnostic Approach

The diagnosis of pericarditis is straightforward, but establishing *M. tuberculosis* as the etiologic agent is more challenging.

Tuberculin skin test. A positive skin test increases the suspicion for tuberculous pericarditis, but a negative skin test does not eliminate the diagnosis.

Chest roentgenogram. Chest radiography reveals cardiomegaly due to pericarditis and pericardial effusions. Approximately 40% of patients with tuberculous pericarditis have an associated pleural effusion. Patients with tuberculous pericarditis may also have findings suggestive of pulmonary or miliary tuberculosis.

Electrocardiogram. The ECG is abnormal in most cases of pericarditis, reflecting pericardial inflammation. ST-segment elevations develop early in the illness. Large pericardial effusions are associated with reduced QRS voltage.

Echocardiogram. Echocardiography detects associated pericardial effusions and pericardial thickening. Patients with tuberculous pericarditis may have nodular densities along the pericardium.

Pericardiocentesis and pericardial biopsy. Acid-fast stains of pericardial fluid are often negative, but pericardial fluid cultures are positive for *M. tuberculosis* in approximately 50% of cases. Polymerase chain reaction testing to detect *M. tuberculosis* has been attempted, but the reliability of this test in pericardial fluid specimens is not clear. Granulomas detected on microscopic examination of pericardial tissue strongly suggest the diagnosis of tuberculous pericarditis. Pericardial tissue is usually acid-fast stain and culture positive and is considered critical to confirming the diagnosis. The most accurate results are obtained if the pericardial tissue sample is acquired before the start of antituberculosis therapy.

Human immunodeficiency virus test. Due to the close association between HIV and tuberculous pericarditis, HIV testing should be performed in all patients diagnosed with tuberculous pericarditis.

VI.　Treatment

If the patient has hemodynamic compromise, pericardiocentesis is indicated. Certainly, in cases of tamponade this is necessary. A second option for drainage is an open surgical procedure, which allows for removal of the pericardial fluid as well as obtaining pericardial tissue for culture and histopathologic studies. Controversy does exist as to whether pericardiocentesis or open drainage should be the procedure of choice in uncomplicated cases of suspected tuberculous pericarditis. Either way, one must strive to prevent the formation of a constrictive pericarditis.

Antibiotic therapy consists of the same regimens as are prescribed for pulmonary tuberculosis. Adjuvant corticosteroid therapy appears to decrease the amount of effusion and reaccumulation of pericardial fluid, reducing the need for repeated interventions.

VII.   References

1. Dooley DP, Carpenter JL, Rademacher S. Adjunctive corticosteroid therapy for tuberculosis: a critical reappraisal of the literature. *Clin Infect Dis* 1997;25:872–877.
2. Gewitz MH, Vetter VL. Cardiac emergencies. In: Fleisher GR, Ludwig S, eds. *Textbook of pediatric emergency medicine,* 4th ed. Baltimore: Lippincott Williams & Wilkins, 2000:659–700.
3. Haas DW. *Mycobacterium tuberculosis.* In: Mandell GL, Bennett JE, Dolin R, eds. *Mandell, Douglas, and Bennett's principles and practice of infectious diseases,* 5th ed. Philadelphia: Churchill Livingstone, 2000:2576–2604.
4. Starke JR. Tuberculosis. In: McMillan JA, DeAngelis CD, Feigin RD, et al., eds. *Oski's pediatrics: principles and practice,* 3rd ed. Philadelphia: Lippincott Williams & Wilkins, 1999:1026–1039.
5. Trautner BW, Darouiche RO. Tuberculous pericarditis: optimal diagnosis and management. *Clin Infect Dis* 2001;33:954–961.

Case 14-3: 20-Year-Old Boy

I. History of Present Illness

A 20-year-old young man with a history of spina bifida presented to the emergency department. Six days earlier, he had reported fatigue and was unable to leave his house. Over the next few days, he had developed a fever, sore throat, and myalgias. Two days before admission, he had noted increasing shortness of breath, which was worse while lying supine. He described a "pounding" discomfort in his chest.

II. Past Medical History

He was born at full term and noted at birth to have a meningomyelocele. He had spina bifida at the L3 level and had surgical correction when he was 4 days old. A ventriculoperitoneal shunt was placed during the first weeks of life. Several shunt revisions had since been required due to obstruction; the last revision was 6 years earlier. Four months before admission, he was diagnosed with pelvic osteomyelitis related to extension of a gluteal ulcer. He was treated with surgical debridement and 3 months of intravenous antibiotics.

He had bilateral club feet. He was able to walk with a brace and had only mild mental retardation. He was not taking any medications. He had had a tattoo placed on his arm 2 weeks before admission. There was a family history of asthma in his mother, and his father died at age 40 years from a myocardial infarction.

III. Physical Examination

T, 41.3°C; RR, 20/min; HR, 138 bpm; BP, 113/80 mm Hg; SpO_2, 98% in room air

In general, he was an obese young man in moderate respiratory distress. His oropharyngeal examination revealed an exudative pharyngitis. His cardiac examination revealed a normal S1 and S2 with no murmur, rub, or gallop. His physical examination was otherwise unremarkable.

IV. Diagnostic Studies

The complete blood count revealed 13,500 WBCs/mm^3, with 42% segmented neutrophils, 26% lymphocytes, 18% atypical lymphocytes, and 1% monocytes. The hemoglobin was 11.3 g/dL, and platelets were 133,000/mm^3. Electrolytes, blood urea nitrogen, and glucose were within normal limits. The serum creatinine concentration was slightly elevated at 1.1 mg/dL. Total bilirubin was elevated at 4.0 mg/dL, with an unconjugated fraction of 2.3 mg/dL. Aspartate aminotransferase (AST) and alanine aminotransferase (ALT) were 246 and 130 U/L, respectively. The erythrocyte sedimentation rate was mildly elevated at 44 mm/hour. A chest roentgenogram revealed normal heart size and no pulmonary infiltrates.

V. Course of Illness

Before arrival at the hospital, the patient was given adenosine twice for heart rates greater than 160 bpm. This did not have any significant effect. On arrival in the emergency department, his chest pain resolved and his ECG abnormalities resolved. An echocardiogram demonstrated a shortening fraction of 28% and no wall motion abnormalities.

He was evaluated for a possible myocardial infarction, given his family history. His cardiac enzymes remained normal. He developed bilious emesis, which was believed to be secondary to his hepatitis. He had a repeat ECG (Fig. 14-2) and echocardiogram on arrival in the intensive care unit. The ECG suggested a diagnostic category, and the spe-

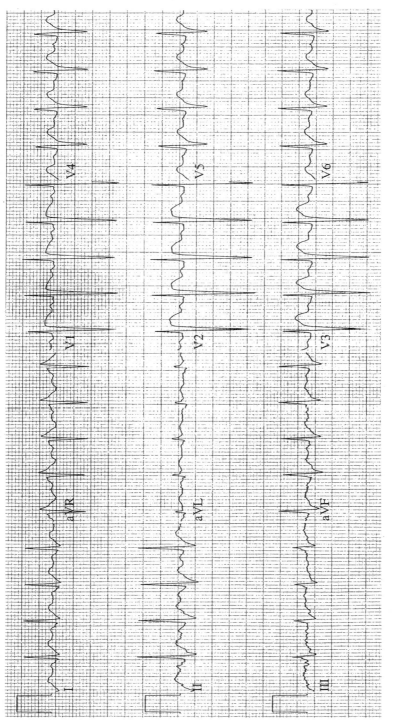

FIG. 14-2. Electrocardiogram (case 14-3).

cific cause was suggested by the initial laboratory testing and confirmed later by sero-logic testing.

DISCUSSION: CASE 14-3

I. Differential Diagnosis

As previously mentioned, the most common causes for chest pain in the adolescent age group are asthma, pneumonia, cough, musculoskeletal causes, psychogenic pain, and idiopathic causes.

The concerning factors in this patient were his positional shortness of breath, his family history of early myocardial infarction, and his abnormal ECG findings. On presentation, he was tachycardic and febrile. The acute nature of his symptoms and the positional nature of his respiratory symptoms should raise the concern for a possible cardiac etiology. Although cardiac causes are rare among all causes of chest pain, they can be the most life-threatening and must be evaluated.

Cardiac causes for chest pain include structural lesions such as aortic or pulmonic stenosis, idiopathic hypertrophic subaortic stenosis (IHSS), and mitral valve prolapse. Patients with IHSS often have a family history of sudden death. Coronary artery disease can also lead to chest pain and may be secondary to anomalous coronary arteries, Kawasaki disease, or long-standing diabetes mellitus. Patients with either corrected or uncorrected congenital heart disease may complain of chest pain, which must be carefully evaluated. Arrhythmias such as supraventricular tachycardia and ventricular tachycardia can also manifest with chest pain and palpitations. Finally, infectious causes such as myocarditis and pericarditis may manifest with chest pain.

II. Diagnosis

The repeat ECG revealed sinus tachycardia at 139 bpm with 2-mm ST-segment elevations in leads V2 and V3 (Fig. 14-2). Repeat echocardiogram revealed a left ventricular ejection fraction of 25% and dilated left and right ventricles. Cardiac catheterization revealed a left ventricle end-diastolic pressure of 16 mm Hg and a cardiac index of 4.4 L/min. The patient was believed to have myocarditis. Soon after admission, he developed congestive heart failure with respiratory distress, diaphoresis, somnolence, and hypotension. He was ultimately treated with dopamine and dobutamine. To help determine the cause of his myocarditis, Epstein-Barr virus (EBV) studies were requested. His Monospot test was positive. He also had hepatitis, thrombocytopenia, and an atypical lymphocytosis. The EBV viral capsid antigen (VCA) IgG was 1:640; early antigen (EA) IgG was 1:80; and Epstein-Barr nuclear antigen (EBNA) IgG was undetectable. **The diagnosis is EBV myocarditis.**

III. Incidence, Epidemiology, and Etiology

EBV is a member of the herpesvirus family. It is a relatively common infectious organism, causing a clinical syndrome of infectious mononucleosis. This syndrome is most frequently seen in adolescents and young adults. Males and females are affected equally, and 90% to 95% of all adults have evidence of past EBV infection. EBV is believed to have low contagiousness, and transmission generally requires intimate contact between individuals. For this reason, infectious mononucleosis has been termed, "the kissing disease."

The classic clinical syndrome consists of fever, sore throat, and adenopathy developing after an incubation period of 3 to 7 weeks. Most cases of EBV infection are self-limited, although rare complications are seen. These complications can be multisystemic and include hematologic, hepatorenal, splenic, dermatologic, immunologic, and cardiopulmonary symptoms.

Myocarditis in EBV infection is rare, with an incidence ranging from 0% to 6%. Viruses are the most common etiologic agents causing myocarditis. Aside from EBV, they include enterovirus (e.g., coxsackie B), adenovirus, cytomegalovirus, herpesvirus, influenza A, varicella, mumps, measles, parvovirus, respiratory syncytial virus (RSV), and HIV. Less commonly, other nonviral infectious agents, such as rickettsiae, bacteria, parasites, fungi, and yeasts, are responsible. Also rare are noninfectious causes such as drugs, hypersensitivity reactions, autoimmune diseases, Kawasaki disease, and sarcoidosis.

IV. Clinical Presentation

Newborns and infants with myocarditis may present with decreased appetite, fever, irritability, and diaphoresis. Sudden death occurs rarely in this age group. Infants with congestive heart failure may not have signs of jugular venous distention and rales on pulmonary examination.

Older children and adolescents typically provide a history of recent viral illness (approximately 2 weeks earlier). Similar to infants, these children exhibit lethargy, fever, and pallor. Diaphoresis, palpitations, rashes, and decreased exercise tolerance may also be present. Occasionally, they complain of abdominal pain. As the disease progresses, respiratory distress may become more prominent. With the development of congestive heart failure, the child may develop jugular venous distention and rales on examination. It is not uncommon for arrhythmias to develop, including supraventricular tachycardia and ventricular tachycardia.

V. Diagnostic Approach

Whenever a patient develops congestive heart failure or arrhythmias of unknown cause, myocarditis should be included in the differential diagnosis.

Chest roentgenogram. With myocarditis, the chest roentgenogram may reveal cardiomegaly with prominent vascular markings. This generally indicates pulmonary edema.

Electrocardiogram. Patients with myocarditis may develop sinus tachycardia with low-voltage QRS complexes. Inverted T waves may also be seen. Q waves and ST-segment elevation indicate myocardial infarction.

Echocardiogram. A dilated, poorly functional left ventricle is seen with myocarditis. This may be accompanied by pericardial effusion. Occasionally, other cardiac chambers are dilated as well.

Cardiac catheterization. This may indicate low cardiac output with elevated end-diastolic pressures. With the use of this procedure, one may obtain endomyocardial biopsies of the right ventricle. In myocarditis, a mononuclear cell infiltrate will be present. Because this procedure carries a relatively significant risk, it is not performed in all cases.

Complete blood count. With EBV infection, there is usually a lymphocytosis that peaks during the second or third week. Classically, the patient has more than 10% atypical lymphocytes. Neutropenia and thrombocytopenia are also seen. An anemia, usually of an autoimmune nature, may develop with EBV infection.

Monospot test. This tests for the presence of heterophile antibodies, which are found in approximately 90% of patients with EBV infection. The heterophile antibody test is often negative in children younger than 4 years of age.

Epstein-Barr virus-specific antibodies. Antibodies to VCA may be seen. VCA IgG antibodies develop rapidly and are present in acute and past infections. However, the presence of VCA IgM is considered diagnostic of acute EBV infection. One may also look for EA antibodies, but 30% of patients do not develop them. Antibodies to EBNA do not develop until late in the infection. The absence of EBNA in the presence of VCA IgG and EA indicates acute EBV infection.

Liver function tests. Most patients develop a hepatitis from an EBV infection, with elevated AST, ALT, and lactic dehydrogenase. Patients may also develop hyperbilirubinemia.

VI.   Treatment

Patients who present with myocarditis may have only mild symptoms of congestive heart failure. They can be monitored with no specific immediate intervention. It is not uncommon for bed rest to be prescribed, because this is thought to possibly decrease intramyocardial viral replication.

However, some patients have poor cardiac output and poor tissue perfusion. In these cases, digitalis and diuretics may be prescribed. One should also consider anticoagulation medications including aspirin, warfarin, and heparin to prevent thromboembolic disease.

With EBV myocarditis, some would advocate the use of steroids and even acyclovir. However, this combination has not been extensively studied, because the disease entity is relatively rare.

VII.   References

1. American Academy of Pediatrics. Epstein-Barr virus infections. In: Pickering LK, Peter G, Baker CJ, et al., eds. *2000 Red Book: Report by the Committee on Infectious Diseases,* 25th ed. Elk Grove Village, IL: American Academy of Pediatrics; 2000: 238–240.
2. Baykurt C, Caglar K, Ceviz N, et al. Successful treatment of Epstein-Barr infection associated with myocarditis. *Pediatr Int* 1999;41:389–391.
3. Graziano JN, Ludomirsky A, Goldberg CS. Acute myocardial ischemia in a healthy male child: an atypical presentation of acute Epstein-Barr virus infection. *Clin Pediatr* 2001;40:277–281.
4. Schooley RT. Epstein-Barr virus (infectious mononucleosis). In: Mandell GL, Bennett JE, Dolin R, eds. *Mandell, Douglas, and Bennett's principles and practice of infectious diseases,* 5th ed. Philadelphia: Churchill Livingstone, 2000:1599–1608.
5. Towbin JA. Myocarditis. In: Allen HD, Gutgesell HP, Clark EB, et al., eds. *Moss and Adams' heart disease in infants, children, and adolescents,* 6th ed. Philadelphia: Lippincott Williams & Wilkins, 2001:1197–1215.

Case 14-4: 17-Year-Old Boy

I. History of Present Illness

A 17-year old boy presented with left-sided chest pain. He was well until 8 days before presentation, when he developed left axillary and shoulder pain. The pain was worse with inspiration. He denied fever, nausea, vomiting, and diarrhea. He reported that he had had rhinorrhea and a dry cough 2 weeks earlier. He had mild shortness of breath with exercise. He had no history of trauma.

II. Past Medical History

He had a history of depression with no history of suicide attempts. He denied a history of asthma or other chronic illnesses. His family and social histories were noncontributory. He denied any drug use but did admit to having smoked cigarettes in the past.

III. Physical Examination

T, 36.6°C; RR, 18 to 20/min; HR, 108 bpm; BP, 120/60 mm Hg; SpO_2, 95% in room air
Weight, 50th to 75th percentile; height, 75th to 90th percentile

In general, he was in no acute respiratory distress. His chest examination revealed no chest wall deformity, and the chest was nontender to palpation. Breath sounds were decreased at the bases, left greater than right. No wheezes or rales were appreciated. His cardiac examination revealed normal S1 and S2, with no murmurs, rubs, or gallops heard. The remainder of his physical examination was normal.

IV. Diagnostic Studies

A complete blood count revealed 5,600 WBCs/mm^3, with 55% segmented neutrophils, 31% lymphocytes, 11% monocytes, and 3% eosinophils. Electrolytes were normal.

V. Course of Illness

A chest roentgenogram was considered diagnostic (Fig. 14-3).

DISCUSSION: CASE 14-4

I. Differential Diagnosis

The differential diagnosis for chest pain in this adolescent boy focused on the acute nature of his pain. In general, the most common causes for chest pain in the adolescent age group are psychogenic pain, cough, asthma, musculoskeletal pain, and pneumonia. These causes most often produce a subacute and subtle type of chest pain.

Therefore, the acute onset of chest pain in this boy should focus the differential diagnosis on a number of other causes. Certainly, tobacco use or the abuse of cocaine or methamphetamine could cause the acute onset of chest pain secondary to vasospasm of the coronary arteries. Pneumothorax or pneumomediastinum commonly manifest with the acute onset of chest pain. Some abdominal processes, such as pancreatitis or cholecystitis, may manifest with acute chest pain. Cardiovascular causes are less common but are life-threatening. With acute chest pain, one should consider coronary artery disease, arrhythmias, structural cardiac defects, and infections.

II. Diagnosis

A chest roentgenogram revealed a left pneumothorax (Fig. 14-3). **The diagnosis is left spontaneous pneumothorax.**

III. Incidence, Epidemiology and Pathophysiology

Pneumothoraces are divided into three groups: spontaneous, traumatic, and iatrogenic. Spontaneous pneumothoraces can be either primary, in which there is no underlying lung

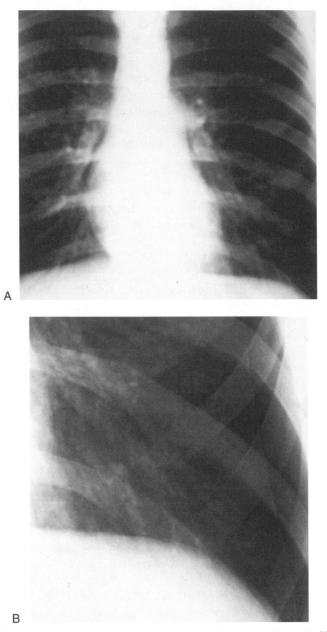

A

B

FIG. 14-3. Chest radiograph **(A)** and close-up view of chest radiograph **(B)** (case 14-4).

disease, or secondary, in which underlying lung pathology is present. The incidence of primary spontaneous pneumothorax ranges between 7.4 and 18 cases per 100,000 males and between 1.2 and 6 cases per 100,000 females. It is most common in tall, thin males between 10 and 30 years of age. Cigarette smoking increases the risk of developing a primary spontaneous pneumothorax in a dose-dependent fashion.

Secondary spontaneous pneumothoraces occur in patients with underlying lung disease. The major causes include airways disease (e.g., cystic fibrosis), infection (e.g.,

Pneumocystis carinii pneumonia), interstitial lung disease, connective tissue disease, malignancy, and thoracic endometriosis. The incidence of secondary spontaneous pneumothorax is 6.3 cases per 100,000 males and 2 cases per 100,000 females. Secondary spontaneous pneumothoraces have a later peak incidence, at 60 to 65 years of age.

Subpleural bullae are seen in 76% to 100% of children who are taken to video-assisted thoracoscopic surgery. There is some speculation as to the mechanism of bullae formation. It is likely that elastic fibers are degraded in the lung, which ultimately leads to an imbalance in the protease/antiprotease system and the development of bullae. A pneumothorax then develops as alveolar pressure increases and air subsequently leaks into the interstitium.

IV. Clinical Presentation

Primary spontaneous pneumothorax usually develops while the patient is at rest. Patients describe pleuritic ipsilateral chest pain and dyspnea. With a small pneumothorax, the physical examination may be completely normal. Tachycardia may be noted. In patients with a large pneumothorax, there may be poor chest wall movement, a hyperresonant chest, and decreased breath sounds on the side with the pneumothorax. Tachycardia and hypotension indicate that the patient has developed tension physiology and requires emergency intervention.

With a large pneumothorax, the patient develops decreased vital capacity and an increased alveolar–arterial oxygen gradient. In patients with primary spontaneous pneumothoraces, the underlying lung function is normal; therefore, they do not develop hypercapnia. In contrast, patients with secondary spontaneous pneumothoraces by definition have underlying lung disease and often develop hypercapnia.

V. Diagnostic Approach

Chest roentgenogram. A posterior-anterior chest roentgenogram reveals the presence of a pneumothorax. Small apical pneumothoraces may be difficult to detect in this fashion, and on occasion an expiratory roentgenogram is necessary.

Chest computed tomography. A chest CT scan may be necessary to differentiate a bulla from a pneumothorax.

VI. Treatment

A variety of treatment options exist for management of a pneumothorax, ranging from observation to simple aspiration with a catheter, chest tube insertion, pleurodesis, thoracoscopy with a single port, video-assisted thoracoscopic surgery, and thoracotomy.

Patients with small primary spontaneous pneumothoraces may be observed without intervention if there is no respiratory distress. They may be treated with supplemental oxygen to hasten the reabsorption of air. With supplemental oxygen, the air is reabsorbed at a rate of 2% per day. With larger primary spontaneous pneumothoraces, needle aspiration or chest tube insertion is required. Secondary spontaneous pneumothoraces are likely to require intervention, because patients are usually ill due to their underlying lung disease.

The main debate with spontaneous pneumothoraces is the ability to prevent recurrences. With a primary spontaneous pneumothorax, the recurrence rate is about 30%, and most recur 6 months to 2 years after the initial event. Smoking and younger age are risk factors for recurrent disease. The recurrence rate with secondary spontaneous pneumothoraces is similar at 39% to 47%.

The general consensus is to recommend preventative therapy after the second ipsilateral pneumothorax. However, patients who participate in risky activities such as scuba diving or flying should be considered for intervention after their first spontaneous pneumothorax. Options for recurrence prevention include the instillation of sclerosing agents through a chest tube and mechanical pleurodesis. With video-assisted thoracoscopic procedures, blebs can also be identified and oversewn.

VII.   References

1. Baumann MH, Strange C, Heffner JE, et al. Management of spontaneous pneumothorax: an American College of Chest Physicians Delphi Consensus Statement. *Chest* 2001;119:590–602.
2. Sahn SA, Heffner JE. Spontaneous pneumothorax. *N Engl J Med* 2000;342:868–874.
3. Weissberg D, Refaely Y. Pneumothorax: experience with 1,199 patients. *Chest* 2000; 117:1279–1285.
4. Montgomery M. Air and liquid in the pleural space. In: Chernick V, Boat TF, eds. *Kendig's disorders of the respiratory tract in children.* Philadelphia: WB Saunders, 1998:403–409.

Case 14-5: 3-Year-Old Girl

I. History of Present Illness

A 3-year old girl was brought to the emergency department crying and clutching her chest. She was extremely difficult to console. She had had poor oral intake over the previous day, with decreased urine output. On the evening of admission, she was found sitting in bed whimpering and holding her chest. She did not have a history of vomiting or diarrhea. Her temperature had not been measured, but she did not feel subjectively warm.

II. Past Medical History

She had been seen in the emergency department 3 weeks earlier, at which time she was diagnosed with viral stomatitis. Culture of the lesions grew herpes simplex virus I (HSV I), and the lesions had resolved since then. She had been taking only ibuprofen at home. The remainder of her past medical history was unremarkable.

III. Physical Examination

T, 38.2°C; RR, 30/min; HR, 130 bpm; BP, 98/60 mm Hg; SpO$_2$, 95% in room air
Weight, 75th to 90th percentile

In general, she was crying and difficult to examine, holding her chest with both arms. She was not in significant respiratory distress. Her chest examination revealed no apparent bony tenderness over her sternum or ribs. She had decreased aeration at the left base, with no wheezes or rales appreciated. Her eyes were slightly sunken and she had some crusty nasal discharge. Her lips and other mucous membranes were dry. The remainder of her physical examination was normal.

IV. Diagnostic Studies

The complete blood count revealed 19,000 WBCs/mm^3 (8% band forms, 81% segmented neutrophils, and 11% lymphocytes). The hemoglobin was 12.8 g/dL, and the platelet count was 402,000/mm^3. Electrolytes and liver function tests were normal.

V. Course of Illness

She was given a 40 mL/kg normal saline fluid bolus. She refused to drink and was given maintenance intravenous fluids. A chest roentgenogram revealed the diagnosis (Fig. 14-4).

DISCUSSION: CASE 14-5

I. Differential Diagnosis

As with adolescents, chest pain in the school age child is very rarely a life-threatening condition. Common causes of chest pain in this age group include cough, asthma, pneumonia, and musculoskeletal causes (muscle strain, trauma, costochondritis.) It is quite common as well for chest pain to be deemed idiopathic. Less commonly, a child with gastroesophageal reflux, pneumothorax or pneumomediastinum, and pleural effusion presents with chest pain. As in older children, the history and physical examination are crucial in guiding the appropriate workup.

Rarely, one sees a child with chest pain and cardiovascular disease. However, because this is the diagnosis that most families are concerned about, it must be addressed. Certainly, children with palpitations, syncope, or chest pain with exertion should have a thorough evaluation. Finally, toddlers are always at risk for foreign body ingestion. Although aspirated foreign bodies are not likely to give chest pain, esophageal foreign bodies commonly cause chest pain.

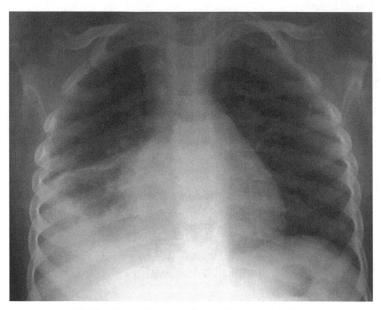

FIG. 14-4. Chest radiograph (case 14-5).

II.   Diagnosis

The chest roentgenogram revealed a right lower lobe opacity with a moderate right pleural effusion (Fig. 14-4). **The diagnosis is pneumonia, and pleural effusion.**

III.   Incidence and Epidemiology

In children younger than 5 years of age, the yearly incidence of community-acquired pneumonia is 34 to 40/1,000; in adolescents, the incidence is 7/1,000. It is fairly difficult to develop a consensus definition of a case of pneumonia. Some define it based on an abnormal chest roentgenogram, whereas others will require only the presence of clinical symptoms.

A large number of organisms can cause community-acquired pneumonia in children. The most common etiologic agents are viruses (RSV, influenza A and B, parainfluenza, adenovirus, and rhinovirus), *Mycoplasma pneumoniae, Chlamydia* spp. (*Chlamydia trachomatis, Chlamydia pneumoniae*), and bacteria (*Streptococcus pneumoniae, M. tuberculosis, Staphylococcus aureus, Haemophilus influenzae* type b, and nontypeable *H. influenzae)*. Less common causes are other viruses (varicella, enteroviruses, cytomegalovirus, EBV), *Chlamydia psittaci*, less common bacteria (*Streptococcus pyogenes*, anaerobic mouth flora, *Bordetella pertussis, Klebsiella pneumoniae,*and *Legionella*), and fungi (*Coccidioides immitis, Histoplasma capsulatum*, and *Blastomyces dermatitidis.*)

Often, the difficulty lies in differentiating a bacterial from a nonbacterial pneumonia. Classically, lobar infiltrates, cavitary lesions, and large pleural effusions suggest either a bacterial or a mycobacterial etiology. Viral pneumonias typically show diffuse radiologic involvement, but focal infiltrates can be seen. Laboratory data have been used in an attempt to differentiate viral from bacterial pneumonia, with C-reactive protein and WBC counts more significantly elevated in bacterial pneumonias. Ultimately, when attempting to determine the etiologic agent for pneumonia, one must determine the underlying immunologic function of the patient. Certainly, immunocompromised patients are susceptible to a whole host of other infectious etiologies that are often life-threatening.

One must also consider that some noninfectious processes can cause a similar clinical picture. These include gastroesophageal reflux, chemical aspiration, asthma, hypersensitivity pneumonitis, and pulmonary hemosiderosis.

IV. Clinical Presentation

Typically, viral pneumonia commences with symptoms of upper respiratory tract infection, fever, rhinorrhea, and cough. Respiratory symptoms may be insidious. This is in contrast to most bacterial pneumonias, where there is often an acute onset with fever, cough, and chest pain.

On physical examination, patients may have signs suggestive of consolidation (dullness to percussion, bronchial breath sounds, and egophony). This is more suggestive of a bacterial process. In contrast, patients with *Mycoplasma* or viral infections may have unimpressive physical examination findings but very distinct infiltrates noted on their chest roentgenograms. Furthermore, patients with *Mycoplasma* infection may have a concurrent bullous myringitis.

V. Diagnostic Approach

Chest roentgenogram. As mentioned previously, the difficulty in diagnosing a pneumonia is differentiating a bacterial from a viral process. Lobar consolidation, cavitation, and large pleural effusions suggest a bacterial or mycobacterial process. Small, bilateral pleural effusions are present in approximately 20% of children with *M. pneumoniae* pneumonia. Pneumococcal pneumonia is the most common bacterial cause of lobar consolidation. However, approximately 10% of cases of *Mycoplasma* pneumonia present with lobar consolidation. Pneumatoceles are detected in two thirds of children with pneumonia caused by *S. aureus*. Viral pneumonias typically have a diffuse appearance that may be either interstitial or alveolar. Disease confined to the lower lobes, or to the upper lobes in supine patients, may suggest aspiration pneumonia.

Chest computed tomography. For an uncomplicated pneumonia, chest CT is not necessary. However, it is useful in cases of recurrent pneumonia and in recalcitrant cases. Furthermore, in the immunocompromised patient, a chest CT may reveal subtle parenchymal disease. In children with unilateral pleural effusion, the chest CT can detect loculations and distinguish pleural effusions from anatomic abnormalities such as pulmonary lobe sequestration.

Sputum examination. Sputum culture may help identify the bacterial cause of pneumonia in adolescents, but it is not predictive of the cause of pneumonia in younger children due to the difficulty in obtaining an adequate sputum sample.

Bronchoscopy. As with chest CT, a bronchoscopy is not necessary in uncomplicated pneumonia. However, a pneumonia that does not respond to appropriate antibiotic therapy may require bronchoscopy to obtain appropriate samples for culture. With this technique, a bronchoalveolar lavage is performed, and the fluid is analyzed for culture of causative organisms. Bronchoscopy is often indicated for immunocompromised patients who are at risk for opportunistic infections in addition to common bacterial and viral infections.

VI. Treatment

In the majority of cases, the causative organism is hypothesized but not verified. Therefore, therapy must be empiric. In the newborn period, the most common organisms are group B streptococci, gram-negative bacteria (particularly *Escherichia coli* and *Klebsiella* spp.), and *Listeria monocytogenes.* Therefore, a combination of ampicillin and either gentamicin or cefotaxime is often used. There is no consensus as to when the newborn period is over, but after 2 to 3 months of age, the causative organisms tend to switch to *C. trachomatis*, viruses, *S. pneumoniae*, *B. pertussis,* and *S. aureus*. Currently, the prevailing opinion is to treat these children (who are generally in the 3- to 4-month age group) with amoxicillin, ampicillin, or cefotaxime.

From 4 months to approximately 4 years of age, the causative organisms tend to include viruses, *S. pneumoniae, H. influenzae, M. pneumoniae,* and *M. tuberculosis.* In a study of 3,475 *S. pneumoniae* isolates by Whitney and colleagues, ampicillin was effective against 98% of isolates with intermediate sensitivity against penicillin, whereas erythromycin and second-generation cephalosporin antibiotics were effective against only 65% of those same isolates. For these reasons, many clinicians commence treatment with either amoxicillin or ampicillin for lobar pneumonia and consider a switch to a macrolide only if the child does not improve clinically, raising their suspicion for a *Mycoplasma* infection. Children with antecedent influenza infection are at higher risk for pneumonia due to *S. aureus.* An agent with activity against both *S. pneumoniae* and *S. aureus,* such as amoxicillin-clavulanate, clindamycin, or azithromycin, is preferred to treat pneumonia in the child with influenza.

Finally, in the 5- to 15-year-age group, *Mycoplasma* spp. and *C. pneumoniae* are more common than other etiologic agents, including *S. pneumoniae* and *M. tuberculosis.* Therefore, the prevailing opinion for this age group is to commence treatment with either macrolide or fluoroquinolone antibiotics. Certainly, in any age range, one should pursue the diagnosis of *M. tuberculosis* if it is at all clinically suspected.

VII. References

1. Campbell PW, Hazinski TA. Acute pneumonia. In: Hoekelman RA, Friedman SB, Nelson NM, et al., eds. *Primary pediatric care,* 3rd ed. St. Louis: Mosby, 1997: 1521–1253.

2. Donowitz GR, Mandell GL. Acute pneumonia. In: Mandell GL, Bennett JE, Dolin R, eds. *Mandell, Douglas, and Bennett's principles and practice of infectious diseases,* 5th ed. Philadelphia: Churchill Livingstone, 2000:717–735.

3. Ferwerda A, Moll HA, de Groot R. Respiratory tract infections by *Mycoplasma pneumoniae* in children: a review of diagnostic and therapeutic measures. *Eur J Pediatr* 2001;160:483–491.

4. Franquet T. Imaging of pneumonia: trends and algorithms. *Eur Respir J* 2001;18: 196–208.

5. McIntosh K. Community-acquired pneumonia in children. *N Engl J Med* 2002;346: 429–437.

6. Whitney CG, Farley MM, Hadler J, et al. Increasing prevalence of multidrug-resistant *Streptococcus pneumoniae* in the United States. *N Engl J Med* 2000;343:1917–1924.

Case 14-6: 15-Year-Old Boy

I. History of Present Illness

A 15-year old boy with a history of asthma and chronic sinusitis presented with a 2-day history of shortness of breath and chest pain. He described the pain as an ache with an occasional squeezing feeling. He developed wheezing that required increasing use of his albuterol inhaler. However, this did not relieve his symptoms. He also developed a productive cough. His mother believed that he had had increasing fatigue since the morning of his presentation, as well as a decreased appetite. He denied fever, vomiting, or diarrhea.

II. Past Medical History

He was diagnosed with asthma at the age of 7 years and required multiple emergency department visits and hospitalizations. Two years before presentation, he had had one asthma admission that lasted for 1 month. He had never needed endotracheal intubation or intensive care. He had recently been started on a leukotriene inhibitor for his asthma. Many of his prior admissions for asthma exacerbations included cardiology evaluations for chest pain. He also had a history of chronic sinusitis requiring six sinus surgeries over the last 3 years, as well as a somatization disorder diagnosed by psychiatry. His daily medications included montelukast and inhaled fluticasone.

The patient had recently been admitted to the hospital for an asthma exacerbation and gastroenteritis. During that admission, he was seen by cardiology staff for bradycardia and chest pain. An echocardiogram at that time revealed a shortening fraction of 24% and a left ventricular end-diastolic pressure of 5.5 mm Hg. A Holter monitor and exercise test were both normal.

III. Physical Examination

T, 37.0°C; RR 26/min; HR, 110 bpm; BP, 85/60 mm Hg; SpO_2, 91% in room air

In general, he was an uncomfortable boy in moderate respiratory distress. He was short of breath and was able to speak only in fragmented sentences. He was sitting up for comfort. His oropharynx was dry. His chest examination revealed diffuse rales and wheezes with fair aeration throughout. His cardiac examination indicated an active precordium and tachycardia with regular rhythm. No murmurs or rubs were noted, but an intermittent gallop was appreciated. His liver was palpable 3 cm below the right costal margin. His extremities were cool, with weak pulses and slightly delayed capillary refill.

IV. Diagnostic Studies

Laboratory analysis revealed 7,500 WBCs/mm^3. Electrolytes, blood urea nitrogen, creatinine, and liver function tests were all within normal limits. ECG revealed a normal sinus rhythm at a rate of 100 bpm. There was possible right atrial enlargement and some ST-segment depression.

V. Course of Illness

A chest roentgenogram suggested the diagnosis (Fig. 14-5).

DISCUSSION: CASE 14-6

I. Differential Diagnosis

The most common causes for chest pain in the adolescent age group are cough, asthma, pneumonia, musculoskeletal causes, and idiopathic causes. With this patient's past medical history of asthma, it was natural for asthma to be the initial focus of con-

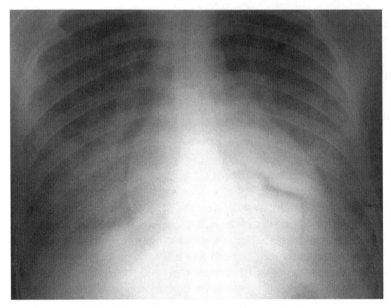

FIG. 14-5. Chest radiograph (case 14-6).

cern. However, because the patient's physical examination was not consistent with an asthma exacerbation, other diagnoses were appropriately considered. The concerning features on this patient's physical examination included signs of congestive heart failure: bilateral rales, a gallop, and a palpable liver edge 3 cm below the right costal margin. Furthermore, his shortness of breath was significantly worse while lying down. Dyspnea with an asthma exacerbation is not usually positional in nature to this extent.

The differential diagnosis for heart failure in this adolescent includes congenital heart disease—both pressure overload (e.g., aortic stenosis) and volume overload (e.g., aortic regurgitation, arrhythmias); acquired heart disease (myocarditis, cardiomyopathy, pericarditis, cor pulmonale, endocarditis); hypoglycemia; storage diseases; and ingestions such as cardiac toxins (e.g., digitalis) and arrhythmogenics (e.g., tricyclic antidepressants).

II. Diagnosis

His chest roentgenogram revealed pulmonary edema with cardiomegaly (Fig. 14-5). An echocardiogram was performed and demonstrated a shortening fraction of less than 20%, with left-ventricular end-diastolic pressure of 6.4 mm Hg. The left ventricle was noted to be dilated. **The diagnosis is a dilated cardiomyopathy.** He was initially treated with intravenous Lasix (furosemide). He was then started on a milrinone infusion. Multiple laboratory studies were requested, including infectious serologies and thyroid function tests, which did not reveal a cause for his cardiomyopathy. Ultimately, a cardiac catheterization was performed, which revealed a cardiac index of 2.81 and superior vena cava saturation of 75%. A biopsy was performed which demonstrated an eosinophilic and monocytic infiltrate.

III. Incidence and Epidemiology

By definition, cardiomyopathy is a structural or functional abnormality of the ventricular myocardium that does not involve coronary artery disease, hypertension, or valvular or congenital heart disease. Cardiomyopathy in children can be divided into primary and secondary forms. Primary cardiomyopathies are either dilated, hypertrophic, restrictive, or arrhythmogenic. Secondary cardiomyopathies have multiple causes, including infection, metabolic disorders, general systemic diseases, hereditary forms, and toxic reactions.

This patient presented with a dilated cardiomyopathy of no definitive cause. Idiopathic dilated cardiomyopathy has a prevalence of 36.5 cases per 100,000 persons and accounts for 50% of the total cases of dilated cardiomyopathy. Idiopathic cardiomyopathy has survival rates of 63% to 90% at 1 year and 20% to 80% at 5 years.

IV. Clinical Presentation

Patients with a dilated cardiomyopathy most often have an insidious onset to their symptoms. The most common complaints in adolescents are shortness of breath and poor exercise tolerance, which are the result of decreased cardiac output and pulmonary edema. Because infants are not able to complain of these same symptoms, their presentation often includes more subtle symptoms, such as tachypnea, irritability, and difficulty with feeding.

Patients often are tachycardiac, tachypneic, and nervous. Hypotension may be seen with poor cardiac output, and fever may indicate an infection that has brought the patient to medical attention. Quite often, patients have orthopnea, preferring to remain in the upright position. With pulmonary edema, many patients wheeze but are unresponsive to traditional asthma therapies.

On chest wall palpation, there may be a laterally displaced point of maximal impulse. With auscultation of the cardiac sounds, a prominent pulmonic segment of the S2 or a gallop, or both, may be appreciated. Many patients with congestive heart failure have a liver edge that is abnormally below the right costal margin.

V. Diagnostic Approach

Chest roentgenogram. Patients generally have an increased heart size noted. This is secondary to left-sided dilation. Accompanying signs include pulmonary edema and possibly pleural effusions.

Electrocardiogram. Sinus tachycardia is the most common finding, with supraventricular or ventricular tachycardia possible as well. Signs of left ventricular hypertrophy and nonspecific ST-segment and T-wave abnormalities may also be seen.

Echocardiogram. The left atrium and left ventricle are generally noted to be enlarged. There may be increased end-diastolic and systolic volumes. Poor wall movement may be seen secondary to ischemic injury. With this imaging modality, pericardial and pleural effusions may also be noted.

Cardiac catheterization. One can obtain hemodynamic data on pressures in the aorta, left ventricle, pulmonary capillary wedge, and pulmonary artery. The cardiac output can be calculated and will be decreased. A endomyocardial biopsy can be performed and may be useful to determine the cause of the cardiomyopathy.

VI. Treatment

Inotropic agents such as the sympathomimetic drugs dopamine, dobutamine, and epinephrine are often required to support the poor cardiac output. Milrinone and amrinone are inotropes that can be used to treat patients with signs of congestive heart failure. Digoxin is used for long-term therapy and increased cardiac contractility.

Because fluid overload is quite common in this clinical scenario, diuretics such as furosemide are often necessary. Peripheral vasodilators, including nitroprusside and hydralazine, may be used to decrease afterload and thereby increase cardiac output. Angiotensin-converting enzyme (ACE) inhibitors can have similar effects to reduce afterload.

With dilation of the cardiac chambers, the patient is at risk for thrombus formation. Use of anticoagulants or antiplatelet drugs should be considered. If the underlying cause of the cardiomyopathy is determined, a more specific therapy may be warranted.

Finally, in severe cases, cardiac transplantation is required. It is difficult to determine which children or adolescents should be considered for transplantation. Certainly, this option should be explored for those children who are still quite ill despite maximal intervention.

VII. References

1. Gewitz MH, Vetter VL. Cardiac emergencies. In: Fleisher GR, Ludwig S, eds. *Textbook of pediatric emergency medicine.* Baltimore: Williams & Wilkins, 1993: 533–572.
2. Olson TM, Chan DP. Dilated congestive cardiomyopathy. In: Driscoll DJ, eds. *Moss and Adams' heart disease in infants, children, and adolescents,* 6th ed. Philadelphia: Lippincott Williams & Wilkins, 2001:1187–1195.
3. Paquet M, Hanna BD. Cardiomyopathy. In: Oski FA, DeAngelis CD, Feigin RD, et al., eds. *Principles and practice of pediatrics,* 2nd ed. Philadelphia: JB Lippincott, 1994: 1606–1614.

15

Jaundice

Eric J. Frehm

APPROACH TO THE PATIENT WITH JAUNDICE

I. Definition of the Complaint

Jaundice is the yellow discoloration of the skin, mucous membranes, and sclerae that is caused by increased serum levels of bilirubin, a byproduct of heme breakdown. As a lipophilic pigment, bilirubin must bind to plasma albumin for carriage to the liver. It is taken up by hepatocytes for conjugation with solubilizing sugars to form bilirubin diglucuronides (and, less commonly, monoglucuronides), thus allowing for excretion into bile. Not all jaundice is pathologic. Indeed, the vast majority of clinically encountered hyperbilirubinemia occurs as physiologic jaundice in neonates.

II. Complaint by Cause and Frequency

Neonatal jaundice can be caused by conjugated or unconjugated hyperbilirubinemia (Table 15-1). The differential diagnosis of cholestatic jaundice in the older child differs from diseases that present early in life. Young infants are more likely to have congenital anatomic anomalies, such as biliary atresia, or inborn metabolic disorders, such as galactosemia. Older children are more likely to experience acquired or secondary liver diseases, such as autoimmune or toxic hepatitis, or liver impairment related to inflammatory bowel disease. Infectious hepatitis is among the most common causes of liver disease in older children and adolescents. Viruses causing hepatitis and jaundice in these children include: hepatitis A, B, C, D and E; Epstein-Barr virus; cytomegalovirus; varicella; human herpesvirus 6 (HHV-6); and herpes simplex virus (HSV). Other infectious diseases associated with jaundice include schistosomiasis, leptospirosis, Rocky Mountain spotted fever, ehrlichiosis, and malaria.

Obstructive, extrahepatic causes of conjugated hyperbilirubinemia in children and adolescents to consider include cholelithiasis, choledochal cysts, sclerosing cholangitis, pancreatitis, and tumors and other anatomic abnormalities along the choledocho-pancreatico-duodenal path.

III. Clarifying Questions

• Is the elevated bilirubin level all unconjugated? Is the process a conjugated hyperbilirubinemia?

— Separating a total bilirubin measurement into its conjugated and unconjugated components is a critical step in the evaluation of hyperbilirubinemia in a child. Conjugated hyperbilirubinemia is present when the conjugated fraction is at least 1.5 mg/dL or accounts for more than 15% of the total bilirubin measurement. Conjugated hyperbilirubinemia is abnormal and merits prompt evaluation, particularly in infants, in whom diseases such as biliary atresia require urgent therapy. An increased unconjugated bilirubin level suggests a very different differential diagnosis but can also be a medical emergency if very high: unconjugated bilirubin is able to cross the blood-brain barrier and directly injure the brain.

TABLE 15-1. *Causes of Neonatal Jaundice*

Unconjugated
  Physiologic jaundice
  Breast-feeding jaundice
  Bacterial infection
  Polycythemia
  Hemolytic disease
    Isoimmune
    Red blood cell enzyme defects
    Red blood cell membrane defects
  Endocrinopathies
  Extravascular blood collections
  Genetic/familial disorders
  Increased enterohepatic circulation
    Upper gastrointestinal obstruction
    Delayed meconium passage
Conjugated
  Extrahepatic/obstructive
    Biliary atresia
    Choledochal cysts
    Paucity of intrahepatic bile ducts (e.g., Alagille syndrome)
  Bacterial infection
  TORCH infection
  Neonatal hepatitis
    Idiopathic
    Viral, bacterial, or parasitic
  Metabolic disorders
    α_1-Antrypsin deficiency
    Inborn errors of metabolism
    Endocrinopathies
    Cystic fibrosis
    Neonatal iron storage disease
    Bile acid synthesis defects
  Cholestasis syndromes
    Byler disease
    Dubin-Johnson syndrome
  Toxic
    Hyperalimentation

Sometimes the terms "direct" and "indirect" bilirubin are used interchangeably with the terms "conjugated" and "unconjugated." The former terms derive from the van den Bergh reaction, in which the conjugated bilirubin component is measured *directly* (by colorimetric analysis after reaction with a diazo compound). The subsequent addition of methanol allows for a measurement of total bilirubin, after which unconjugated fraction is determined *indirectly,* by subtracting the conjugated bilirubin level from the total bilirubin level. Of note, measurement of the direct bilirubin fraction detects not just bilirubin diglucuronides and monoglucuronides but also "delta" bilirubin, which forms when conjugated bilirubin seeps retrograde into the serum and binds covalently to albumin. Because of the delta component's long half-life, the "direct fraction" can remain deceptively elevated even as a conjugated hyperbilirubinemia improves.

• Does the jaundiced baby have other concerning physical findings?

— A significant unconjugated hyperbilirubinemia can result from the increased bilirubin of a cephalohematoma or extensive bruising. A newborn afflicted with a TORCH infection might have microcephaly, growth retardation, hepatosplenomegaly, chorioretinitis, or petechiae. A heart murmur is often heard in children with Alagille syndrome, whereas a baby with Zellweger syndrome is hypotonic and dysmorphic. Of course, serious bacterial infection must always be considered in any case of significant bilirubinemia.

* Is there a family history of jaundice?

— Many of the disorders that manifest with jaundice are heritable. α_1-Antitrypsin deficiency, Crigler-Najjar syndrome type I and II, galactosemia, and tyrosinemia are just a few of the autosomal recessive diseases associated with neonatal jaundice. On the other hand, Alagille syndrome is an autosomal dominant disorder (but with variable penetrance and expressivity). The inheritance of glucose-6-phosphate dehydrogenase (G6PD) deficiency is X-linked but so highly polymorphic that it should be considered in the evaluation of boys and girls alike.

* Were there changes in the child's diet or other new "exposures" that preceded the onset of jaundice?

— Deficiencies in the metabolism of galactose or fructose can lead to jaundice in infants. Likewise, children with G6PD deficiency can have hemolytic crises triggered by certain foods (e.g., fava beans), medications (e.g., antimalarial agents), or other compounds (e.g., mothballs).

* Are neonatal hyperbilirubinemia risk factors present?

— Risk factors for neonatal jaundice that derive from the mother include ethnicity (e.g., Asian, Native American) and pregnancy complications such as gestational diabetes or blood group incompatibility. Birth trauma that results in extravascular blood collections is also a risk factor for jaundice. Other independent risk factors for the infant include polycythemia, prematurity, breast-feeding, perinatal infections, and a long, heterogenous list of genetic disorders.

IV. References

1. D'Agata ID, Balistreri WF. Evaluation of liver disease in the pediatric patient. *Pediatr Rev* 1999;20:376–389.

2. Dennery PA, Seidman DS, Stevenson DK. Neonatal hyperbilirubinemia. *N Engl J Med* 2001;344:581–590.

3. Gourley GR. Neonatal jaundice and disorders of bilirubin metabolism. In: Suchy FJ, Sokol RJ, Balistreri WF, eds. *Liver disease in children,* 2nd ed. Philadelphia: Lippincott Williams & Wilkins, 2001:275–314.

4. Maisels MJ. Jaundice. In: Avery GB, Fletcher MA, MacDonald MG, eds. *Neonatology: pathophysiology and management of the newborn,* 5th ed. Philadelphia: Lippincott Williams & Wilkins, 1999:765–819.

5. Maller ES. Jaundice. In: Altschuler SM, Liacouris CA. *Clinical pediatric gastroenterology.* New York: Churchill Livingstone, 1998:49–61.

Case 15-1: 14-Day-Old Boy

I. History of Present Illness

A 14-day-old, full-term male infant was transferred from a local community hospital for further evaluation and management of sepsis and hyperbilirubinemia. He had been discharged home from the well-baby nursery on the fourth day of life with a bilirubin concentration of 16.7 mg/dL. Two days later, his bilirubin level was 19.4 mg/dL and he was admitted for phototherapy. Within 48 hours after admission, he developed emesis and temperature instability. A blood culture and lumbar puncture were performed, and ampicillin and gentamicin were started. Additional bilirubin measurements revealed the direct fraction to be 5.2 mg/dL. An ultrasound study, performed to assess hepatomegaly, revealed a nondilated biliary system, small gall bladder, and diffuse hepatic enlargement. A nuclear medicine liver scan did not show bile excretion after 4 hours, prompting initiation of phenobarbital therapy.

The baby continued to receive breast milk feedings (with nasogastric tube supplementation required because of poor oral intake) until he experienced blood-tinged emesis. Coagulation studies at that time revealed the prothrombin time (PT) to be greater than 50 seconds and the partial thromboplastin time (PTT) to be greater than 200 seconds; for this reason, vitamin K and a dose of fresh-frozen plasma were given. By report, the baby's abdomen was soft and his stool quantity and quality were unremarkable. Transfer to a tertiary care center was arranged.

II. Past Medical History

The baby was born to a 27-year-old gravida 1 parity 0 mother with unremarkable prenatal laboratory values. Delivery was via cesarean section at 37 weeks because of breech presentation. The baby's birth weight was 3.04 kg. He was discharged with his mother on the fourth day of life and was breast-feeding every 3 hours.

III. Physical Examination

T, 36.4°C; RR, 48/min; HR, 140 bpm; BP, 83/50 mm Hg
Weight, 2.7 kg

Physical examination revealed a 2-week-old term boy who was listless but arousable. His skin demonstrated a yellow-green jaundice but no petechiae, rash, or bruising. He was nondysmorphic and normocephalic, with an open, flat fontanel. His pupils were equal, round, and reactive with red reflexes present bilaterally. Mucous membranes were yellow-pink and slightly dry. His respirations were slightly rapid but otherwise unlabored with clear breath sounds bilaterally. The heart examination was normal. The abdomen was soft and nondistended, with a smooth, firm liver edge palpable 3 cm below the right costal margin. Examinations of the genitalia and extremities were normal. His tone, power, and primitive reflexes all appeared to be within normal limits.

IV. Diagnostic Studies

A complete blood count revealed the following: white blood cells (WBCs), 9,400/mm^3 (1% band forms, 41% segmented neutrophils, and 45% lymphocytes); hemoglobin, 16.0 g/dL; and platelets, 66,000/mm^3. PT and PTT were markedly prolonged at 50 and 112 seconds, respectively. Fibrinogen was 127 mg/dL, and fibrin split products were negative. Serum bicarbonate was 17 mEq/L, but the remainder of the serum electrolytes, calcium, magnesium, and phosphorus were normal. Serum glucose was 52 mg/dL. A hepatic function panel revealed the following: alanine aminotransferase (ALT), 115 U/L aspartate aminotransferase (AST), 126 U/L; alkaline phosphatase, 730 U/L; γ-glutamyl transferase

(GGT), 55 U/L; and albumin, 3.5 mg/dL. The unconjugated bilirubin concentration was 13.1 mg/dL, and the conjugated bilirubin was 5.9 mg/dL.

V. Course of Illness

On admission, the infant received intravenous fluids and antibiotics. In addition, he required a second dose of fresh-frozen plasma for treatment of his coagulopathy. A repeat liver ultrasound examination was consistent with the earlier study. An ophthalmology examination was unremarkable. In light of the illness as described and mild hypoglycemia, the baby ultimately received a full 10 days of antibiotic therapy for presumed sepsis. The blood culture from the referring hospital remained negative.

Further testing revealed a specific underlying diagnosis. This determination guided the infant's subsequent inpatient management.

DISCUSSION: CASE 15-1

I. Differential Diagnosis

The differential diagnosis for the systemically ill neonate is quite broad. Infectious causes are often considered first, especially common bacterial pathogens (e.g., group B *Streptococcus,* staphylococci, *Escherichia coli, Listeria monocytogenes*) and viruses (e.g., HSV, enterovirus). Less often, fungi (e.g., *Candida* species) and other classes of organisms (e.g., parasites) are implicated. Congenital heart disease is another critically important consideration in sick neonates; ductal-dependent anatomic lesions (e.g., coarctation of the aorta, hypoplastic left heart syndrome) and tachydysrhythmias may manifest early in life with profound cardiovascular compromise. Shock can also be seen in severely anemic infants—for instance, after a placental catastrophe or even a major intracranial hemorrhage. Multiorgan dysfunction can also result from perinatal asphyxia, neonatal surgical emergencies, and a multiplicity of endocrine and metabolic abnormalities (including congenital adrenal hyperplasia, glucose and electrolyte derangements, and numerous inborn errors of metabolism).

Conjugated hyperbilirubinemia in the neonate, such as that seen in the patient described here, also has a multiplicity of causes. Among the possibilities are idiopathic neonatal hepatitis, α_1-antitrypsin deficiency, hypopituitarism, hypothyroidism, bile acid synthesis deficiency, exposure to intravenous hyperalimentation, and long lists of infections and disorders of hepatobiliary anatomy. Similarly, neonatal hepatomegaly is seen in a wide variety of settings, including infections—either congenitally acquired (e.g., TORCH) or acute-onset (e.g., sepsis); neonatal hepatitis; liver or gall bladder disease (e.g., α_1-antitrypsin deficiency, biliary atresia, choledochal cyst); hydrops or congestive heart failure; tumors; and metabolic disease (e.g., glycogen storage diseases, galactosemia, tyrosinemia).

In addition to jaundice and hepatomegaly, the baby in this case study had elevated liver enzymes and possible liver synthetic dysfunction (as a potential contributing factor in his coagulopathy). In addition, his hepatobiliary scintigraphic examination was concerning for its lack of excretion at 4 hours.

II. Diagnosis

Shortly after interhospital transfer, this baby's state newborn screening results revealed him to have **galactosemia.**

III. Incidence and Pathophysiology

Galactosemia is a rare inborn error of metabolism that occurs in 1 of every 60,000 infants. It is caused by the absence of an enzyme of galactose metabolism. Presenting signs in the galactose-exposed, affected neonate can include jaundice, hepatomegaly, seizures, lethargy, vomiting, hypoglycemia, cataracts, and failure to thrive. In addition, babies with galactosemia exhibit a heightened susceptibility to bacterial infection, particularly *Escherichia coli* sepsis. Although galactosemia is widely assessed in state newborn screening programs, the onset of life-threatening clinical illness may precede the completion of testing.

The hydrolysis of dietary lactose produces glucose and galactose. Galactose is subsequently phosphorylated to galactose-1-phosphate. This compound, in turn, is converted by the galactose-1-phosphate uridyl transferase enzyme to uridine diphosphate (UDP)-galactose. These conversions enable galactose to enter the glycolytic pathway of the cell. If the transferase enzyme is missing, as it is in "classic" galactosemia, galactose-1-phosphate accumulates in the tissues, and signs and symptoms of the disease become evident. Classic galactosemia is caused by a mutation in the *GALT* gene, which codes for the galactose-1-phosphate uridyl transferase enzyme. In addition, there are two other types of "nonclassic" galactosemia. Galactokinase deficiency, a deficiency of the enzyme necessary for the phosphorylation of galactose, can cause jaundice, cataracts, and elevations of plasma galactose levels but does not result in mental deficiency. A second and still rarer type of galactosemia is caused by uridyl diphosphogalactose 4-epimerase deficiency. This condition behaves very much like classic galactosemia.

IV. Clinical Presentation

Classic galactosemia is an autosomal recessive disease. If not recognized and treated, it can be fatal in the neonatal period. Some of the more common presenting clinical signs have already been discussed (jaundice, hepatomegaly, vomiting, and encephalopathy); more fulminant clinical courses may represent superimposed bacterial sepsis. Among the laboratory findings seen with classic galactosemia are conjugated (or combined) hyperbilirubinemia, liver function test and coagulation study abnormalities, elevations of serum and urine amino acids, and a renal tubulopathy with galactosuria, glycosuria, proteinuria, and metabolic acidosis. Not surprisingly, plasma galactose and erythrocyte galactose-1-phosphate levels are also elevated.

Disappointingly, even galactosemic children whose diets were restricted very early are at increased risk for developmental delays and learning disabilities, compared with their healthy counterparts. Although many children have IQs in the normal range, cognitive, speech, and motor impairments are, nevertheless, more common. Longer delays before initial diagnosis and treatment of galactosemia correlate with worse neurodevelopmental sequelae.

Hypergonadotropic hypogonadism is often observed in girls with galactosemia, and most are infertile as adults. Galactosemic males demonstrate normal puberty and fertility.

The gene for the galactose-1-phosphate uridyl transferase enzyme has been localized to chromosome 9, and multiple variations at that locus have been described. Some African-Americans with galactosemia have a milder clinical course because of a different transferase variant. Still another variant, known as the Duarte variant, is usually clinically insignificant. Prenatal diagnosis of galactosemia is available.

V. Diagnosis

Definitive diagnosis of galactosemia is established by laboratory assay of the glucose-1-phosphate uridyl transferase enzyme in erythrocytes. If clinical suspicion for galactosemia exists, preliminary evidence for that diagnosis can be obtained by testing the infant's urine for nonglucose reducing substances (provided that the infant had recently been exposed to lactose). Caution must be taken to employ the appropriate urine tests, because glucose-oxidase strips (e.g., Clinistix) are sensitive only to glucose, whereas

Clinitest tablets detect all reducing substances, including glucose, galactose, and fructose. An ill-appearing, jaundiced neonate with nonglucose reducing substances present in the urine should be presumed to have galactosemia until definitive testing is available.

VI. Treatment

The removal of galactose from the diet remains the first principle of therapy for galactosemia. The exclusion of milk (including breast milk) and dairy products is necessary for the patient's lifetime.

Depending on the degree of illness at the time of presentation, galactosemic neonates often require supportive care measures such as intravenous fluids and antibiotics. Liver synthetic function may be compromised, and the sick infant may require supplemental vitamin K or even transfusion of fresh-frozen plasma.

VII. References

1. Chen YT. Defects in metabolism of carbohydrates. In: Behrman RE, Kleigman RM, Jenson HB, eds. *Nelson textbook of pediatrics,* 16th ed. Philadelphia: WB Saunders, 2000:405–420.
2. D'Agata ID, Balistreri WF. Evaluation of liver disease in the pediatric patient. *Pediatr Rev* 1999;20:376–389.
3. Gotoff SP. Infections of the neonatal infant. In: Behrman RE, Kleigman RM, Jenson HB, eds. *Nelson textbook of pediatrics,* 16th ed. Philadelphia: WB Saunders, 2000: 538–552.
4. Walter JH, Collins JE, Leonard JV. Recommendations for the management of galactosaemia. *Arch Dis Child* 1999;80:93–96.

Case 15-2: 2-Year-Old Boy

I. History of Present Illness

A 2-year-old Asian-American boy presented with a 3-day history of "looking yellow" according to family description. In addition, there was a 1-day history of darker urine and somewhat decreased oral intake. The patient had had symptoms of an upper respiratory tract infection for 1 week but no fever, vomiting, diarrhea, localizing pain, rashes, bleeding, or bruising. He had not recently traveled or taken medications; his diet has not changed except for the recent additions of chocolate from Hong Kong and broad beans. He was evaluated by his pediatrician and referred to the emergency department.

II. Past Medical History

The patient was a full-term infant with a history of hyperbilirubinemia (total bilirubin concentration, greater than 20 mg/dL), for which he required phototherapy, but no intercurrent episodes of jaundice until now. He was hospitalized at age 10 months for bacteremia. He was born in the United States to Chinese parents; because his parents worked in another state, he stayed with his grandmother during the week. There was no family history of anemia, transfusions, gallstones, liver problems, or spleen problems.

III. Physical Examination

T, 37.6°C; RR, 24/min; HR, 150 bpm; BP, 100/66 mm Hg; SpO_2, 99% in room air
Weight, 13 kg

The physical examination revealed a jaundiced and somewhat pale child who was active and in no apparent distress. There was scleral icterus and conjunctival pallor. There was no nasal discharge, and the oropharynx was clear with moist mucous membranes. His neck was supple without lymphadenopathy. Breath sounds were clear and unlabored. His pulse was regular, with a II/VI systolic ejection murmur. First and second heart sounds (S_1 and S_2, respectively) were normal, and there was no gallop. The abdomen was soft, nontender, nondistended, and free of masses. A smooth liver edge was palpable 1 cm below the right costal margin, and the spleen was nonpalpable. The remainder of the examination was unremarkable.

IV. Diagnostic Studies

The complete blood count showed 22,700 WBCs/mm³, with 3% band forms, 32% segmented neutrophils, and 55% lymphocytes. The hemoglobin was 5.9 g/dL with a reticulocyte count of 11.9%. The peripheral blood smear revealed "bite cells." The direct Coombs test was negative. Serum electrolytes revealed the following: sodium, 139 mEq/mL; potassium, 4.5 mEq/mL; chloride, 21 mEq/mL; and bicarbonate, 21 mEq/mL. Blood urea nitrogen (BUN) and creatinine concentrations were normal. Serum glucose was 166 mg/dL. Serum transaminases and alkaline phosphatase were normal, but total bilirubin was 11.2 mg/dL, unconjugated bilirubin was 11.7 mg/dL, and conjugated bilirubin was 0.2 mg/mL. Urine dipstick analysis revealed 2+ blood, but there were no WBCs or red blood cells (RBCs) by microscopy.

V. Course of Illness

The patient was admitted to the hospital for further evaluation of his anemia and jaundice. He did not require RBC transfusion. Additional laboratory studies revealed the diagnosis.

DISCUSSION: CASE 15-2

I. Differential Diagnosis

The toddler described had an unconjugated hyperbilirubinemia and evidence of a non-immune hemolysis (including anemia with reticulocytosis and peripheral smear abnormalities with a negative direct Coombs test). The differential diagnosis should focus on conditions that result in an increased bilirubin load's being presented to the liver (as opposed to a familial disorder of bilirubin metabolism, such as Gilbert syndrome).

Disorders that result in an increased bilirubin load include acquired hemolytic anemias, either autoimmune or drug-induced; sepsis with disseminated intravascular coagulation; transfusion reactions; paroxysmal nocturnal hemoglobinuria; and a multitude of intrinsic RBC abnormalities, including hemoglobinopathies (e.g., sickle cell disease, thalassemia), enzyme defects (e.g., G6PD deficiency, pyruvate kinase deficiency), and defects of the RBC membrane (e.g., hereditary spherocytosis, hereditary elliptocytosis, hereditary pyropoikilocytosis).

II. Diagnosis

G6PD deficiency testing was performed, and the level was 1.4 IU/g hemoglobin (normal range, 7 to 10 IU/g hemoglobin), consistent with a **diagnosis of G6PD deficiency.**

III. Incidence and Epidemiology

G6PD deficiency is an enzymopathy that affects hundreds of millions of people worldwide. The disease has especially high prevalence in parts of Africa, Asia, and areas surrounding the Mediterranean Sea. The major clinical manifestations of G6PD deficiency are nonphysiologic neonatal hyperbilirubinemia and hemolytic anemia, both chronic and episodic. It is a disorder of an enzyme of the hexose monophosphate pathway (HMP), the pathway through which erythrocytes convert oxidized nicotinamide adenine dinucleotide phosphate (NADP+) to the reduced form (NADPH), a critical biochemical reductant. This conversion is necessary for maintaining the tripeptide glutathione in a reduced state, which is essential to the erythrocyte's self-protection from oxidant stressors such as hydrogen peroxide.

The particular sensitivity of RBCs to G6PD deficiency derives from many factors, including the erythrocyte's exclusive dependence on the HMP to produce NADPH, the RBCs' continuous exposure to oxygen and oxidant stressors, and the inability of those nonnucleated RBCs to make new enzyme, even an enzyme with diminished activity.

Of the many identified mutant enzymes, the most common clinically significant variants are G6PD-A− in African Americans; G6PD-B− (or G6PD-Mediterranean) in Italian, Greek, Middle Eastern, Asian, and African peoples; and G6PD-Canton in Chinese individuals. (G6PD-B+ is the most common normal enzyme, and G6PD-A+ is the designation of a common normal variant found among African-Americans.) Because the genes for erythrocyte G6PD production are located on the X chromosome, G6PD deficiency manifests with much greater frequency in males than females. Heterozygous females have two distinct RBC populations—one normal and one G6PD deficient—as a result of lyonization; most of these females remain asymptomatic. Clinically affected females may be G6PD-deficient heterozygotes or even homozygotes.

IV. Clinical Presentation

G6PD deficiency is a heterogeneous disorder. A 1967 World Health Organization classification of G6PD-deficiency phenotypes delineated the following subtypes: class 1, hereditary nonspherocytic hemolytic anemia; class 2, severe enzyme deficiency (e.g.,

G6PD-Mediterranean); class 3, mild enzyme deficiency (e.g., G6PD-A−); and class 4, nondeficient variants (e.g., G6PD-A+).

The episodic hemolytic anemia of G6PD deficiency, as in the case described here, is typically precipitated by an infection or exposure to an oxidant stress. Identified oxidant stressors include certain medications, including sulfonamides (e.g., trimethoprim-sulfamethoxazole), nitrofurantoin, and primaquine (as well as several other antimalarial agents); chemical stressors (e.g., mothballs); and fava beans. *Favism* is the term designating the acute hemolytic anemia precipitated by exposure to fava beans, also known as broad beans (like those consumed by the patient in this case). Although not every patient with G6PD deficiency is susceptible to favism, only patients with G6PD deficiency can get it.

Signs of G6PD deficiency-mediated hemolytic anemia typically appear within 1 to 2 days after exposure to an oxidant stress, when evidence of hemolysis and falling hemoglobin are observable. The relative severity of derangements depends on the nature of the oxidant crisis and the patient's G6PD-deficiency variant; severe cases may manifest jaundice, hemoglobinuria, and anemia severe enough to require transfusion. Hemoglobin levels can continue to fall for many days after an oxidant exposure and should be monitored closely. Removal of any identified oxidant stressors and treatment of any identified infections are other mainstays of therapy for an acute hemolytic episode.

In addition to causing hemolytic anemia, G6PD deficiency is an important cause of severe neonatal hyperbilirubinemia and, in the extreme, the devastating and potentially lethal complication of kernicterus. The hyperbilirubinemia seen with G6PD deficiency appears to result from dysfunctional hepatic bilirubin elimination rather than frank hemolysis. Jaundice requires aggressive therapy and may be severe enough to necessitate exchange transfusion. Severe jaundice is more common with some enzyme variants (e.g., G6PD-Mediterranean) than with others (e.g., G6PD-A−, the variant common among African-Americans). Nevertheless, G6PD deficiency should be considered in all cases of severe jaundice, especially in infants of East Asian, Mediterranean, or West African descent. Consideration should not be limited to male children alone. In one study of *female* Sephardic Jewish infants at high risk of inheriting the G6PD-Mediterranean mutation, both the homozygous *and heterozygous* girls were at higher risk for clinically significant neonatal hyperbilirubinemia. It is concerning that many of the heterozygote females who developed jaundice had normal G6PD deficiency screening tests. They were diagnosed as G6PD-Mediterranean heterozygotes only after sophisticated DNA polymerase chain reaction (PCR) testing.

V.   Diagnostic Approach

Glucose-6-phosphate dehydrogenase level. Several possibilities for laboratory evaluation of G6PD deficiency exist. Fluorescent spot testing, the simplest method, is useful for screening male patients without a recent history of hemolysis. Direct, quantitative measurement of enzyme function is also easy to perform, although false-negative results are frequently obtained if the testing is done in the setting of hemolysis or reticulocytosis, or both. Hemolysis results in the removal of the most G6PD-deficient RBCs from the circulation. This triggers increased production of reticulocytes, which, because of their youth, naturally contain higher levels of G6PD. Both of these factors can mask the detection of G6PD deficiency by quantitative assay analysis. Even more definitive diagnosis of G6PD deficiency is now possible with DNA analysis, which is particularly useful for detecting heterozygotes.

Hemoglobin, reticulocyte count, and peripheral blood smear. These studies raise the suspicion for hemolytic anemia. Typical findings include mild to moderate anemia, elevated reticulocyte count, and the presence of burr cells, blister cells, helmet cells, and schistocytes on peripheral blood smear.

Other studies. Other studies supporting acute hemolysis include elevated serum lactate dehydrogenase and unconjugated bilirubin levels. Mean corpuscular volume (MCV) may be normal or mildly elevated, but the RBC distribution width is usually high due to the presence of normal RBCs and the larger reticulocytes.

VI. Treatment

Treatment of acute hemolytic episodes should center on removing inciting stressors (e.g., stopping an offending medication, treating a triggering infection) and, in cases of severe anemia, transfusion of packed RBCs to support the circulation. Prevention is, of course, the best medicine. In cases of significant neonatal hyperbilirubinemia, early detection and aggressive treatment are critical, including intensive phototherapy and possibly double-volume exchange transfusion. Promising new research offers evidence that G6PD deficiency-related, severe neonatal hyperbilirubinemia may be preventable with pharmacologic inhibition of the enzyme heme oxygenase with synthetic metalloporphyrins.

VII. References

1. Beutler E. G6PD deficiency. *Blood* 1994;84:3613–3636.
2. Balint JP, Balistreri WF. Jaundice. In: Kliegman RM, ed. *Practical strategies in pediatric diagnosis and therapy.* Philadelphia: WB Saunders, 1996:360–379.
3. Kaplan M, Beutler E, Vreman HJ, et al. Neonatal hyperbilirubinemia in glucose-6-phosphate dehydrogenase-deficient heterozygotes. *Pediatrics* 1999;104:68–74.
4. Kappas A, Drummond GS, Valaes T. A single dose of Sn-mesoporphyrin prevents development of severe hyperbilirubinemia in glucose-6-phosphate-dehydrogenase-deficient newborns. *Pediatrics* 2000;108:25–30.
5. Maisels MJ. Jaundice. In: Avery GB, Fletcher MA, Macdonald MG, eds. *Neonatology: pathophysiology and management of the newborn,* 5th ed. Philadelphia: Lippincott, Williams & Wilkins, 1999:765–819.
6. Segel GB. Enzymatic defects. In: Behrman RE, Kleigman RM, Jenson HB, eds. *Nelson textbook of pediatrics,* 16th ed. Philadelphia: WB Saunders, 2000:1488–1491.

Case 15-3: 2-Month-Old Boy

I. History of Present Illness

A 2-month-old male infant was admitted for further evaluation of his jaundice and poor growth.

II. Past Medical History

The baby was born via spontaneous vaginal delivery after an uncomplicated, full-term pregnancy and weighed 3.0 kg at birth. On the second day of life, he was transferred to the special care nursery because of hypoglycemia requiring intravenous dextrose. A sepsis evaluation was performed, and the baby received 7 days of ampicillin and gentamicin. On the third day of life, his total bilirubin level was noted to be 18.6 mg/dL (with a direct bilirubin concentration of 2.8 mg/dL), and he received phototherapy for 4 days. His complete blood count, blood type and antibody screen, abdominal ultrasound, and state newborn screen were all normal. The birth hospital reported that the baby was taken home on the ninth day of life against medical advice; his prefeed blood sugar measurement that day was 33 mg/dL.

The baby had been seen by his pediatrician three times for weight and bilirubin checks; blood sugar measurements at those visits were described as "borderline." His feeding regimen was about 2.5 ounces every 3 hours of cow's milk formula. Because of poor growth and persistent hyperbilirubinemia, he was referred to the hospital's gastroenterology clinic and subsequently admitted for additional evaluation.

III. Physical Examination

T, 37.3°C; RR, 24/min; HR, 140 bpm; BP, 96/60 mm Hg

Weight, 3.6 kg (less than 3rd percentile); length, 52 cm (less than 3rd percentile); head circumference, 38 cm (10th percentile)

Physical examination revealed a cachectic, somewhat icteric 2-month-old boy in no apparent distress. There was scleral icterus and a 5×5 cm anterior fontanel; the oropharynx was clear, with moist mucous membranes. His neck was supple without lymphadenopathy or masses. Breath sounds were clear and unlabored. His pulse was regular, and there was no murmur. The abdomen was soft, nontender, and nondistended; the liver edge was palpable just below the right costal margin, and a small umbilical hernia was present. The testes were palpable (but not fully descended) bilaterally; the penis appeared small, with a stretched penile length of 2.0 cm. The baby appeared alert with grossly normal tone and reflexes. The remainder of the examination was unremarkable.

IV. Diagnostic Studies

Serum electrolyte measurement revealed the following: sodium, 131 mEq/L; potassium, 4.1 mEq/L; chloride, 100 mEq/L; bicarbonate, 22 mEq/L; BUN, 14 mg/dL; creatinine; 0.2 mg/dL; and glucose, 50 mg/dL. The complete blood count revealed 8,000 WBCs/mm^3 with 5% band forms, 30% segmented neutrophils, and 52% lymphocytes. The hemoglobin was 9.2 g/dL, and the reticulocyte count was 1.7%. The total bilirubin measured 10.5 mg/dL; the direct and unconjugated bilirubin levels were 1.5 and 9.0 mg/dL, respectively. Serum albumin was normal. ALT was 46 U/L, AST was 87 U/L, and GGT was 125 U/L.

Abdominal ultrasound examination of the liver revealed normal size, slightly increased echogenicity, and a small, nondistended gall bladder without biliary dilatation. The spleen and kidneys were normal. A sweat test was attempted, but an insufficient amount of sweat was obtained to properly interpret the test.

V. Course of Illness

The infant was admitted to the hospital and given intravenous fluids containing dextrose to maintain the blood sugar concentration greater than 60 mg/dL. Serum amino acids, α_1-antitrypsin testing, and serology analyses for hepatitis B and C were performed, as was a liver biopsy. None of this testing revealed a specific hepatic or intestinal abnormality.

DISCUSSION: CASE 15-3

I. Differential Diagnosis

The susceptibility of neonates to unconjugated hyperbilirubinemia is favored by a number of factors, including relative increases in bilirubin production and enterohepatic circulation along with relative decreases in hepatic uptake and conjugation. Unconjugated hyperbilirubinemia is a very common occurrence in the newly born and is usually self-limited and benign. However, if the serum concentration of bilirubin exceeds 17 mg/dL, the jaundice can no longer be regarded as physiologic.

Given this predisposition of newborns to an imbalance between bilirubin generation and hepatic excretory capacity, pathologic or prolonged neonatal hyperbilirubinemia is often attributable to conditions that exacerbate the imbalance. For instance, hemolytic diseases (e.g., ABO incompatibility), polycythemia, and extravascular blood collections (e.g., cephalohematoma, subgaleal blood, ecchymoses) are conditions that favor increased bilirubin production. Decreased bilirubin clearance can result from inherited bilirubin metabolism disorders (e.g., Crigler-Najjar syndrome, Gilbert disease), hypothyroidism, and circumstances that increase enterohepatic reuptake (e.g., breast-feeding, delayed meconium passage). As for older children, Gilbert syndrome (a genetic disorder of the uridine diphosphoglucuronate glucuronosyltransferase enzyme system that occurs in about 6% of adults) and hemolytic anemias are the most common causes of unconjugated bilirubinemia.

II. Diagnosis

The baby's persistent hypoglycemia prompted an endocrinology service consultation. Among the array of examinations requested were thyroid function tests, which revealed a thyroid-stimulating hormone (TSH) concentration of 1.00 mIU/mL (normal range, 0.6 to 10.0) and a thyroxine (T4) level of 5.0 μg/dL (normal range, 5.5 to 17 μg/dL). These results—a low T4 with a TSH in the low-normal range—were deemed typical for central hypothyroidism, and T4 replacement was begun. A magnetic resonance imaging (MRI) study revealed an atrophic anterior pituitary gland and an ectopic posterior pituitary with arrested descent. More sophisticated biochemical testing was subsequently performed and indicated global pituitary dysfunction consistent with **a diagnosis of panhypopituitarism.**

III. Incidence and Epidemiology

Congenital hypothyroidism has been estimated to occur in about 1 of every 4,000 newborns, and about one third of these infants demonstrate prolonged hyperbilirubinemia. It appears that T4 is necessary to the bilirubin conjugating process. The baby in this case had hypothyroidism and protracted unconjugated bilirubinemia as dominant features of an even rarer endocrinopathy, congenital hypopituitarism. Of note, the hyperbilirubinemia seen in panhypopituitarism can also be *cholestatic,* particularly when growth hormone or corticotropin (ACTH) deficiencies dominate the pathophysiology.

IV. Clinical Presentation

Prolonged neonatal jaundice may be the first sign of congenital hypothyroidism and hypopituitarism. Feeding difficulties, apnea, noisy breathing, and overall sluggishness are other common manifestations. Physical findings specifically attributable to hypothyroidism can include a relatively large head, anterior fontanel, tongue, and abdomen; umbilical hernia; edema; and a lower-than-expected pulse and temperature. Mental and physical development become increasingly retarded over time when hypothyroidism goes undetected and uncorrected.

Among the physical findings that may be detected in patients with congenital hypopituitarism are micropenis, midline craniofacial defects (e.g., cleft lip or palate), a single central incisor, and signs of hypoglycemia or hypocortisolism, such as lethargy or apnea. The possibility of septo-optic dysplasia should be considered whenever congenital hypopituitarism is diagnosed. In addition to the neuroendocrine deficiency, these patients have optic nerve hypoplasia and agenesis of the septum pellucidum.

V.   Diagnostic Approach

Testing for deficiencies of pituitary hormones and MRI of the brain are crucial steps in evaluating suspected hypopituitarism. Standard newborn screening programs do not always detect pituitary hypothyroidism. Thyroid function tests in particular must be interpreted carefully. A TSH in the low-normal range, for instance, is not appropriate when the T4 level is borderline. Because presenting signs and symptoms of these endocrinopathies can often be quite subtle at first, an index of suspicion and appropriate, targeted testing are key to making the diagnosis.

VI.   Treatment

Replacement of the hormones produced by the pituitary's target organs is the cornerstone of hypopituitarism therapy. Thyroid hormone replacement should begin as soon as confirmatory testing is completed; delays in therapy can result in increased risk of cognitive impairment. Jaundice improves as the underlying endocrine disorder is treated.

VII.   References

1. Balint JP, Balistreri WF. Jaundice. In: Kleigman RM, ed. *Practical strategies in pediatric diagnosis and therapy.* Philadelphia: WB Saunders, 1996:360–379.
2. Dennery PA, Seidman DS, Stevenson DK. Neonatal hyperbilirubinemia. *N Engl J Med* 2001;344:581–590.
3. Gourley GR. Neonatal jaundice and disorders of bilirubin metabolism. In: Suchy FJ, Sokol RJ, Balistreri WF, eds. *Liver disease in children,* 2nd ed. Philadelphia: Lippincott Williams & Wilkins, 2001:275–314.
4. Kaplan M, Hammerman C, Maisels MJ. Bilirubin genetics for the nongeneticist: hereditary defects of neonatal bilirubin conjugation. *Pediatrics* 2003;111:886–893.
5. MacMahon JR, Stevenson DK, Oski FA. Unconjugated hyperbilirubinemias. In: Taeusch HW, Ballard RA, eds. *Avery's diseases of the newborn,* 7th ed. Philadelphia: WB Saunders, 1998:1014–1033.
6. Moshang T, Grimberg A. Neuroendocrine disorders. In: McMillan JA, DeAngelis CD, Feigin RD, et al., eds. *Oski's pediatrics: principles and practice,* 3rd ed. Philadelphia: Lippincott Williams & Wilkins, 1999:1787–1793.

Case 15-4: 6-Week-Old Girl

I. History of Present Illness

A 6-week-old, full-term female infant was brought to the hospital by her mother because of persistence of scleral icterus. The infant had been seen during the first week of life after the mother noted she "looked yellow." At that time, she was otherwise doing well and the pediatrician diagnosed physiologic jaundice. At 2 weeks of age, the baby began having blood-tinged stools. She was changed first from cow's milk to soy milk formula, and then to an elemental formula, after which the bleeding resolved.

The baby had lately been acting well, taking her feedings without difficulty, and making a normal number of wet diapers. There was no recent history of emesis, excessive fussiness, bleeding, or bruisability. The mother did report that the baby's stools had become increasingly white and pasty.

II. Past Medical History

The child was born by an uncomplicated, repeat cesarean section at 38 weeks. Her birth weight was 3.6 kg. Her hospital stay was unremarkable, and she was discharged home with her mother on the third day of life.

The infant had a healthy 3-year-old brother. There was no family history of jaundice, liver disease, anemia, or familial blood disorders.

III. Physical Examination

T, 37.0°C; RR, 32/min; HR, 136 bpm; BP, 88/60 mm Hg

Weight, 4.1 kg (10th to 25th percentile); length, 56 cm (25th to 50th percentile)

On examination, the infant was resting quietly in her mother's arms and was observed to have a mild "muddy" jaundice in her face. She was nondysmorphic and normocephalic, with an open, flat fontanel. Scleral icterus was pleasant. There was no nasal discharge or flaring. The oropharynx was clear, with moist mucous membranes. The lung and cardiac examinations were normal. Her abdomen was soft and nondistended, and a smooth, firm liver edge palpable 2 cm below the right costal margin. The genitourinary, extremity, and neurologic examinations were all normal.

IV. Diagnostic Studies

The complete blood count revealed the following: 6,900 WBCs/mm^3 (43% segmented neutrophils and 48% lymphocytes); hemoglobin, 9.2 g/dL; and 332,000 platelets/mm^3. Total bilirubin was 9.5 mg/dL, and the direct bilirubin concentration was 8.4 mg/dL. ALT and AST were 267 and 288 U/L, respectively. Albumin was 3.2 g/dL, and the alkaline phosphatase was 641 U/L. Serum electrolytes, BUN, creatinine, and glucose were normal. Calcium was also normal. Urinalysis revealed a specific gravity of 1.015 and 1+ blood but no nitrites, leukocyte esterase, protein, or urobilinogen.

V. Course of Illness

Abdominal ultrasound studies demonstrated mild hepatomegaly but normal-appearing kidneys, spleen, and adrenal glands. The infant was admitted for urgent evaluation of her cholestatic hyperbilirubinemia.

DISCUSSION: CASE 15-4

I. Differential Diagnosis

The differential diagnosis for cholestatic jaundice in the infant is quite broad, and many excellent and detailed reviews exist. General categories of disease entities to be considered include *infections,* such as hepatitis viruses, TORCH infections, and serious bacterial infections; *idiopathic neonatal hepatitis*; a long list of *metabolic and endocrine diseases,* including galactosemia, α_1-antitrypsin deficiency, cystic fibrosis, hypothyroidism, hypopituitarism, and bile acid synthesis defects; *genetic cholestatic syndromes,* such as Byler disease; *obstructions to bile flow,* including biliary atresia, Alagille syndrome, choledochal cysts, and cholelithiasis; and *iatrogenic causes,* such as drug-induced cholestasis or cholestasis related to total parenteral nutrition.

II.   Diagnosis

The infant was sent for a hepatic scintigraphic study (diisopropyl iminodiacetate [DISIDA] scan). It showed good tracer uptake but no intestinal excretion at 4 or 24 hours. An obstructive etiology of cholestasis was feared, and the baby was taken to the operating room. An intraoperative cholangiogram confirmed the **diagnosis of extrahepatic biliary atresia (EHBA).**

III.   Incidence and Etiology

Biliary atresia occurs in about 1 in every 10,000 to 15,000 infants worldwide. The disease is characterized by postinflammatory obliteration of some or all of the extrahepatic biliary ducts. The extent of biliary tree involvement varies. If the disease is limited to the distal segment, surgical correction may be possible. Far more common, however, is diffuse involvement of the extrahepatic biliary ducts, for which hepatic portoenterostomy (the Kasai procedure) or liver transplantation is required.

The etiology of EHBA remains a mystery. It is presumably caused by an insult, perhaps viral or ischemic, to the developing biliary tree. Not even the timing of the disease onset is clear. Some children with biliary atresia are born with other true congenital anomalies (e.g. malrotation, polysplenia, heart defects). On the other hand, most infants with EHBA have no other malformations and are clinically well until several weeks of age, suggesting a progressive, acquired process with relatively late onset. Likewise, the range of histopathologic findings seen in biliary atresia is heterogeneous. Therefore, it seems likely that multiple etiologies of biliary atresia exist.

IV.   Clinical Presentation

Infants with biliary atresia often present in the first 2 to 6 weeks of life with acholic stools, hepatomegaly, and jaundice. Over time the urine darkens, the jaundice persists, the liver grows (as bile stasis worsens), and even the spleen may enlarge. In the early weeks and months, these children often appear well and have unremarkable medical histories. If the disease goes untreated, malnutrition, growth retardation, and liver dysfunction emerge. Portal hypertension, coagulopathy, and hypersplenism may develop. In untreated patients, average expected survival time is about 1 year.

In this case, the baby presented with a direct hyperbilirubinemia but also a mild elevation of liver enzymes suggestive of hepatocellular injury. This is common in EHBA, although these findings may also be seen with neonatal hepatitis or other disease entities, and indeed there can be considerable overlap in clinical and laboratory findings among the various etiologies of conjugated hyperbilirubinemia. The complete blood count was not suggestive of acute infection, and the urinalysis appeared benign. The absence of urobilinogen is actually consistent with an obstructive cholestasis, because its formation requires entry of conjugated bilirubin into the intestine for degradation by gut bacteria. The presentation of a jaundiced but otherwise well-appearing 6-week-old infant with conjugated hyperbilirubinemia prompted an immediate search for an obstructive process, and hepatic scintigraphy strongly suggested the diagnosis that was confirmed by intraoperative cholangiogram.

V.   Diagnostic Approach

The differentiation of biliary atresia from other common causes of cholestatic jaundice in the young infant (particularly "neonatal hepatitis") can be complex. Prompt diagnosis of biliary atresia is critical because of the declining success of hepatic portoenterostomy performed beyond 2 months of age. Among the other causes of cholestatic jaundice for which urgent intervention is required are galactosemia, hormone deficiency states (specifically, hypothyroidism and hypopituitarism), and acute infections, notably with gram-negative organisms.

Once cholestatic jaundice has been diagnosed (with a fractionated bilirubin measurement) and a thorough history and physical examination have been performed, laboratory assessment of liver function should be made (e.g., prothrombin time, glucose, ammonia, albumin). Simultaneously, infectious and metabolic causes of cholestasis for which immediate therapy might be necessary, such as those mentioned previously, should be excluded. This evaluation should include cultures of blood and urine, assessment of thyroid function, and a measurement of urine reducing substances (in infants receiving lactose) or other appropriate assay for galactosemia. Other helpful first-line tests include liver enzymes (e.g., ALT, AST, alkaline phosphatase, GGT), complete blood count, and an abdominal ultrasound study.

Abdominal ultrasonography. Although abdominal ultrasonography does not diagnose biliary atresia, it can identify anomalies (e.g., polysplenia) that are specifically associated with some cases of EHBA, as well as gall bladder sludge or stones, choledochal cysts, ascites, and other disease states.

Hepatic scintigraphy. If abdominal ultrasonography is nondiagnostic, hepatic scintigraphy (e.g., DISIDA scan) may demonstrate biliary tract patency. A scintigraphic examination that *fails* to show hepatic excretion of the isotope, however, neither diagnoses EHBA nor excludes intrahepatic bile duct obstruction and neonatal hepatitis. Sampling of nasoduodenal tube aspirates for bile pigments—or even for radioactivity, if scintigraphy was performed—can also provide evidence of bile duct patency.

Other studies. Magnetic resonance cholangiography and endoscopic retrograde cholangiography are among the newer modalities for assessing the biliary tract anatomy. Liver biopsy is highly sensitive and specific for biliary atresia and can also differentiate EHBA from intrahepatic bile duct obstruction. Ultimately, if continuity between the liver and duodenum remains unproved, exploratory laparotomy with cholangiography is required.

If evaluation for obstructive processes and potential medical emergencies (e.g., galactosemia, sepsis, an endocrinopathy) is nondiagnostic, the scope of the evaluation must be widened. Once the extrahepatic diseases are excluded, the remainder of the differential diagnosis can be conceptualized as being related to either *hepatocellular* or *intrahepatic bile duct* etiologies. Multiple tests on blood and urine (in addition to sweat testing to rule out cystic fibrosis) are available to assess for specific disease entities. Among these are plasma amino acids, urine amino and organic acids, α_1-antitrypsin phenotype, plasma iron and ferritin (to rule out neonatal iron storage disease), serum and urine bile acid profile, and serologic analyses for the hepatitis virus, TORCH infections, syphilis, cytomegalovirus, human immunodeficiency virus (HIV), HHV-6, Epstein-Barr virus, and parvovirus B19. Liver biopsy is a safe and straightforward procedure, and the histopathologic data it provides can discriminate among diseases of intrahepatic bile duct hypoplasia or paucity.

VI. Treatment

The hepatic portoenterostomy (Kasai procedure) for biliary atresia involves the anastomosis of a limb of small intestine to hepatic ducts in the region of the porta hepatis (where the portal vein and hepatic artery enter the liver and the hepatic ducts exit). It relies on the patency of tiny duct remnants to allow for bile drainage from the liver. Cholangitis is among the most worrisome of the postoperative complications of hepatic portoenterostomy; its signs and symptoms include fever, diminished bile flow, and the return of hyperbilirubinemia. Over time, survivors of hepatic portoenterostomy are also at risk for liver dysfunction, portal hypertension, esophageal varices, hypersplenism, and hepatopulmonary syndrome, in which arteriovenous shunts form within the lung. Liver transplantation is often required for patients who have undergone portoenterostomy for EHBA, and it is sometimes necessary as a primary operation if liver disease is far advanced at the time of diagnosis. Estimates of 10-year survival for patients with EHBA range from 40% to 70%. Approximately 25% to 40% of patients survive 10 years without requiring transplantation.

VII.　References

1. Balistreri WF. Cholestasis. In: Behrman RE, Kleigman RM, Jenson HB, eds. *Nelson textbook of pediatrics,* 16th ed. Philadelphia: WB Saunders, 2000:1203–1207.
2. D'Agata ID, Balistreri WF. Evaluation of liver disease in the pediatric patient. *Pediatr Rev* 1999;20:376–388.
3. MacMahon JR, Stevenson DK, Oski FA. Obstructive jaundice due to biliary atresia and neonatal hepatitis. In: Taeusch HW, Ballard RA, eds. *Avery's Diseases of the Newborn,* 7th ed. Philadelphia: WB Saunders, 1998:1021–1029.
4. Nio M, Ohi R. Biliary atresia. *Semin Pediatr Surg* 2000;9:177–186.
5. Suchy FJ. Approach to the infant with cholestasis. In: Suchy FJ, Sokol RJ, Balistreri WF, eds. *Liver disease in children,* 2nd ed. Philadelphia: Lippincott Williams & Wilkins, 2001:187–194.
6. Witzleben CL, Piccoli DA. Extrahepatic bile ducts. In: Walker WA, Durie PR, Hamilton JR, et al., eds. *Pediatric gastrointestinal disease,* 3rd ed. Hamilton, Ontario: BE Decker, 2000:915–926.

Case 15-5: 12-Year-Old Boy

I. History of Present Illness

A 12-year-old boy presented with recent onset of scleral icterus. He had been in his usual state of good health until 3 weeks earlier, at which time his parents noticed yellowing of his eyes. The patient also noted occasional itching of his arms and legs. He reported having a good appetite but was experiencing earlier-than-usual satiety; his parents agreed that he was eating smaller meals. His stool output had not changed in quantity or quality, and there was no history of bloody or dark stool. Urine output was unchanged. There was no history of abdominal pain, vomiting, diarrhea, anorexia, weight loss, fever, fatigue, bleeding, or easy bruisability. There was no joint pain. There was no history of travel, tattooing, or unusual exposures. The boy was seen in his pediatrician's office, where a midline abdominal mass was detected. He was referred to the hospital for further evaluation.

II. Past Medical History

The boy had no history of hospitalization, surgery, or chronic medical problems. He was a full-term baby. He was taking no medications, had no allergies, and was up to date with immunizations. The family history was noncontributory. His three siblings were healthy. The boy was a seventh-grader who liked school and did well there.

III. Physical Examination

T, 37.2°C; RR, 20/min; HR, 96 bpm; BP, 110/64 mm Hg

Weight, 37 kg (5th percentile); height, 144 cm (5th percentile)

Physical examination revealed a smiling, pleasant, and cooperative boy. His examination was notable for mildly icteric sclerae and some injection of his conjunctivae. The oropharynx was clear. There was no lymphadenopathy. His lungs were clear with unlabored respirations. Cardiac examination revealed a regular rate and rhythm with a soft I/VI systolic ejection murmur at the left sternal border; peripheral pulses were normal. The abdomen was soft with mild right upper quadrant tenderness and a 8 × 5 cm midline mass extending 8 cm below the xyphoid process. In addition, there was splenomegaly to the level of the umbilicus, and the liver edge was palpable 2 cm below the right costal margin. A rectal examination was normal. On genitourinary examination, he was a Tanner I male without hernia or scrotal swelling. His extremities were warm and well perfused without edema. Neurologically, he was alert and entirely appropriate, with a grossly normal examination. His skin examination revealed only multiple chest nevi and some faint scratch marks on his arms.

IV. Diagnostic Studies

There were 4,800 WBCs/mm^3, with 41% segmented neutrophils and 44% lymphocytes. Hemoglobin was 12.1g/dL, and there were 160,000 platelets/mm^3. Serum electrolytes, BUN, and creatinine were normal. Serum glucose was 86 mg/dL. Calcium was 9.4 mg/dL. Total and conjugated bilirubin were 3.0 and 2.5 mg/dL, respectively. ALT was 176 U/L, and AST was 228 U/L. GGT was elevated at 345 U/L. Amylase was 67 U/L, and lipase was 178 U/dL. The uric acid was 3.2 mg/dL, and the lactate dehydrogenase was 664 U/L.

Chest radiography revealed borderline cardiomegaly but no infiltrates. An abdominal radiograph revealed a midline abdominal mass without calcifications. There was no evidence of bowel obstruction.

V. Course of Illness

Additional laboratory studies were obtained and revealed the following: erythrocyte sedimentation rate, 80 mm/hour; PT, 12.7 seconds; PTT, 31 seconds; and α$_1$-antitrypsin,

520 mg/dL (reference range, 95 to 224 mg/dL). Hepatitis B surface antibody was positive. Hepatitis B surface antigen, hepatitis B core antibody, hepatitis A immunoglobulin M, and hepatitis C PCR were all negative. Computed tomography of the chest was normal; the abdominal study showed an enlarged left lobe of the liver, macronodular changes in the liver parenchyma consistent with cirrhosis, a very enlarged spleen, minimal scattered adenopathy, and dilatation of the left bile duct. The child was admitted to the hospital for further evaluation of his hyperbilirubinemia, cirrhosis, and bile duct dilatation.

DISCUSSION: CASE 15-5

I. Differential Diagnosis

The differential diagnosis of cholestatic jaundice in the older child is very different from the list of diseases that manifest in the first few months of life. Whereas infants are more likely to have congenital anatomic anomalies (e.g., biliary atresia, cystic malformations) or inborn metabolic disorders (e.g., galactosemia, Zellweger syndrome, bile acid metabolism deficiencies), older children are more likely to experience acquired or secondary liver diseases, such as autoimmune or toxic hepatitis or liver impairment related to inflammatory bowel disease. One area where broad overlap does exist is infectious diseases: infectious hepatitis is among the most common causes of liver disease in older children and adolescents. Viruses causing hepatitis and jaundice in these children include hepatitis A, B, C, D and E; Epstein-Barr virus; cytomegalovirus; varicella; HHV-6; and HSV. Parasitic infections (e.g., schistosomiasis, leptospirosis) can also manifest with liver involvement, as can bacterial sepsis.

This youngster presented with conjugated hyperbilirubinemia, evidence of liver injury (reflected in the elevated transaminases), and left bile duct dilatation. The biochemical tests indicate a cholestatic disorder, whereas the bile duct dilatation suggests a structural, extrahepatic etiology.

Obstructive, extrahepatic causes of conjugated hyperbilirubinemia to consider in children and adolescents include cholelithiasis, choledochal cysts, sclerosing cholangitis, pancreatitis, and tumors or other anatomic abnormalities along the choledocho-pancreatico-duodenal path. (Cystic dilatation of *intrahepatic* bile ducts occurs in Caroli disease and in congenital hepatic fibrosis, conditions that usually manifest in younger children.)

II. Diagnosis

An open biopsy of the liver and surrounding lymph nodes was performed. It revealed cirrhosis, bile duct proliferation, patchy lymphocytic infiltrates, and concentric fibrosis around the bile ducts; the lymph node pathology was consistent with a reactive adenitis. Endoscopic retrograde cholangiopancreatography (ERCP) revealed irregularity and "beading," findings consistent with **sclerosing cholangitis.**

III. Incidence and Pathophysiology

Sclerosing cholangitis, an inflammatory disease of the hepatobiliary system, is characterized by intrahepatic and extrahepatic bile duct inflammation that progresses to areas of obliteration and dilatation. Ultimately, biliary cirrhosis and portal hypertension may develop and liver failure ensues.

Sclerosing cholangitis is considered to be *secondary* when it occurs in the setting of cholelithiasis, cystic fibrosis, Langerhans histiocytosis, neoplasia (e.g., Hodgkin's disease, ductal carcinoma), anatomic abnormalities (e.g., congenital disorders, postsurgical conditions), immunodeficiencies, and chronic ascending infection. *Primary* sclerosing cholangitis (PSC), on the other hand, is diagnosed when no such underlying disease exists. PSC is strongly associated with, but is not caused by, inflammatory bowel disease;

indeed, the onset of hepatobiliary disease can precede the development of intestinal disease by years. The etiology of PSC is not known.

IV. Clinical Presentation

PSC can develop at any age, including infancy, though young adulthood is the most common period of presentation. Early, insidious symptoms often include malaise, anorexia, abdominal pain, diarrhea, and weight loss. Pruritus is another common symptom of extrahepatic cholestasis, though the precise nature of the pruritogen is not well understood. Frank cholangitis may manifest with right upper quadrant pain, jaundice, and fever.

As PSC progresses, biliary obstruction worsens and secondary biliary cirrhosis develops. One complication of worsening liver disease is portal hypertension with varices. PSC has an unfavorable prognosis and is a common indication for liver transplantation. PSC is a risk factor for cholangiocarcinoma in adults.

V. Diagnostic Approach

Clinical and biochemical evidence of cholestasis may suggest the possibility of PSC, but these findings alone do not differentiate this disease from entities such as hepatitis (acute and chronic), α_1-antitrypsin deficiency, Wilson disease, cholelithiasis, and many other causes of cholestatic jaundice. Furthermore, the diagnosis of PSC in patients with established Crohn's disease or ulcerative colitis can be confounded by the chronic hepatitis that sometimes accompanies inflammatory bowel disease.

Cholangiography. The definitive diagnosis of sclerosing cholangitis is made by cholangiography. Characteristic hepatobiliary changes include strictures, irregular narrowing of bile ducts, and decreased peripheral branching of intrahepatic ducts. Histologic changes may include the dilatation and obliteration of bile ducts with concentric, periductal fibrosis ("onion-skin fibrosis").

VI. Treatment

There is no known effective medical treatment for PSC. Attention must be paid to nutrition and to the prevention of fat-soluble vitamin deficiencies. Ursodeoxycholic acid is useful for reducing pruritus but does not appear to alter the disease course. Some patients with focal, dominant biliary tract strictures have benefited from endoscopic balloon dilatation. Nevertheless, for most patients, no specific medical or surgical therapy is available. Liver transplantation is the only effective treatment for PSC patients with progressive liver disease. Recurrence of disease in the graft is possible.

VII. References

1. Balint JP, Balistreri WF. Sclerosing cholangitis. In: Suchy FJ, Sokol RJ, Balistreri WF, eds. *Liver disease in children.* Philadelphia: Lippincott Williams & Wilkins, 2001:443–461.
2. Balint JP, Balistreri WF. Jaundice. In: Kleigman RM, ed. *Practical strategies in pediatric diagnosis and therapy.* Philadelphia: WB Saunders, 1999:360–379.
3. D'Agata ID, Balistreri WF. Evaluating liver disease in the pediatric patient. *Pediatr Rev* 1999;20:376–388.
4. Piccoli DA, Witzleben CL. Intrahepatic bile ducts. In: Walker WA, Durie PR, Hamilton JR, et al., eds. *Pediatric gastrointestinal disease,* 3rd ed. Hamilton, Ontario: BC Decker, 2000:895–914.

Case 15-6: 5-Week-Old Girl

I. History of Present Illness

A 5-week-old girl was referred to the hospital for evaluation of her jaundice and poor weight gain. Her father stated that she had been "yellow her whole life," starting before she left the newborn nursery. Except for some nasal congestion, the baby seemed to be acting and sleeping normally. She had been feeding on cow's milk formula, taking 2 to 3 ounces every 3 hours, and made five to six wet diapers per day. The father described the baby's stool output as two to four "loose" and "pasty" bowel movements per day. There was no history of fever, emesis, diarrhea, travel, or unusual exposures.

II. Past Medical History

The baby weighed 3.25 kg at birth; she was the product of a full-term gestation, delivered via cesarean section to a mother with a history of osteoporosis and back pain. The mother took no medications and denied use of drugs or alcohol. The baby was discharged home with her mother on the second day of life. She lived at home with both parents. There was no family history of cystic fibrosis, cardiac or gastrointestinal disease, or other pediatric illnesses.

III. Physical Examination

T, 37.2°C; RR, 28/min; HR, 120 bpm; BP, 80/56 mm Hg

Weight, 3.35 kg (5th percentile); length, 51 cm; head circumference, 36 cm

The infant appeared small but comfortable in her father's lap. She had an open, flat fontanel and a broad forehead; equal and round pupils; and scleral icterus. The oropharynx was clear with moist mucous membranes. Respirations were clear and unlabored. Cardiac examination revealed a II/VI systolic murmur that was loudest at the left sternal border; the rate, rhythm, and distal pulses were all normal. Her abdomen was soft and nondistended, with a smooth liver edge palpable 3 cm below the right costal margin; no spleen or other masses were appreciated. The genitourinary, extremity, and neurologic examinations were all normal.

IV. Initial Diagnostic Studies

A complete blood count revealed the following: 16,700 WBCs/mm^3 (31% segmented neutrophils and 61% lymphocytes); hemoglobin, 9.6 g/dL; and 625,000 platelets/mm^3. The BUN and creatinine concentrations were 26 and 1.1 mg/dL, respectively. Serum electrolytes were normal. The total bilirubin concentration was 11.0 mg/dL; unconjugated and conjugated bilirubin were 8.0 and 3.1 mg/dL, respectively. The remainder of the hepatic function panel was as follows: ALT, 190 U/L; AST, 94 U/L; albumin, 3.0 mg/dL; and alkaline phosphatase, 450 U/L. Blood and urine cultures were obtained and were negative. Evaluations for toxoplasmosis, rubella, cytomegalovirus, and HIV were also negative.

V. Course of Illness

The baby was admitted to the hospital for further evaluation. A renal ultrasound study showed two somewhat small but otherwise unremarkable kidneys, and biochemical measurements of her renal function (e.g., BUN, creatinine, non–anion gap metabolic acidosis) trended toward normal during the hospitalization without specific therapy. Echocardiography revealed a structurally normal heart. An extensive investigation of her cholestatic jaundice culminated in a liver biopsy and intraoperative cholangiogram. The biopsy showed prominent cholestasis, occasional giant hepatocytes, and a ratio of bile ducts to portal tracts of about 0.5 (normal, 0.9 to 1.8); the cholangiogram was normal.

DISCUSSION: CASE 15-6

I. Differential Diagnosis

This infant presented with the following signs: a nonobstructive conjugated hyper-bilirubinemia; renal insufficiency with a mild, non–anion gap metabolic acidosis; poor weight gain; and a heart murmur. Her liver biopsy revealed cholestasis and bile duct paucity.

Interlobular bile duct paucity is the characteristic, but not unvarying, pathologic finding in Alagille syndrome; biopsies performed early in the disease's course might simply reveal findings of cholestasis, inflammation, or even ductal proliferation. In addition, bile duct paucity is sometimes seen in diseases other than Alagille syndrome. So-called non-syndromic bile duct paucity can be a feature of congenital infections (e.g., CMV, rubella, syphilis), metabolic disorders (e.g., α_1-antitrypsin deficiency, defects of bile acid synthesis), sclerosing cholangitis, and idiopathic cholestasis.

II. Diagnosis

As part of an extensive evaluation, the baby was seen by a geneticist, who noted hyper-telorism and a pointed mandible in addition to the broad forehead noted on initial examination. The recommended ophthalmology examination revealed the baby to have posterior embryotoxon, and a review of her admission chest radiograph detected butterfly vertebrae. The baby's constellation of clinical and pathologic findings led to a **diagnosis of Alagille syndrome.**

III. Pathology

Alagille syndrome (also known as arteriohepatic dysplasia) is an uncommon disorder of intrahepatic bile duct paucity associated with well-defined anomalies of the heart, eyes, kidneys, and skeleton. The inheritance is autosomal dominant with variability in expression, although many cases appear to arise from new mutations. The disease has been mapped to chromosome 20, specifically to mutations in *JAGGED1,* which is part of a cell signaling pathway important in embryogenesis.

IV. Clinical Presentation

Alagille syndrome typically manifests as cholestasis in the first months of life. Clinical and laboratory findings of the liver disease include jaundice, acholic stools, pruritus, growth failure, conjugated hyperbilirubinemia, and elevations of hepatic enzymes. Most patients with Alagille syndrome also have heart murmurs, and the underlying heart conditions range in severity from benign (e.g., mild peripheral pulmonary stenosis) to complex disease requiring surgery (e.g. tetralogy of Fallot). The most common ocular finding in Alagille syndrome is posterior embryotoxon, a dysgenesis of the anterior chamber of the eye (best seen on slit-lamp examination) in which there is prominence of Schwalbe's ring, a ridge of collagenous fibers surrounding the periphery of Descemet's membrane.

Patients with Alagille syndrome often have a distinctive facies that may be detectable as early as infancy. Features can include a triangular face with a broad forehead and pointed chin, deeply set eyes, and a long nose with a bulbous tip. Xanthomas are another physical finding common to patients with Alagille syndrome.

Other problems associated with Alagille syndrome include renal anomalies (both structural and functional), pancreatic insufficiency, intracranial hemorrhage, and cognitive impairments. Assessments of renal function and anatomy (i.e., ultrasonography) should be performed. The patient presented in this case, for example, demonstrated slow but spontaneous improvement in her renal function and never required alkali supplementation.

V.   Diagnostic Approach

Patients with known or suspected Alagille syndrome require a multidisciplinary initial assessment. The diagnosis is based on the histopathologic demonstration of bile duct paucity in the setting of well-recognized clinical associations as described later. Early evaluation and follow-up by specialists in gastroenterology and nutrition is critical. In addition, cardiology and ophthalmology evaluations should be performed as early as possible.

Chest radiography. Radiographs of the chest are necessary to assess for vertebral anomalies (butterfly vertebrae and hemivertebrae).

Ophthalmologic evaluation. Ophthalmologic evaluation detects posterior embryotoxon.

Echocardiography. Recognized cardiac involvement includes peripheral pulmonary artery stenosis and tetralogy of Fallot.

Genetic consultation. As previously noted, most patients with Alagille syndrome have a characteristic facial appearance. Early evaluation by a geneticist can help guide diagnosis and provide appropriate genetic counseling. In addition, genetic testing is now available for *JAGGED1* mutations. The testing is far from perfect, however, and a significant percentage of patients with Alagille syndrome have no demonstrable mutation.

VI.   Treatment

Treatment of Alagille syndrome focuses on the medical management of cholestasis, promotion of growth and development, and treatment of any comorbidities (e.g., congenital heart disease). Children with Alagille syndrome suffer from malabsorption and require supplementation of fat-soluble vitamins and provision of sufficient calories for growth, which may necessitate tube feeding. Infants should receive formulas containing medium-chain triglycerides, which are absorbable without bile salts. Medications that may benefit Alagille patients (for example, by promoting bile flow or reducing pruritus) include phenobarbital, cholestyramine, ursodeoxycholic acid, and antihistamines.

Long-term follow-up of patients with Alagille syndrome includes monitoring for the development of cirrhosis, portal hypertension, ascites, and liver failure. The 20-year life expectancy for patients with Alagille syndrome is about 75% overall, although rates are lower for those patients who require liver transplantation and for those with severe associated abnormalities (e.g., congenital heart disease).

VII. References

1. Emerick KM, Rand EB, Goldmuntz E, et al. Features of Alagille syndrome in 92 patients: frequency and relation to prognosis. *Hepatology* 1999;29:822–829.
2. Krantz ID, Piccoli DA, Spinner NB. Alagille syndrome. *J Med Genet* 1997;34: 152–157.
3. Piccoli DA. Alagille syndrome. In: Suchy FJ, Sokol RJ, Balistreri WF, eds. *Liver disease in children,* 2nd ed. Philadelphia: Lippincott Williams & Wilkins, 2001:327–342.
4. Piccoli DA, Witzleben CL. Intrahepatic bile ducts. In: Walker WA, Durie PR, Hamilton JR, et al., eds. *Pediatric gastrointestinal disease,* 3rd ed. Hamilton, Ontario: BC Decker, 2000:895–914.
5. Suchy FJ. Anatomy, histology, embryology, developmental anomalies, and pediatric disorders of the biliary tract. In: Feldman M, ed. *Sleisenger and Fordtran's gastrointestinal and liver disease,* 7th ed. Philadelphia: WB Saunders, 2002:1019–1042.

16

Abnormal Gait, Including Refusal to Walk

Jeanine Ronan

APPROACH TO THE PATIENT WHO REFUSES TO WALK

I. Definition of the Complaint

When a child refuses to walk, the list of possible causes is very extensive, consisting of both benign and life-threatening conditions. A systematic approach is necessary to complete a thorough evaluation.

A normal gait is a "smooth, mechanical process that advances the center of gravity with a minimum expenditure of energy." The stance phase is the time period when the heel strikes the ground and the ball of the other foot leaves the ground. This requires very strong abductor muscles in order to stabilize the pelvis. The swing phase is defined as the time when the foot leaves the ground until the next heel strike.

There are many types of abnormal walking patterns. An *antalgic gait* is the pattern used to minimize pain. In this pattern, the patient shortens the stance phase of the affected limb and also shortens the stride length. A patient with a fracture, soft tissue injury, or infection will use an antalgic gait. *Circumduction* is the pattern used to shorten a limb and improve limb clearance. This is commonly seen in patients with excessive joint stiffness secondary to spasticity. A *Trendelenburg gait* is present when the muscles on one side of the pelvis are weak, causing pelvic instability; if both sides are involved, a *waddling gait* is seen. An *unsteady gait* suggests the presence of ataxia. A *steppage gait* is seen in cases of peripheral neurologic weakness. The foot slaps the ground as the patient walks due to decreased ankle dorsiflexion.

II. Complaint by Cause and Frequency

When a child refuses to walk, the most common causes vary based on the child's age (Table 16-1). The primary causes of limp are pain, weakness, and mechanical factors. These can be further grouped by the following types of mechanisms: traumatic, infectious, inflammatory, congenital, developmental, neurologic, neoplastic, hematologic, and metabolic (Table 16-2).

III. Clarifying Questions

When evaluating a child who refuses to walk or a child with an abnormal gait, a thorough history and physical examination are crucial. Consideration of the patient's age, duration of symptoms, and presence of systemic complaints allow the examiner to

TABLE 16-1. *Common Causes of Refusal to Walk in Childhood by Age*

Infant/toddler	School age	Adolescent
Developmental dysplasia of the hip	Toxic synovitis	Slipped capital femoral epiphysis
Torsional deformities	Septic arthritis	Patellofemoral problems
Toddler's fracture	Osteomyelitis	Stress fracture
Foreign bodies	Legg-Calvé-Perthes disease	Arthritis
Tumor	Tumor	Tumor

TABLE 16-2. *Causes of Abnormal Gait in Childhood by Mechanism*

Trauma	Fractures (accidental or child abuse)
	Contusions/soft tissue injuries
	Foreign bodies/splinters/poorly fitting shoes
	Patellofemoral pain
	Spondylolisthesis
Infectious	Septic arthritis
	Osteomyelitis
	Toxic synovitis or reactive arthritis
	Diskitis
	Lyme arthritis
Inflammatory	Rheumatologic disease
	Ankylosing spondylitis
	Psoriatic arthritis
	Arthritis related to inflammatory bowel disease
	Rheumatic fever
	Serum sickness
Congenital	Congenital limb abnormalities
	Spinal dysraphism
Developmental or acquired	Developmental dysplasia of hips
	Blount's disease
	Limb length discrepancy
	Avascular necrosis (Legg-Calvé-Perthes)
	Slipped capital femoral epiphysis
	Osgood-Schlatter disease
Neurologic	Cerebral palsy
	Peripheral neuropathies
	Charcot-Marie-Tooth disease
	Guillan-Barré syndrome
	Cerebellar problems
Neoplastic	Benign bone tumors
	Osteoid osteoma
	Malignant bone tumors (osteosarcoma, Ewing sarcoma, neuroblastoma)
	Leukemia
Metabolic	Rickets
	Hyperparathyroidism
Hematologic	Sickle cell disease
	Hemophilia

develop the appropriate differential diagnosis for the problem. The following list of questions may help guide the clinician to the ultimate diagnosis.

- Is the child's refusal to walk due to pain?

  — Trauma is the most common etiology that results in a child's refusing to walk. The cause may be repetitive or overuse injury, accidental injury, or child abuse. Clues to differentiating between accidental and abuse-related injuries include understanding the mechanism of the injury. Does the explained mechanism for the incident seem appropriate for the developmental age of the child? In addition, pain may be present because of inflammation and swelling in the bone or joint. Septic arthritis and osteomyelitis are other common causes for limping. A child with juvenile rheumatoid arthritis (JRA) or reactive arthritis also complains of pain in the joints and may refuse to walk. If a child is unable to walk but denies the presence of pain, one must look hard for neuromuscular, metabolic, or congenital and developmental abnormalities. Developmental dysplasia of the hip may result in limb length discrepancy and an abnormal walking pattern. A child with appendicitis may refuse to walk due to referred pain from the abdomen.

- How did the symptoms evolve? Was there a sudden or a gradual onset?

  — In some cases, the parents notice that the child initially develops an abnormal gait and as symptoms worsen ultimately refuses to walk. This suggests the presence of an inflammatory condition or mechanical cause. In other cases, a child abruptly is unable to walk; this may suggest the presence of an injury or septic joint.

- Are there any associated symptoms?

  — The presence of other symptoms, including fever, weight loss, abdominal pain, diarrhea, and rash, may be suggestive of other causes. Children with leukemia commonly complain of bone pain as well as weakness, malaise, and fever. A child with undiagnosed inflammatory bowel disease may have diarrhea, weight loss, and isolated joint swelling. Systemic JRA manifests commonly with fever, weight loss, and rash in a school age child.

- Are joint swelling and erythema present?

  — Associated signs of infection, including toxic appearance; fever; chills; and joint redness, swelling, warmth, and decreased mobility, accompany septic arthritis. Many inflammatory causes will result in joint swelling and increased joint warmth.

- How could the limp be characterized?

  — Does the child refuse to walk due to the presence of pain? Does the child's abnormal walking pattern represent an attempt to minimize the amount of time spent on the involved leg? Is the child able to bear weight? Abnormalities in the structure of the lower extremity, such as torsional deformities or leg length discrepancies, also cause an abnormal walking pattern. In addition, any abnormalities in the muscle, such as an increase in tone or the presence of contractures, will generate an abnormal walking pattern. A child may also refuse to walk due to weakness. Weakness may be found in the muscle, or there may be a problem with the peripheral nerves of central nervous system.

- Are there localizing signs on physical examination of the child?

  — If pain is present, the clinician should try to localize the area of maximum tenderness. In some cases, a child refuses to walk due to referred pain. The child may have an acute abdomen or torsion of the testes and may refuse to walk to minimize pain.

IV. References

1. Kost S. Limp. In: Fleisher GR, Ludwig S, eds.*Textbook of pediatric emergency medicine*. Philadelphia: Lippincott Williams & Wilkins, 2000:369–374.
2. Myers M, Thompson GH. Imaging the child with a limp. *Pediatr Clin North Am* 1997; 44:637–667.
3. Dabney KW, Lipton G. Evaluation of limp in children. *Curr Opin Pediatr* 1995;7: 88–94.
4. Flynn JM. Evaluation of the limping child (lecture). *Pediatric Refresher Course,* 2000.

The following cases illustrate the approach to a patient with abnormal gait.

Case 16-1: 4-Year-Old Boy

I. History of Present Illness

A 4-year-old white male child presented to the emergency department after a 1-week history of leg pain. Initially, the pain was described as bilateral, primarily surrounding his knees. However, the pain gradually became more diffuse and consistently woke the patient from sleep. In addition, the parents noted that their son was more clumsy. He had difficulty walking and he was dropping objects from both of his hands. Review of systems was significant for constipation, urinary incontinence, and fatigue. Three weeks earlier, the patient had had an upper respiratory tract infection, which was resolved by the time of presentation.

II. Past Medical History

There was no significant prior medical history. He had reached all his developmental milestones, and he had been walking since 9 months of age.

III. Physical Examination

T, 36.3°C; RR, 24/min; HR, 120 bpm; BP, 120/70 mm Hg

Height, less than 5th percentile; weight, 10th percentile

Initial examination revealed an alert and interactive young boy. His neurologic examination was remarkable for decreased strength in his lower extremities. Deep tendon reflexes were not elicited in the upper and lower extremities. He was unable to perform rapid alternating movements or finger-to-nose proprioception. His cranial nerves were intact, including a normal gag reflex. The remainder of the examination was unremarkable.

IV. Diagnostic Studies

Laboratory analysis included a normal complete blood count and ESR. Computed tomography (CT) of the head demonstrated mild mucosal thickening of the maxillary sinus. Cerebral spinal fluid demonstrated 1 white blood cell (WBC)/mm^3 and 25 red blood cells/mm^3. The protein concentration was 106 mg/dL, and the glucose level was 69 mg/dL. The boy was admitted to the hospital for further evaluation.

V. Course of Illness

What is the most likely diagnosis?

DISCUSSION: CASE 16-1

I. Differential Diagnosis

The combination of symptoms including refusal to walk, pain, and areflexia suggests a peripheral neuropathy. There are many causes of peripheral neuropathies. Guillain-Barré syndrome is the most common cause. But this may be the presentation of a progressive form, chronic inflammatory demyelinating polyneuropathy. Many drugs have been implicated in inducing neuropathies, including isoniazid, vincristine, heavy metals (mercury and lead), and organophosphates. In addition, there could be involvement of the spinal cord, as is seen in transverse myelitis or a compressive myelopathy. Myopathies may manifest with similar symptoms but with hyporeflexia.

II. Diagnosis

In this case, the physical finding of absent deep tendon reflexes was very important in leading to the proper diagnosis. The elevated cerebrospinal fluid protein with a normal number of WBCs (cytoalbuminemic dissociation) was also consistent with the diagnosis of Guillain-Barré syndrome. Electromyography (EMG) showed prolonged distal motor latencies in all motor nerves and a slowed conduction velocity that was consistent with a demyelinating process. **The diagnosis of Guillain-Barré syndrome was made.** At this point, the patient did not show any signs of respiratory compromise. Intravenous gamma globulin (IVIG) therapy was started. Gradually his symptoms began to improve.

III. Incidence and Epidemiology

Guillain-Barré syndrome, the most common cause of acute generalized paralysis, has prevalence of 0.4 to 1.7 cases per 100,000 children. It is an acquired disease of the peripheral nervous system whose exact cause is not known. It may be mediated by an immune response against antigens or themyelin sheath axons of peripheral nerves, which leads to demyelination of motor and sensory nerves. Many cases are postinfectious; in these cases, there is a history of gastrointestinal or respiratory illness within 4 weeks of the appearance of symptoms. Infections associated with the development of Guillain-Barré syndrome include *Campylobacter jejuni,* varicella, cytomegalovirus, hepatitis, measles, mumps, and *Mycoplasma* species.

IV. Clinical Presentation

The diagnosis of Guillain-Barré syndrome requires the presence of progressive and ascending motor weakness of more than one limb, as well as areflexia. There is also the presence of sensory loss, including paresthesias, numbness, and diminished position and vibratory sensation. Ataxia is another common finding.

Pain is a surprisingly common finding in children. A review of 29 children hospitalized with Guillain-Barré syndrome demonstrated the presence of pain in 79%. However, in many cases the presence of pain obscured the proper diagnosis. The pain hindered accurate neurologic examination and usually caused clinicians to initially suspect a rheumatologic or inflammatory disorder. Adults typically classify the pain as a deep lower limb pain, exacerbated by straight leg raises.

Fever is not a common sign. However, there may be signs of autonomic dysfunction, including labile blood pressure, tachycardia or bradycardia, and bladder or bowel dysfunction. Respiratory failure can be fairly rapid in onset and is seen in 20% of patients.

The Miller-Fisher variant involves ophthalmoplegia and is caused by a specific immunoglobulin G directed at a ganglioside.

V. Diagnostic Approach

The important step in making the diagnosis is to consider Guillain-Barré as a possible etiology.

Lumbar puncture. Cerebrospinal fluid demonstrates an elevated protein content with only minimal pleocytosis (fewer than 10 WBCs/mm^3).

Electromyography. The diagnosis is usually supported by EMG studies, which demonstrate slowed or blocked motor conduction. Within 2 weeks after illness onset, the EMG is abnormal in approximately 50% of patients. Ultimately, 85% of patients with Guillain-Barré syndrome have an abnormal EMG.

Magnetic resonance imaging (MRI) of the spine. Although MRI is not usually required for diagnosis, it should be performed if spinal compression is suspected. In patients with Guillain-Barré syndrome, MRI frequently reveals spinal nerve root enhancement.

VI. Treatment

A large part of treatment is supportive care. Monitoring for autonomic dysfunction and respiratory failure are key components to effective treatment. Plasmapheresis and intravenous gammaglobulin (IVIG) are the current treatment modalities. In general, IVIG is thought to be as effective as plasmapheresis and may have a quicker onset of action. A recent study concluded that 23% of children continued to have evidence of mild muscle weakness after IVIG therapy, but in many cases this weakness had no impact of daily function. Children who were young and who had a rapid progression of symptoms were more likely to have long-term weakness.

Most patients recover spontaneously within 6 months. Recovery is made in a descending manner. Physical therapy is important for all patients.

VII. Reference

1. Evans OB, Vedanarayanan V. Guillain-Barré syndrome. *Pediatr Rev* 1997;18:10–16.
2. Gordon PH, Wilbourn AJ. Early electrodiagnostic findings in Guillain-Barré syndrome. *Arch Neurol* 2001;58:913–917.
3. Nguyen DK, Agenarioti-Belanger S, Vanasse M. Pain and the Guillain-Barré syndrome in children under 6 years old. *J Pediatr* 1999;134:773–776.
4. Vajsar J, Fehlings D, Stephens D. Long-term outcome in children with Guillain-Barré syndrome. *J Pediatr* 2003;142:305–309.

Case 16-2: 3-Year-Old Boy

I. History of Present Illness

A healthy 3-year-old boy presented to the emergency department with significant left ankle swelling and inability to walk. Over the past several months, he had had swelling and tenderness of multiple joints, including his knees, wrists, fingers, and hips. He had also had daily fevers with associated night sweats and an 8-pound weight loss. His mother noted a rash that appeared on his face, back, chest, and lower extremity.

II. Past Medical History

His past medical history was unremarkable.

III. Physical Examination

T, 38.2°C; RR, 24/min; HR, 106 bpm; BP, 102/64 mm Hg

Height, 50th percentile; weight, 10th percentile

In general, the boy appeared tired. Musculoskeletal examination revealed multiple painful and swollen joints with limited range of motion, including his right hip, right wrist, and left third digit. His neurologic examination was nonfocal; however, the child refused to walk. A salmon-colored rash was noted on the lower extremity. The remainder of the examination was normal.

IV. Diagnostic Studies

Initial laboratory data revealed 14,600 WBCs/mm³, with 54% segmented neutrophils, 6% band forms, and 36% lymphocytes. The hemoglobin was 7.9 g/dL, and there were 997,000 platelets/mm³. The erythrocyte sedimentation rate (ESR) was 63 mm/hour. Electrolytes, blood urea nitrogen, and creatinine were normal. Liver function tests were normal, except for an albumin concentration of 2.9 mg/dL. Blood cultures were subsequently sterile. Lyme antibodies and anti-streptolysin O (ASO) titers were also negative. Radiologic studies were normal, including hip and abdominal radiographs.

V. Course of Illness

A septic arthritis was considered unlikely, given the number of joints involved and the chronicity of the problem. Throughout his hospital stay, the patient continued to have fevers and joint swelling. A salmon-colored rash appeared with each temperature elevation and suggested the diagnosis (Fig. 16-1).

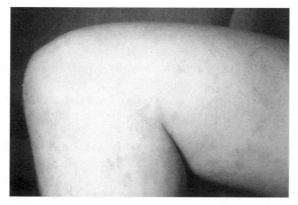

FIG. 16-1. Photograph of the patient's rash (case 16-2).

DISCUSSION: CASE 16-2

I. Differential Diagnosis

In a child with fever and refusal to bear weight on an extremity, infectious causes such as septic arthritis and osteomyelitis must be considered. Children with septic arthritis may have systemic symptoms including irritability and malaise. The affected joint acutely appears erythematous, edematous, and tender. Range of motion is typically limited. In more than 90% of cases, only a single joint is affected. Children with acute hematogenous osteomyelitis manifest symptoms for a period of less than 2 weeks. On physical examination, erythema, edema, and tenderness over the affected bone are often present. However, the degree of tenderness is out of proportion to the other findings. The femur, tibia, humerus, and fibula are most commonly involved. Laboratory findings in both septic arthritis and osteomyelitis include leukocytosis and elevation of the ESR and C-reactive protein (CRP) concentration.

Acute rheumatic fever may also manifest with fever, but in this case the arthritis is extremely painful and migratory. In addition, there must be evidence of a recent group A *Streptococcus* infection. The constellation of fever, rash, and joint pain also suggests systemic-onset juvenile rheumatoid arthritis (JRA). The presentation of systemic-onset JRA can be elusive and is sometimes confused with that of leukemia or lymphoma. The patient with systemic-onset JRA may have lymphadenopathy and hepatosplenomegaly. The arthritis and joint symptoms may not be apparent initially.

II. Diagnosis

In this case, the evanescent salmon-colored rash strongly suggested the **diagnosis of systemic JRA** (Fig. 16-1).

III. Incidence and Epidemiology

JRA is the most common rheumatic disease of childhood. The incidence is 1:10,000, with a prevalence of 1:1,000. In general, these disorders are more common among children of European descent. Based on the symptoms present within the first 6 months of illness, JRA is classified as systemic, pauciarticular, or polyarticular. Systemic JRA represents about 10% of all cases, is seen equally among boys and girls, and has no peak in the age at onset. Pauciarticular JRA is the most common type, accounting for about 50% of the cases. It is seen more commonly in girls, with a 5:1 ratio. Most children with pauciarticular JRA present between 1 and 6 years of age. Polyarticular JRA comprises the remaining 40% of cases. It is also seen more commonly in girls, but with a ratio of only 3:1. Age at onset of polyarticular JRA has two peaks, between 1 and 4 years of age and between 7 and 10 years of age.

IV. Clinical Presentation

As previously discussed, the clinical presentation of JRA is extremely diverse, depending of the type of JRA. In general, JRA represents a group of diseases that involve infiltration and proliferation of the synovial membrane, which results in joint swelling. This type of pain is associated with morning stiffness and a gait disturbance, in contrast to musculoskeletal pain due to mechanical or overuse injuries. Patients with musculoskeletal pain have worsening of symptoms during the day or with exercise and have no associated joint effusion.

Systemic-onset juvenile rheumatoid arthritis. Systemic-onset JRA manifests with high spiking fevers, a salmon-colored rash that begins in the groin or axilla and extends to the trunk and extremities, hepatosplenomegaly, and lymphadenopathy, with or without the arthritis. Supporting laboratory data show an elevated WBC count, anemia, thrombocytosis, and signs of disseminated intravascular coagulation due to the macrophage activation syndrome. The ESR is typically greater than 80 mm/hour. The disease is managed with systemic corticosteroids, nonsteroidal antiinflammatory drugs (NSAIDs), or methotrexate. Chronic iriditis is not typically seen.

Pauciarticular juvenile rheumatoid arthritis. In pauciarticular JRA, the patient presents with fewer than five joints involved. In early-onset or type I disease, the typical patient is a preschool girl with isolated knee swelling and difficulty with walking. Most patients have a positive antinuclear antibody (ANA) titer, which puts them at high risk for silent uveitis. Treatment may include NSAIDs or intraarticular steroid injections. These patients are most likely to go into permanent remission. In contrast, patients with late-onset or type II disease have joint involvement of the axial skeleton, namely the hips and sacroiliac joints. This is seen more commonly in boys older than 6 years of age. Many are positive for the human leukocyte antigen HLA-B27 and go on to have continued symptoms and enthesitis.

Polyarticular juvenile rheumatoid arthritis. Polyarticular JRA affects five or more joints at the time of presentation. Usually the joints involved are symmetric and include the small joints of the hands, the temporomandibular joint, or the cervical spine. Rheumatoid factor may be present in some cases. This represents a poorer prognosis, with a disease course similar to that of adult rheumatoid arthritis. If the ANA titer is positive, these patients are also at risk for chronic iriditis.

V. Diagnostic Approach

For a diagnosis of JRA, by definition the patient must have had symptoms for at least 6 weeks. The history and physical examination should be directed at eliciting clues to changes in gait, the presence of joint effusions, and pain in the joints. It is important to examine all joints, including the temporomandibular joint and the cervical spine, for subtle changes. Associated symptoms, including fever, rash, and adenopathy, must be assessed. Laboratory data may be a helpful adjunct.

Complete blood count. Patients with systemic JRA often have leukocytosis with neutrophil predominance, thrombocytosis, and anemia. Many patients with polyarticular JRA have anemia.

Rheumatoid factor. For the most part, a positive rheumatoid factor is not helpful in making the diagnosis. In most cases of JRA the test is negative, with the exception of approximately 15% of cases of polyarticular JRA. In this instance, a positive rheumatoid factor is important for prognosis but is not required for the diagnosis.

Anti-nuclear antibody. ANA studies are not required for the diagnosis of JRA but are helpful in classifying patients. ANA is positive in approximately 80% of children with pauciarticular JRA and 50% of children with polyarticular JRA. If JRA patients are ANA positive, their risk for chronic uveitis is higher. Because chronic uveitis is an asymptomatic condition with devastating complications, including cataracts, glaucoma, and loss of visual acuity, these patients require close ophthalmologic follow-up.

Radiography. Radiographs are normal early in the course of illness, but persistent arthritis may lead to bone demineralization and loss of articular cartilage.

Other studies. ESR and CRP may be elevated in systemic and polyarticular JRA.

VI. Treatment

The goals of treatment for JRA are to maintain functional mobility, by controlling inflammation and increasing joint range of motion, and to limit the side effects of medications. The mainstay of treatment is NSAIDs. Naproxen is commonly used, because it is a twice-a-day medication. The chronic use of NSAIDs requires monitoring of certain data, including urinalysis, complete blood count, and renal and liver function tests. A particular skin rash called pseudoporphyria is associated with use of naproxen. This photosensitive eruption results in small facial vesicles that may lead to permanent scar formation.

Corticosteroids are also used as a means of controlling inflammation, particularly in children with systemic JRA who present with high fevers. The side effects of systemic corticosteroids make them less appealing for chronic control of inflammation. In patients with pauciarticular JRA, intraarticular injections may be very effective.

Methotrexate, considered a second line of therapy, is particularly useful for patients with systemic or polyarticular JRA. Methotrexate is usually very safe, but it can be associated with liver toxicity, so hepatic function must be tested every 4 to 8 weeks. In addition, folic acid supplementation once a week decreases the incidence of side effects.

Newer agents currently available include Etanercept, a tumor necrosis factor inhibitor. These agents are used in methotrexate-resistant cases.

VII.   References

1. Gottlieb B, Ilowite N. Meeting the challenges of rheumatologic diseases in teens. *Contemp Pediatr* 2000;17:61–98.
2. Jarvis J. Juvenile rheumatoid arthritis: a guide for pediatricians. *Pediatr Ann* 2002;31: 437–446.
3. Rapoff M. Assessing and enhancing adherence of medical regimens for juvenile rheumatoid arthritis. *Pediatr Ann* 2002;31:373–379.

Case 16-3: 2-Year-Old Boy

I. History of Present Illness

A 2-year-old boy presented with the chief complaint of refusing to walk. The child was in his usual state of health until the previous day and was outside playing with his older brother. The mother was looking outside and noticed that her son had fallen while running on the grass, but he got right up and continued trying to keep up with his older brother. Over the remainder of the day he seemed to be acting normally. However, when he woke up the next morning there was significant swelling over the right lower leg, and he was walking with a limp. There was no history of fever or viral infections.

II. Past Medical History

The past medical history was unremarkable. He met all his developmental milestones appropriately.

III. Physical Examination

T, 36.9°C; RR, 28/min; HR, 125 bpm; BP, 96/70 mm Hg

Height, 75th percentile; weight, 50th percentile

In general, the child appeared to be a happy, well-developed boy. His physical examination was normal with the exception of the right lower extremity. There was an area of focal swelling and discrete tenderness along the lower third of the tibial shaft. His neurologic examination was normal, but he refused to bear weight on his right leg. His skin examination did not demonstrate any bruises or unusual marks.

IV. Diagnostic Studies

The complete blood count revealed 8,200 WBCs/mm^3, with 54% segmented neutrophils, no band forms, 38% lymphocytes, and 8% monocytes. The ESR and CRP were normal.

V. Course of Illness

A radiograph of the right leg revealed the diagnosis (Fig. 16-2).

DISCUSSION: CASE 16-3

I. Differential Diagnosis

When a child presents with the abrupt onset of refusal to walk, it is important to evaluate for the presence of child abuse. In many cases, the physician must decide whether a traumatic injury was accidental or the result of physical abuse. In the case of a fracture in a toddler, a significant traumatic event may not have occurred. Fracture may result from a minor accident involving a fall while walking or running. A toddler's fracture typically involves the distal portion of the tibia, resulting in a spiral or oblique fracture. In contrast, a fracture that results from abuse usually involves the midshaft of the tibia, because of the large amount of force inflicted while the child's foot is held and the leg twisted. In the case of child abuse, the history often does not seem plausible in relation to the injury or the developmental age of the child. If abuse is considered, a skeletal survey should be done to evaluate for any other injuries. Fractures involving the metaphysis and epiphysis (bucket-handle fractures); fractures of the thoracic cage, scapula, or spine; and complex skull fractures should raise the suspicion of child abuse.

II. Diagnosis

The radiograph of the right leg demonstrated a spiral fracture involving the tibia (Fig. 16-2). **The diagnosis is a toddler's fracture.**

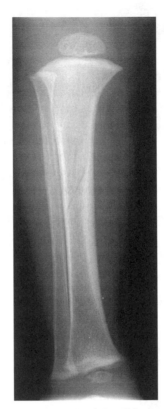

FIG. 16-2. Radiograph of the tibia (case 16-3).

III.   Incidence and Epidemiology

Toddler's fractures are common injuries seen in children between 9 months and 3 years of age. Developmentally, as children start to master walking, they are prone to fall while walking or running. They can easily twist their lower leg, because the foot is fixed on the ground. Their rapid increases in linear growth also contribute to the incidence of this problem. A toddler's fracture in a nonambulatory child is very unusual and should raise the suspicion of a nonaccidental injury.

IV.   Clinical Presentation

When a child presents with refusal to walk with isolated swelling of the tibial shaft, one must suspect a toddler's fracture. In many cases there is no definitive history of trauma. In some cases, the incident seemed so minor that the parents are unable to recall a fall or injury. On physical examination, there may be minimal swelling, increase in warmth, and tenderness. Typically, pain can be elicited by gentle twisting of the extremity.

V.   Diagnostic Approach

Radiography. Approximately 75% of toddler's fractures are seen on plain film. The anteroposterior and lateral projections show a spiral or oblique fracture extending downward and medially in the distal third of the tibia. If these projections are negative, an internal oblique view should be ordered, because it may be able to demonstrate more subtle findings. If the index of suspicion remains high and plain films are normal, a triple-phase bone scan can be performed. Twenty-five percent of toddler's fractures are initially radiographically occult; a repeat radiograph 10 to 14 days later reveals subperiosteal reaction and new bone formation, confirming the diagnosis.

VI. Treatment

Treatment primarily involves immobilization via casting if the fracture is discovered within 2 weeks after symptom onset. Orthopedic surgery colleagues should be consulted in the management of these fractures.

VII. References

1. Bachman D, Santora S. Orthopedic trauma. In: Fleisher GR, Ludwig S, eds. *Textbook of pediatric emergency medicine.* Philadelphia: Lippincott Williams & Wilkins, 2000: 1470–1471.
2. Cooperman DR, Merten DF. Skeletal manifestations of child abuse. In: Reece RM, Ludwig S, eds. *Child abuse medical diagnosis and management,* 2nd ed. Philadelphia: Lippincott Williams & Wilkins, 2001:135–139.
3. Kling TF, Hensingesr RN. Angular and torsional deformities of the lower limbs in children. *Clin Orthop* 1983;176:136–147.

Case 16-4: 2-Year-Old Boy

I. History of Present Illness

A 2-year-old boy was well until 2 days before admission, when he slipped and fell on his right side. After the injury, the parents stated, he began limping. Later that evening he developed fevers to 39.4°C. He was treated with ibuprofen. Over the course of the night, he became irritable, particularly when his parents attempted to carry him. He refused to stand. He was taken a nearby emergency department for evaluation. Radiographs of the right lower extremity were negative, and he was sent home with the diagnosis of knee contusion. The following day, he was able to walk for brief periods but continued to limp. However, over the course of the next few hours, he again stopped walking and became very clingy. He was taken to the hospital for reevaluation.

II. Past Medical History

This child was a healthy boy with no significant past medical history. His immunizations were up to date. His developmental history was also normal.

III. Physical Examination

T, 38.3°C; RR, 24/min; HR, 110 bpm; BP, 98/75 mm Hg

Height, 25th percentile; weight, 50th percentile

On physical examination, the child was crying and difficult to console. Heart, lungs, and abdomen were normal. There was mild swelling and erythema of the right lower extremity. There was significant tenderness over the length of the tibia. Range of motion was normal at the hip, knee, and ankle. Deep tendon reflexes were present. Perfusion to the right foot was normal. He would walk only with assistance, but he was able to crawl.

IV. Diagnostic Studies

The complete blood count revealed 17,400 WBCs/mm^3 (18% band forms, 77% segmented neutrophils, and 5% lymphocytes); hemoglobin, 10.7 g/dL; and a platelet count of 578,000/mm^3. The ESR was 75 mm/hour, and the CRP was 9.2 mg/dL. A blood culture was obtained. Repeat radiography of the right tibia was normal.

V. Course of Illness

MRI of the right lower extremity confirmed the diagnosis (Fig. 16-3).

DISCUSSION: CASE 16-4

I. Differential Diagnosis

Diagnosing the cause of limp or refusal to walk in a toddler is challenging. A history of overt trauma may be absent, or, as in this case, the history of trauma may be misleading. Furthermore, localizing pain in young children may be difficult, and the location of the pain may not accurately represent the area of pathology. In these children, the differential diagnosis can be narrowed by assessing associated symptoms. In this child, who also had fever, infectious causes must be considered. Septic arthritis was unlikely given the normal examination of the hip, knee, and ankle joints. However, osteomyelitis remained a concern, particularly with associated leg swelling. Cellulitis and myositis were also possible. In addition, this could be the presentation of a neoplasm, such as leukemia, neuroblastoma, or osteoblastoma. Rheumatologic diseases, including JRA and reactive arthritis, also manifest with joint pain and fever.

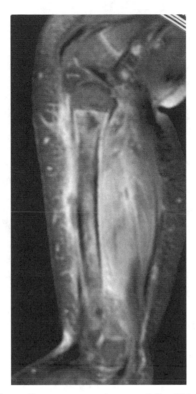

FIG. 16-3. Magnetic resonance image of the tibia (case 16-4).

II. Diagnosis

MRI of the lower extremity revealed significant soft tissue swelling (Fig. 16-3). There was mixed low signal along the entire diaphysis of the tibia, consistent with small subperiosteal abscesses surrounded by edema. Edema was also seen circumferentially along the fascia, consistent with fasciitis. These findings indicated extensive osteomyelitis of the entire tibia, with one large and numerous small subperiosteal collections. Neither the knee nor the ankle joint was involved. *Staphylococcus aureus* was isolated from the initial blood culture. **The diagnosis was acute hematogenous osteomyelitis of the tibia due to *S. aureus.*** In this case, the diagnosis was suspected based on the combination of findings, including swelling, erythema, and tenderness over the tibia. The elevated ESR and CRP supported the diagnosis. The MRI confirmed the diagnosis. The patient was treated with intravenous oxacillin. A peripherally inserted central venous catheter was placed in the right antecubital fossa after the repeat blood culture was negative for more than 48 hours. The patient was discharged on the sixth day of hospitalization to complete 4 weeks of intravenous antibiotic therapy. The CRP peaked on the second day after initiation of antibiotic therapy and was normal by the seventh day of treatment. The ESR peaked on the fifth day and normalized by 3 weeks after initiation of antibiotics.

III. Incidence and Epidemiology

Osteomyelitis in young children is usually caused by hematogenous spread of bacteria. Most cases occur within the first 5 years of life, probably due to the rich vascular blood supply at the sites of rapid growth near the growth plates. In order of decreasing frequency, the affected bones include the femur, tibia, humerus, fibula, and pelvis. The most common organisms causing osteomyelitis vary by age. In neonates, *S. aureus*, group B streptococci, and enteric gram-negative bacteria predominate. In infants and toddlers, *S. aureus* predominates. Fungal osteomyelitis due to *Candida* species occurs in premature neonates and in intravenous drug abusers. Tuberculous osteomyelitis due to hematogenous or lymphatic dissemination occurs in fewer than 1% of children with active tuberculosis. The spine, femur, and small bones of the hands and feet may be involved with tuberculous osteomyelitis.

Nonhematogenous osteomyelitis usually develops from open fractures, decubitus ulcers, implanted orthopedic equipment, or puncture wounds. In the case of puncture wounds through sneakers, *Pseudomonas aeruginosa* and *S. aureus* are likely pathogens.

IV. Clinical Presentation

The presenting signs and symptoms in children with osteomyelitis depend on the site of infection. The typical presentation for patients with osteomyelitis is fever and bone pain. In many cases, there is a history of trauma. Trauma is believed to be a risk factor because of the increase in blood flow to the injured area that occurs after an injury.

Systemic symptoms include fever, malaise, and poor appetite. On physical examination, there may be swelling and erythema of the affected extremity. Often there is point tenderness rather than diffuse bone tenderness. In most cases, the metaphyses of the long bones are the sites of infection. Range of motion should be intact, in comparison with septic arthritis. However, patients may have some limited mobility due to pain or muscle spasm. The osteomyelitis may extend to involve an adjacent joint, but joint infection rarely extends to cause secondary osteomyelitis.

V. Diagnostic Approach

Laboratory data may be helpful in supporting the diagnosis of osteomyelitis.

Blood culture. Blood cultures demonstrate the responsible organism in up to 50% of cases. Blood cultures should be obtained in all cases of suspected osteomyelitis.

Complete blood count. The peripheral WBC count can be normal or elevated. If symptoms have been present for several days, thrombocytosis may also be noted.

Markers of inflammation. The CRP concentration is elevated at presentation in more than 95% of cases, as is the ESR in approximately 90%. Once the diagnosis is made, the CRP and ESR can be used to monitor response to therapy (see later discussion).

Bone biopsy or aspiration of subperiosteal collections. The gold standard for diagnosis is bone aspiration and culture. In 80% of cases, an organism is identified from blood, bone, or joint fluids.

Radiologic studies. A plain radiograph shows lytic lesions and periosteal elevation approximately 10 to 14 days after onset of symptoms. A triple-phase technetium bone scan localizes the bony involvement in cases involving (a) vertebral or pelvic osteomyelitis; (b) neonates, toddlers, and other children who may have difficulty localizing pain; or (c) multifocal involvement. Although the sensitivity of the technetium bone scan is high (80% to 100%), it does not delineate the anatomy and cannot differentiate among trauma, fracture, infection, and infarction and therefore has a low specificity. MRI has the highest sensitivity, at 92% to 100%, for demonstrating osteomyelitis. MRI also detects secondary osteomyelitis. MRI is clearly the imaging modality of choice when symptoms are localized.

VI. Treatment

Appropriate antibiotic selection depends on many factors, including the patient's age and the mechanism of acquisition. For neonates with osteomyelitis, appropriate therapy includes the combination of an antistaphylococcal penicillin (oxacillin, nafcillin) with an aminoglycoside (gentamicin, amikacin) or cefotaxime. In older children, either oxacillin, nafcillin, or a first-generation cephalosporin (e.g., cefazolin).would be appropriate. Children with allergies to those antibiotics can receive ceftriaxone, cefotaxime, clindamycin, vancomycin, or linezolid. Children with underlying hemoglobinopathies should receive cefotaxime or ceftriaxone empirically, given the high risk for *S. aureus* and *Salmonella* infections. Additional antibiotics can be added to these regimens based on clinical presentation and mechanism of infection. Definitive therapy should be based on clinical response and culture results.

Response to therapy can be monitored by checking serial CRP and ESR levels. The CRP peaks on the second day after initiation of appropriate antibiotic therapy and returns to normal between the seventh and the ninth day. The ESR usually peaks on the fifth day after initiation of antibiotics and returns to normal by the third or fourth week. If these markers of inflammation increase during therapy or fail to return to normal, additional evaluation is warranted. Usually, the CRP and ESR are monitored on a weekly basis.

Therapy typically continues for 3 to 6 weeks but depends on the causative organism, the severity of illness, and the clinical and laboratory response. Historically, treatment of *S. aureus* bone infections for less than 4 weeks has led to an unacceptably high rate of relapse. Sequential parenteral-oral therapy can be used successfully. After the CRP is normal and the signs of acute inflammation have improved, oral therapy may be used. The willingness of the child to take oral medications and the ability of the parents to administer them must also be taken into account. The doses for oral treatment are generally two or three times the doses used for minor infections. Sequential parenteral-oral therapy should be performed in conjunction with a pediatric infectious disease specialist or other physician with experience in managing pediatric bone and joint infections.

VII. References

1. Roy DR. Osteomyelitis. *Pediatr Rev* 1995;16:380–384.
2. Erdman WA, Tamburro F, Jayson HT, et al. Osteomyelitis: characteristics and pitfalls of diagnosis with MR imaging. *Radiology* 1991;180:553–559.
3. Roine I, Arguedas A, Faingezicht I, et al. Early detection of sequela: prone osteomyelitis in children with use of simple clinical and laboratory criteria. *Clin Infect Dis* 1997;24:849–853.
4. Peltola H, Unkila-Kallio L, Kallio MJ. Simplified treatment of acute staphylococcal osteomyelitis of childhood. *Pediatrics* 1997:99:846–850.
5. Jacobs RF, McCarthy RE, Elser JM. *Pseudomonas* osteochondritis complicating puncture wounds of the foot in children: a 10-year evaluation. *J Infect Dis* 1989;160: 657–661.
6. Tetzlaff TR, McCracken GH, Nelson JD. Oral antibiotic therapy for skeletal infections of children. *J Pediatr* 1978;92:485–490.
7. Unkila-Kallio L, Kallio MJ, Eskola J, et al. Serum C-reactive protein, erythrocyte sedimentation rate and white blood cell count in acute hematogenous osteomyelitis of children. *Pediatrics* 1994;93:59–62.

Case 16-5: 1-Year-Old Boy

I. History of Present Illness

A 1-year-old male child presented to the emergency department 1 day after sustaining a fall. His mother was carrying him when she tripped over a footstool and fell with him in her arms. The child fell forward and landed on a carpet with his stomach and chest. There was no loss of consciousness, and the toddler cried immediately. That day, he remained very fussy and refused to use his right leg. He cried with all diaper changes. Soon the mother noticed some increased swelling over the boy's right lower extremity. There was no history of any recent viral infections or skin changes.

II. Past Medical History

The birth history was remarkable for a baby that was small for gestational age, born at 39 weeks via emergency cesarean section. The birth weight was 4 pounds 5 ounces. He remained hospitalized for 1 week, in part due to a severe snowstorm that swept through the area shortly after his birth. The child had been treated in the past with iron supplementation for anemia diagnosed at 10 months of age. His developmental history was appropriate. He crawled up steps and cruised holding onto furniture. He was not walking by himself yet. He was able to take off his own socks. His current diet consisted of breast milk. He did not take many solid foods. He did not receive any medications.

III. Physical Examination

T, 37.4°C; RR, 24/min; HR, 138 bpm; BP, 90/50 mm Hg

Height, 63 cm (less than 5th percentile); weight, 8.26 kg (less than 5th percentile)

In general, the child appeared tearful but consolable. His forehead was prominent. His cardiorespiratory examination was normal. The abdominal examination was benign. The musculoskeletal examination revealed some swelling around the distal end of the right femur and some widening of the wrists. His neurologic examination was unremarkable, including normal strength and deep tendon reflexes.

IV. Diagnostic Studies

His complete blood cell count revealed 11,400 WBCs/mm^3 (16% segmented neutrophils, 71% lymphocytes, and 3% eosinophils); hemoglobin, 11.8g/dL; and platelets, 260,000 cells/mm^3. His serum electrolytes, blood urea nitrogen, and creatinine values were normal. The calcium level was 8.4 mg/L; phosphorus, 2.2 mg/dL; and magnesium, 2.2 mg/dL. His liver function tests were remarkable for a low serum albumin at 3.3 mg/dL and an elevated serum alkaline phosphatase at 1,077 U/L. A skeletal survey was otherwise normal.

V. Course of Illness

A radiograph of the swollen leg revealed both the primary and the underlying diagnosis (Fig. 16-4).

DISCUSSION: CASE 16-5

I. Differential Diagnosis

In this case, the differential diagnosis is particularly narrow. The normal WBC count and absence of fever made acute osteomyelitis less likely. In this case, fracture due to the trauma described was the most likely diagnosis.

II. Diagnosis

Radiologic films of the right lower extremity showed osteopenia, widened metaphyses, irregular metaphyseal and physeal borders, and an incomplete nondisplaced fracture of

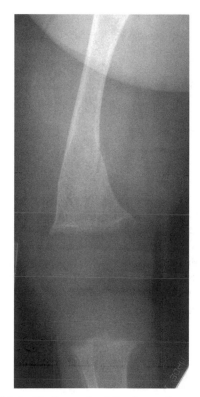

FIG. 16-4. Radiograph of the femur (case 16-5).

the distal right femur (Fig. 16-4). After obtaining further history, it was discovered that the child received very little sunlight exposure and that his diet was very limited, consisting only of juice and breast milk. The findings on radiography, in conjunction with an extremely elevated alkaline phosphatase concentration, raised the suspicion of rickets. **The diagnosis of rickets was confirmed by a low level of 25-hydroxycholecalciferol (25(OH)D$_3$) and a normal level of 1,25-dihydroxycholecalcierol (1,25(OH)$_2$D$_3$). This child had a femur fracture precipitated by trauma in conjunction with nutritional rickets.** There was no evidence of an underlying renal or hepatic disease that could have contributed to the development of rickets. An electrocardiogram revealed a normal sinus rhythm and normal intervals. He was placed on vitamin D and calcium supplements orally.

III. Incidence and Epidemiology

Rickets is defined as inadequate mineralization of growing bone or osteoid tissue caused by a deficiency of vitamin D. Vitamin D receptors are found on the kidney, intestine, bone osteoblasts, and parathyroid gland. Vitamin D$_2$ is available in the diet, and cholecalciferol (vitamin D$_3$) is naturally present in human skin in provitamin form. Vitamins D$_2$ and D$_3$ are hydroxylated in the liver (25-hydroxylation) to form 25(OH)D$_3$ (*calcidiol*) and again in the renal cortical cells (1-hydroxylation) to produce 1,25-(OH)$_2$D$_3$ (*calcitriol*). Rickets develops due to nutritional deficiency of vitamin D or vitamin D transport or metabolism defects (vitamin D–dependent rickets). Nutritional rickets is seen in infants who are exclusively breast-fed. Typically, these babies are not started on other foods. In addition, a limited exposure to sunlight increases the risk of rickets in these patients. As children become older, nutritional rickets may be seen in patients on vegetarian diets. Vitamin D may be found in liver and fish oils. Many cereals are fortified with vitamin D.

For some patients, there is an impaired absorption of vitamin D. This is seen in patients with malabsorption (e.g., celiac sprue, cystic fibrosis). Also, bile salt depletion decreases the absorption of vitamin D.

Nutritional rickets develops because the body tries to maintain a normal serum calcium level. When vitamin D is not present, less calcium is absorbed through the intestine. A lower calcium level causes the secretion of parathyroid hormone and mobilization of calcium from the bone. Therefore, as the body tries to preserve a normal calcium level, the parathyroid hormone concentration becomes elevated, the serum phosphorus level is low, and the alkaline phosphatase enzyme is extremely elevated.

Other causes of rickets occur when there is difficulty with the metabolism of vitamin D. Liver disease may decrease the production of 25-OH cholecalciferol. Certain medications, including phenobarbital, cause rickets by affecting liver metabolism of vitamin D. Vitamin D–dependent rickets type I develops from the absence of renal hydroxylase. Laboratory data are similar to those of nutritional rickets, with the exception of low calcitriol levels. Symptoms can be overcome with high doses of vitamin D. Vitamin D–dependent rickets type II (vitamin D receptor mutations) occurs when there is a low affinity for vitamin D at the level of receptor. In this case, the calcitriol level is very high. This too can be overcome by high doses of vitamin D.

Rickets may also occur in conditions that cause chronic acidosis, because bone is resorbed to buffer the acid load. Excess phosphate excretion due to defects in renal tubular resorption of phosphate (e.g., primary hyperphosphaturia, Fanconi syndrome) may also lead to rickets (vitamin D–resistant rickets), because phosphate is important in bone formation. In these patients, the calcitriol levels are also decreased.

IV.   Clinical Presentation

Most patients with rickets are asymptomatic. A thorough social and dietary history allows the clinician to identify children who may be at risk for development of rickets. The clinical findings vary based on the child's age, the underlying disorder, and the duration of the problem. Patients with rickets may present with multiple abnormalities of the musculoskeletal system. Children with congenital rickets and those who develop symptoms at a young age may have significant frontal bossing, because the head grows rapidly early in life. Delayed dentition and enamel disruption may be present. In slightly older children, the upper extremities and ribs grow quickly, so findings involving the wrist and ribs may be more common during the first year of life. The child may experience painful and tender bones. The wrists and ankles may be broad and swollen. A rachitic rosary occurs when there is enlargement of the costochondral junctions of the anterior lateral ribs. There is a prominence of bowing of the lower extremities in an ambulatory child. Some children have trouble reaching some gross motor milestones, including possible delay in ambulation. Children with underlying chronic acidosis may present with failure to thrive. If rickets has been present for a long time, signs of hypocalcemia may develop, including stridor or carpopedal spasm.

V.   Diagnostic Approach

Radiography. Rickets may be diagnosed based on radiographic findings. Radiographs of the wrists are usually the most revealing. The metaphysis demonstrates cupping and widening, with an increase in the width of radiolucency between the metaphysis and epiphysis. Bone density is decreased, and the cortical bone is thin. A Milkman's pseudofracture is a ribbon-like radiolucency that extends transversely across the concave side of the long bones. Pathologic fractures may be present. Occasionally, children are diagnosed with rickets by incidental findings on chest radiography during evaluation of a first episode of bronchiolitis. Chest radiography findings include demineralization of the skeleton with cupping of the distal end of the ribs and humerus.

Laboratory studies can be used to determine the cause of rickets (Table 16-3). Some important values are discussed here.

Calcium, magnesium, and phosphorus. Calcium is typically mildly depressed (7 to 8 mg/dL). Phosphorus may be particularly low in children with defective tubular resorption of phosphate. Hypocalcemia may be seen with hypomagnesemia.

Alkaline phosphatase. Alkaline phosphatase is elevated before development of hypocalcemia.

Vitamin D metabolites. Both $25(OH)D_3$ and $1,25(OH)_2D_3$ should be determined. In nutritional rickets, the $25(OH)D_3$ is low and the $1,25(OH)_2D_3$ may be low or normal depending on the severity of the rickets.

Other studies. Intact parathyroid hormone and serum creatinine are helpful in determining the cause of rickets (Table 16-3). Urinary calcium, pH, creatinine, and amino acids can be used to exclude (or diagnose) Fanconi syndrome and proximal renal tubular acidosis.

Once rickets is considered in the diagnosis, then one must determine the exact cause. Laboratory evaluation helps in this determination and thus leads to the proper treatment (Table 16-3).

VI. Treatment

Depending on the cause, the treatment of rickets is aimed at restoring the serum calcium and phosphorus levels and increasing the mineralization of bone. In the case of nutritional rickets, supplementation with vitamin D and calcium is the treatment of choice.

Currently, emphasis is placed on prevention of nutritional rickets. Breast-fed infants should receive vitamin D supplementation while nursing. Other natural sources of vita-

TABLE 16-3. *Classification of Laboratory Values in Causes of Rickets*

Disorder[a]	Calcium	iPTH	Phosphate	Creatinine	25(OH)D3	1,25(OH)2D3
Mild nutritional vitamin D deficiency	Normal/low	Normal	Normal/low	Normal	Low	Normal
Severe nutritional vitamin D deficiency	Low	Very high	Low	Normal	Very low	Low
Anticonvulsant-induced rickets	Low	High	Low	Normal	Low	Normal/low
Liver disease	Normal/low	Normal	Normal	Normal	Normal	Normal/low
Chronic renal failure	Normal/low	Very high	High	High	Normal	Very low
Vitamin D receptor mutation	Low	High	Low	Normal	Normal	Very high

[a]Alkaline phosphatase concentration is elevated early in all disorders.
iPTH, intact parathyroid hormone; $25(OH)D_3$, calcidiol; $1,25(OH)_2D_3$, calcitriol.

min D include liver, fish, and fortified breakfast cereals. Sunlight remains another source to increase the amount of vitamin D.

If the patient has signs of symptomatic hypocalcemia, it is important also to monitor the patient's heart rate and rhythm and to evaluate for prolonged QT syndrome. This should improve as the calcium level is restored to normal.

VII.   References

1. Bergstrom WH. Twenty ways to get rickets in the 1990's. *Contemp Pediatr* 1991:8: 88–106.
2. Carpenter TO. Disorders of calcium and bone metabolism in infancy and childhood. In: Becker KL. *Principles and practice of endocrinology and metabolism.* Philadelphia: Lippincott Williams & Wilkins, 1996:631–637.
3. Ryan S. Nutritional aspects of metabolic bone disease in the newborn. *Arch Dis Child* 1996;74:145–148.

Case 16-6: 2-Year-Old Boy

I. History of Present Illness

A 2-year-old boy with a past medical history of asthma initially presented to the emergency department with a fever, cough, and difficulty breathing. The toddler also complained intermittently of back pain. At this time, the physical examination was remarkable only for cervical adenopathy and a mild diffuse expiratory wheeze. He was treated with albuterol by metered-dose inhaler and discharged home. One week later, he returned to the hospital with a history of unsteady gait for 2 days. At the time of presentation, he was refusing to walk. He had continued to have fevers over the past few days. His activity level was drastically diminished. In addition, he appeared to have focal pain over his lower back. There was no discomfort over any of his extremities. There was no history of trauma. There was no weight loss, night sweats, emesis, or diarrhea.

II. Past Medical History

His birth history was complicated by meconium aspiration syndrome that necessitated mechanical ventilation for 1 week. He had a history of asthma. He had had several exacerbations requiring albuterol. He had never received corticosteroids or required hospitalization. The family history was unremarkable.

III. Physical Examination

T, 38.5°C; RR, 24/min; HR, 111 bpm; BP, 120/70 mm Hg
Weight, 25th percentile

In general, he appeared comfortable lying with his parents but expressed significant discontent when asked to sit or stand. There was no lymphadenopathy. The heart and lungs were normal. There was no splenomegaly or hepatomegaly. There was mild focal tenderness over the lumbosacral spine with palpation. He was able to flex and extend both lower extremities without difficulty. Deep tendon reflexes were 2+ and symmetric. Cranial nerves appeared intact. His motor strength was symmetric in all extremities. Sensation appeared intact. There were no cerebellar signs.

IV. Diagnostic Studies

His complete blood cell count revealed 5,500 WBCs/mm^3 (65% segmented neutrophils and 33% lymphocytes); hemoglobin, 11.2 g/dL; and platelets, 225,000 cells/mm^3. The ESR was elevated at 70 mm/hour. The CRP was also elevated at 8.5 mg/dL. The lactate dehydrogenase level was high at 2,276 U/L (normal range, 470 to 900 U/L).

V. Course of Illness

The patient was hospitalized to evaluate for possible vertebral osteomyelitis and diskitis. Given the focal findings on examination, MRI of the lumbar spine was performed (Fig. 16-5). The MRI suggested a diagnostic category, and biopsy of the lesion confirmed the final diagnosis.

DISCUSSION: CASE 16-6

I. Differential Diagnosis

In this case, the initial concern was to evaluate the patient for possible osteomyelitis and diskitis. When this toddler presented with fever, refusal to walk, and elevated markers of inflammation, an infectious etiology had to be considered. The most common cause of vertebral osteomyelitis is *S. aureus.* Less common causes include group A *Streptococcus, Streptococcus pneumoniae,* and enteric gram-negative rods. Tuberculosis can

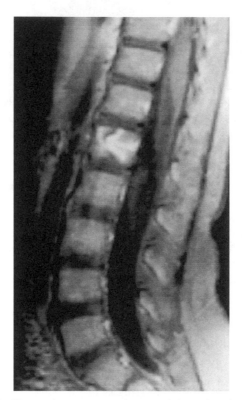

FIG. 16-5. Magnetic resonance image of the spine (case 16-6).

cause vertebral osteomyelitis. Malignancies should also be considered in this setting. Leukemia and lymphoma often manifest with nonspecific findings, including fever, weight loss, malaise, and refusal to walk. Bone tumors, including osteosarcoma or Ewing's sarcoma, are other possible etiologies. Metastatic neuroblastoma often manifests with bone pain and fever. Neuroblastoma can also manifest with local effects, including an isolated thoracic or abdominal mass.

II. Diagnosis

The MRI (Fig. 16-5) demonstrated a heterogeneous bone marrow signal, with marked contrast enhancement of approximately 1 cm in the anterior aspect of the vertebral body. The lesion did not extend into or disrupt the disk space. There was no associated soft tissue edema or abscess. These MRI findings were not consistent with osteomyelitis. With an infectious cause, soft tissue edema and disk space involvement should be seen. Given these concerns, biopsies of the vertebral lesion and bone marrow were performed. **The pathology results showed metastatic neuroblastoma.** Further radiologic studies, including CT of the head, abdomen, and chest, were unable to determine a primary lesion. The patient received chemotherapy for stage 4 neuroblastoma.

Neuroblastoma is a tumor derived from the neural crest cells that form the sympathetic ganglia and adrenal medulla. As in this case, the diagnosis is suspected based on the history and radiographic findings but is confirmed by pathology. Histologically, neuroblastoma typically is made up of areas of calcification and hemorrhage surrounding small round cells with cytoplasmic granules. The cells may form together into rosette-like shapes, which are called Homer Wright rosettes.

III. Incidence and Epidemiology

Neuroblastoma, the most common extracranial solid tumor of childhood, accounts for about 10% of all childhood cancers. There are about 500 new cases in the United States every year. Most cases are diagnosed before 4 years of age, with the median age at diagnosis being 2 years. Most tumors (80%) are located below the diaphragm, and approximately 50% of all neuroblastoma tumors arise from the adrenal gland.

IV. Clinical Presentation

Neuroblastoma manifests in a wide variety of ways, depending on the tumor location and extent of disease. A thoracic mass may be seen as a hard, painless lump in the neck or chest, or it may manifest with signs of superior vena cava syndrome due to compression from large mediastinal tumors. In some cases, a young child presents with an enlarging abdominal mass. Depending on its location, the patient may be asymptomatic or may show signs of bowel obstruction or liver involvement. If compression occurs on renal vasculature due to an enlarging adrenal tumor, the patient may develop hypertension. If the tumor involves cells from the sympathetic ganglia, a paraspinal mass may be present. These patients may experience back pain and nerve compression resulting in bladder or bowel dysfunction or gait disturbance. If cervical sympathetic ganglia are involved, a unilateral Horner's syndrome may be seen. About two thirds of patients present with metastatic disease initially. Common sites of metastatic disease include the liver, bone marrow, skin, and lymph nodes.

There are some unique presentations with neuroblastoma. A paraneoplastic syndrome, called opsoclonus–myoclonus or "dancing eyes," may develop. This involves jerky and chaotic eye movements and myoclonic jerks. If this is detected, it is important to look for the primary source of the tumor. In most cases, the opsoclonus and myoclonus improve with treatment. However, some patients continue to have issues even after tumor eradication. Occasionally, metastases deposit in the periorbital region, causing proptosis and periorbital ecchymosis. This finding resembles "raccoon eyes." Excess secretion of catecholamines from the tumor leads to other systemic signs, including flushing, tachycardia, hypertension, and diarrhea.

V. Diagnostic Approach

The first step to the diagnostic approach is to consider the possibility of neuroblastoma. This diagnosis should be considered in patients who have nonspecific systemic signs and bone pain. Physical examination findings may involve a palpable abdominal mass and lymphadenopathy. It is also important to pay attention to the patient's blood pressure.

Complete blood count. Pancytopenia suggests bone marrow involvement.

Urinary catecholamines. In more than 90% of cases, urine catecholamines, such as homovanillic acid (HVA) and vanillylmandelic acid (VMA), are elevated. A 24-hour urine collection should be analyzed, because random "spot" samples may yield false-positive results.

Bone marrow biopsy. Bone marrow aspiration is necessary to determine metastatic disease of the bone marrow.

Radiologic studies. Skeletal radiography or a technetium bone scan should be performed to detect metastatic bone lesions. CT should be performed to detect the primary site and possible metastatic sites of involvement.

VI. Treatment

As with many oncologic diseases, the treatment and prognosis are determined based on the patient's stage at presentation. The International Neuroblastoma Staging System (INSS) was developed based on clinical, radiographic, and surgical evaluation of children with neuroblastoma. Stage 1 represents localized tumor with complete gross excision. Stage 4 refers to any primary tumor with dissemination to distant lymph nodes, bone, bone marrow, liver, skin, or other organs (except as defined for stage 4S). Stage 4S refers to localized primary tumor with dissemination limited to skin, liver, or bone marrow in infants younger than 1 year of age. When patients present with localized disease (all stage 1 and most stage 2 cases), surgical removal of the tumor is usually curative. Patients with stage 4S disease are frequently classified into the low-risk category.

In patients with disseminated disease and poor prognostic factors due to histologic findings, the treatment regimen involves surgery, chemotherapy, and radiation therapy. Occasionally, patients require bone marrow transplantation for adequate treatment. Factors that are important in predicting prognosis include patient age, histology, serum ferritin level, DNA content of the tumor, and the amplification of the *N-myc* oncogene. The 5-year survival rate exceeds 95% in those children categorized as low risk and approaches 90% in those children categorized as intermediate risk; those considered to be at high risk have a survival rate of only 20%.

VII. References

1. Castleberry RP. Biology and treatment of neuroblastoma. *Pediatr Clin North Am* 1997;44:919–937.
2. Hogarty M, Lange BJ. Oncologic emergencies. In: Fleisher GR, Ludwig S, eds. *Textbook of pediatric emergency medicine.* Philadelphia: Lippincott, Williams & Wilkins, 2000:1157–1190.
3. Santana VM. Neuroblastoma. In: Behrman RE, Kliegman RM, Arvin AM. *Nelson textbook of pediatrics.* Philadelphia: WB Saunders, 1996:1460–1463.

17

Diarrhea

Christina Lin Master

APPROACH TO THE PATIENT WITH DIARRHEA

I. Definition of the Complaint

Diarrhea is one of the most common reasons for which patients seek medical care. It is a condition that continues to be associated with significant morbidity and mortality worldwide despite medical advances. It is characterized by an increase in the frequency, volume, or liquid content of stool in a given individual, compared with his or her usual pattern.

Diarrhea may be further characterized by the duration of the symptoms, with acute episodes of diarrhea resolving anywhere from 72 hours to 2 weeks and chronic diarrhea generally lasting longer than 2 weeks. Another important distinction in the type of diarrhea is whether it is secretory or osmotic in nature. Agents that disrupt the normal absorption of intestinal luminal fluid at the cellular level cause a profuse and voluminous secretory diarrhea that continues regardless of the patient's oral intake. Osmotic diarrhea, on the other hand, is the result of poorly absorbed substances that draw fluid into the intestinal lumen. This type of diarrhea tends to improve with fasting.

The most common causes of diarrhea are infectious, with viral etiologies occurring more frequently than bacterial. The differential diagnosis of diarrhea, however, is quite long and includes some rare causes. Many cases of diarrhea occur in children who are otherwise well-appearing, whereas some cases occur in children who are ill-appearing because of poor nutrition, lack of hydration, or other systemic reasons.

II. Complaint by Cause and Frequency

The myriad causes of diarrhea can be stratified by age (Table 17-1) or by diagnostic category (Table 17-2).

TABLE 17-1. *Causes of Diarrhea by Age*

Prevalence	Neonate/infant	School age child/adolescent
Common	Systemic infections	Infectious gastroenteritis
	Infectious gastroenteritis	Nonspecific diarrhea of childhood
	Necrotizing enterocolitis	Antibiotic-associated
	Antibiotic-associated	Encopresis
	Overfeeding	Carbohydrate malabsorption
	Carbohydrate malabsorption	Food poisoning
Less common	Hirschsprung's enterocolitis	Inflammatory bowel disease
	Milk protein allergy	Lactose intolerance
	Cystic fibrosis	Cystic fibrosis
	Celiac disease	Laxative abuse
Uncommon	Congenital lactase deficiency	Secretory tumors
	Congenital villous atrophy	Hyperthyroidism
	Secretory tumors	Intestinal lymphangiectasia
	Congenital adrenal hyperplasia	

TABLE 17-2. *Causes of Diarrhea by Diagnostic Category*

Diagnostic category	Specific cause
Infectious	Viral
	Rotavirus
	Adenovirus
	Enterovirus
	Norwalk agent
	Calicivirus
	Bacteria
	Salmonella species
	Shigella species
	Escherichia coli
	Campylobacter jejuni
	Yersinia enterocolitica
	Vibrio cholerae
	Clostridium difficile
	Parasitic
	Giardia lamblia
	Cryptosporidium species
Dietary	Sorbitol
	Fructose
	Food poisoning
Malabsorptive	Celiac disease
	Cystic fibrosis
	Carbohydrate malabsorption, postinfectious
Oncologic	Neuroblastoma
	Ganglioneuroma
Endocrine	Hyperthyroidism
	Hyperparathyroidism
	Congenital adrenal hyperplasia
	Adrenal insufficiency
Toxicologic	Medication side effect
	Antibiotic-associated
	Laxatives
Allergic	Milk protein allergy
Immunologic	Immune deficiencies
	Acquired immunodeficiency syndrome
	Inflammatory bowel disease
Anatomic	Short bowel syndrome
	Malrotation
	Hirschsprung's disease
Congenital	Congenital lactase deficiency
	Congenital villous atrophy
Vasculitis	Henoch-Schönlein purpura
	Hemolytic-uremic syndrome
Miscellaneous	Irritable bowel syndrome
	Chronic nonspecific diarrhea of childhood
	Overfeeding
	Encopresis

III. Clarifying Questions

A thorough history can provide clues to facilitate accurate diagnosis for the child who presents with diarrhea. Consideration of the age and appearance of the patient, the length and course of the illness, and associated clinical features provides a useful framework for creating a differential diagnosis. The following questions may help provide clues to the diagnosis.

- How long has the diarrhea lasted?

    — Diarrhea that has lasted less than 2 weeks is acute diarrhea, rather than chronic. Acute diarrhea is more likely to be infectious (viral or bacterial) in origin. Chronic diarrhea raises the concern for other diagnoses such as malabsorptive conditions (e.g., cystic fibrosis, celiac disease), although infectious causes (e.g., parasitic) and postinfectious conditions (e.g., postinfectious carbohydrate malabsorption) are still possible.

- Is there any blood or mucus in the stool?

  — In the acute setting, blood or mucus in the stool increases the possibility of an enteroinvasive agent (e.g., enteroinvasive *Escherichia coli, Salmonella* spp., *Shigella* spp.). In the chronic setting, inflammatory bowel disease should be considered. In a systemically ill-appearing child, hemolytic-uremic syndrome (HUS) must be considered.

- Is there abdominal pain or cramping? Is tenesmus present?

  — Acute infectious gastroenteritis can manifest with abdominal cramping, whereas a chronic history of cramping or tenesmus raises the possibility of inflammatory bowel disease.

- Is there any vomiting?

  — Vomiting may be associated with acute infectious gastroenteritis. However, if bilious vomiting is noted, especially in a neonate or an infant, an anatomic condition (e.g., malrotation, incarcerated hernia) must be considered.

- Is fever present?

  — Presence of a fever acutely may indicate either an enteroinvasive infectious agent or systemic illness (e.g., pneumonia) with an associated nonspecific diarrhea. In a toxic-appearing child, sepsis and toxic shock syndrome must be considered. In a patient with a history of chronic diarrhea with acute exacerbations associated with fever, inflammatory bowel disease is a distinct possibility.

- Does the patient appear systemically ill?

  — In acute diarrhea, a systemically ill-appearing child should raise the concern for sepsis (e.g., *Salmonella* spp., *E. coli*), especially in a neonate or infant. If oliguria is also present, HUS must be considered in addition to simple dehydration associated with diarrheal losses. In patients who have a history of chronic diarrhea and failure to thrive, superimposed episodes of acute diarrhea can make them appear systemically ill, as in cases of inflammatory bowel disease, celiac disease, or cystic fibrosis.

- Is there failure to thrive?

  — A chronic history of diarrhea associated with failure to thrive raises the concern for malabsorptive conditions such as cystic fibrosis and celiac disease. Neuroendocrine tumors that cause a secretory diarrhea may manifest with significant weight loss. Inflammatory bowel disease also commonly manifests with linear growth arrest in addition to poor weight gain.

- Are there ill contacts with diarrhea?

  — The existence of close contacts with similar symptoms may indicate an outbreak with a common source of contamination (e.g., day care, family reunion, restaurant), either toxin-associated food poisoning or fecal-oral contamination.

- Has there been any unusual food exposure?

  — In particular, undercooked foods, specifically beef, are of concern as a source for *E. coli* O157:H7 infection resulting in HUS. Improperly stored food is another potential source for food poisoning. New foods may not be tolerated well and may be the source of transient diarrhea, or they may cause bloody diarrhea, as in the case of milk-protein allergy in infants.

- Is there any history of recent travel?

  — Foreign travel increases the concern for travelers' diarrhea, often due to strains of *E. coli,* or unusual organisms, such as *Entamoeba histolytica,* as a cause of chronic diarrhea. Other parasites, such as *Giardia lamblia,* and agents such as hepatitis A may also be acquired during travel.

- What is the water source?

  — Untreated or contaminated water sources can harbor *G. lamblia* or *Cryptosporidium.* Cases of *E. coli* O157:H7 transmission have also been known to occur with exposure in water sources such as swimming pools or lakes.

- Are there any pets? Has there been any exposure to animals?

  — Unusual pets, such as lizards, can harbor *Salmonella,* which can then cause diarrhea in children who play with them. Farm animals and petting zoos are also potential sources for *E. coli* O157:H7 and epidemic cases of HUS.

- Is there a history of recent antibiotic use?

  — *Clostridium difficile* colitis is a common sequela to antibiotic use in children.

- Is there any significant past medical history?

  — Failure to thrive is of particular concern with superimposed diarrhea, either acute or chronic. Former premature infants who had surgical necrotizing enterocolitis may subsequently have chronic diarrhea due to short-bowel syndrome. Diarrhea may also be associated with other immune compromising conditions (e.g., human immunodeficiency virus [HIV] infection) or with endocrinologic disorders (e.g., hyperthyroidism).

- Is there a significant family history?

  — Patients with inflammatory bowel disease may present with family members who have the same symptoms. Cystic fibrosis and celiac disease have traditionally been associated with northern European ancestry, although patients of other ethnicities can also carry these diagnoses.

- Is the diarrhea worse with oral intake? Is it improved with fasting?

  — This question helps to differentiate osmotic diarrhea, which characterizes most cases of diarrhea, from secretory diarrhea, which is much less common and is often associated with otherwise occult oncologic conditions.

- Is there a rash?

  — A petechial, purpuric rash is indicative of Henoch-Schönlein purpura, although, in an ill-appearing child, sepsis would also have to be considered. Other rashes, such as dermatitis herpetiformis, can be seen in chronic conditions such as celiac disease. Rashes may also develop due to nutritional deficiencies.

- Is the weight loss intentional?
  - Teenagers who are overly concerned with body image may be using laxatives to lose weight.

Case 17-1: 2-Month-Old Boy

I.   History of Present Illness

A 2-month-old male child presented with vomiting and diarrhea. He had been discharged from the hospital 3 days earlier, with a diagnosis of gastroesophageal reflux based on a pH probe and an upper gastrointestinal radiographic series. He was discharged to home on ranitidine and metoclopramide and had been doing well until the evening before presentation, when he developed vomiting and diarrhea. He had 12 episodes of nonbloody, nonbilious vomiting and 8 episodes of loose stools. There was no fever or associated upper respiratory tract symptoms. He had normal urine output. His mother reported that he was more fussy than usual, and she noted a lump in his groin on the day of presentation to the hospital.

II.   Past Medical History

The patient was a full-term baby with an uncomplicated pregnancy, labor, and delivery history. He had been hospitalized only once, diagnosed with gastroesophageal reflux, and prescribed ranitidine and metoclopramide.

III.   Physical Examination

T, 36.9C; RR, 32/min; HR, 136 bpm; BP, 100/54 mm Hg

Weight, 5th percentile

On examination, the infant was alert and in no acute distress. His head, neck, cardiac, and respiratory examinations were unremarkable. He was well hydrated with a nontender and nondistended, soft abdomen. There was no hepatosplenomegaly. There were no abdominal masses. He had normal male genitalia, with bilaterally descended testicles. A tender, firm, and erythematous mass measuring 5 × 3 cm was palpable in the right inguinal region.

IV.   Diagnostic Studies

The complete blood count revealed 10,100 white blood cells (WBCs)/mm³, with 11% segmented neutrophils and 76% lymphocytes). The hemoglobin was 10.8 g/dL with a mean corpuscular volume of 87 fL, and the platelet count was 387,000 mm³. Serum electrolytes, blood urea nitrogen (BUN), and creatinine values were normal.

V.   Course of Illness

An abdominal radiograph obtained on his previous admission suggested a cause of the current complaint (Fig. 17-1). A surgical consultation was requested.

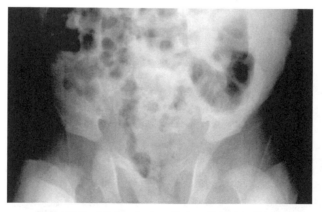

FIG. 17-1. Abdominal radiograph (case 17-1).

DISCUSSION: CASE 17-1

I. Differential Diagnosis

In this case, diarrhea was associated with vomiting and a critical physical finding, that of an inguinal mass. This essential finding directed the differential diagnosis toward causes of inguinal or scrotal swelling. An important distinction to make is between a painful and a painless mass. A hydrocele is a common entity that causes painless inguinal or scrotal swelling. It is primarily differentiated from an inguinal hernia by the ability to palpate above the mass, revealing discontinuity between the mass and the inguinal canal. The mass, as a result, does not change in size with straining or crying. In addition, a hydrocele is not reducible and usually transilluminates, although the ability to transilluminate the mass does not exclude the possibility of an incarcerated hernia.

Another cause of a painful scrotal mass is testicular torsion. There often is no history of a prior scrotal mass, and in fact there may be a history of undescended testis. This mass is very tender and does not extend into the inguinal canal.

Torsion of the appendix testis results in a painful scrotal mass that may appear as a tender blue nodule on the upper pole of the testis, which itself is not tender. Inguinal lymphadenopathy may be tender or painless, but the key to diagnosis is the lateral and inferior location of these nodes in relation to the inguinal canal. Signs of infection in the area of lymphatic drainage are also important in making this diagnosis. An inguinal hernia is usually characterized by a painless swelling in the inguinal area that often increases in size with crying or straining. Incarceration of the hernia results in extreme pain and signs of bowel obstruction. If strangulation occurs, bloody diarrhea may result.

II. Diagnosis

A thorough history and physical examination are the keys to this diagnosis. In this case, the painful nature and inguinal location of this mass are the essential findings. An abdominal radiograph from the previous admission revealed a right inguinal hernia (Fig. 17-1) that had now become incarcerated. **The diagnosis is incarcerated inguinal hernia.** The hernia was reduced in the emergency department by pediatric surgical staff. No hernia was noted on the left side on physical examination. The patient was admitted for administration of intravenous fluids and observation, to allow the bowel edema from the incarceration to resolve. The patient manifested no signs or symptoms of bowel necrosis during 2 days in the hospital, after which he was taken to the operating room. Intraoperatively, bilateral inguinal hernias were found and repaired without any complications.

III. Incidence and Epidemiology

The incidence of inguinal hernia is estimated to be between 1% and 5%, or approximately 10 to 20 cases per 1,000 live births. The incidence in premature infants is significantly higher, approaching 30%. The ratio of boys to girls is 6:1. In boys, the right side is more frequently involved than the left, presumably due to the embryologic origin of inguinal hernias through a patent processus vaginalis and the fact that the right testis descends later during gestation than the left. In both boys and girls, 60% of inguinal hernias occur on the right, 30% on the left, and 10% bilaterally. Inguinal hernias are usually diagnosed during the first year of life, most frequently during the first month. There is often a family history of inguinal hernia. Undescended testes may be associated with inguinal hernias. Other conditions associated with inguinal hernias include Ehlers-Danlos syndrome, cystic fibrosis, congenital cytomegalovirus infection, and testicular feminization. There is no apparent ethnic or racial predisposition to inguinal hernia. Incarcerated inguinal hernias occur most frequently before 6 months of age, are less common after 2 years of age, and are rare after 5 years of age.

IV. Clinical Presentation

An inguinal hernia usually manifests as an asymptomatic swelling in the scrotal or labial area that increases in size with any increase in intraabdominal pressure, as occurs with crying or straining. Reducible hernias disappear spontaneously or with minimal pressure. An incarcerated hernia develops when a loop of bowel becomes trapped, and it is accompanied by severe pain and signs of bowel obstruction, such as bilious emesis. Strangulation of the herniated loop of bowel occurs when the blood supply to the bowel is compromised and may develop within 2 hours after incarceration. Urgent medical attention is required in cases of incarceration, and emergency surgical intervention may be necessary in cases of strangulation.

V. Diagnostic Approach

The key to diagnosis of inguinal hernia lies in maintaining an index of suspicion in the appropriate historical context, which is then confirmed by physical examination. In distinguishing an incarcerated hernia, awareness of the other important entities in the differential diagnosis is important. The diagnosis itself is founded primarily on the history and physical examination as well as a thorough knowledge of the disease process.

Abdominal radiography. An abdominal radiograph may show signs of bowel obstruction and may serve as an adjunctive and supportive piece of evidence in making the diagnosis.

VI. Treatment

In cases of incarcerated hernia, time is of the essence. Compromised blood flow to the affected loop of bowel can result in strangulation and bowel necrosis within 2 hours, so medical intervention is necessary. Reduction of the incarcerated hernia by experienced pediatric surgical staff is optimal. A gentle attempt at reduction using pressure on the scrotum with simultaneous counterpressure above the external inguinal ring is indicated but should never be forcefully done. Intravenous hydration and nasogastric tube decompression, in anticipation of definitive surgical management, are also indicated. Emergency surgery is sometimes required if the incarcerated hernia is not reducible. If the incarcerated loop of bowel is reduced, surgery may be postponed 12 to 36 hours so that the bowel edema can resolve.

Elective repair of an asymptomatic inguinal hernia should be performed as soon as possible after diagnosis, to avoid complications such as incarceration. All inguinal hernias require surgical intervention, because they do not resolve spontaneously. In boys, undescended testes may be associated with inguinal hernia, requiring orchiopexy. There is still some debate as to the importance of surgical exploration of the contralateral side in search of an occult inguinal hernia not detected by physical examination, as was the case in this patient. This decision is left to the individual surgeon, but contralateral exploration is commonly performed.

VII. References

1. Kapur P, Caty M, Glick P. Pediatric hernias and hydroceles. *Pediatr Clin North Am* 1998;45:773–789.
2. Irish M, Pearl R, Caty M, et al. The approach to common abdominal diagnoses in infants and children. *Pediatr Clin North Am* 1998;45:729–772.
3. Pillai S, Besner G. Pediatric testicular problems. *Pediatr Clin North Am* 1998;45: 813–830.
4. Kelly C, Kelly R. Lymphadenopathy in children. *Pediatr Clin North Am* 1998;45: 875–888.
5. Davenport D. ABC of general paediatric surgery: inguinal hernia, hydrocele and the undescended testis. *BMJ* 1996;312:564–567.
6. Katz D. Evaluation and management of inguinal and umbilical hernias. *Pediatr Ann* 2001;30:729–735.

Case 17-2: 2-Year-Old Boy

I. History of Present Illness

A 2-year-old boy presented to the hospital with a 3-day history of watery diarrhea and decreased appetite. Two days before presentation, he also developed vomiting and was seen by his primary physician, who treated him with trimethobenzamide hydrochloride (Tigan) suppositories, which provided no relief. The symptoms progressed to 20 episodes of diarrhea, now with blood and mucus and abdominal cramping, on the day of presentation. The patient was admitted to an outside hospital for presumed bacterial gastroenteritis. There were no known ill contacts, no known ingestion of undercooked foods, no recent travel, no recent course of antibiotics.

II. Past Medical History

His past history was significant only for one hospital admission for exacerbation of a reactive airways disease. There was no surgical history, and he was taking no medications. His mother had a history of irritable bowel syndrome.

III. Physical Examination

T, 37.5°C; RR, 30/min; HR, 150 bpm; BP, 105/50 mm Hg
Weight, 50th percentile

The patient was alert but quiet and ill-appearing. His eyes were mildly sunken. He had dry mucous membranes. There was no lymphadenopathy. The remainder of his head and neck examination was unremarkable. His cardiac examination revealed tachycardia but no murmur or gallop. Tachypnea was present, but there were no rales or wheezing. His neurologic examination was nonfocal. His skin turgor was diminished.

IV. Diagnostic Studies

A complete blood count revealed 16,600 WBCs/mm^3 with a differential of 62% segmented neutrophils, 24% band forms, 10% lymphocytes, 3% monocytes, and 1% atypical lymphocytes. Hemoglobin was 14.2 g/dL, and the platelet count was 381,000 cells/mm^3. Stool Gram stain was positive for WBCs. Routine bacterial and viral stool cultures were sent and eventually returned negative. Serum electrolytes were significant for a chloride concentration of 100 mmol/L and a bicarbonate level of 19 mmol/L. BUN was 73 mg/dL, and the creatinine concentration was 1.2 mg/dL

IV. Course of Illness

The patient was admitted to the hospital and for intravenous fluid rehydration and was given nothing by mouth after failing repeated clear liquid challenges by mouth and continuing to have diarrhea. A Foley catheter was placed to monitor urine output (Fig. 17-2). On the second day of hospitalization, he developed a fever to 39°C with increased abdominal pain, especially in the periumbilical region and in the right lower quadrant. His abdominal examination now revealed hypoactive bowel sounds, and an abdominal radiograph demonstrated ileus. An abdominal ultrasound study showed a small amount of ascites. Ampicillin, gentamicin, and clindamycin were started intravenously. A sigmoidoscopy was performed to 50 cm, and the colon appeared normal. A biopsy was obtained which showed signs of chronic inflammation. Later that day, the patient was taken for an exploratory laparotomy due to worsening abdominal pain and signs of an acute abdomen. Surgery revealed a leathery thickening of the descending colon, possibly consistent with chronic inflammation, without involvement of the transverse colon or distal sigmoid. A large amount (500 mL) of clear yellow ascitic fluid was removed. A central venous catheter was placed, given the anticipated need for prolonged intravenous fluids and medications.

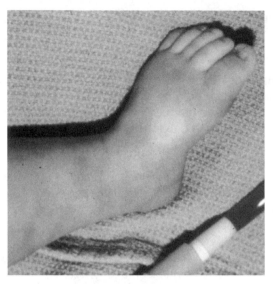

FIG. 17-2. Photograph of patient (case 17-2).

DISCUSSION: CASE 17-2

I.   Differential Diagnosis

The key to this diagnosis is having the appropriate level of suspicion in the right clinical context. During the initial prodrome of bloody diarrhea, any of the other bacterial causes of enteroinvasive diarrhea would be on the list of differential diagnoses, including *Salmonella, Shigella,* and *Campylobacter* species. HUS has been associated with *Shigella* infection, as a result of elaboration of Shiga toxin. All of these bacterial causes are routinely screened for in most stool cultures; however, *E. coli* O157:H7 may not be routinely screened for, even though it may now be the most common cause of bloody diarrhea in the United States. *C. difficile* colitis could also manifest in this manner, and assay for toxins A and B would be important in distinguishing this entity, as would a prior history of recent antibiotic use.

Inflammatory bowel disease could also manifest in this fashion, especially in terms of an acute flare with signs of systemic toxicity and abdominal symptoms severe enough at times to warrant surgical exploration.

II.   Diagnosis

The Foley catheter revealed bloody urine. The patient's lower extremity, also included in the photograph in Fig. 17-2, revealed evidence of poor perfusion. Postoperatively, the patient was noted to be edematous while receiving maintenance intravenous fluids. Repeat laboratory studies revealed the following: serum sodium, 133 mmol/L; chloride, 114 mmol/L; bicarbonate, 11 mmol/L; BUN, 24 mg/dL; and creatinine, 3.0 mg/dL. The hemoglobin had decreased to 11.3 g/dL, and the platelet count was 118,000 cells/mm^3. The peripheral smear showed the presence of schistocytes, suggesting a hemolytic process. Liver function tests were significant for an aspartate aminotransferase (AST) of 532 U/L; alanine aminotransferase (ALT), 287 U/L; lactate dehydrogenase, 4,290 U/L; and albumin, 1.7 g/dL. The partial thromboplastin time (PTT) was slightly elevated at 37.4 seconds.

Over the next 3 hours, the patient's urine output stopped completely. He was given 25% albumin intravenously with intravenous fluids followed by furosemide, which resulted in only 10 mL of urine output. At this point, the patient was transferred to another institution for continuous arteriovenous hemoperfusion. A stool culture sent specifically for detection of *E. coli* O157:H7 returned positive. **This culture confirmed the diagnosis of hemolytic-uremic syndrome secondary to infection with *E. coli* O157:H7, otherwise known as D(+) HUS, in that it is associated with diarrhea.**

During his 4-week hospitalization, his BUN level peaked at 101 mg/dL and creatinine at 9.9 mg/dL. His hemoglobin nadir was 4.7 g/dL, and the platelet count nadir was 103,000/mm^3. He required continuous arteriovenous hemoperfusion for most of the remainder of his hospitalization. On discharge, his BUN was 74 mg/dL and his creatinine concentration was 5.5 mg/dL.

III. Incidence and Epidemiology

HUS is one of the most common causes of acute renal failure in children, and *E. coli* O157:H7 infection is the most common cause of HUS. As a member of the enterohemorrhagic group of *E. coli,* this serotype causes a hemorrhagic colitis and elaborates a verotoxin that is similar to Shiga toxin, produced by *Shigella dysenteriae* type 1. Based on retrospective studies and the apparent recent emergence of HUS as a clinical entity, it appears that *E. coli* O157:H7 is a relatively newly evolved serotype. In the United States, it is one of the most common causes of bloody diarrhea. Cases can occur on a sporadic as well as an epidemic basis, and the incidence of sporadic cases appears to have increased in the last decade. There is a seasonal pattern to infection, in that cases are more common in the summer months, although they do sometimes occur in the winter. This may also be associated with the fact that cattle and their undercooked meat products or unpasteurized dairy products are the most significant factors in transmission and are more likely to be consumed in the summertime.

The highest attack rates are at the extremes of the age spectrum: the very old and the very young appear to be at greatest risk. In particular, children younger than 4 years of age are at great risk of contracting *E. coli* O157:H7 infection and are also at greater risk for developing HUS as a result. HUS occurs in approximately 10% of patients who acquire sporadic infection with *E. coli* O157:H7, and it appears to occur at a higher attack rate of up to 40% among patients infected in an outbreak. The mortality rate is approximately 5%, and another 5% of patients develop severe neurologic sequelae or end-stage renal failure. Extremely poor prognostic factors include a high leukocyte count, a severe gastrointestinal prodrome, age younger than 2 years, and early onset of anuria.

IV. Clinical Presentation

Infection with *E. coli* O157:H7 begins as a nonbloody diarrhea that progresses to bloody diarrhea, often within a few days after the onset of illness. Vomiting occurs in half of patients and a fever in approximately one third. Fecal leukocytes are often present. The hemorrhagic colitis is otherwise nonspecific and may appear indistinguishable clinically from many other colitides. Abdominal symptoms may become severe enough to mimic those of an acute abdomen, prompting surgical intervention. Complications include intussusception, perforation, and stricture. The classic triad of microangiopathic hemolytic anemia, thrombocytopenia, and acute renal failure follows the gastrointestinal prodrome. Leukocytosis develops, as can cerebral edema with seizure activity. Irritability progressing to stupor and coma may also develop. Cortical blindness and stroke may occur as well.

HUS may manifest in a D(−) form, which is not associated with diarrhea. Cases of D(−) HUS, otherwise known as atypical HUS, have been associated with use of medications, familial patterns of inheritance, recurrent episodes of HUS, and bacterial infections, such as *Streptococcus pneumoniae*. In general, patients with D(−) HUS have a higher incidence of neurologic sequelae in addition to the renal sequelae, and overall they have worse outcomes than patients with D+ HUS.

V. Diagnostic Approach

Clinical and laboratory findings. The key to diagnosis is recognition of the clinical syndrome in the appropriate context. An abnormal complete blood count with thrombocytopenia and anemia with schistocytes and red blood cell fragments on the peripheral smear, in the context of fluid overload and oliguria or anuria with a rising serum creatinine, confirm the diagnosis of this syndrome.

Microbiology. Stool culture is important to exclude other infectious causes of colitis, but the specific biochemical tests that are necessary to identify the specific serotype, O157:H7, may not be routinely performed in some laboratories and must be specifically requested.

Enzyme immunoassays. New, rapid methods to detect *E. coli* O157:H7 lipopolysaccharide and Shiga toxin are very useful in diagnosing infection in a timely fashion.

VI. Treatment

Current therapy remains supportive in nature, so prevention is essential by ensuring complete cooking of all beef products, particularly ground beef; thorough hand-washing after interaction with animals that may be known carriers; and avoidance of unpasteurized dairy or other products. Patients who develop HUS require significant volume support with careful fluid and electrolyte management. Transfusion may be necessary due to significant gastrointestinal blood loss and microangiopathic hemolytic anemia. Hypertension and renal failure must be anticipated in the clinical management, and patients often require dialysis. Neurologic complications, such as seizures, may require antiepileptic therapy. There is no evidence that antibiotics are helpful, and they may be potentially harmful, by causing increased release of toxin. Antimotility agents are also contraindicated because of the increased absorption of toxin. SYNSORB Pk is a promising new therapy undergoing clinical trials; preliminary data suggest that the use of this synthetic molecule, which binds Shiga toxin, may decrease the risk of developing HUS in patients who are infected with *E. coli* O157:H7.

VII. References

1. Cohen M. *Escherichia coli* O157:H7 infections: a frequent cause of bloody diarrhea and the hemolytic-uremic syndrome. *Adv Pediatr* 1996;43:171–207.
2. Trachtman H, Christen E. Pathogenesis, treatment, and therapeutic trials in hemolytic uremic syndrome. *Curr Opin Pediatr* 1999;11:162–168.
3. Boyce T, Swerdlow D, Griffin P. *Escherichia coli* O157:H7 and the hemolytic-uremic syndrome. *N Engl J Med* 1995;333:364–368.
4. Neuhaus T, Calonder S, Leumann E. Heterogeneity of atypical haemolytic uraemic syndromes. *Arch Dis Child* 1997;76:518–521.
5. Siegler R. The hemolytic uremic syndrome. *Pediatr Clin North Am* 1995;42: 1505–1529.
6. Taylor C, Monnens L. Advances in haemolytic uraemic syndrome. *Arch Dis Child* 1998;78:190–193.

Case 17-3: 17-Year-Old Boy

I. History of Present Illness

A 17 year-old boy was well until 1 week before presentation, when he developed a fever to 39.5°C, severe abdominal pain, and bloody diarrhea. The diarrhea occurred with any oral intake. There was no nausea or vomiting, no upper respiratory tract symptoms, no history of recent travel, no known ingestion of undercooked food. He had been treated with clarithromycin for sinusitis the previous week. For the last 7 months, he had had nonbloody diarrhea with no mucus. The stools were watery and occurred three to four times per week. He had attributed this to eating out frequently. During that time there was no associated nausea, vomiting, fever, or abdominal pain. He had had a 7-pound weight loss during that time.

II. Past Medical History

His past history was significant for seasonal allergic rhinitis, for which he was taking Claritin (loratadine) as needed. There was no known family history of any gastrointestinal disease.

III. Physical Examination

T, 37°C; RR, 18/min; HR, 60 bpm; BP, 120/65 mm Hg

Weight, 10th percentile; height, 25th percentile

Physical examination revealed a thin patient who was anicteric with moist mucous membranes. Cardiac and respiratory examinations were normal. His abdomen was soft, without hepatosplenomegaly. Rectal examination revealed heme-positive stool with no masses and no skin tags. His extremity examination revealed mild digital clubbing. There were no rashes. The neurologic examination was normal.

IV. Diagnostic Studies

Serum electrolytes, serum glucose, BUN, and serum creatinine concentrations were all normal. A complete blood count revealed 23,700 WBCs/mm^3; hemoglobin, 11.7 g/dL; and platelets, 302,000/mm^3. The erythrocyte sedimentation rate (ESR) was 5 mm/hour. The serum albumin concentration was low at 2.4 g/dL, and the serum alkaline phosphatase concentration was also low at 58 U/L. The serum lactate dehydrogenase was elevated at 540 U/L. A stool sample was negative for *C. difficile* toxin, and a routine stool culture was negative for bacterial pathogens. A stool sample for ova and parasites was negative.

V. Course of Illness

The patient was admitted to an outside hospital, where he underwent flexible sigmoidoscopy, which reportedly showed inflammation consistent with inflammatory bowel disease. Mesalamine and prednisone were started, with some improvement of diarrhea in terms of frequency and consistency. He was discharged after a 12-day hospitalization but was readmitted 5 days later with bloody diarrhea and abdominal pain. A colonoscopy was performed and showed villous adenomatous polyposis versus inflammatory bowel disease. Mesalamine and prednisone were continued, and oral meprazole and mesalamine enemas were added. He did not improve, and weight loss progressed to a total of 15 pounds lost over the preceding month. The patient was transferred to another institution for further evaluation.

A complete blood count revealed 10,700 WBCs/mm^3 (71% segmented neutrophils, 1% band forms, and 17% lymphocytes). The hemoglobin was 11.9 g/dL, with a low mean corpuscular volume of 77 fL and an increased red blood cell distribution width of 17.4.

The ESR was 8 mm/hour. Total protein concentration was low at 5.6 g/dL, as was serum albumin at 2.9 g/dL. Serum cholesterol was elevated at 255 mg/dL. Retinal examination suggested a diagnosis.

DISCUSSION: CASE 17-3

I. Differential Diagnosis

In this patient, the significant duration of diarrhea (7 months) and the associated weight loss (7 pounds) led to consideration of multiple causes of chronic diarrhea. Inflammatory bowel disease was a serious consideration, given the weight loss and the recent acute presenting episode with fever and bloody diarrhea. Colonoscopy would be useful in making this diagnosis. Causes of infectious gastroenteritis that result in chronic diarrhea and must be excluded include *C. difficile, G. lamblia,* and other parasites. Specific microbiologic culture assays would be necessary to evaluate for these etiologies. Secretory causes of diarrhea, such as tumor-secreting intestinally active peptides, must also be considered. Fasting on the part of the patient is helpful in this instance, as are stool samples for various peptide assays.

II. Diagnosis

The normal ESR was believed to be inconsistent with the diagnosis of inflammatory bowel disease in the context of persistent symptoms. Formal ophthalmologic examination revealed retinal pigment epithelial clumping with nevi. Further review of the pathology findings was believed to be suggestive of adenomatous polyposis with carcinoma *in situ.* Steroids were tapered off. **The diagnosis is Gardner syndrome.** Computed tomography of the chest, abdomen, and pelvis showed thickening of the polyps but no signs of metastasis. A gastrointestinal barium study revealed multiple polyps but no areas of thickened bowel or intestinal strictures. Small-bowel enteroclysis was performed, which revealed no polyps of the small bowel. Stool examination for ova and parasites was positive for *Blastocystis hominis,* for which he received metronidazole treatment. A peptide panel revealed normal levels of gastrin, calcitonin, somatostatin, and substance P. Carcinoembryonic antigen level was elevated at 13.9 ng/dL (normal, less than 2.5 ng/dL). He was scheduled to have surgery, but due to his religious beliefs as a Jehovah's Witness, he did not want to have any blood transfusions. He was sent home on erythropoietin-α and was readmitted 1 month later to have a total colectomy with ileostomy and ileoanal pull-through, J-pouch, and loop-diverting ileostomy, which he tolerated well. Two months later, his ileostomy was taken down.

III. Incidence and Epidemiology

Gardner syndrome is a phenotypic variant of familial adenomatous polyposis, which has a prevalence between 1:5,000 and 1:17,000. Patients may have anywhere from only a few adenomatous polyps to thousands. The average age at onset of adenomatous polyps is 16 years, and progress to carcinoma is likely to occur by the fifth decade of life. The presence of upper gastrointestinal polyps is associated with an increased risk of carcinoma.

In addition to adenomatous colonic polyps, Gardner syndrome is characterized by the presence of a number of extraintestinal manifestations, such as exostoses involving the skull, mandible, or long bones. Congenital hypertrophy of the retinal pigment epithelium may be found on funduscopic examination. Lipomas and fibromas may be associated, as may epidermoid or sebaceous cysts. Dental abnormalities such as impacted or supernumerary teeth or mandibular cysts have also been associated with Gardner syndrome. Desmoid tumors, characterized by fibromatosis of the mesentery, can be found in approximately 8% to 13% of patients with Gardner syndrome. These tumors can cause bowel obstruction or perforation as well as intraabdominal abscesses. The association of malignant brain tumors in patients with Gardner syndrome or familial adenomatous polyposis is known as Turcot syndrome and is often associated with high morbidity and mortality.

Gardner syndrome is inherited in an autosomal dominant fashion, although spontaneous mutations can be seen in about one third of cases. The molecular defect causing the occurrence of the multiple adenomatous colonic polyps is a mutation in the adenomatous polyposis coli (*APC*) tumor suppressor gene located on chromosome 5q21. This mutated gene encodes for a truncated version of the cytoplasmic protein, β-catenin.

IV. Clinical Presentation

The clinical presentation of Gardner syndrome can vary greatly, from painless rectal bleeding to chronic abdominal pain with diarrhea. Colocolic intussusception is possible, with the adenomatous polyps serving as a lead point. Otherwise asymptomatic iron deficiency anemia due to occult gastrointestinal blood loss is another possible presentation. Extraintestinal manifestation is likely in children, because the polyps may not become symptomatic for decades. Exostoses of the mandible or long bones and dental abnormalities such as supernumerary teeth should raise the index of suspicion for Gardner syndrome.

V. Diagnostic Approach

Endoscopy. Colonoscopy and upper endoscopy for direct visualization with removal of polyps provides a pathologic specimen which can be used to confirm the presence of adenomatous polyps or even, as in this case, carcinoma *in situ*. Evaluation of the upper gastrointestinal tract for polyps is important both therapeutically and prognostically, in terms of future risk of neoplasia. Accurate review of the pathologic specimen is essential, because confusion may occur with polyps that arise secondary to a chronic inflammatory process.

Upper gastrointestinal series with small-bowel follow-through and small-bowel enteroclysis. This radiologic study may show upper gastrointestinal polyps, but it is not necessary, because endoscopy provides both diagnostic and therapeutic results in the removal of polyps for pathologic analysis.

Roentgenograms of long bones and mandible. These radiographs can help identify the exostoses often associated as extraintestinal manifestations of Gardner syndrome.

Computed tomography. Computed tomography of the abdomen may be helpful in identifying associated desmoid tumors or metastases from carcinoma that has arisen from the adenomatous polyps.

Complete ophthalmologic examination. A thorough retinal examination is important in detecting the presence of congenital hypertrophy of the pigment epithelium, which is often found in Gardner syndrome and, as in this case, may confirm the clinical diagnosis in conjunction with the pathologic findings from endoscopy specimens.

Genetic testing. Genetic testing is available using peripheral blood lymphocytes in an *in vitro* protein truncation assay; 80% to 90% of affected patients are detected by this assay. However, 10% to 20% of patients who have a negative result on this assay may be considered truly negative for the *APC* mutation only if another affected family member has had a positive test.

VI. Treatment

For patients with Gardner syndrome, prophylactic total proctocolectomy is the treatment of choice, because of the unavoidable progression to neoplasia. Colectomy is recommended shortly after the diagnosis of polyposis is confirmed. Although nonsteroidal antiinflammatory drugs have been used to decrease the size and number of polyps in these patients, this is currently not the treatment of choice because it has not been shown to decrease the cancer risk. Studies are currently underway to evaluate the usefulness of cyclooxygenase-2 inhibitors in these patients.

Once an individual has been diagnosed with Gardner syndrome, screening of other family members should take place. Genetic testing is the method of choice under these circumstances. The general consensus is that children should undergo genetic testing at age 8 to 10 years. Once a mutant allele of *APC* has been identified in a patient, annual flexible sigmoidoscopy is recommended. If colonic polyps are found, upper endoscopy is also recommended. If there is a family history of malignant brain tumors, indicating the presence of Turcot syndrome, then magnetic resonance imaging of the head is indicated. In cases of Gardner syndrome, radiographs of the skull, long bones, and mandible, as well as a full ophthalmologic examination, may be warranted. Family members who test negative are presumed to have a cancer risk comparable to that of the general population, although screening sigmoidoscopy is still recommended at least every 10 years, starting in adolescence.

VII. References

1. Corredor J, Wambach J, Barnard J. Gastrointestinal polyps in children: advances in molecular genetics, diagnosis, and management. *J Pediatr* 2001;138:621–628.
2. Rustgi A. Hereditary gastrointestinal polyposis and nonpolyposis syndromes. *N Engl J Med* 1994;331:1694–1702.

Case 17-4: 15-Month-Old Boy

I. History of Present Illness

A 15-month-old boy presented with a 3-month history of watery diarrhea associated with weight loss. At 12 months of age, he developed diarrhea characterized by six to eight watery brown stools per day accompanied by significant flatulence. There was no associated emesis or blood in the stool. He had continued to have a good appetite despite the frequent stooling. Dietary changes, including a BRAT (bananas, rice, apples, toast) diet and a lactose-free diet, had been introduced but did not improve the diarrhea. Occasional low-grade fevers had been noted. There was no history of foreign travel or ill contacts. There were two cats and one dog in the home. He had lost 3 pounds in the last 3 months.

II. Past Medical History

He was a full-term infant with a birth weight of 6 lb, 11 oz who was fed Similac without any problems. He had normal weight gain and developmental milestones. He had been introduced to rice cereal, baby foods, and adult table foods without any problems. He was taking no medications.

III. Physical Examination

T, 36.8°C; RR, 26/min; HR, 100 bpm; BP, 102/53 mm Hg

Weight, less than 5th percentile (50th percentile for a 6-month-old child); height, 10th percentile

The initial examination revealed a quiet, gaunt-appearing child. His eyes were sunken, but the rest of the head, eyes, ears, nose, mouth, and throat examination was unremarkable. His cardiac and respiratory examinations were normal. His abdominal examination revealed no masses. His liver edge was palpable at the right costal margin. There was no clubbing of the fingers. He had dry skin around his nose and lips. He had very little subcutaneous fat. His neurologic examination was nonfocal.

IV. Diagnostic Studies

Laboratory analysis revealed 11,100 WBCs/mm^3 with 29% segmented neutrophils, 66% lymphocytes, and 5% monocytes. The hemoglobin was 12.2 g/dL, and there were 492,000 platelets/mm^3. Electrolytes were significant for a potassium concentration of 2.8 mmol/L and a bicarbonate concentration 16 mmol/L. His ESR was 4 mm/hour. Urinalysis was negative, with a urine specific gravity of 1.005. The serum alkaline phosphatase level was low at 115 U/L, whereas ALT was elevated at 59 U/L, AST at 64 U/L, and lactate dehydrogenase at 845 U/L.

V. Course of Illness

The patient was admitted and hyperalimentation was started for his nutritional status and to correct his hypokalemia. Blood culture and stool culture were both negative. A sweat test was normal. A stool sample tested negative for *C. difficile* toxins. Stool for ova and parasites revealed Indian meal moth larvae. Colonoscopy was performed on the sixth day of hospitalization and revealed nonspecific lymphoid hyperplasia. Despite taking nothing by mouth, he continued to have mucusy diarrhea which became heme positive. Stool osmolality was normal at 298 mOsm/kg H$_2$O. Chest radiography (Fig. 17-3) suggested a diagnosis, which was confirmed by biopsy.

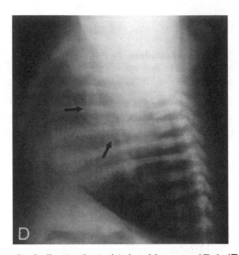

FIG. 17-3. Chest radiograph similar to that obtained in case 17-4. (From Swischuk LE. *Imaging of the newborn, infant, and young child,* 4th ed. Baltimore: Williams & Wilkins, 1997:144.)

DISCUSSION: CASE 17-4

I.   Differential Diagnosis

The chronic nature of his diarrhea for the last 3 months, associated with weight loss, moved the differential diagnosis away from the diagnosis of acute infectious diarrhea due to either bacterial or viral causes. A prolonged bout of postinfectious diarrhea due to disaccharidase deficiency was possible but unlikely. Chronic diarrhea due to infection with *C. difficile* or ova and parasites was a possibility even without a history of antibiotic use, bloody diarrhea, foreign travel, or use of untreated water sources. The key observation in making this diagnosis occurred while the patient was in the hospital: he took nothing by mouth but continued to produce profuse voluminous watery diarrhea. This finding indicated the presence of secretory, rather than osmotic, diarrhea. In this differential diagnosis, the list is rather brief and includes rare congenital and paraneoplastic conditions. Congenital defects in chloride or sodium transport are more likely to manifest in infancy. Infectious causes of secretory diarrhea include small-bowel overgrowth or infection with immuno adherent *E. coli* stimulating gastrointestinal secretions. Any cause of villous atrophy, whether congenital, autoimmune, or secondary to immune deficiency (e.g., HIV infection, severe combined immunodeficiency) may also result in this presentation. Neuroblastoma or other tumors of neural crest origin (e.g., ganglioneuroma) may secrete vasoactive intestinal peptide (VIP), resulting in secretory diarrhea.

II.   Diagnosis

Chest radiography revealed a large posterior mediastinal mass (Fig. 17-3). Computed tomography of the chest performed on the seventh day of hospitalization confirmed a 4 × 4 cm right posterior mediastinal mass. The urine vanillylmandelic acid level was 498 mg/g of creatinine, and the homovanillic acid level was 245 mg/g of creatinine, both extremely elevated. Surgical excision revealed neuroblastoma with a favorable histology. **These findings were consistent with the diagnosis of neuroblastoma causing secretory diarrhea.**

III. Incidence and Epidemiology

The annual incidence of neuroblastoma is approximately 8 per 1 million children younger than 15 years of age. The median age at diagnosis is 22 months, and 95% of cases are diagnosed by the age of 10 years. Neuroblastoma accounts for approximately 6% of all pediatric tumors. There is a slight male preponderance, with a ratio of 1.2:1. There also appear to be cases that are familial in nature and manifest at a younger age, with a median age of 9 months at diagnosis. These tumors derive from postganglionic sympathetic cells found in the paraspinal sympathetic ganglia and in the adrenal chromaffin cells. Neuroblastoma and ganglioneuroblastoma represent the malignant forms of these neural crest tumors, whereas ganglioneuroma represents the most benign form, with no metastatic potential.

IV. Clinical Presentation

Most pediatric patients with neuroblastoma are diagnosed by 5 years of age, and most tumors are intraabdominal in location. However, patients older than 1 year of age have a higher incidence of intrathoracic and cervical tumors, compared with younger patients. Among children older than 1 year of age, 75% present with a disseminated, advanced stage of disease and account for a significant proportion of neuroblastoma-associated mortality. Infants younger than 1 year of age tend to present with lower-stage disease and have much higher cure rates. Some of the tumors in this latter group even undergo spontaneous regression. One percent of patients have no detectable primary tumor. In 35% of children, neuroblastoma metastases occur to the regional lymph nodes, qualifying as disseminated disease. Hematogenous spread to bone, bone marrow, liver, and skin also occurs. Late metastases are seen in the brain and lung. Patients may present with a large abdominal mass or with respiratory distress secondary to the intraabdominal mass. Intrathoracic tumors are often incidentally found. Opsoclonus-myoclonus is an well-defined presenting syndrome for neuroblastoma. Presentation as severe secretory diarrhea, as in this case, is known as Verner-Morrison syndrome.

V. Diagnostic Approach

Clinical observation. The observation of continued, intractable watery diarrhea while the patient takes nothing by mouth is key to the ultimate diagnosis. Whether this is accomplished by obtaining a very thorough history or by observation while in the hospital, this piece of information is vital to making the ultimate diagnosis.

Radiography. Radiographs may localize calcifications, and often they provide the first indication of the presence of a tumor as an incidental finding. Skeletal surveys may show bone involvement and are used in tumor staging.

Computed tomography or magnetic resonance imaging. Three-dimensional imaging more accurately delineates the location of the tumor, which is usually retroperitoneal or adrenal, and also assists in staging. Occasionally, tumors are found along the sympathetic chain in the thoracic or cervical region.

Vasoactive intestinal peptide level. Plasma VIP may be elaborated by tumors of neural crest origin and may cause secretory diarrhea.

Urinary (or serum) catecholamine levels. Elevation of urinary homovanillic or vanillylmandelic acid, in conjunction with diagnostic pathologic features, is diagnostic for neuroblastoma. These levels may also be used to monitor disease activity.

Surgical removal. Complete surgical excision provides a pathologic specimen for further identification and characterization of the tumor and is also therapeutic, especially with regard to the secretory diarrhea. It is also important in the staging process, especially in assessing lymph node involvement.

Bone scintigraphy. A bone scan is important in detecting possible metastases and is used in the staging process.

Radionuclide scan. Radiolabeled metaiodobenzylguanidine (MIBG) is taken up by catecholamine-secreting cells and is useful for staging (i.e., detecting bone and soft tissue involvement).

VI.   Treatment

Surgical resection is usually performed. Low-risk patients may not need any additional therapy. Radiotherapy and chemotherapy are used, depending on the stage of the disease. Patients with high-risk disease may have some improvement in short-term survival with autologous bone marrow transplantation, but longer-term outcome is still poor. Surgical removal of the tumor usually cures the secretory diarrhea. The use of somatostatin analogues also has a therapeutic effect on the secretory diarrhea, but the definitive therapy for the diarrhea remains surgical.

VII.   References

1. Castleberry R. Biology and treatment of neuroblastoma. *Pediatr Clin North Am* 1997;44:919–937.
2. Bown N. Neuroblastoma tumour genetics: clinical and biological aspects. *J Clin Pathol* 2001;54:897–910.
3. Castleberry R. Paediatric update: neuroblastoma. *Eur J Cancer* 1997;33:1430–1438.
4. Alexander F. Neuroblastoma. *Urol Clin North Am* 2000;27:383–392.

Case 17-5: 5-Year-Old Girl

I. History of Present Illness

A 5-year-old girl with a recent diagnosis of cystic fibrosis presented to the pulmonary clinic with a 1-week history of watery stools. Her pancreatic enzyme dosages had been increased without effect on her diarrhea. There had also been no improvement with a clear liquid diet. Two days before admission, oral metronidazole was started for possible parasitic infection. Recent tests for *C. difficile* toxins A and B had been negative. Symptoms were worsening, with increased abdominal distention and lethargy. She had lost 2 kg over the previous 3 weeks. She had had no fever or vomiting. She had normal urine output and a mild cough.

II. Past Medical History

She was the product of a full-term, uncomplicated pregnancy. She did not have meconium ileus at birth. She was diagnosed with cystic fibrosis 9 weeks before this admission. She presented at that time with failure to thrive and with foamy, foul-smelling stools. Her diagnosis was delayed due to the finding of *Dientamoeba fragilis,* which was treated with iodoquinol, and also *B. hominis,* which was treated with metronidazole. Despite treatment and follow-up stool tests, which were negative, she did not gain weight, although her stool symptoms had resolved. She had 6 weeks with no diarrhea before this admission. Her current medications included trimethoprim-sulfamethoxazole, metronidazole, albuterol, nebulized cromolyn sodium, inhaled *N*-acetylcysteine, pancrelipase capsules, and vitamins A, D, E, and K. Her family history was significant for an older sibling who had a history of constipation and poor growth.

III. Physical Examination

T, 37°C; RR, 32/min; HR, 147 bpm; BP, 109/68 mm Hg

Weight and height, both far below the 5th percentile

Physical examination revealed a thin girl with no rhinorrhea and slightly dry mucous membranes. The remainder of her head and neck examination was normal. Her cardiac and respiratory examinations were normal except for mild tachycardia. Her abdomen was distended but otherwise unremarkable. Her rectal examination revealed a minimal amount of stool, which was heme negative. Her extremities were wasted with very little subcutaneous fat. There were no skin rashes. Her neurologic examination was nonfocal.

IV. Diagnostic Studies

Chest radiography revealed mildly increased interstitial markings but no infiltrates. A complete blood count revealed 13,100 WBCs/mm^3 (40% segmented neutrophils, 46% lymphocytes, 14% monocytes), a hemoglobin of 12.7 g/dL, and a platelet count of 472,000 cells/mm^3. Her ESR was 5 mm/hour. Serum electrolytes, BUN, serum creatinine, and serum glucose were normal. Her serum ALT was mildly elevated at 56 U/L, as was her AST at 68 U/L. Her serum alkaline phosphatase was low at 72 U/L, as was serum albumin at 1.9 g/dL and total protein at 3.8 g/dL. Her stool pH was 6.0, and her routine stool cultures were negative. Stool examination was negative for ova and parasites, and assays for *C. difficile* toxins A and B were negative. Tests for *G. lamblia* antigen and *Cryptosporidium* were negative.

V. Course of Illness

All feeding attempts resulted in abdominal distention and pain. Abdominal radiographs showed the presence of stool and dilated loops of small bowel with air–fluid levels. An upper gastrointestinal barium study with small-bowel follow-through suggested the diagnosis (Fig. 17-4).

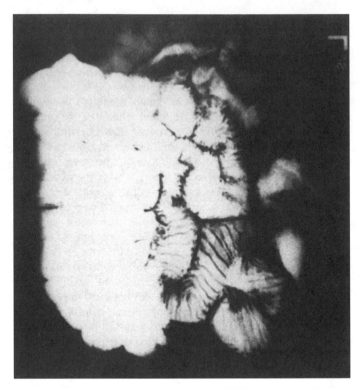

FIB. 17-4. Upper gastrointestinal study with small-bowel follow-through similar to that obtained in case 17-5. (From First LR. Pediatric medicine. In: Avery ME, First LR, eds. Baltimore: Williams & Wilkins, 1989:435.)

DISCUSSION: CASE 17-5

I. Differential Diagnosis

In the context of her recent diagnosis of cystic fibrosis, this patient had many symptoms of chronic malabsorption, including poor weight gain, chronic diarrhea, and abdominal distention. Inadequate management of her cystic fibrosis could account for her symptoms, as could infectious causes of chronic diarrhea superimposed on the diagnosis of cystic fibrosis. *C. difficile, G. lamblia,* and *Cryptosporidium* are potential culprits. Celiac sprue should be considered in the differential due to reports of an association with cystic fibrosis.

II. Diagnosis

The upper gastrointestinal barium study revealed thickened, dilated small-bowel loops with prominent valvulae conniventes resulting from the dilatation (Fig. 17-4). This finding suggested the diagnosis of celiac sprue. Duodenal bulb biopsies showed intense lamina propria inflammatory cells with villous blunting and ulceration, with almost complete villous flattening and inspissated secretions in some crypts. Anti-gliadin immunoglobulin G (IgG) was found to be greater than 140 mg/dL (normal, less than 15 mg/dL), and IgA was greater than 136 mg/dL (normal, less than 4 mg/dL). The anti-endomysial IgA titer was 1:320. **The diagnosis is celiac sprue in the setting of cystic fibrosis.**

III. Incidence and Epidemiology

Celiac sprue is also known as celiac disease or gluten-sensitive enteropathy. The prevalence of celiac sprue in the United States has been estimated at 1 per 3,000 in the population, but recent seroprevalence studies indicate that the prevalence may be as high as 1 in 120 to 1 in 300 persons in Europe and North America. There is an ethnic predisposition in western Europeans and their descendants. It appears to be a rare condition among people from an African-Caribbean, Chinese, or Japanese background. Females are slightly more frequently affected than males. There is a familial predisposition, with approximately 10% of patients having affected first-degree relatives and more than 95% of patients with celiac sprue expressing a specific human leukocyte antigen HLA-DQ heterodimer.

IV. Clinical Presentation

Celiac sprue is a malabsorptive condition caused by an autoimmune T cell–mediated response against gluten that results in severe inflammation in small-bowel mucosa. The classic presentation is in infants who develop diarrhea, abdominal distention, and failure to thrive as cereals are introduced into their diets. Vomiting and abdominal pain may be associated. The infants may develop iron deficiency anemia and rickets secondary to the malabsorption. Older children and adolescents may not present with malabsorptive symptoms but rather with hypertransaminasemia, short stature, pubertal delay, or recurrent aphthous ulcers. Adults may present with a history of symptoms that date back to childhood, or they may have had no previous symptoms whatsoever. Diarrhea with lactose intolerance and steatorrhea are common. Weight loss with flatulence and abdominal distention also occur. Adults may be otherwise asymptomatic and may present with only iron deficiency anemia or recurrent aphthous ulcers.

Conditions that are associated with celiac disease include dermatitis herpetiformis, which is a pruritic papulovesicular rash on the extensor surfaces of the extremities and the trunk. Biopsy of these lesions reveal the presence of IgA deposits, and the lesions resolve with gluten withdrawal from the diet. Autoimmune thyroiditis and type 1 diabetes mellitus are also are associated with celiac sprue.

Patients with refractory sprue are at increased risk for development of enteropathy-associated T-cell lymphoma. These patients have severe symptoms despite adherence to a gluten-free diet for at least 6 months. This condition often requires treatment with corticosteroids or immunosuppressants. A recent study showed that strict adherence to a diet free from gluten can decrease the risk of cancers associated with celiac sprue.

V. Diagnostic Approach

Endoscopy. Endoscopy with biopsy of the small intestine remains the gold standard in diagnosis. Pathologic specimens reveal the presence of absent or flattened villi with hyperplastic crypts, with a significant presence of inflammatory lymphocytes and plasma cells. These findings usually resolve after withdrawal of gluten from the diet, but the resolution of pathologic findings generally lags behind signs of clinical improvement. Repeat biopsies are not necessary due to the highly accurate nature of the serologic tests that are now available.

Serologic tests. The serologic tests are highly specific and sensitive and are key to the diagnosis of celiac sprue. Measurement of IgA anti-endomysial antibodies is reported to be 85% to 98% sensitive and 97% to 100% specific. Anti-gliadin IgA and IgG are much less specific and have moderate sensitivity; increased levels can be seen in adults with nonspecific gastrointestinal inflammation and therefore are not as useful. In children younger than 2 years of age, these may be false negative results in assays for IgA anti-endomysial antibodies. All of these markers respond to withdrawal of gluten, and they often become undetectable within 3 to 6 months after initiation of the appropriate dietary regimen.

Radiographic studies. Abdominal radiographs and upper gastrointestinal radiographic series using barium are no longer necessary to make the initial diagnosis, given the extreme sensitivity and specificity of serologic tests and endoscopy findings. However, radiographic imaging, including computed tomography, may be helpful in evaluating patients with refractory celiac sprue, especially for signs of intestinal lymphoma.

Tests of malabsorption. Measurement of fecal fat or oral D-xylose absorption are not specific and therefore not necessary; they merely serve to confirm the malabsorptive nature of the condition.

Gluten withdrawal. Empiric elimination of gluten from the diet is not indicated, because the results of intestinal biopsy after this intervention may be equivocal, and serologic tests are far superior in making the definitive diagnosis in the appropriate clinical context.

VI.   Treatment

The definitive therapy for celiac sprue is lifetime avoidance of gluten in the diet. Complete avoidance is probably impossible due to the widespread presence of gluten in processed foods, but elimination of products that contain wheat gluten, barley, or rye is important. Oats should also be avoided initially; they may be slowly reintroduced in some patients without serious consequences. Dairy products are also initially avoided due to a secondary lactase deficiency; they may be reintroduced in the diet after a few months. A multivitamin is also important, in addition to correction of any severe vitamin deficiencies that may be present. Patients with hyposplenism should receive antibiotic prophylaxis for invasive procedures and should consider receiving the pneumococcal vaccine.

VII.   References

1. Farrell R, Kelly C. Current concepts: celiac sprue. *N Engl J Med* 2002;346:180–188.
2. Valletta E, Mastella G. Incidence of celiac disease in a cystic fibrosis population. *Acta Paediatr Scand* 1989;78:784–785.
3. Fasano A, Catassi C. Current approaches to diagnosis and treatment of celiac disease: an evolving spectrum. *Gastroenterology* 2001;120:636–651.
4. Troncone R, Greco L, Auricchio S. Gluten-sensitive enteropathy. *Pediatr Clin North Am* 1996;43:355–373.
5. Taminiau J. Celiac disease. *Curr Opin Pediatr* 1996;8:483–486.

Case 17-6: 2-Year-Old Boy

I. History of Presenting Illness

A 2 year-old boy was well until 5 months before admission, when he developed intermittent watery diarrhea. He had had more than 3, and sometimes up to 10, large watery stools per day. As an outpatient, he was seen and examined; a stool culture was negative, as were tests for *C. difficile* and ova and parasites. Other blood tests obtained at that time were also normal, according to his mother. Since then, he had been seen once in an emergency department, where he was treated for an intestinal parasite without any improvement in his symptoms. He had been otherwise well-appearing during these last 5 months until the day before presentation to the hospital, when he had significantly decreased oral intake and decreased activity and was acting cranky. On the day of admission to the hospital, he had three episodes of nonbloody, nonbilious emesis. He had also developed a tactile temperature and was refusing to walk. He had not had any rash or weight loss, according to his mother. She was unsure about his urine output.

II. Past Medical History

He was a former premature infant who was born at 33 weeks gestation and did not require endotracheal intubation. He had had a patent ductus arteriosus ligation, hernia repair and a vocal cord cyst removal. He was hospitalized 6 months before admission for pneumonia and had recurrent otitis media six times. His only medication was a multivitamin. His family history was significant only for diabetes and asthma.

III. Physical Examination

T, 38.5°C; RR, 24/min; HR, 117 bpm; BP, 108/54 mm Hg

Weight, 25th percentile

His examination revealed an ill-appearing but responsive toddler. His head and neck examinations were significant only for tacky mucous membranes. His cardiac and respiratory examinations were normal. His abdomen was soft and nontender, without any organomegaly. His rectal examination was normal, and the stool was heme negative. His extremity examination was unremarkable and his neurologic examination was nonfocal, but he continued to refuse to walk.

IV. Diagnostic Studies

A complete blood count revealed 9,600 WBCs/mm^3, with 66% segmented neutrophils, 24% lymphocytes, 9% monocytes, and 1% eosinophils. The hemoglobin was 15.1 g/dL, and the platelet count was 291,000 cells/mm^3. Serum electrolytes were significant for potassium, 2.1 mmol/L; bicarbonate, 11 mmol/L; and alkaline phosphatase, 214 U/L. Cerebrospinal fluid analysis revealed no WBCs and 4 red blood cells/mm^3; protein and glucose were normal. His urinalysis was significant for moderate blood, with 5 to 10 red blood cells and 0 to 2 white blood cells per high-power field.

V. Course of Illness

The patient took nothing by mouth while in the hospital but continued to make more than 2 L/day of diarrhea for the next 3 days. Despite fluid repletion, his serum bicarbonate never rose above 18 mmol/L. Repeat stool cultures for bacteria and viruses, stool examination for ova and parasites, and assays for *C. difficile* toxins A and B were all negative. An abdominal radiograph (Fig. 17-5) and computed tomogram (Fig. 17-6) directed further testing.

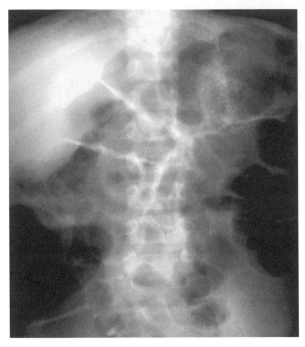

FIG. 17-5. Abdominal radiograph (case 17-6).

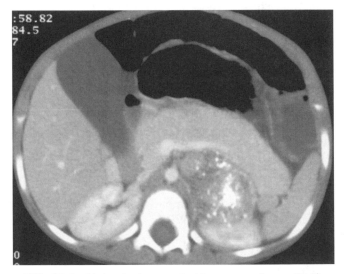

FIG. 17-6. Abdominal computed tomogram (case 17-6).

DISCUSSION: CASE 17-6

I. Differential Diagnosis

The chronic nature of his diarrhea for the last 5 months made acute infectious diarrhea, from either bacterial or viral causes, highly unlikely. Lactase or other disaccharidase deficiency secondary to an episode of infectious gastroenteritis was possible, but other entities must also be considered. Infectious enteritis caused by unusual organisms (e.g., *C. difficile*) and ova and parasites must be considered, although there was no history of antibiotic use, bloody diarrhea, foreign travel, or use of untreated water sources. He was too ill-appearing to consider toddler's diarrhea as a cause. Other entities that cause chronic diarrhea, such as inflammatory bowel disease or celiac disease, were possible considerations, but there was a key finding during the patient's hospital stay that quickly directed the investigation down another path. While in the hospital, the patient took nothing by mouth but continued to produce profuse voluminous watery diarrhea. This indicated the presence of secretory, rather than osmotic, diarrhea. In this differential diagnosis, the list is rather brief and includes rare congenital and paraneoplastic conditions. Congenital defects in chloride or sodium transport are unlikely to manifest in a 2-year old in this fashion. Infectious causes of secretory diarrhea include small-bowel overgrowth and infection with immuno-adherent *E. coli* stimulating gastrointestinal secretions. Any cause of villous atrophy, whether congenital, autoimmune, or secondary to immune deficiency (e.g., HIV infection, severe combined immunodeficiency) may also result in this presentation. Neuroblastoma and other tumors of neural crest origin, such as ganglioneuroma, may secrete VIP, resulting in secretory diarrhea.

II. Diagnosis

An abdominal radiograph showed calcifications above the left kidney (Fig. 17-5), and subsequent computed tomography revealed a large left adrenal mass (Fig. 17-6). Surgery was performed, and the mass was completely resected. It was identified as a ganglioneuroblastoma on pathology. The VIP level was 195 pg/mL (normal, less than 70 pg/mL). **These findings were consistent with the diagnosis of VIP-secreting ganglioneuroblastoma causing secretory diarrhea.** Immediately after surgery, his diarrhea resolved and a repeat VIP level was normal.

III. Incidence and Epidemiology

Most VIP-secreting tumors in childhood are neurogenic in origin; in contrast, most of those in adults are of pancreatic islet cell origin. Pediatric patients usually present during the first 10 years of life. Most pediatric tumors are adrenal or retroperitoneal in location, and ganglioneuromas or ganglioneuroblastomas are common.

IV. Clinical Presentation

Generally speaking, pediatric patients present, as this child did, with profuse, watery, secretory diarrhea and not with a palpable mass. The biochemical profile is that of hypokalemia and achlorhydria due to the effect of VIP on the gastrointestinal tract to promote secretion of water and electrolytes and inhibit gastric acid secretion. Calcifications may also be noted incidentally on radiographs, prompting further investigation.

V. Diagnostic Approach

Clinical observation. The observation of continued, intractable watery diarrhea while the patient takes nothing by mouth is key to the ultimate diagnosis. Whether this is accomplished by obtaining a very thorough history or by observation while in the hospital, this piece of information is vital to making the ultimate diagnosis.

Radiography. Radiographs may localize calcifications and often provide the first indication of the presence of such a tumor as an incidental finding.

Computed tomography. Computed tomography more accurately delineates the location of the tumor, which is usually retroperitoneal or adrenal. Occasionally, tumors are found along the sympathetic chain in the thoracic region.

Peptide panel. Elevated plasma VIP levels are diagnostic. Other peptides that are tested include gastrin, somatostatin, calcitonin, and serotonin. These peptides are elaborated by tumors not commonly found in the pediatric population (gastrinoma, carcinoid syndrome, medullary thyroid carcinoma, mastocytosis, and villous adenoma of the rectosigmoid colon).

Surgical removal. Complete surgical excision provides a pathologic specimen for further identification and characterization of the tumor and is also therapeutic, especially with regard to the secretory diarrhea.

VI.   Treatment

Complete surgical excision is necessary and sufficient to cure the secretory diarrhea. Somatostatin analogues have been shown to decrease diarrhea due to their inhibitory effect on gastrointestinal secretions, but surgery remains the definitive treatment. Subsequent chemotherapy is then determined based on the type of tumor, tissue pathology findings, and other information, such as the presence of molecular amplification of oncogenes.

VII.   References

1. Rodriguez M, Regalado J, Zaleski C, et al. Chronic watery diarrhea in a 22-month-old girl. *J Pediatr* 2000:136:262–265.
2. Murphy M, Sibal A, Mann JR. Persistent diarrhoea and occult vipomas in children. *BMJ* 2000;320:1524–1526.

18

Syncope

Phillip Spandorfer

APPROACH TO THE PATIENT WITH SYNCOPE

I. Definition of the Complaint

Syncope is generally thought of as a temporary, but sudden, loss of consciousness and postural tone. It is caused by a reversible interruption of cerebral function, typically due to a deficit of cerebral oxygen or glucose delivery. The deficit in oxygen delivery may be caused by decreased cardiac output, peripheral vasodilatation, or obstruction of cerebral blood flow. It is important to differentiate the episode of syncope from other etiologies that appear like syncope, such as seizure and near-syncopal episodes. Painful events, episodes of micturition or defecation, and stress frequently precede syncope. Sweating and nausea before the episode are common as well. Seizures frequently have no prodromal period, but they may be associated with an aura before the event. Seizures are frequently associated with tonic-clonic movements during the event; however, syncopal events that last 20 seconds or longer can also be associated with very brief tonic-clonic movements. Confusion after the event, prolonged return to normal state of consciousness, and unconsciousness lasting longer than 5 minutes suggest seizure activity. During near-syncopal episodes, patients feel as if they are about to lose consciousness but do not actually become unconscious.

Syncope is a common complaint in pediatrics. Approximately 15% of children have a syncopal episode by the time they reach adulthood.

II. Complaint by Cause and Frequency

Pediatric causes of syncope are generally benign, but syncope may signal serious, life-threatening causes, particularly if it is recurrent or there is a family history of sudden cardiac arrest. In children, common causes of syncope include vasovagal episodes, orthostatic hypotension, and breath-holding spells (Table 18-1). In contrast, most adult syncope has a cardiac origin. The goal in evaluating syncope is to differentiate benign causes from more worrisome etiologies (Table 18-2).

TABLE 18-1. *Differential Diagnosis of Syncope by Age*

Disease prevalence	Neonate/infant	School age child	Adolescent
Common	Breath-holding spell Arrhythmia Mimickers of syncope	Vasovagal Breath-holding spell Anemia Arrhythmia Mimickers of syncope	Vasovagal Mimickers of syncope Anemia Arrhythmia Pregnancy
Uncommon	Structural heart disease Hypoglycemia Hypoxemia	Structural heart disease Hypoglycemia Hypoxemia	Structural heart disease Hypoglycemia Hypoxemia

TABLE 18-2. *Differential Diagnosis of Syncope by Etiology*

Autonomic	Vasovagal syncope
	Increased vagal tone
	Orthostatic hypotension (volume depletion)
	Breath-holding spell
	Situational syncope (cough, micturition, defecation)
	Pregnancy
Structural heart disease	Outflow obstruction (idiopathic hypertrophic subaortic stenosis, valvular aortic stenosis, primary pulmonary hypertension, Eissenminger syndrome, atrial myxoma)
	Dilated cardiomyopathy
	Pericarditis with tamponade
Arrhythmias	Long QTc syndrome (congenital or acquired)
	Supraventricular tachycardia
	Ventricular tachycardia
	Atrioventricular block
	Sinus node disease
Vascular	Vertebrobasilar insufficiency
Metabolic	Hypoglycemia
	Hypoxia
	Hyperammonemia
	Carbon monoxide poisoning
Mimickers of syncope	Seizures
	Migraines
	Hysteric faints
	Malingering
	Hyperventilation
	Panic disorder
	Depression

III. Clarifying Questions

• Were there any palpitations or unusual heartbeats?

— If the child reports palpitations, then a cardiac dysrhythmia should be considered.

• Did the syncope occur with activity?

— Syncope that occurs with activity is particularly concerning for idiopathic hypertrophic cardiomyopathy (HCM).

• Was there a prodrome?

— Migraines and some seizure types may cause symptoms before the actual episode.

• Did the syncope happen on standing?

— Orthostatic hypotension is associated with syncope on standing.

• Was there pain, fear, or some disturbing visual sight before the syncope?

— Strong emotional impulses may stimulate a vasovagal response and ultimately syncope.

• Was there any seizure-like activity?

— Brief seizure-like motor activity can occur with vasovagal syncope. Prolonged seizure activity should prompt a more thorough seizure workup. There is no significant postictal period with the seizure-like activity associated with syncope.

- How long did it take to return to baseline?

  — Vasovagal syncope is associated with a relatively quick (minutes) return to baseline mental status as soon as cerebral blood flow is restored. If there is a delay in assuming a recumbent position, there may be a longer delay in return to baseline mental status.

- Is there a history of trauma?

  — A recent history of head trauma raises concern for intracranial hemorrhage.

- Is there a history of anemia?

  — Anemic patients may be more likely to have a syncopal episode because of decreased cerebral oxygen delivery.

Case 18-1: 17-Year-Old Girl

I. History of Present Illness

A 17-year-old girl presented to the emergency department after her second episode of passing out in a week. The first episode happened 7 days earlier, while she was walking home from school. She experienced a prodromal period in which everything around her became black and then awoke on the sidewalk with her friends around her. Her friends took her home that day. The next episode occurred shortly before presentation. She had just finished dinner and was walking into another room when a similar episode of darkening occurred and then she awoke on the floor. On review of systems, she was found to have had occasional episodes of shaking chills, tactile temperatures, and a 5-pound weight loss over a 2-week period. She was a senior in high school and planned on going to college. She was sexually active but had used protection every time. Her last menstrual period was 1 week before presentation and was normal.

II. Past Medical History

She was a healthy child and had never been hospitalized. She had three brothers who were also healthy. Her immunizations were up to date.

III. Physical Examination

T, 38.2°C; RR, 20/min; HR, 90 bpm; BP, 95/58 mm Hg

Weight, 75th percentile; height, 20th percentile

On examination she was alert and cooperative in no distress. She did not appear pale. Her head and neck examination was normal. Her lungs were clear to auscultation. Her cardiac examination was normal. Her abdomen was soft, with no organomegaly or masses detected. Her neurological examination was normal. Her skin examination revealed a rash all over her body (Fig. 18-1).

IV. Diagnostic Studies

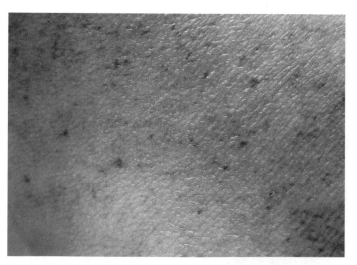

FIG. 18-1. Photograph of patient's rash (case 18-1).

A complete blood count revealed the following: 12,000 white blood cells (WBCs)/mm³ (6% bands, 30% segmented neutrophils, 42% lymphocytes, 19% atypical lymphocytes, and 3% monocytes); hemoglobin, 12.2 g/dL; and platelets 14,000/mm³.

V. Course of Illness

She was admitted to the hospital for further evaluation. Due to the thrombocytopenia, fever, and weight loss, the hematology/oncology service was consulted. A bone marrow aspiration was performed.

DISCUSSION: CASE 18-1

I. Differential Diagnosis

The low platelet count and diffuse petechial rash associated with intermittent fevers and a 5-pound weight loss over the past 2 weeks were concerning for a neoplastic disorder such as leukemia or lymphoma. Frequently, the atypical lymphocytes reported in the peripheral smear are actually blasts that are mistaken for atypical lymphocytes. However, they are also a marker for a potential Epstein-Barr virus (EBV) infection. The other causes of thrombocytopenia are numerous and include infections such as cytomegalovirus (CMV), human immunodeficiency virus (HIV), hepatitis B or C, toxoplasmosis, leptospirosis, syphilis, Rocky Mountain spotted fever, and ehrlichiosis. Idiopathic thrombocytopenic purpura is a frequent cause of thrombocytopenia in children that can have either an acute or a chronic course. Autoimmune disorders such as systemic lupus erythematosus, acquired hemolytic anemia, and hyperthyroidism all are associated with thrombocytopenia. Drug-induced thrombocytopenia should be considered if the patient is taking any medications, particularly sulfonamides, digoxin, quinine, quinidine, or chemotherapeutic agents. Important, but less common, causes to remember include any cause of disseminated intravascular coagulation, hemolytic-uremic syndrome, aplastic anemia, and hypersplenism syndromes. Thrombocytopenia can occur after vaccination with measles-mumps-rubella vaccine. Rare genetic disorders such as Fanconi anemia, Hermansky-Pudlak syndrome, thrombocytopenia with absent radii syndrome (TAR), Wiskott-Aldrich syndrome, May-Hegglin anomaly, and Bernard-Soulier disease are possibilities as well.

II. Diagnosis

The petechial rash was consistent with her thrombocytopenia (Fig. 18-1). The bone marrow aspirate revealed a normal marrow with increased megakaryocytes. The interpretation was that this was a clinical picture consistent with viral consumption of platelets. The EBV titers were positive for immunoglobulin M (IgM) and IgG antibody to viral capsid antigen (VCA). No Epstein-Barr nuclear antigen (EBNA) was detected. **The diagnosis is EBV infection.**

III. Incidence and Epidemiology

EBV is close to ubiquitous. It infects more than 90% of the population and persists for the lifetime of the host. Infection occurs at a later age in developed countries than in developing countries, possibly because of improved sanitary conditions. The incidence of EBV infection is 50 per 100,000 individuals overall; however, among those age 15 to 25 years, it is 1 per 1,000 individuals. The incubation period may last up to 30 days.

EBV is linked to infectious mononucleosis, Burkitt's lymphoma, nasopharyngeal carcinoma, and other cancers. The virus is a member of the herpesvirus family. EBV binds to the CD21 molecule on the B cell and gains entry into the cell. After infection of an epithelial cell in the oropharynx, the virus replicates and the cell ultimately dies. When EBV infects the B cell, the virus becomes latent. However, unlike other herpesvirus infections, EBV does not recur. Infection is spread from person to person through contact with oral secretions.

IV.   Clinical Presentation

The majority of EBV infections are asymptomatic or produce relatively nonspecific symptoms (e.g., coryza, fever). Acute EBV infection is not synonymous with infectious mononucleosis ("mono"), but infectious mononucleosis is the most commonly recognized clinical manifestation of EBV infection. Infectious mononucleosis typically manifests with fever, tonsillopharyngitis, lymphadenopathy, increased atypical lymphocytes in the peripheral blood smear, and positive heterophile antibodies or EBV titers. The pharyngitis is typically exudative. The lymphadenitis symmetrically involves the posterior cervical chains. Nausea, vomiting, and anorexia occur frequently, which is probably a reflection of the fact that 90% of patients have a mild hepatitis. About half of patients with EBV infection have splenomegaly; hepatomegaly is much less frequent. Typically, the acute symptoms resolve within 2 weeks, yet the fatigue may persist longer.

Other, less common systemic presentations of EBV infection include the possibility of hematologic changes or neurologic changes. Patients can develop hemolytic anemia, thrombocytopenia, aplastic anemia, or a disseminated intravascular coagulopathy. Neurologically, patients may develop Guillain-Barré syndrome, facial nerve palsy, aseptic meningitis, transverse myelitis, peripheral neuropathy, optic neuritis, or meningoencephalitis.

Complications from EBV infection include the possibility of a diffuse morbilliform rash if the patient is administered a penicillin drug, splenic rupture, upper airway obstruction, or lymphoproliferative disorders. Splenic rupture, which is more common in male patients, has been reported to occur in 1 of every 1,000 cases, typically on day 4 to 21 after the onset of symptoms. It often occurs spontaneously, and the patient presents with left upper abdominal pain that radiates to the left shoulder. Airway obstruction is very rare but carries significant morbidity and mortality. The airway compromise can be treated with steroids if necessary. Lymphoproliferative disorders can occur if there is decreased cellular immunity. It is the T cells and natural killer cells that keep the latent EBV infection in check.

V.   Diagnostic Approach

The diagnosis of an EBV infection is based on the correct clinical picture with supporting laboratory evidence.

Complete blood count. The complete blood count typically reveals a leukocytosis with 50% lymphocytes and greater than 10% atypical lymphocytes. Other viruses that cause atypical lymphocytes include CMV, HIV, hepatitis, and measles; however, only EBV and CMV result in greater than 10% atypical lymphocytes. About 50% of patients with EBV have thrombocytopenia, less than 150,000 platelets/mm^3. Anemia is not typically associated with EBV, but if it is present, autoimmune hemolysis (which occurs in fewer than 1% of patients) or splenic rupture should be considered.

Heterophile antibodies. Heterophile antibodies (e.g., Monospot), which agglutinate sheep or horse red blood cells, may be positive in the older patient.

EBV-specific antibodies. EBV antibody titers may be sent for confirmation of disease. The three antigens that are tested for are VCA, early antigen (EA), and EBNA. The antibodies to VCA are the first to appear; the IgM is transient, and the IgG antibodies persist. The antibodies to EA appear next, and both IgM and IgG are transient. The antibodies to EBNA appear 1 to 2 months after the onset of symptoms but persist for the lifetime of the host.

EBV polymerase chain reaction. EBV polymerase chain reaction (PCR) is a diagnostic test that is available but has limited utility in the acute infectious stage. It may or may not be positive in acute infections, but it is usually positive in those who have had a past EBV infection in whom the current symptoms may be unrelated to EBV. It is most useful in immune-compromised hosts at risk for lymphoproliferative disorders.

VI. Treatment

The mainstay of treatment is supportive care, including adequate rest, fluids, and antipyretics. Antivirals have not been shown to be of long-term benefit. The use of steroids is not routinely recommended but can be considered if there are complications such as airway obstruction, neurologic complications, myocarditis, pericarditis, hemolytic anemia, or thrombotic thrombocytopenic purpura. Because of the possibility of splenic rupture, patients should avoid contact sports for at least 1 month or until resolution of the splenomegaly.

VII. References

1. American Academy of Pediatrics. Epstein-Barr virus infections. In: Pickering LK, ed. *2000 Red Book: Report of the Committee on Infectious Diseases,* 25th ed. Elk Grove Village, IL: American Academy of Pediatrics; 2000:238–240.
2. Cohen JI. Epstein-Barr virus infection. *N Engl J Med* 2000;343:481–492.
3. Durbin WA, Sullivan JL. Epstein-Barr virus infection. *Pediatr Rev* 1994;15:63–68.
4. Straus SE, Cohen JI, Tosato G, et al. Epstein-Barr virus infections: biology, pathogenesis, and management. *Ann Intern Med* 1993;118:45–58.
5. Sumaya CV. Epstein-Barr virus. In: Feigin RD, Cherry JD, eds. *Textbook of pediatric infectious diseases,* 4th ed. Philadelphia: WB Saunders, 1998:1751–1764.

Case 18-2: 15-Year-Old Boy

I. History of Present Illness

A 15-year-old boy felt the acute onset of his heart beating fast while he was on the phone with a friend. He became dizzy and lightheaded and fell backward onto his bed. He was not sure whether he had lost consciousness but remembered calling for his mother to help him. On arrival at the community emergency department, he had some mild midsternal chest pain. He denied fever, nausea, vomiting, diarrhea, and cough. The remainder of his review of systems was negative.

II. Past Medical History

He had been a healthy child with no significant illnesses. He was a good student at school and was active in sports. His family history did not reveal any episodes of sudden unexplained death. Of note, his sister had coarctation of the aorta that required repair in infancy. He did not take any medications. He had completed his childhood immunizations.

III. Physical Examination

T, 37.2°C; RR, 20/min; HR, 230 bpm; BP, 105/68 mm Hg

Weight, 50th percentile; height, 90th percentile

On examination he was awake but anxious-appearing. His head and neck examination was normal. His lungs were clear to auscultation. His cardiac examination was significant for profound tachycardia with a rate that could not be counted manually. There was no jugular venous distention. His perfusion was adequate, with a capillary refill of 1 second at the fingertip. His pulses were palpable throughout. His abdomen was soft without any enlargement of spleen or liver. His extremities were well perfused. His neurologic examination was normal.

IV. Diagnostic Studies

The WBC count was 12,400 cells/mm^3, 54% segmented neutrophils, 1% bands, and 38% lymphocytes. Hemoglobin was 13.2 g/dL, and the platelet count was 278,000/mm^3. Serum chemistry analysis revealed the following: sodium, 138 mEq/L; potassium, 4.3 mEq/L; chloride, 106 mEq/L; bicarbonate, 22 mEq/L; calcium, 9.2 mg/dL; and magnesium, 2.9 mg/dL.

V. Course of Illness

A chest roentgenogram revealed a normal heart size and no pulmonary edema. The initial (Fig. 18-2A) and subsequent (Fig. 18-2B) electrocardiograms (ECG) revealed the acute and underlying diagnoses.

DISCUSSION: CASE 18-2

I. Differential Diagnosis

This patient presented with a narrow complex tachycardia. The differential diagnosis included supraventricular tachycardia (SVT) and sinus tachycardia. Fever, pain, volume loss, use of sympathomimetics, and dehydration could cause the child to be tachycardic and subsequently to have sinus tachycardia.

II. Diagnosis

The initial ECG (Fig. 18-2A) revealed a narrow complex tachycardia at a rate of almost 300 bpm. At the community emergency department, the patient received two doses of adenosine. When that failed to convert his rhythm, he received a loading dose of digoxin.

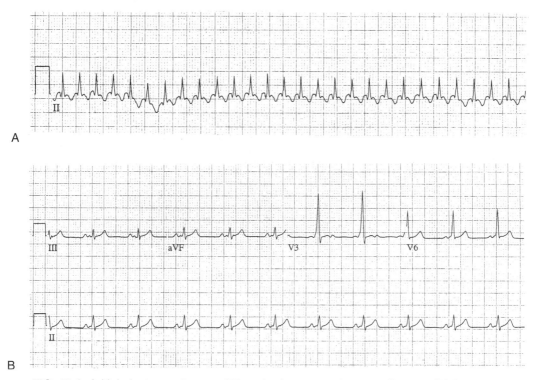

FIG. 18-2. Initial electrocardiogram **(A)** and subsequent electrocardiogram **(B)** for case 18-2.

He was then transferred to the regional children's hospital and admitted to the cardiac intensive care unit. There he was treated with intravenous procainamide, with no response. While he was undergoing induction for cardioversion with propofol, he converted to a sinus rhythm.

This patient presented with SVT. He failed to convert with vagal maneuvers, adenosine, digoxin, and procainamide. On subsequent ECGs, he was found to have a delta wave consistent with Wolff-Parkinson-White syndrome (WPW) (Fig. 18-2B). **The diagnosis is SVT due to WPW syndrome.**

III. Incidence and Epidemiology

SVT encompasses three diagnostic etiologies: atrial tachycardia, nodal tachycardia, and atrioventricular (AV) reentrant tachycardia. The majority of SVTs are caused by AV reentrant tachycardias. Ectopic tachycardias are rare in pediatrics. Nodal tachycardias originate from the AV node and tend to have slower rates (150 to 200 bpm) than do tachycardias that arise from above the node.

WPW syndrome is a form of preexcitation disorder that results from an anomalous conduction pathway between the atrium and the ventricle and can result in a reentrant tachycardia. There is conduction down the accessory pathway that bypasses the normal conduction delay at the AV node. The premature depolarization of a ventricle produces a delta wave (i.e., an initial slurring of the QRS complex) and QRS prolongation. The diagnostic criteria for WPW syndrome include a short PR interval, a delta wave, and a wide QRS. Patients with WPW syndrome are prone to SVT. About 20% of cases of SVT are caused by WPW syndrome, about 20% are due to congenital heart defects such as

Ebstein's anomaly or corrected transposition of the great arteries, 20% are related to medication, and about 50% are considered idiopathic.

IV. Clinical Presentation

WPW syndrome manifests with frequent episodes of SVT. It can be diagnosed by detection of a delta wave in asymptomatic patients on an ECG obtained for another purpose. SVT is the most common arrhythmia in childhood, with 40% of patients presenting in the first 6 months of life and 30% presenting in the school age years. An infant who presents with SVT is typically more fussy than usual, may have difficulty feeding, and may have episodes of grunting. Frequently the infant is in SVT for a longer period, until there are behavioral changes that alert the caretaker that something is wrong with the infant. As the time spent in SVT continues, there is an increased chance that the child will begin to show symptoms of heart failure. When the heart rate is actually measured, it will be in the range of 220 to 320 bpm. An older child who is verbal will be able to report the acute onset of a rapid heartbeat. Many children describe the feeling as having butterflies in their chest.

V. Diagnostic Approach

Electrocardiogram. An ECG obtained during the episode of tachycardia reveals a tachycardia, a narrow QRS complex, and P waves that are either partially obscured by the ST segment or not visible at all. In infants, the typical rates are 220 to 320 bpm. In older children and adolescents, the rates are in the 150 to 250 bpm range. If the SVT is aberrantly conducted, the QRS complex will be wide, resembling ventricular tachycardia. If a wide complex tachycardia is detected, the patient should be treated as if in ventricular tachycardia until proved otherwise.

VI. Treatment

Treatment depends on the hemodynamic stability of the child. If the child has hypotension, decreased mentation, or decreased end-organ perfusion, then the child is considered unstable and synchronized cardioversion is indicated. The energy used is 0.5 to 2 joules/kg. Procedural sedation should be provided as long as doing so does not delay the procedure significantly. If the patient is normotensive and there is no concern about shock, then administration of adenosine is the appropriate next step. Adenosine blocks conduction through the AV node and hence provides pharmacologic cardioversion. Because the half-life of the drug is short, less than 1 minute, it must be administered as a rapid push. Verapamil is used frequently in the adult population for SVT, but it is associated with profound vasodilatation and cardiovascular collapse in pediatric patients and should be avoided. If the patient has recalcitrant SVT or pharmacologic treatment is indicated for chronic SVT, digoxin can be administered. Digoxin slows conduction through the AV node. If the patient is in SVT secondary to WPW syndrome, avoidance of digoxin is important, because it may potentiate conduction down the faster accessory pathway and result in ventricular fibrillation. β-Blockers, such as nadolol and propranolol, are safe to give to patients with SVT due to WPW syndrome. Other alternatives include procainamide and amiodarone. Radiofrequency catheter ablation is a surgical procedure that is available for long-term treatment of WPW syndrome.

VII. References

1. Ganz LI, Friedman PL. Supraventricular tachycardia. *N Engl J Med* 1995;332: 162–173.
2. Kirk CR, Gibbs JL, Thomas R, et al. Cardiovascular collapse after verapamil in supraventricular tachycardia. *Arch Dis Child* 1987;62:1265–1282.
3. Trohman RG. Supraventricular tachycardia: implications for the intensivist. *Crit Care Med* 2000;28:N129–N135.

Case 18-3: 14-Year-Old Boy

I. History of Present Illness

A 14 year-old boy was brought to the emergency department after collapsing at school. He was at basketball practice when he was seen to collapse on the ground. The paramedics were called and brought him to the emergency department. He awoke within a few minutes after the fall. There was no seizure activity reported. He did not complain of shortness of breath, palpitations, or chest pain. He denied fever, cough, and rhinorrhea. He had no complaints at present. He denied having taken any illicit drugs

II. Past Medical History

He had been healthy with no significant past medical history. There was no family history of early cardiac death in children or young adults. He was taking no medications, and all his immunizations were up to date.

III. Physical Examination

T, 37.0°C; RR, 20/min; HR, 112 bpm; BP, 124/78 mm Hg

Weight, 90th percentile; height, 75th percentile

On examination, he was awake and in no acute distress. His mucous membranes were moist. His lungs were clear to auscultation. His cardiac examination revealed a regular rate and rhythm with normal first and second heart sounds (S1 and S2, respectively) and an S3 gallop rhythm. No murmur could be detected. His abdomen was soft without any hepatosplenomegaly. His extremities were warm and well perfused, with strong peripheral pulses. His neurologic examination was normal.

IV. Diagnostic Studies

Because of the syncopal episode, his glucose level was checked at bedside and measured 108 mg/dL. Electrolyte measurements and a complete blood count were normal. Because of the gallop rhythm, an ECG (Fig. 18-3) and chest radiograph were obtained. The chest radiograph revealed a top-normal sized cardiothymic silhouette.

V. Course of Illness

After the studies were performed in the emergency department, the patient was admitted to the cardiology service to further determine the etiology of the syncope. He underwent echocardiography and exercise stress testing.

DISCUSSION: CASE 18-3

I. Differential Diagnosis

This case of syncope probably had a cardiac cause, because of the abnormal physical examination findings and the ECG and chest radiography abnormalities. Of all the abnormalities present, the left ventricular hypertrophy seen on the ECG is the most concerning (Fig. 18-3). Causes to consider include systemic hypertension, aortic valvular stenosis, and HCM. Metabolic disorders such as glycogen storage disease, type II may also cause left ventricular hypertrophy.

II. Diagnosis

Echocardiography revealed a large intraventricular septum and a top-normal sized left ventricular end-diastolic dimension. No left ventricular outflow obstruction was detected. Exercise stress testing did not reveal any arrhythmias, but there was a 3-mm ST-segment depression during maximal exercise. **The diagnosis is hypertrophic cardiomyopathy (HCM).** Treatment with nadolol was started, and discussion with

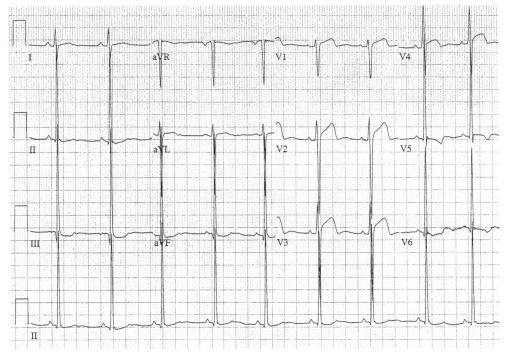

FIG. 18-3. Electrocardiogram (case 18-3).

the family about the possible insertion of an implantable cardiodefibrillator was begun.

III. Incidence and Epidemiology

HCM is a relatively common genetic disease. Ten genes have been identified that code for proteins in the cardiac sarcomere. Any one of these genes may have a mutation that results in HCM. It is considered to be autosomal dominant with variable penetrance. HCM is an important cause of disability and death in patients of all ages; however, the sudden unexpected death of a young patient is one of the more distressing aspects of the disease. There is a large heterogeneity of clinical expression, natural history, and prognosis in patients with HCM. The prevalence of HCM is not well defined in children, but in the adult population several studies have reported an estimate of 1 in 500, or 0.2% of the general adult population. Furthermore, a substantial proportion of patients in the general population probably have a mutant gene for HCM yet are undetected due to lack of clinical symptomatology.

IV. Clinical Presentation

HCM is frequently suspected because of a heart murmur, positive family history, new clinical symptoms (syncope), or an abnormal ECG. The physical examination of patients with HCM is normal for the most part, because more than 75% of the patients with HCM do not have outflow tract obstruction and most of the physical findings are related to outflow obstruction. If an outflow tract obstruction is present, a murmur can be heard. The murmur is louder with increasing outflow obstruction (e.g., Valsalva maneuvers) and softer with relief of the obstruction (e.g., with squatting). There is misleading information about the prognosis of patients with HCM. Older literature reported mortality rates of 3% to 6% annually for the general population and 6% in children. However, these data were biased toward tertiary care centers representing patients with more extreme expressions of the disease. More recent and less biased data indicate annual mortality rates of about 1% in the general population and 2% in children.

V. Diagnostic Approach

Echocardiogram. The diagnosis of HCM is most reliably made with echocardiography that reveals a hypertrophied but not dilated left ventricle. There should be a lack of other clinical diseases that could produce a dilated ventricle, such as hypertension or aortic stenosis.

Electrocardiogram. An ECG can be of benefit in the diagnosis of HCM. It is abnormal in at least 75% of patients and has a wide range of patterns.

Genetic screening. It is not uncommon for children younger than 13 years of age to carry a mutant HCM gene and yet not have a hypertrophied left ventricle. Therefore, negative echocardiography in children younger than 13 years does not exclude the possibility of HCM.

Myocardial biopsy. Biopsy specimens of HCM hearts reveal cellular disarray patterns in sections of the heart that are affected by the disease.

VI. Treatment

The treatment for patients with HCM is as variable as their presentations. It is prudent to consider treatment options based on the patient's subgroup rather than considering the overall disease. If the patient has a positive genotype and a negative phenotype, then follow-up alone is the most prudent course of action. If there are mild or no symptoms with a positive phenotype, then no treatment or drug therapy may be the best option. Drug therapy consists of β-blockers, verapamil, and antiarrhythmic agents. If there is a high risk of sudden death, then implantable cardiodefibrillators are placed in the patient. Patients at high risk for sudden death include those patients with a prior cardiac arrest, sustained ventricular tachycardia, syncope or near-syncope, or a family history of HCM-related death (particularly if sudden or in a young patient); those patients in whom Holter monitoring reveals nonsustained ventricular tachycardia; those who have hypotension with exercise; and those with extreme left ventricular wall thickness (particularly in adolescents and young adults). Patients with severe HCM should be restricted from competitive sports and strenuous activities.

VII. References

1. Arnold R, Kitchiner D. Left ventricular outflow obstruction. *Arch Dis Child* 1995;72: 180–183.
2. Berger S, Dhala A, Friedberg DZ. Sudden cardiac death in infants, children, and adolescents. *Pediatr Clin North Am* 1999;46:221–234.
3. Maron BJ. Hypertrophic cardiomyopathy: a systematic review. *JAMA* 2002;287: 1308–1320.
4. McKenna WJ, Behr ER. Hypertrophic cardiomyopathy: management, risk stratification, and prevention of sudden death. *Heart* 2002;87:169–176.
5. Spirito P, Seidman CE, McKenna WJ, et al. The management of hypertrophic cardiomyopathy. *N Engl J Med* 1997;336:775–785.

Case 18-4: 14-Year-Old Boy

I. History of Present Illness

A 14 year-old boy was taken to the emergency department by paramedics after passing out at school. The history provided by the paramedics was that he had a nosebleed and stood up. Shortly after standing, he became lightheaded and passed out, falling to the ground. The paramedics found him to be unresponsive. They placed him in a cervical collar, inserted an intravenous line, and administered naloxone and dextrose while *en route* to the emergency department. There was no response to either of the medications.

II. Past Medical History

He had been a healthy teenager who suffered only from seasonal allergies. One year before this presentation, he had testicular torsion and underwent an orchioplexy. He was not taking any medications currently and was not allergic to any medications. His immunization status was current. He lived at home with his parents and sister. He was in the eighth grade and was a B/C student. He denied the use of any illicit drugs.

III. Physical Examination

T, 37.9°C; RR, 16/min; HR, 110 bpm; BP, 129/72 mm Hg

Weight, greater than 95th percentile; height, 50th percentile

On examination he was somnolent but arousable to verbal stimuli. Shortly after stimulation, he fell asleep. His head and neck examination revealed 5-mm pupils that were briskly reactive to 2 mm bilaterally. His extraocular muscles were intact. He had dried blood in his right nares and an eschar on the anterior nasal septum. The cervical collar was in place, and no spinal tenderness was elicited. His lungs were clear to auscultation. His cardiac examination revealed no murmurs or abnormal heart sounds. His pulse was regular and strong. His abdominal, rectal, extremity, and skin examinations were entirely normal. On neurologic examination, he was found to be arousable to verbal stimuli. He was oriented to person, time, place, and situation. He followed simple commands and was able to count backward from 100 by sevens. His deep tendon reflexes were 2+ and symmetric. His sensation was intact. However, his motor strength was rated 2/5 in both arms and legs. He was able to move his extremities in the plane of the bed but could not lift them against gravity.

IV. Diagnostic Studies

A complete blood count and basic metabolic panel returned with normal values. His urine and serum drug screens were negative. A head computed tomogram was obtained and revealed no intracranial pathology. A chest radiograph was normal. An ECG revealed a normal sinus rhythm with normal intervals. A lumbar puncture was performed with an opening pressure of 17 cm H_2O; the results showed 1 WBC/mm^3, no red blood cells, normal protein and glucose, and a Gram stain with no bacteria and no WBCs present.

V. Course of Illness

The patient underwent the diagnostic studies described while in the emergency department. He did not regain his strength or return to baseline mental status after several hours and was admitted to the inpatient service.

DISCUSSION: CASE 18-4

I. Differential Diagnosis

This patient presented with a change in mental status and a history of syncope. The differential diagnosis for the change in mental status can be discussed using the mnemonic

VITAMINS. The clinician should consider *vascular events* such as cerebral thromboembolism or intracranial bleeding. *Intussusception* is a frequent cause of depressed mental status in children from about 6 months to 2 years of age. *Trauma* should always be considered a possibility, with resultant cerebral contusion and concussions. *A lot of toxins* can result in depressed mental status. *Metabolic disorders* such as hypoglycemia and other electrolyte abnormalities can manifest with decreased mental status. *Infectious etiologies* such as meningitis and encephalitis should always be considered. *Neoplasms* in the brain can produce depressed mental status as well as a cancer that produces profound anemia. And finally, *seizures* are a frequent cause of depressed mental status whether the patient is postictal or in subclinical status epilepticus.

II. Diagnosis

This patient was admitted to the inpatient service. The sudden and prolonged weakness that began after a syncopal episode was difficult to explain. The neurologists were consulted, and after a thorough evaluation determined that functional signs were present during his examination. On further questioning, it became clear that he was under a significant amount of stress at school. His grades were poor, he had been in several fights recently, and he believed that a group of kids at school were out to get him. The psychiatrists were consulted. **The diagnosis is malingering.**

III. Incidence and Epidemiology

Malingering is described as the intentional production of, or gross exaggeration of, physical or psychological symptoms. It is frequently motivated by external incentives such as avoidance of school, work, or military obligations. Malingering differs from factitious disorder in that there is no external incentive in factitious disorders, where as there is a clearly definable goal for the malingering patient. The actual incidence of malingering is unknown, but it is a rare phenomenon in children. It is more common among patients who are in a restrictive environment such as a prison facility or the armed forces. Malingering represents a conscious attempt to avoid an unpleasant situation. Somatoform disorders, such as conversion disorders, are much more common in children and represent an unconscious attempt to handle unpleasant emotions without an obvious external incentive. Malingering is not considered a mental disorder.

IV. Clinical Presentation

Many malingering patients appear aloof and hostile toward the physician in an attempt to delay the discovery of their deception. They readily submit to painful diagnostic procedures. By contrast, patients who have conversion disorders tend to be very friendly and appropriately concerned about diagnostic procedures.

V. Diagnostic Approach

Psychological evaluation. According to the *Diagnostic and Statistical Manual of Mental Disorders,* 4th edition (DSM-IV), malingering should be suspected if any of the following are noted, particularly in combination: (a) medicolegal context (i.e., the patient was referred to the physician by an attorney); (b) an obvious discrepancy between the patient's claimed stress and disability and the objective findings; (c) lack of cooperation during the examination and with the recommended treatment; and (d) presence of an antisocial personality disorder.

Other studies. Most patients who present with malingering have vague and subjective complaints such as headache, pain in a body part, dizziness, amnesia, anxiety, or depression. These symptoms are difficult to disprove. Objective tests such as audiometry, electromyography, nerve conduction studies, or evoked potential studies may be of benefit for particular symptoms.

VI. Treatment

The patient with suspected malingering should be thoroughly evaluated in an objective manner. Merely linking the symptoms to psychosocial stressors may be therapeutic.

Unfortunately, in the adult patients, confrontation frequently occurs and results in the end of the doctor-patient relationship, or else the patient becomes more on guard, and proof of the deception becomes impossible. Careful evaluation of the patient and environment often reveals the cause of the symptoms without the need for a confrontation. Preservation of the doctor-patient relationship is important to arrive at the correct diagnosis and long-term care of the patient. Of note, in malingering, symptom relief is not obtained by suggestion or hypnosis, as it is in the somatoform disorders. Psychiatric referral may be needed in some cases.

VII. References

1. American Psychiatric Association. *Diagnostic and statistical manual of mental disorders,* 4th ed. Washington, DC: American Psychiatric Association, 1994:683.
2. Prazar G. Conversion reactions in adolescents. *Pediatr Rev* 1987;8:279–286.
3. DeMaso DR, Beasley PJ. The somatoform disorders. In: Klykylo WM, Kay J, Rube D, eds. *Clinical child psychiatry.* Philadelphia: WB Saunders, 1998;429–437.
4. Nemzer ED. Somatoform disorders. In: Lewis M, ed. *Child and adolescent psychiatry: a comprehensive textbook,* 2nd ed. Philadelphia: Williams & Wilkins, 1996: 693–702.

Case 18-5: 13-Year-Old Girl

I. History of Present Illness

A 13-year old girl was brought to the emergency department after having had a syncopal episode when she stood up at home. She related that she was watching television and stood up. On standing, she felt lightheaded and dizzy, and everything went gray and then black; the next thing she remembered was lying on the floor at home. She denied any trauma. This event was not witnessed. She stated that she had had a cold for the past day and feeling as if she had a fever, sore throat, and runny nose. She has not actually taken her temperature. She also stated that her menstrual flow has been heavier than usual. In fact, for the past 2 days she has been soaking through six pads per day and had been passing blood clots as well. She denied ever having been sexually active and also denied genital trauma.

II. Past Medical History

She had been healthy with no previous episodes of abnormal bleeding. She was not described as a child who bruises easily. She had never been hospitalized or undergone a surgical procedure. She was not allergic to any medications, nor was she taking any medications. She had menarche at age 12 years and had been having her periods every month. She had never been pregnant and had never had a sexually transmitted disease.

III. Physical Examination

T, 38.5°C; RR, 26/min; HR 136 bpm; BP, 70/48 mm Hg

Weight, 25th percentile; height, 50th percentile

On examination, she was tired and slightly pale. Her head and neck examination was remarkable for pale conjunctivae and mucous membranes. Her lungs were clear to auscultation. Her cardiac examination was hyperdynamic, with a II/VI systolic ejection murmur heard best at the left lower sternal border. She had a 1-second capillary refill time. Her abdomen was soft with normoactive bowel sounds. Her pelvic examination revealed active menses, no cervical motion tenderness, and no adnexal tenderness. There were no signs of vaginal trauma or lacerations. There were no bruises or petechiae on her skin. Her extremity and neurologic examinations were normal.

IV. Diagnostic Studies

A complete blood count revealed 10,700 WBCs/mm^3 (91% segmented neutrophils, 3% lymphocytes, and 5% monocytes); hemoglobin, 9.4 g/dL; and platelets, 218,000/mm^3. Her prothrombin time was slightly elevated at 15.4 seconds; her partial thromboplastin time was slightly elevated at 37.5 seconds; and her fibrinogen level was slightly decreased at 155 mg/dL. Fibrin split products were negative. Her urine pregnancy test was negative. Blood and urine cultures were sent. Cervical cultures were sent for gonorrhea and chlamydia.

V. Course of Illness

While in the emergency department, her orthostatic vitals signs were checked. When she was lying down, her heart rate was 136 bpm with a blood pressure of 70/48 mm Hg. When she stood up, her heart rate increased to 184 bpm and her blood pressure decreased to 40/26 mm Hg. She immediately had two intravenous catheters placed and received 2 L of saline. She remained hypotensive despite approximately 100 mL/kg of normal saline boluses. Her repeat hemoglobin was decreased to 5.7 g/dL. Subsequently, 2 units of packed red blood cells were administered. Because of the fever and persistent hypotension, she was treated with broad-spectrum antibiotics.

DISCUSSION: CASE 18-5

I. Differential Diagnosis

The differential diagnosis of this adolescent who presented with a syncopal episode focused on the vaginal bleeding. The presumption was that this patient was anemic; however, she appeared to be more symptomatic than a hemoglobin of 9.4 g/dL would suggest. The reason behind this degree of symptomatology was hemoconcentration; when volume replacement was accomplished by fluid resuscitation, her hemoglobin dropped. Her vaginal bleeding could be a result of anovulation, pregnancy-related conditions, infection (pelvic inflammatory disease, vaginitis, cervicitis), a coagulation disorder (von Willebrand's disease, idiopathic thrombocytopenic purpura), trauma (accidental, coital-related, sexual abuse, foreign body), endometriosis, neoplasms, systemic diseases (hepatic disease, renal disorders, diabetes mellitus), or other endocrinologic disorders (thyroid disease, prolactinoma).

II. Diagnosis

This patient was admitted to the inpatient service and monitored very closely. She was started on oral hormone replacement therapy with a combination of estrogen and progesterone. Her bleeding resolved over the next 24 hours. The hypotension resolved after transfusion with packed red blood cells. Her posttransfusion hemoglobin increased to 9.0 g/dL. Her coagulation studies returned to normal, and assays for clotting factors all returned within normal limits. She was treated for presumed sepsis because of the fever and hypotension; however, no culture was able to document an infection. Because she was still within her first year after menarche and her menstrual periods were nonpainful (i.e., there was no associated cramping), she was determined to be having anovulatory cycles. **The diagnosis is dysfunctional uterine bleeding (DUB) due to anovulatory cycles.**

III. Incidence and Epidemiology

Approximately 50% to 80% of menstrual cycles within the first 2 years after menarche are anovulatory cycles. There is an interval of approximately 14 months from the start of menarche and regular periods. There is a 24-month interval from menarche to painful and presumably ovulatory periods. The later the age at menarche, the longer the interval before 50% of cycles become ovulatory. Specifically, if menarche occurs before 12 years of age, 50% of cycles are ovulatory within 1 year. If menarche occurs between the ages of 12 and 13 years, then 50% of cycles are ovulatory by about 3 years after menarche. If menarche occurs after the 13th birthday, the average time interval until 50% of the cycles are ovulatory is 4.5 years.

DUB occurs when there is abnormal uterine bleeding that is not the result of an acquired or congenital cause. The bleeding is either excessive in amount or lasts longer than usual. DUB can occur at any time during the reproductive years, but it is most commonly caused by anovulatory cycles. During an anovulatory cycle, there is unopposed estrogen, which can lead to endometrial hyperplasia. The endometrium sloughs off if it reaches an unstable thickness or if estrogen levels drop. Because of the lack of progesterone production, endometrial hemostasis is deficient and DUB can occur. DUB is the most common cause of abnormal uterine bleeding in adolescents.

IV. Clinical Presentation

The clinical presentation of DUB is variable. There may be an increased duration in the regular bleeding patterns, there may be heavier flow, or there may be a combination of alterations. Menorrhagia occurs when there is increased flow with normal intervals; metrorrhagia refers to increased flow with abnormal intervals.

V. Diagnostic Approach

DUB is a diagnosis of exclusion in adolescents. A complete history and physical examination should be performed. The history should exclude thyroid, renal, hepatic, and hematologic abnormalities. It is important to obtain an accurate menstrual, sexual, and pregnancy history. A complete physical examination should also be performed, including orthostatic vital signs. A pelvic examination should be performed in all sexually active females and perhaps a limited pelvic examination in all patients with DUB.

Other studies. Laboratory testing includes cultures for gonorrhea and chlamydia, a pregnancy test, a complete blood count, and coagulation studies if the bleeding is severe. Additional testing can be performed if necessary.

VI. Treatment

The main goal of therapy for the patient with DUB is to stop the bleeding. For adolescents who are having DUB due to anovulation but have normal hemoglobin values, menstrual calendars, iron supplementation, and close follow-up are all that is necessary. Patients with mild anemia who are not actively bleeding can be started on oral contraceptive pills, particularly an estrogen-progesterone combination pill if the bleeding has been prolonged. If the bleeding is heavy and the patient is anemic, then an oral contraceptive with a higher estrogen content, such as norgestrel, can be used. Frequently it is prescribed as one pill taken four times a day for 4 days, one pill three times a day for 3 days, one pill twice a day for 2 weeks, and then 1 week off. Nausea is a significant side effect from this higher-dose estrogen and needs to be addressed to ensure patient compliance. After this 1-month regimen, the patient should be started on an oral contraceptive pill with a lower dose of estrogen. Inpatient therapy is indicated for patients who have hemoglobin values lower than 7 g/dL, orthostatic changes, or heavy bleeding and hemoglobin lower than 10 g/dL. The prognosis for DUB is considered to be excellent; the condition typically resolves as the patient grows older. Patients with polycystic ovary syndrome may have chronic anovulation and should be maintained on oral contraceptive therapy to decrease the risk of endometrial carcinoma.

VII. References

1. Lavin C. Dysfunctional uterine bleeding in adolescents. *Curr Opin Pediatr* 1996;8: 328–332.
2. Munro MG. Dysfunctional uterine bleeding: advances in diagnosis and treatment. Curr Opin Obstet Gynecol 2001;13:475–489.
3. Bravender T, Emans SJ. Menstrual disorders: dysfunctional uterine bleeding. *Pediatr Clin North Am* 1999;46:545–553.

19

Seizures

Samir S. Shah

APPROACH TO THE PATIENT WITH SEIZURES

I. Definition of the Complaint

Seizures, a common neurologic disorder of childhood, occur in 4% to 6% of all children. A seizure is defined as a transient, involuntary alteration of consciousness, behavior, motor activity, sensation, and/or autonomic function that is caused by an excessive rate and hypersynchrony of discharges from a group of cerebral neurons. A seizure disorder, or epilepsy, is a condition of susceptibility to recurrent seizures. This chapter discusses possible causes of seizures. The classification of seizure types can be found in standard pediatrics textbooks.

The first step in formulating a differential diagnosis for a child who presents with "seizures" is to characterize the type of event that has occurred. Seizures should be differentiated from other childhood paroxysmal events that can mimic seizure activity. Syncope is the most common alternative diagnosis given to patients who present for evaluation of a suspected seizure episode. Gastroesophageal reflux with opisthotonic posturing (Sandifer syndrome) frequently mimics seizures in infancy. Breath-holding spells, which occur in approximately 4% of infants, can resemble seizures and are also associated with cyanosis. A variety of movement disorders, such as benign myoclonus of infancy and Tourette syndrome, may also be mistaken for seizures. Additionally, seizure activity is often subtle, making seizures difficult to diagnose. For example, in the neonatal period seizures may manifest with horizontal eye movements, repetitive sucking, or pedaling and stepping motions that are difficult to distinguish from normal newborn infant activity.

II. Complaint by Cause and Frequency

A seizure does not constitute a diagnosis but is a symptom of an underlying pathologic process that requires a thorough evaluation. The causes of seizures in childhood vary by age (Table 19-1) and may also be grouped by etiology (Table 19-2): (a) infectious, (b) toxicologic, (c) metabolic, (d) vascular, (e) oncologic, (f) endocrine, (g) traumatic, (h) congenital, and (i) idiopathic.

III. Clarifying Questions

Thorough history taking is essential to arriving at an accurate diagnosis in a child who presents with seizures. Consideration of seizure type, precipitating factors, and associated clinical features provides a useful framework for creating a differential diagnosis. The following questions may help provide clues to the diagnosis.

- Did the seizure involve the entire body or only a portion?

  — Partial, or focal, seizures reflect initial involvement limited to one cerebral hemisphere and are further classified based on whether consciousness is impaired. Partial seizures are less common in children than in adults. Although partial seizures are more likely to be associated with focal hemispheric lesions than are general-

TABLE 19-1. *Causes of New-Onset Seizures in Childhood by Age*

Disease prevalence	Neonate	Infant and school age child	Adolescent

Common	CNS infection
	  Bacterial meningitis
	  Viral meningitis
	Drug withdrawal
	Hypoxic-ischemic injury
	Idiopathic
	Intracranial hemorrhage
	Metabolic abnormalities
	  Hypoglycemia
	  Hyponatremia
	  Hypernatremia
	  Hypomagnesemia
	  Hypocalcemia
		Toxic ingestion
		CNS infection
		  Bacterial meningitis
		  Viral meningitis
		  Parasitic infestation
		  Cat-scratch
		    encephalitis
		Febrile seizure
		Head trauma
		Idiopathic
			CNS infection
			  Bacterial meningitis
			  Viral meningitis
			  Parasitic infestation
			Head trauma
			Idiopathic
			Intentional toxic ingestion

Less common	Developmental
	  abnormalities
	Incontinentia pigmenti
	Neurocutaneous
	  syndromes
	Metabolic disorders
	  Aminoacidopathy
	  Organic aciduria
	  Urea cycle defects
	  Galactosemia
		Developmental
		  abnormalities
		Intracranial birth injury
		Neurocutaneous
		  syndromes
		Dilutional hyponatremia
		Heavy metal poisoning
		Postinfectious
			Juvenile myoclonic
			  epilepsy

Uncommon	Benign neonatal seizures
	Congenital cerebral
	  malformation
	  Cerebral agenesis/
	    dysgenesis
	  Holoprosencephaly,
	    lissencephaly
	Kernicterus
	Adrenoleukodystrophy
	Pyridoxine dependency
		Congenital cerebral
		  malformation
		Hypertensive
		  encephalopathy
		Metabolic disorders
		Rett syndrome
		Tumors
		  Primary
		  Metastatic
			Drug withdrawal
			Tumors
			  Primary
			  Metastatic
			Vasculitis

CNS, central nervous system.

ized seizures, such structural causes are only found in 30% to 50% of cases. Children with congenital heart disease or right-to-left shunts may have cerebral emboli resulting in neurologic deficits and partial seizures. Herpes simplex virus (HSV) can cause seizures with a temporal lobe focus. Partial seizures occur later in childhood in individuals with heritable familial degenerative disorders that are characterized by storage abnormalities, such as GM1 and GM2 gangliosidoses. Parasitic infections such as echinococcosis and cysticercosis also cause focal brain lesions predisposing to partial seizures.

• Was there a preceding illness or fever?

— Febrile seizures occur most commonly in children younger than 5 years of age. Infectious causes must be excluded, because seizures are often the initial manifestation of bacterial meningitis in infants and children.

• Has there been an ingestion or toxin exposure?

— Many medications and environmental toxins can lead to seizures, including anticonvulsant medications, hypoglycemic agents, isoniazid, lithium, methylxanthines, heavy metals (lead), and tricyclic antidepressants.

TABLE 19-2. *Causes of Seizures in Childhood by Etiology*

Infectious	Brain abscess
	Encephalitis
	Febrile
	Meningitis
	Parasites (central nervous system)
	Echinococcosis (*Echinococcus granulosus*)
	Neurocysticercosis (*Taenia solium*)
	Syphilis
Toxicologic	Ingestion
	Anticonvulsants
	Carbon monoxide
	Cocaine
	Heavy metals (lead)
	Hypoglycemic agents
	Isoniazid
	Lithium
	Methylxanthines
	Pesticides (organophosphates)
	Topical anesthetics
	Tricyclic antidepressants
	Withdrawal
	Alcohol
	Anticonvulsants
Metabolic	Electrolyte abnormalities
	Hypocalcemia
	Hypoglycemia
	Hyponatremia
	Hypomagnesemia
	Hepatic failure
	Hypoxic-ischemic injury
	Inborn errors of metabolism
	Pyridoxine dependency
	Uremia
Vascular	Cerebrovascular accident
	Hypertensive encephalopathy
Oncologic	Primary brain tumor
	Metastatic central nervous system disease
Endocrine	Addison's disease
	Hypothyroidism or hyperthyroidism
Traumatic	Intracranial hemorrhage
Congenital	Developmental brain abnormalities
Idiopathic	

- Is there a history of recent headache, vomiting, lethargy, weakness, or alteration in gait?

  — These symptoms suggest underlying central nervous system (CNS) pathology and the need for neuroimaging. In the neonate, the early onset of lethargy, vomiting, and seizures should prompt an evaluation for an underlying metabolic disorder such as an aminoacidopathy, organic aciduria, or urea cycle defect; examples include phenylketonuria and maple syrup urine disease.

- Is there a history of previous seizures (febrile or afebrile) or neurologic abnormality?

  — One third of children with a simple febrile seizure have a second episode. A previous afebrile seizure or existing neurologic abnormality increases the likelihood of a seizure disorder or epileptic syndrome.

- Is there a history of head trauma?

  — Head trauma can result in epilepsy at any age. Seizures can occur within 1 to 2 weeks after the injury (early posttraumatic seizures), as an acute reaction to head trauma, or after intervals of several months or even years (late posttraumatic seizures). The risk of developing seizures is related to the severity of the head injury. The child with a mild head injury (transient loss of consciousness without evidence of skull fracture or neurologic abnormality) is not at significantly higher risk than the general population. Moderate head injuries are associated with an incidence of epilepsy ranging from 2% to 10%. Children with severe head injuries, such as intracerebral hematoma or a history of unconsciousness lasting longer than 24 hours, have a 30% risk of developing epilepsy.

- Is there a history of a remote neurologic insult?

  — A history of anoxic birth injury, cerebral palsy, stroke, intracranial hemorrhage, or meningitis places the child at increased risk for seizure disorder. Intrauterine infection with cytomegalovirus, toxoplasma, or rubella is known to cause abnormal brain development and to predispose the child to seizures.

- Are there skin findings on physical examination, such as café-au-lait spots, ash leaf spots, or cutaneous vascular malformations?

  — These findings suggest an underlying neurocutaneous disorder such as neurofibromatosis, tuberous sclerosis, ataxia-telangiectasia, or Sturge-Weber syndrome.

- What is the child's head morphology?

  — Microcephaly suggests an underlying neurologic abnormality. A full or bulging fontanel can signify elevated intracranial pressure due to meningitis, trauma, or malignancy.

- Is there a family history of seizures?

  — Both febrile and afebrile seizures can be hereditary.

The following cases represent less common causes of seizures in childhood.

Case 19-1: 8-Day-Old Girl

I. History of Present Illness

An 8-day-old girl presented to the emergency department after an episode of irregular, rapid breathing followed by stiffening of her body and shaking of her extremities that lasted several seconds. On arrival, the infant was lethargic, cyanotic, and bradycardic with minimal spontaneous respirations. She underwent emergency endotracheal intubation and received multiple boluses of normal saline, with improvement in her perfusion and heart rate.

She then had a generalized seizure and received intravenous lorazepam. Ampicillin and cefotaxime were administered after a blood culture was obtained. According to the family, she had fed poorly that day and had been sleeping more than usual. The infant had been afebrile and had had normal stooling and urine output. There was no vomiting, diarrhea, or rashes. There were no ill contacts.

II. Past Medical History

The infant weighed 3,400 g at birth and was the product of a full-term gestation. She was born by spontaneous vaginal delivery after an uncomplicated pregnancy. Maternal serology was negative. The infant's postnatal course was remarkable only for mild jaundice that did not require phototherapy. The mother denied a history of genital HSV infection. There was no family history of seizures.

III. Physical Examination

T, 39.0°C; RR, 20/min; HR, 180 bpm; BP, 86/45 mm Hg; SpO$_2$, 100% in room air
Weight, 25th percentile; head circumference, 50th percentile

Examination revealed a mechanically ventilated infant. She was sedated but withdrew in response to painful stimuli. The fontanel was bulging. There were no head lacerations or skull depressions. The sclerae were anicteric, and the pupils were 1.5 mm and symmetrically reactive. There were no cardiac murmurs, and the femoral pulses were weakly palpable. The lungs were clear to auscultation. The abdomen was soft, and the umbilical stump was well healed without erythema or discharge. There were two pustules in the perineal area.

IV. Diagnostic Studies

Laboratory results were as follows: sodium, 132 mEq/L; potassium, 3.3 mEq/L; chloride, 99 mEq/L; bicarbonate, 23 mEq/L; glucose, 73 mg/dL; calcium, 8.9 mg/dL; and magnesium, 2.1 mg/dL. The complete blood count revealed 8,000 WBCs/mm^3, including 33% band forms, 18% segmented neutrophils, 35% lymphocytes, and 10% monocytes. The hemoglobin and platelet count were normal. On cerebrospinal fluid (CSF) examination, there were 879 WBCs/mm^3 (48% segmented neutrophils, 19% lymphocytes, and 33% monocytes) and 1,739 red blood cels/mm^3; no organisms were seen on Gram staining. The CSF glucose concentration was 36 mg/dL, and the protein concentration was 400 mg/dL. CSF was sent for bacterial culture and detection of HSV by polymerase chain reaction (PCR). There were no abnormalities on chest radiograph.

V. Course of Illness

In the intensive care unit, the patient received ampicillin, gentamicin, and acyclovir. A head computed tomogram (CT) was normal, and the patient's neurologic examination improved quickly over the next day. She was extubated on the second day of hospitalization but required replacement of the endotracheal tube due to multiple episodes of apnea.

Electroencephalography (EEG) revealed status epilepticus. Sustained seizure control was observed only after the addition of phenobarbital and phenytoin. Because HSV was not detected in the CSF by PCR, acyclovir was discontinued. Growth of an organism from the CSF on the third day of hospitalization guided additional therapy.

DISCUSSION: CASE 19-1

I. Differential Diagnosis

Seizures are a feature of almost all brain disorders in the newborn. The time of onset of the first seizure is helpful in determining the cause. The causes of neonatal seizures that occur after the first 72 hours of life include intracranial infection, intracranial hemorrhage, metabolic abnormalities, developmental defects, and drug withdrawal. Intracranial infections occur in 5% to 10% of neonatal seizures, and after 72 hours of life group B streptococci and *Listeria monocytogenes* are common bacterial causes. Seizures with HSV typically occur during the second week of life, and 30% of infected infants present with a vesicular rash. Intracranial hemorrhages are frequently associated with hypoxic-ischemic or traumatic birth injury. Intraventricular hemorrhages principally occur in the premature infant, and subarachnoid and subdural hemorrhages usually occur in the term infant. Metabolic abnormalities include disturbances of glucose, calcium, magnesium, and sodium. Hypocalcemia is associated with low birth weight, asphyxia, maternal diabetes, transient neonatal hypoparathyroidism, and microdeletions of chromosome 22q11. Other metabolic abnormalities include inborn errors of metabolism, especially aminocidurias, because protein and glucose feedings have been initiated. Aberrations of brain development are usually related to a disturbance of neuronal migration such as lissencephaly, pachygyria, or polymicrogyria. Passive addiction of the newborn and drug withdrawal may involve narcotic-analgesics (methadone), sedative-hypnotics (shorter-acting barbiturates), cocaine, alcohol, or tricyclic antidepressants. In the case described, the results of CSF analysis were suggestive of intracranial infection, but interpretation of the Gram stain was misleading.

II. Diagnosis

The diagnosis is meningitis due to *L. monocytogenes,* a gram-positive rod. On the fourth day of hospitalization, the organism was noted to have only intermediate susceptibility to ampicillin. The patient was switched to intravenous vancomycin, and gentamicin was continued. CSF from the lumbar puncture, repeated on the sixth day of hospitalization, was sterile. Head CT was repeated on the eighth day of hospitalization and revealed bilateral frontal, parietal, and temporal lobe infarcts but no ventriculomegaly. Mechanical ventilation was required until the ninth day of hospitalization. The infant was discharged after 21 days of antibiotic therapy.

III. Incidence and Epidemiology

L. monocytogenes, a motile gram-positive rod, was first isolated in 1926 during an investigation of epidemic perinatal infection among a colony of rabbits. It is a common veterinary pathogen that causes meningoencephalitis in sheep and cattle. It is widespread in the environment and is found commonly in soil and decaying vegetation. Many foods are contaminated with this organism; it has been recovered from raw vegetables, fish, poultry, unpasteurized milk, and certain types of cheese. The organism has been isolated from the stools of 5% of healthy adults, and higher rates of recovery have been reported for household contacts of patients with clinical infection. Infection in humans is uncommon but occurs most frequently in neonates, pregnant women, and elderly or immunosuppressed patients. Approximately 30% of all *L. monocytogenes* infections occur in neonates.

IV. Clinical Presentation

Neonatal *L. monocytogenes* infection, like group B streptococcal infection, manifests in both an early- and a late-onset form. Clinical manifestations of *L. monocytogenes* infection are similar to those of other neonatal bacterial infections. Signs of infection include temperature instability, respiratory distress, irritability, lethargy, and poor feeding. In early-onset disease, transplacental transmission after maternal bacteremia or ascending spread from vaginal colonization leads to intrauterine infection with *L. monocytogenes*. Preterm labor is common among infants with early-onset *L. monocytogenes* infection; length of gestation is less than 35 weeks in approximately 70% of cases. There is often evidence of an acute febrile maternal illness, with symptoms of fatigue, arthralgias, and myalgias preceding delivery by 2 to 14 days. Blood cultures are positive for *L. monocytogenes* in 35% of mothers of infants with early-onset listeriosis.

Early-onset infection classically develops within the first or second day of life. Bacteremia (75%) and pneumonia (50%) are usually seen with early-onset infection. Meningitis is seen in 25% of early-onset cases. In severe infection, a granulomatous rash is associated with disseminated disease (granulomatosis infantisepticum). The mortality rate, including stillbirths, is 40% for early-onset infection. In late-onset infection, modes of transmission unrelated to maternal carriage may be involved. Late-onset infection develops during the second to eighth week of life. The most common form *of L. monocytogenes* infection over this period is meningitis, which is present in approximately 95% of cases. Bacteremia (20%) and pneumonia (10%) are less common. Mortality of late-onset infection is generally low (15%) if the infection is diagnosed early and treated appropriately.

A nosocomial outbreak occurred when nine newborn infants were bathed in mineral oil contaminated with *L. monocytogenes*. The affected infants developed bacteremia (two cases), meningitis (two cases), or both (five cases); one infant died. Signs of infection developed within 1 week after exposure to the mineral oil.

V. Diagnostic Approach

Lumbar puncture. Isolation of the organism from culture of CSF is the only reliable means of diagnosing meningitis due to *L. monocytogenes*. The finding of short, sometimes coccoid, gram-positive rods on microscopic examination of the CSF strongly supports the diagnosis of *L. monocytogenes* meningitis. However, because of the low concentration of organisms, most (60%) Gram-stained smears of CSF from infants with *L. monocytogenes* meningitis do not reveal bacteria, as occurred with the infant in this case. Furthermore, *L. monocytogenes* sometimes does not stain clearly as gram positive. In such cases, variable decoloration on Gram staining may cause the organism to appear as a gram-negative rod and be confused with *Haemophilus influenzae*, especially with long-standing disease or when the patient has received prior antibiotics. In other instances, *Listeria* has been mistaken for *Streptococcus pneumoniae* or for *Corynebacterium* spp. CSF glucose is normal in more than 60% of cases. Mononuclear cells predominate in one third of cases.

Additional studies. PCR probes and antibodies to listeriolysin O, the major virulence factor of the organism, have not proved useful for acute diagnosis of invasive disease.

VI. Treatment

Ampicillin is the preferred agent in the treatment of *L. monocytogenes* infections. Based on synergy studies *in vitro* and in animal models, most authorities suggest adding gentamicin to ampicillin for the treatment of meningitis due to *L. monocytogenes*. There appears to be partial synergy with combinations of ampicillin or vancomycin with rifampin. Vancomycin alone has been used successfully in a few penicillin-allergic adult patients, but others have developed listerial meningitis while receiving the drug. Trimethoprim-sulfamethoxazole is effective for penicillin-allergic patients but should not be used in neonates because of the concern of bilirubin toxicity. Cephalosporins are not active against *L. monocytogenes*. Once susceptibility studies become available, changes in therapy may be necessary. Treatment of *L. monocytogenes* meningitis should continue for a minimum of 3 weeks.

Corticosteroids should be avoided, if possible, because impairment of cellular immunity due to corticosteroid therapy is a major risk factor for the development of listeriosis. A maternal history of a previous infant with perinatal listeriosis is not an indication for intrapartum antibiotics.

VII. References

1. Bortolussi R, Schlech WF III. Listeriosis. In: Remington JS, Klein JO, eds. *Infectious diseases of the fetus and newborn infant.* Philadelphia: WB Saunders, 2001; 1157–1177.
2. Lorber B. Listeriosis. *Clin Infect Dis* 1997;24:1–11.
3. Schuchat A, Lizano C, Broome CV, et al. Outbreak of neonatal listeriosis associated with mineral oil. *Pediatr Infect Dis J* 1991;10:183–189.
4. Southwick FS, Purich DL. Mechanisms of disease: intracellular pathogenesis of listeriosis. *N Engl J Med* 1996;334:770–776.

Case 19-2: 10-Day-Old Boy

I. History of Present Illness

A 10-day-old boy was well until the day of admission, when he was noted by his mother to have the sudden onset of left arm and leg shaking while sleeping. The episode lasted about 1 minute and was accompanied by eyelid fluttering. After spontaneous cessation of the episode, the infant continued sleeping but aroused easily. He was brought to the emergency department for evaluation. He did not have fever or cyanosis. There was no recent vomiting or diarrhea. His oral intake had been unchanged over the past several days and consisted exclusively of cow milk-based formula every 2.5 to 3 hours. The parents were uncertain about urine output because the maternal grandmother had cared for the infant on the day before admission.

II. Past Medical History

The infant weighed 3,600 g at birth. He was born by spontaneous vaginal delivery after an uncomplicated pregnancy. He required phototherapy briefly on the second day of life for hyperbilirubinemia with a peak total bilirubin level of 15.5 mg/dL. The mother had vaginal colonization with group B *Streptococcus* and received two doses of penicillin during labor. She also had a history of genital HSV infection. Although no lesions were noted at delivery, she did develop lesions on the seventh postpartum day.

III. Physical Examination

T, 37.5°C; RR, 40/min; HR, 124 bpm; BP, 75/45 mm Hg; SpO_2, 100% in room air

Weight, 50th percentile; length, 25th percentile; head circumference, 25th percentile

The infant appeared alert. There were no vesicles on the scalp or skin. His anterior fontanel was open and flat. His conjunctivae were pink and anicteric. Red reflex was present bilaterally. There was no murmur on cardiac examination, and femoral pulses were strong. The spleen tip was just palpable, and there was no hepatomegaly. The Moro reflex was symmetric. The remainder of the examination was also normal.

IV. Diagnostic Studies

A complete blood count revealed 8,800 WBCs/mm^3 (16% segmented neutrophils, 70% lymphocytes, 11% monocytes, and 3% atypical lymphocytes); hemoglobin, 13.4 g/dL; and platelets, 511,000/mm^3. Serum chemistry values included sodium, 139 mmol/L; potassium, 5.5 mmol/L; chloride, 104 mmol/L; and bicarbonate, 28 mmol/L. The blood urea nitrogen and creatinine concentrations were normal. Serum alanine and aspartate aminotransferases were normal. Serum albumin was 3.3 g/dL. Examination of the CSF revealed the following: WBCs, 12/mm^3; red blood cells, 1,834/mm^3; glucose, 45 g/dL; and protein, 124 g/dL. There were no bacteria on Gram staining.

V. Course of Illness

The infant was treated empirically with ampicillin, cefotaxime, and acyclovir while the results of CSF bacterial culture and CSF HSV PCR were awaited. An ECG (Fig. 19-1) suggested a cause of the seizures, which was confirmed by additional blood tests in both the infant and his mother.

DISCUSSION: CASE 19-2

I. Differential Diagnosis

Many neonatal seizures are idiopathic. The most common definable etiologic agents are asphyxia, intracranial infection, trauma, nontraumatic hemorrhage, strokes, metabolic

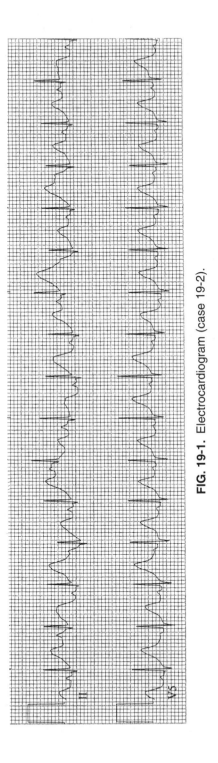

FIG. 19-1. Electrocardiogram (case 19-2).

disorders, CNS malformations, and maternal drug abuse. Seizures due to perinatal asphyxia typically occur within the first 24 hours of life. Common infectious causes in the first week of life include bacterial meningitis due to group B *Streptococcus* and *Escherichia coli*. Neonates with HSV meningitis typically present during the second week of life, but up to 40% develop symptoms within the first 5 days of life. Intracranial hemorrhage of any cause can provoke seizures. Neonatal seizures related to birth trauma with subsequent subarachnoid hemorrhage or subdural and epidural hematomas usually occur within the first 72 hours of life. Nontraumatic causes of intracranial hemorrhage, including ruptured arteriovenous malformations and underlying disorders of coagulation, can occur at any time. Metabolic disorders include hypocalcemia, hypoglycemia, and pyridoxine dependency. Neonatal hypocalcemia occurring after the third day of life is usually caused by transient relative hypoparathyroidism. The immature neonatal parathyroid may be unable to handle an excessive phosphate load, particularly if the infant is fed a formula with a relatively low ratio of calcium to phosphorus. Rarely, prolonged phototherapy induces hypocalcemia. Phototherapy decreases melatonin secretion, which decreases glucocorticoid secretion, which in turn leads to an increase in bone calcium uptake with subsequent hypocalcemia. Multiple defects in urea cycle and organic acid metabolism may cause seizures in the neonatal period. Infants with these disorders usually have unexplained stupor, coma, and vomiting in addition to seizures. Infants born to mothers who have used heroin or methadone may have seizures, although other symptoms, such as poor feeding, diarrhea, sweating, jitteriness, and irritability, are more common.

II. Diagnosis

Bacterial cultures and HSV PCR of the CSF were negative. The ECG demonstrated QTc prolongation (QTc = 0.47 seconds) characteristic of hypocalcemia (Fig. 19-1). The infant's serum calcium concentration was 6.6 mg/dL (normal range, 8.8 to 10.1 mg/dL); ionized calcium was 0.83 mmol/L (normal, 1.00 to 1.17 mmol/L); phosphate, 10.6 mg/dL (normal, 4.8 to 8.2 mg/dL); and magnesium, 1.1 mg/dL (normal, 1.5 to 2.5 mg/dL). Additional testing included intact parathyroid hormone (PTH), 9.7 pg/mL (normal, 10 to 55 pg/mL); 25-hydroxyvitamin D (25-hydroxycholecalciferol [25(OH)D$_3$]), 7 ng/mL (normal, 5 to 42 ng/mL); and active vitamin D (1,25-dihydroxycholecalciferol [1,25(OH)$_2$D$_3$]), 114 pg/mL (normal, 8 to 72 pg/mL). Although the mother was asymptomatic, her calcium level was elevated to 12.8 mg/dL. The mother was subsequently diagnosed with hyperparathyroidism related to a parathyroid adenoma. **The diagnosis is transient neonatal hypoparathyroidism secondary to maternal hyperparathyroidism.** The infant was initially treated with intravenous calcium gluconate followed by oral calcium and vitamin D supplementation, which were weaned over the subsequent 3 weeks.

III. Incidence and Epidemiology

Hyperparathyroidism has a prevalence rate of 0.15%, with a peak incidence between 30 and 50 years of age. Approximately 80% of cases are due to a solitary adenoma that requires resection, and 15% are due to chief cell hyperplasia. Maternal symptoms are not apparent until the serum calcium level exceeds 12 to 13 mg/dL. However, even mild maternal hypercalcemia leads to chronic fetal hypercalcemia, which in turn suppresses fetal production of PTH. After birth, calcium levels decrease but PTH production cannot be rapidly increased. In this condition, neonatal hypoparathyroidism is transient, lasting only several days to several weeks. Eventually, as the parathyroids become more active, increasing PTH levels stimulate vitamin D production and extra calcium absorption from the plentiful supply in the gut. Clinically detectable hypocalcemia develops in 15% to

25% of infants born to mothers with hyperparathyroidism. As in this case, neonatal seizures or tetany often leads to a search that identifies a maternal parathyroid adenoma.

IV.   Clinical Presentation

Signs of hypocalcemia usually develop within the first 3 weeks of life. Signs of neonatal hypocalcemia are often nonspecific and may be seen in a variety of other conditions. Tremors and jitteriness are most commonly seen. Other signs include irritability, hyperreflexia, facial twitching, carpopedal spasm, seizures, cyanosis, and, rarely, laryngospasm. More importantly, other disorders that can manifest with hypocalcemia should be considered. Features of 22q11 deletion syndromes include cleft palate, micrognathia, ear anomalies, bulbous nasal tip, and conotruncal heart defects. Findings associated with Albright hereditary osteodystrophy (pseudohypoparathyroidism type Ia) include round face, short distal phalanges of the thumbs, subcutaneous calcifications, and a family history of developmental delay and dental hypoplasia. Sensorineural deafness, renal dysplasia, and mental retardation are also associated with syndromes that include hypoparathyroidism.

V.   Diagnostic Approach

Serum calcium and ionized calcium (Ca^{2+}). Both calcium and Ca^{2+} levels are low with symptomatic hypocalcemia.

Serum albumin. Because approximately 45% of serum calcium is protein bound, low serum albumin levels lead to low serum calcium levels with normal Ca^{2+} levels. Symptoms of hypocalcemia develop only when Ca^{2+} is low. The following correction factor is used to indicate whether a low measured serum calcium level is due solely to hypoalbuminemia:

$$\text{Corrected serum calcium} = \text{Measured serum calcium} + [(\text{Normal serum albumin} - \text{Measured serum albumin}) \times 0.8]$$

If the corrected serum calcium is less than normal (i.e., less than 8.8 mg/dL), the Ca^{2+} may also be low, increasing the likelihood of symptomatic hypocalcemia. In this patient described, the corrected serum calcium was calculated as follows:

$$\text{Corrected calcium} = 6.6 \text{ mg/dL} + (4.0 \text{ mg/dL} - 3.3 \text{ mg/dL}) \times 0.8] = 7.1 \text{ mg/dL}$$

Serum magnesium. Magnesium deficiency can lead to neonatal hypocalcemia through functional hypoparathyroidism and pseudohypoparathyroidism. In most cases, it is seen in neonates born to magnesium-deficient mothers, such as those with poorly controlled diabetes mellitus. In magnesium deficiency, magnesium replenishment leads to increases in both calcium and PTH levels. In hypoparathyroidism of any other cause, magnesium administration does not lead to changes in the calcium and PTH levels.

Serum phosphorus. Phosphorus levels are elevated with both phosphate-induced neonatal hypocalcemia and hypoparathyroidism.

Serum parathyroid hormone. PTH levels are low with hypoparathyroidism. However, in phosphate-induced neonatal hypocalcemia, serum PTH is appropriately elevated.

Active vitamin D. Levels of $1,25(OH)_2D_3$ are low with hypocalcemia due to vitamin D deficiency but normal or high with underlying hypoparathyroidism.

Other tests. Infants who were treated with bicarbonate or other alkali to correct acidosis can develop very significant hypocalcemia; therefore, an arterial blood gas determination should be considered. A chest radiograph can document a normal thymic shadow in neonates if 22q11 deletion syndromes are a concern. If neonatal risk factors for hypocalcemia are absent, measurement of maternal serum calcium, phosphorus, and PTH levels should be considered.

VI. Treatment

Emergency treatment for neonatal hypocalcemia consists of intravenous 10% calcium gluconate infusion with continuous ECG monitoring. Additionally, $1,25(OH)_2D_3$ (calcitriol) should be given. Once the QTc interval on ECG is normal, therapy can be continued with oral calcium and vitamin D_2 (ergocalciferol), which is less costly than calcitriol. Serum calcium levels should be measured frequently in the early stages of treatment to determine the appropriate dosing. If hypercalcemia occurs, therapy should be discontinued and resumed at a lower dose after the serum calcium level has returned to normal. When maternal hyperparathyroidism is the cause of neonatal hypoparathyroidism and hypocalcemia, supplementation with calcium and vitamin D analogues is required for only 3 to 4 weeks.

VII. References

1. Hsieh YY, Chang CC, Tsai HD, et al. Primary hyperparathyroidism in pregnancy: report of three cases. *Arch Gynecol Obstet* 1998;261:209–214.
2. Kaplan EL, Burrington JD, Klementschitsch P, et al. Primary hyperparathyroidism, pregnancy, and neonatal hypocalcemia. *Surgery* 1984;96:717–722.
3. Mimouni FB, Root AW. Disorders of calcium metabolism in the newborn. In: Sperling MA, ed. *Pediatric endocrinology.* Philadelphia: WB Saunders, 1996;95–115.
4. Morrison A. Neonatal seizures. In: Pomerance JJ, Richardson CJ, eds. *Neonatology for the clinician.* Norwalk, CT: Appleton & Lange, 1993;411–423.
5. Romagnoli C, Polidori G, Cataldi L, et al. Phototherapy induced hypocalcemia. *J Pediatr* 1979;94:815–816.

Case 19-3: 8-Month-Old Boy

I. History of Present Illness

An 8-month-old boy was well until 1 week before admission, when he was found by his mother having a "seizure." He had shaking and jerking of all extremities that did not stop when his extremities were held. He did not respond to touch or stimulation. There was no cyanosis. The episode lasted approximately 15 minutes. By the time Emergency Medical Services personnel arrived, the patient was alert and feeding on a bottle. He was not taken to the hospital. His last feeding had been approximately 3 hours before the event. Two days later, he was evaluated by his primary physician, who performed the following laboratory evaluations: glucose (during feeding), 121 mg/dL; alanine aminotransferase (ALT), 73 U/L; aspartate aminotransferase (AST), 93 U/L; γ-glutamyl transferase (GGT), 28 U/L; and cholesterol, 423 mg/dL. These laboratory studies were repeated 2 days later, with similar results except the glucose was 16 mg/dL. Head CT and EEG were normal. He was hospitalized for additional evaluation.

II. Past Medical History

The patient was born at 38 weeks' gestation with a birth weight of 3,400 g. His delivery was complicated by meconium aspiration. He was treated with supplemental oxygen and empiric antibiotics for 3 days. He also had hypoglycemia requiring intravenous dextrose and bottle feedings every 1.5 hours. This resolved, and he was discharged home on the fourth day of life. At 3 months of life, he had been diagnosed with otitis media and received oral antibiotics. There was no family history of seizures or mental retardation.

III. Physical Examination

T, 36.2°C; RR, 20/min; HR, 90 to 110 bpm; BP, 120/55 mm Hg; SpO_2, 100% in room air

Height, 25th percentile; weight, 10th percentile; head circumference, 25th percentile

On examination, he was thin but playful and interactive. The anterior fontanel was open and flat. His pupils were symmetrically reactive to light. The heart sounds were normal, and the lungs were clear to auscultation. His abdomen was slightly protuberant, with a liver edge that was firm and palpable 6 cm below the right costal margin. The spleen tip was just palpable below the left costal margin. There was no ascites or palpable abdominal mass. The infant was circumcised and had normal male genitalia. The neurological examination was normal. He was able to sit without support and maintained good head control. Deep tendon reflexes were 2+ and symmetric. The gag reflex was intact. There were no hyperpigmented or hypopigmented skin lesions.

IV. Diagnostic Studies

Serum chemistry values included sodium, 137 mmol/L; potassium, 5.5 mmol/L; chloride, 100 mmol/L; bicarbonate, 13 mmol/L; calcium, 10.5 mg/dL; phosphorous, 6.5 mg/dL; and serum glucose 20 mg/dL. The cholesterol and triglyceride concentrations were 465 and 4,070 mg/dL, respectively. Hepatic function tests included AST, 125 U/L; ALT, 155 U/L; GGT, 564 U/L; total bilirubin, 0.6 mg/dL; and albumin, 4.0 g/dL. Serum and urinary ketones were present. The WBC count, hemoglobin, and platelet count, as well as prothrombin and partial thromboplastin times, were normal. Blood, urine, and stool cultures were obtained.

V. Course of Illness

The patient underwent a fasting study that revealed the diagnosis within approximately 4 hours.

DISCUSSION: CASE 19-3

I. Differential Diagnosis

This infant had seizures related to hypoglycemia. Hypoglycemia in an infant, defined as a blood glucose concentration of 40 mg/dL or less, warrants immediate treatment followed by appropriate investigation. Many inborn errors of metabolism responsible for hypoglycemia manifest during the first year of life, whereas milder defects of glycogen degradation and gluconeogenesis manifest in childhood only after prolonged periods of fasting. Causes of hypoglycemia in an infant include hyperinsulinism, hormone deficiency, and defects in branched-chain amino acid metabolism, fatty acid oxidation, and hepatic enzymes.

Urinary ketones are absent or low in children with hyperinsulinism and fatty acid oxidation defects who present with hypoglycemia. Hypoglycemia secondary to hyperinsulism most commonly appears during the first year of life. It is usually associated with islet-cell dysplasia and rarely with islet-cell adenomas. Insulin is elevated (greater than 5 μU/mL), and injection of glucagon elicits a rapid rise in blood glucose levels. Children with disorders of fatty acid metabolism can present with hypoglycemia and profound disturbance of consciousness that may not improve when the plasma glucose is normalized. In addition to hypoketonemia, they have high plasma free fatty acid concentrations, elevated ALT and AST, rhabdomyolysis, cardiomyopathy, and cerebral edema.

The presence of urinary ketones usually suggests hormone deficiency, glycogen storage disease (GSD), or defects in gluconeogenesis. Hypoglycemia is a common presentation for infants with panhypopituitarism, isolated growth hormone deficiency, and absolute (adrenal hypoplasia, Addison's disease, adrenal leukodystrophy) or relative (congenital adrenal hyperplasia) glucocorticoid deficiency. Midline defects such as cleft lip or palate, optic dysplasia, and microphallus suggest anterior pituitary hormone deficiency. Hyperpigmentation associated with Addison's disease rarely occurs in young children. Addison's disease is occasionally associated with hypoparathyroidism (hypocalcemia). Severely compromised adrenal function, as in congenital adrenal hyperplasia, may lead to serum electrolyte disturbances or ambiguous genitalia.

Children with branched-chain ketonuria (maple syrup urine disease) excrete urinary ketoacids that impart the characteristic odor of maple syrup. Clinically, these infants have frequent hypoglycemic episodes, lethargy, vomiting, and muscular hypertonia. GSDs are inherited autosomal recessive defects that are characterized by either deficient or abnormally functioning enzymes involved in the formation or degradation of glycogen. Hepatomegaly, growth failure, hyperlipidemia, and hyperuricemia are common clinical features. Other disorders to consider include galactosemia, especially in children with hepatosplenomegaly, jaundice, and mental retardation; and fructose-1,6-diphosphatase deficiency, in children with hepatomegaly due to lipid storage but only mildly abnormal liver function studies.

II. Diagnosis

After 4 hours, the child's glucose concentration was 16 mg/dL; lactate, 32 mg/dL (normal range, 5 to 18 mg/dL); and uric acid, 14.2 mg/dL (normal range, 2 to 7 mg/dL). He received intravenous glucagon (30 μg/kg), after which the blood glucose concentration was 22 mg/dL and the lactate level was 44 mg/dL. He then received oral glucose, which increased his blood glucose concentration to 65 mg/dL and decreased the lactate concentration to 24 mg/dL. **These findings suggested type IA glycogen storage disease (von Gierke disease).** Liver biopsy demonstrated increased glycogen content and deficient glucose-6-phophatase (G6P) enzyme activity (2 nmol/min per milligram of protein; normal range, 20 to 70 nmol/min per milligram of protein).

III.   Incidence and Epidemiology

The GSDs, or glycogenoses, comprise several inherited diseases caused by deficiency in one of the enzymes that regulate the synthesis or degradation of glycogen. The end result is abnormal accumulation of glycogen in various tissues. GSD type I has an estimated incidence of 1 in 200,000 births. GSD IA is caused by deficiency of the enzyme G6P, which catalyzes the breakdown of stored glycogen into glucose for use by the body. At least 56 different mutations in the gene for G6P (chromosome 17q21) have been found in patients with GSD IA. Failure of the G6P transporter (GSD IB) or of the microsomal phosphate transporter (GSD IC) also ultimately impair G6P activity. The three types of GSD result in similar clinical and biochemical disturbances. G6P is expressed in the liver, kidneys, and intestines.

IV.   Clinical Presentation

GSD type I is characterized by severe hypoglycemia occurring within 3 to 4 hours after a meal. Although symptomatic hypoglycemia may appear soon after birth, most patients are asymptomatic as long as they receive frequent feeds that contain sufficient glucose to prevent hypoglycemia. Symptoms of hypoglycemia appear only when the interval between feedings increases, such as when the child begins to sleep through the night or when an intercurrent illness disrupts normal feeding patterns.

Patients may have hyperpnea from lactic acidosis. Untreated patients have poor weight gain and growth retardation. Most patients have a protuberant abdomen and hepatomegaly due to glycogen deposition and fatty infiltration. Social and cognitive development are normal unless the infant suffers neurologic impairment after frequent hypoglycemic seizures. Xanthomas may appear on the extensor surfaces of the extremities and buttocks. Older children develop gout.

V.   Diagnostic Approach

Fasting study. In GSD, the liver is not able to release sufficient glucose from hepatic stores to meet peripheral tissue demands. The consequence of this "fasting state" is hypoglycemia, which causes lipolysis and protein breakdown. Therefore, in GSD, hypoglycemia is accompanied by elevated lactic acid, elevated uric acid, and metabolic acidosis. The serum insulin level is low, but serum and urinary ketones are markedly elevated. Glucagon does not significantly alter the glucose level and actually increases the lactic acid level. An oral glucose load increases serum glucose and decreases lactic acid. At the time of hypoglycemia, serum should be collected for determinations of insulin, C-reactive peptide, growth hormone, β-hydroxybutyrate, lactate, and free fatty acids. Urine may be analyzed for organic acids, ketones, and reducing substances. This combination of studies allows diagnosis of GSD as well as exclusion of other disorders that manifest with hypoglycemia.

Liver function tests. Mild elevations of AST and ALT occur.

Lipid profile. Markedly elevated serum triglycerides, free fatty acids, and apolipoprotein C-III are seen. Infants with triglyceride levels greater than 1,000 mg/dL are at high risk for development of acute pancreatitis. Despite the hypertriglyceridemia, the risk for cardiovascular disease is not increased.

Complete blood count. Neutropenia develops with GSD IB but not with GSD IA.

Bleeding time. Although this test is not routinely performed, most children with GSD type I have impaired platelet function due to systemic metabolic abnormalities. This bleeding tendency, manifested by recurrent epistaxis and prolonged bleeding after surgery, resolves with correction of the metabolic abnormalities.

Urinalysis. Glucosuria and proteinuria indicate proximal renal tubular dysfunction that improves with correction of metabolic abnormalities.

Abdominal ultrasound. Hepatic adenomas occur in the majority of patients by the second decade of life but may be noted before puberty. Women also usually have polycystic ovaries, a finding whose clinical significance remains unclear.

Other studies. Measurement of G6P enzyme activity in a fresh liver biopsy specimen can be used to diagnose GSD IA. Molecular analysis to identify mutations on the G6P gene is a reliable alternative to liver biopsy.

VI. Treatment

Treatment consists of providing a continuous dietary source of glucose to prevent hypoglycemia. When hypoglycemia is prevented, the biochemical abnormalities and growth improve and liver size decreases. Infants require frequent feedings, approximately every 2 to 3 hours during the day and every 3 hours at night. A variety of methods can be used to provide a continuous source of glucose at night in older children, including intravenous dextrose infusion, continuous intragastric feeding via a nasogastric or gastrostomy tube, and the use of low glycemic index foods such as cornstarch. Orally administered uncooked cornstarch seems to act as an intestinal reservoir of glucose that is slowly absorbed into circulation. It has been used successfully in infants as young as 8 months of age and may obviate the need for continuous intragastric infusion of formula overnight. It can be mixed with water, formula, or artificially sweetened fluids in 4- to 6-hour intervals overnight. The optimal schedule requires validation by serial glucose monitoring. Allopurinol and lipid-lowering agents are used for severe uric acid and lipid abnormalities. Hepatocyte infusion and liver transplantation may be curative, but the long-term complications in children with GSD are not yet known.

VII. References

1. Lee PJ, Patel A, Hindmarsh PC, ct al. The prevalence of polycystic ovaries in the hepatic glycogen storage diseases: its association with hyperinsulinism. *Clin Endocrinol* 1995;42:601–606.
2. Rake JP, ten Berge AM, Visser G, et al. Glycogen storage disease type Ia: recent experience with mutation analysis, a summary of mutations reported in the literature and a newly developed diagnostic flow chart. *Eur J Pediatr* 2000;159:322–330.
3. Sperling MA, Finegold DN. Hypoglycemia in the child. In: Sperling MA, ed. *Pediatric endocrinology.* Philadelphia: WB Saunders, 1996;265–279.
4. Willi SM. Glycogen storage diseases. In: Altschler SM, Liacouras CA, eds. *Clinical pediatric gastroenterology.* Philadelphia: Churchill Livingstone, 1998:377–383.
5. Wolfsdorf JI, Holm IA, Weinstein DA. Glycogen storage diseases. *Endocrinol Metab Clin* 1999;28:801–823.

Case 19-4: 3-Year-Old Boy

I. History of Present Illness

A 3-year-old boy with a history of developmental delay was in his usual state of health until 1 day before admission, when he developed a tactile fever and had one episode of nonbloody, nonbilious emesis. On the day of admission, he was noted to have poor oral intake and decreased activity. On the evening of admission, he was found lying on the kitchen floor. He had abnormal eye movements and twitching of his mouth. According to his mother, this episode lasted for 20 minutes and was followed by a period of somnolence. He was taken to a nearby hospital, where he was lethargic, responding only to noxious stimuli. There he had several generalized seizures that were treated with lorazepam. He was noted to have very poor respiratory effort. An arterial blood gas analysis obtained at that time revealed the following: pH, 6.9; carbon dioxide tension ($PaCO_2$), 146 mm Hg; oxygen tension (PaO_2), 311 mm Hg; and base deficit, 6.4 mmol/L. The patient was transferred to another institution after endotracheal intubation. There was no history of trauma or ingestion. Additional history revealed that he had required evaluation by his primary physician for irritability and poor appetite approximately 2 weeks before admission but was otherwise well.

II. Past Medical History

The patient was the full-term product of an uncomplicated pregnancy and weighed 3,100 g at birth. He had speech delay and a history of pica. He had received mineral oil periodically over the past 2 months due to constipation, but he did not require any other medications. His immunization status was not known. There was no family history of mental retardation or seizures.

III. Physical Exam

T, 37.5°C; RR, 10/min; HR, 110 bpm; BP, 130/80 mm Hg

Height, 25th percentile (estimated); weight, 50th percentile

On examination the patient was sedated, endotracheally intubated, and minimally responsive to stimulation. His pupils were sluggishly reactive. The optic discs were sharp, and there was no papilledema. The left tympanic membrane was mildly erythematous without bulging or retraction. The oropharynx was moist. The neck was supple. Heart sounds and femoral pulses were normal. Auscultation of the lungs revealed symmetric air entry without wheezing or rales. The Glasgow Coma Score was 7. His gag reflex was intact. Deep tendon reflexes were 3+ but symmetric. There was sustained left ankle clonus, and his toes were upgoing on Babinski testing.

IV. Diagnostic Studies

The complete blood count revealed 11,300 WBCs/mm^3 (74% segmented neutrophils, 20% lymphocytes, 5% monocytes, and 1% eosinophils), a hemoglobin of 6.6 g/dL, and 473,000 platelets/mm^3. The reticulocyte count was 5.1%. Serum electrolytes and calcium were normal. The blood urea nitrogen concentration was 15 mg/dL, and the creatinine level was 0.3 mg/dL. Serum glucose was 170 mg/dL. Serum ALT and AST were 83 and 118 U/L, respectively. Ammonia was mildly elevated at 64 µg/dL. Urinalysis revealed moderate amounts of glucose and protein (2+), 5 to 10 WBCs per high-power field, no red blood cells, and no ketones. Head CT showed diffuse cerebral edema and decreased grey/white differentiation but no masses or intracranial hemorrhage. Opening pressure measured during lumbar puncture was 46 mm H_2O. CSF analysis revealed 15 WBCs/mm^3 and 15 red blood cells/mm^3. CSF glucose was 85 mg/dL, and protein was 42

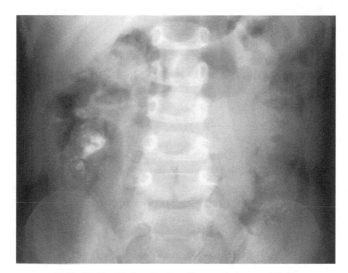

FIG. 19-2. Abdominal radiograph (case 19-4).

mg/dL. No bacteria were seen on Gram staining. Urine and serum toxicology screens were negative.

V. Course of Illness

EEG showed paroxysmal epileptiform activity with generalized slowing of the background electrical activity. The seizures were controlled with phenytoin infusion. Examination of the abdominal radiograph suggested a diagnosis (Fig. 19-2).

Discussion: Case 19-4

I. Differential Diagnosis

Encephalopathy refers to a diffuse neurologic disturbance in the absence of CNS inflammation. Acute encephalopathy may manifest with seizures, delirium, or coma. The diagnosis of encephalopathy is usually inferred from clinical examination. The ultimate distinction between encephalopathy and encephalitis requires neuropathologic examination, but CSF pleocytosis is generally absent in children with encephalopathy. The differential diagnosis of encephalopathy and seizures in this patient includes CNS infection. Viral causes to consider include HSV, influenza virus, and enteroviruses, the most common cause of CNS infection in children. Bacterial causes in this age group may be suggested by appropriate exposures and include *Bartonella henselae* (cat-scratch disease, or CSD), *Rickettsia rickettsii* (Rocky Mountain spotted fever), and *Borrelia burgdorferi* (Lyme disease). Children with *Mycoplasma pneumoniae* encephalitis may have a concurrent respiratory infection. *Salmonella* species, *Shigella* species, and *Campylobacter jejuni* have all been reported to cause toxic encephalopathy accompanied by diarrhea. Postinfectious encephalitis may be seen with measles, mumps, rubella, and varicella, but knowledge of the patient's immunization history is important. Substrate deficiencies such as hypoglycemia are possible but were not suggested by the laboratory findings in this case. Ingestion of medications or toxins (e.g. phenothiazine, anticonvulsants, lead, organophosphates) can cause an acute encephalopathy. Organ failure causing hepatic coma or hypertensive encephalopathy should be considered. Diabetes mellitus should be considered but is unlikely in this case due to the absence of urinary ketones. Trauma with accompanying intracranial hemorrhage must always be excluded as a cause of seizures and encephalopathy in an infant. Anemia with reticulocytosis makes sickle cell disease with stroke, coagulopathy with intracranial hemorrhage, and lead intoxication possible. The absence of rash, ketonuria, diarrhea, and exposure to pets makes several of these diagnostic considerations unlikely.

II. Diagnosis

In this case, the abdominal radiograph revealed a radiodensity in the right lower quadrant in the area of the cecum, consistent with ingestion of lead or another foreign substance (Fig. 19-2). **This finding raised the possibility of lead ingestion and subsequent lead encephalopathy.** Additional findings on complete blood count included a mean corpuscular volume of 50 fL and a red cell distribution width of 12.4. The serum lead level was 375 µg/dL, and the free erythrocyte protoporphyrin level was 260 µg/dL. Other findings of lead poisoning were present, including glucosuria, aminoaciduria, reticulocytosis, mild CSF pleocytosis, elevated CSF protein, and elevated opening pressure on lumbar puncture.

III. Incidence and Epidemiology

Although the hazards of lead exposure have been recognized for some time, lead intoxication remains the most common metal poisoning encountered today. Sources of lead that contribute to poisoning include interior paint removal in older homes and soil contamination from lead pipes and leaded fuel (lead was a gasoline additive until 1996). Folk medicines (azarcon in Mexican cultures) and cosmetics (kohl in Asian-Indian cultures) may also contain substantial quantities of lead. The frequent hand-to-mouth activity of young children renders them particularly vulnerable to lead ingestion.

Before 1991, lead levels of 25 µg/dL were considered elevated. Metaanalyses of epidemiologic studies found that blood lead levels as low as 10 to 20 µg/dL were associated with attentional impairment, aggressive behavior, and cognitive deficits, suggesting that the public health significance of low-level lead exposure may be substantial. In 1991, these findings prompted the Centers for Disease Control and Prevention to consider a childhood blood lead concentration of 10 µg/dL or higher to be a level of concern. The percentage of children younger than 6 years of age with lead levels of 10 µg/dL or higher varies by state and ranges from 2.7% to 14.9%.

IV. Clinical Presentation

The signs and symptoms of lead poisoning depend on the blood lead level and the age of the patient. Most children with mildly increased lead levels are asymptomatic. Some may have mild neurocognitive deficits or behavioral problems. As the lead level increases above 50 µg/dL, young children gradually develop anorexia, apathy, lethargy, anemia, irritability, poor coordination, constipation, abdominal pain, and sporadic emesis. Regression of newly acquired skills, especially speech, may be reported. These complaints increase in severity over 3 to 6 weeks. Children with lead levels greater than 80 µg/dL are most susceptible to encephalopathy. The onset of encephalopathy is heralded by the development of ataxia, persistent emesis, periods of lethargy, and, finally, intractable seizures.

Physical examination findings include ataxia, tremor, and peripheral motor weakness, particularly in the extensors of the fingers and wrists. Pallor of the skin and mucosa develops with severe anemia. Children with chronic lead exposure may develop dark deposits of lead sulfide at the interface of the teeth and gums, resulting in the gingival "lead line." This finding can be an important clue to the presence of high lead exposure but must be differentiated from normal pigmentation in dark-skinned children.

V. Diagnostic Approach

Blood lead. Because blood samples obtained by fingerstick may be contaminated by exogenous lead on the finger, elevated capillary blood lead levels should be confirmed in blood obtained by venipuncture.

Free erythrocyte protoporphyrin (FEP) and zinc protoporphyrin (ZPP). Elevated FEP and ZPP concentrations reflect lead-induced inhibition of heme synthesis. FEP and ZPP levels are increased 2 to 6 weeks after elevation of lead levels above approximately 15 µg/dL.

Complete blood count and reticulocyte count. Hemolysis occurs after acute, high-dose lead exposure. Chronic lead exposure causes a slowly developing hypochromic, microcytic or normocytic anemia. Anemia usually develops when the lead level is greater than 40 to 50 µg/dL. Microscopic inspection of the peripheral blood smear may reveal basophilic stippling (aggregation of ribosomal fragments) as a consequence of lead-induced inhibition of cellular ribonucleases. Reticulocytosis is usually present.

Renal function tests. Urinalysis may be unremarkable or may reveal mild to moderate proteinuria. A Fanconi-like syndrome with aminoaciduria, glucosuria, and hypophosphatemia with relative hyperphosphaturia occurs after acute, high-dose lead exposure. Interstitial nephritis is occasionally detected on renal biopsy in patients with lead-induced renal dysfunction.

Lumbar puncture. Elevated opening pressure and increased CSF protein are characteristic of lead encephalopathy. The CSF WBC count may be normal or mildly elevated (up to 15 cells/mm^3).

Head computed tomography or magnetic resonance imaging (MRI). CNS imaging reveals symmetrically narrowed ventricles and effacement of the cerebral gyri consistent with diffuse cerebral edema.

Other tests. Abdominal radiographs may reveal radiopaque lead fragments within the gastrointestinal tract. Radiographs of long bones reveal transverse linear opacities at the metaphyseal ends, which represent hyperdense calcium deposits that accumulate due to lead-induced inhibition of calcified cartilage reabsorption. These "radiographic lead lines" are seen in children 2 to 6 years of age who have lead levels greater than approximately 70 µg/dL. They do not persist, and do not first develop, during late childhood.

VI. Treatment

Lead encephalopathy constitutes a medical emergency requiring management in the intensive care unit. Optimal treatment of lead poisoning combines decontamination, supportive care, and chelation. Whole-bowel irrigation for inorganic lead compounds and activated charcoal after recent ingestion should be considered. Surgical or endoscopic removal of solitary lead objects in the gastrointestinal tract is important, especially if there is evidence of ongoing lead absorption. Goals of supportive care include (a) normalization of intracranial pressure; (b) transfusion of packed red blood cells, if clinically indicated, for severe anemia; (c) treatment of seizures; and (d) maintenance of adequate urine output to permit renal lead excretion.

Chelating agents are used to decrease the blood lead concentration and increase urinary lead excretion. Children with lead encephalopathy require combination therapy with dimercaprol (British anti-Lewisite), 75 mg/m^2, and calcium disodium edetate (EDTA), 1,500 mg/m^2/24 hours. Lead levels appear to decrease more rapidly in children with lead encephalopathy who are given the combination, rather than calcium EDTA alone. The duration of dimercaprol plus calcium EDTA therapy is limited to 5 days to diminish the risk of nephrotoxicity. In one series of 130 children with lead poisoning who were treated with the combination of dimercaprol and calcium EDTA, 13% developed nephrotoxicity and 3% developed reversible acute renal failure. After completion of combination parenteral therapy, children should receive succimer (dimercaptosuccinic acid, or DMSA), an orally-administered water-soluble analogue of dimercaprol, for 14 days.

Blood levels are measured again after 24 to 48 hours to ensure that they are declining. Failure of levels to decline by at least 20% over 48 hours suggests ongoing external lead exposure, significant lead retention in the gastrointestinal tract, renal insufficiency, or noncompliance with chelation therapy. Blood lead levels should be determined at weekly intervals during and after succimer therapy. Children with lead encephalopathy have a high body lead burden, and redistribution of lead from bone to soft tissues after cessation of chelation often results in a rebound of the blood lead concentration to within 20% of pretreatment values. Repeat courses of chelation are often necessary.

VII. References

1. American Academy of Pediatrics, Committee on Drugs. Treatment guidelines for lead exposure in children. *Pediatrics* 1995;96:155–160.
2. Bellinger DC, Stiles KM, Needleman HL. Low-level lead exposure, intelligence and academic achievement: a long-term follow-up study. *Pediatrics* 1992;90:855–861.
3. Centers for Disease Control and Prevention. Blood lead levels in young children—United States and selected states, 1996–1999. *MMWR Morb Mortal Wkly Rep* 2000;49:1133–1137.
4. Chisolm JJ Jr. The use of chelating agents in the treatment of acute and chronic lead intoxication in childhood. *J Pediatr* 1968;73:1–38.
5. Kosnett MJ. Lead. In: Ford MD, Delaney KA, Ling LJ, et al., eds. *Clinical toxicology.* Philadelphia: WB Saunders, 2001;723–736.
6. Moel DI, Kumar K. Reversible nephrotoxic reactions to a combined 2,3-dimercapto-1-propanol and calcium disodium ethylenediaminetetraacetic acid regimen in asymptomatic children with elevated blood lead levels. *Pediatrics* 1982;70:259–262.

CASE 19-5: 11-YEAR-OLD BOY

I. History of Present Illness

An 11-year-old boy was well until the day of admission, when he stood up and fell, striking his head on a desk at school. Approximately 1 hour later, he developed head twitching, eye blinking, and tonic-clonic movements of his right arm that lasted approximately 20 minutes. During this episode, he had bowel and bladder incontinence. The school nurse found him confused, combative, and unable to follow simple commands. He was taken to the emergency department for evaluation. His family reported that he had been intermittently febrile over the past 2 weeks but denied any history of headache, vomiting, rash, visual problems, alteration in gait, travel, ill contacts, or use of alcohol or illicit drugs.

II. Past Medical History

He did not have any underlying medical conditions. His growth and development had been normal. His older brother had died from complications related to acquired immunodeficiency syndrome several years earlier, after becoming infected with the human immunodeficiency virus (HIV) through intravenous drug use. There was no family history of seizures, metabolic disorders, or sickle cell disease. His maternal grandmother and father had both died of complications related to hypertension. He lived at home with his mother and stepfather. They had two healthy kittens at home but no reptiles or birds. He had received all required immunizations. He did not require any medications.

III. Physical Examination

T, 38.6°C; RR, 18/min; HR, 110 bpm; BP, 136/80 mm Hg; SpO$_2$ 96% in room air
Weight, 50th percentile; height, 75th percentile

On examination, he was agitated and combative. There was a small contusion over his left eyebrow but no other signs of trauma. There were no scleral hemorrhages. There was no hemotympanum. Pupils were symmetrically reactive (6 mm to 4 mm). His neck was supple. There were no murmurs or rubs on cardiac examination. The lungs were clear to auscultation. There was a 2-cm right axillary lymph node without surrounding erythema or drainage. No other lymphadenopathy was appreciated. His abdomen was soft without hepatosplenomegaly. He was incontinent of urine and stool. There were no petechiae. Neurologic assessment was difficult to obtain. The child cried and shouted but was unintelligible. He did not follow simple commands. He thrashed his arms and legs spontaneously and purposefully.

IV. Diagnostic Studies

Complete blood count revealed 5,300 WBCs/mm^3 (50% segmented neutrophils, 32% lymphocytes, 13% monocytes, and 5% eosinophils); hemoglobin, 11.6 g/dL; and platelets, 333,000/mm^3. Serum ALT and AST were 152 and 114 U/L, respectively. Serum electrolytes, blood urea nitrogen, calcium, magnesium, phosphorus, creatinine, and albumin were normal. Serum glucose was 106 mg/dL. Serum and urine toxicology screens were negative. CT of the head did not reveal any hemorrhage, mass lesions, or ventriculomegaly. Examination of the CSF revealed 24 WBCs/mm^3; 1 red blood cell/mm^3; glucose, 77 mg/dL; and protein, 19 mg/dL. There were no organisms found on Gram staining of the CSF.

V. Course of Illness

The patient was admitted to the intensive care unit and received vancomycin, cefotaxime, and acyclovir as empiric therapy for encephalitis while the results of additional

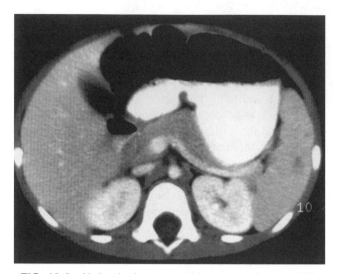

FIG. 19-3. Abdominal computed tomogram (case 19-5).

CSF testing were pending. Two hours after admission, he had several additional right-sided motor seizures with occasional generalization. He received phenytoin and multiple doses of lorazepam, with resolution of each seizure. He ultimately required endotracheal intubation for respiratory failure. The EEG showed a right temporal focus that spread mostly through the right hemisphere, with occasional spread to the left hemisphere. Continuous EEG monitoring demonstrated a total of 75 clinical and subclinical seizures over the next 24 hours, despite the addition of Tegretol (carbamazepine), valproate, and phenobarbital. CSF PCR for *B. burgdorferi* (Lyme disease), HSV (repeated twice), and enterovirus were negative, as were cultures for bacteria and stains for fungi and acid-fast bacilli. Viral culture of the CSF was also ultimately negative. Serum acute and convalescent immunoglobulin M (IgM) and IgG titers were undetectable for Lyme disease, Rocky Mountain spotted fever, and human granulocytic ehrlichiosis. Metabolic studies including serum and urine organic acids, serum amino acids, and serum and CSF lactate and pyruvate were within normal limits. Findings on abdominal CT suggested a diagnosis (Fig. 19-3).

DISCUSSION: CASE 19-5

I. Differential Diagnosis

Encephalitis occurs in 0.5 per 100,000 individuals in the United States. In late childhood, a variety of agents cause encephalitis, although viruses are most commonly implicated. HSV is a serious but potentially treatable cause of viral encephalitis. Viral culture is frequently negative in cases of HSV encephalitis; therefore, HSV PCR is considered the gold standard diagnostic test. Enteroviruses are the most common cause of CNS infection in children, but predominant encephalitis without meningitis is an unusual manifestation. Encephalitis occurs in approximately 1 of every 1,000 cases of Epstein-Barr virus-associated mononucleosis; children frequently have a history of antecedent fatigue and pharyngitis. Other viral causes of encephalitis in the United States include human herpesvirus 6, arboviruses (Eastern and Western equine encephalitis), hepatitis viruses A and B, HIV, and rabies virus. Postinfectious encephalitis often occurs after respiratory infections, especially those caused by influenza virus or *M. pneumoniae.* The incidence of encephalitis related to measles, mumps, and varicella has declined due to widespread immunization. Encephalitis in the summer months should raise suspicion for Rocky Mountain spotted fever, Lyme neuroborreliosis, and enterovirus infection. Exposure to kittens raises the possibility of *B. henselae* encephalitis. Few pyogenic bacteria cause encephalitis without overt meningitis. Syphilis, leptospirosis, brucellosis, tuberculosis, and listerosis are rare causes of encephalitis but should be considered when an appropriate exposure has been documented.

II. Diagnosis

The abdominal CT revealed multiple hypodense hepatic and splenic lesions (Fig. 19-3). These findings, in conjunction with axillary lymphadenopathy and history of contact with a kitten, suggested infection with *B. henselae,* the causative agent of CSD. *B. henselae* antibody titers were 1:2,048. **These findings supported the diagnosis of hepatosplenic cat-scratch disease with encephalitis.** The patient's seizures continued for more than 1 week despite aggressive anticonvulsant therapy. He received rifampin and macrolide antibiotics for his CSD. Unfortunately, his hospital course was complicated by disseminated fungal infection, including *Candida albicans* retinitis and meningitis, and chronic respiratory failure requiring a tracheostomy. He was discharged after 8 months of hospitalization with impaired vision, developmental delay, and recurrent seizures. His poor neurologic outcome was most likely related to prolonged seizures and disseminated candidiasis.

III. Incidence and Epidemiology

CSD, a well-recognized and self-limited cause of regional lymphadenitis in children, is often associated with systemic symptoms such as fever and malaise. Approximately 24,000 cases are reported in the United States each year; the highest age-specific incidence occurs in children younger than 10 years of age. CSD predominantly occurs in the fall and winter, possibly related to temporal changes in animal behavior and reproduction. History of contact with a cat can be established in more than 90% of cases of CSD. The infection may be transmitted through licks, scratches, or bites. Cats who transmit CSD are not ill and have no distinctive features, although most are kittens (younger than 1 year of age). In a study of 1,200 patients with CSD, 64% reported contact with only a kitten, and 25% reported contact with both kittens and adult cats.

Approximately 10% of children with CSD develop atypical features, including Parinaud's oculoglandular syndrome, neuroretinitis, erythema nodosum, pulmonary nodules, osteomyelitis, and encephalitis or encephalopathy. Encephalitis or encephalopathy complicates 3 to 10 of every 1,000 cases of CSD.

IV. Clinical Presentation

The clinical manifestations of CSD depend on the site of inoculation and infection. Children with hepatosplenic CSD often complain of fever, malaise, and abdominal pain. Physical examination findings include hepatomegaly (30%), hepatosplenomegaly (16%), and lymphadenopathy (25%)—usually a single enlarged lymph node. A scratch or papule identifies the probable site of inoculation in 60% to 90% of cases.

Children with CSD-associated encephalitis often present with complaints of fever, malaise, and lymphadenopathy. Two to three weeks later, they develop headache, alterations in mental status, and seizures. Less common manifestations of this rare event include hallucinations, hemiplegia, aphasia, cerebellar ataxia, and sixth cranial nerve palsy. In Florida, a cluster of five children with acute CSD encephalopathy occurred within a 6-week period in 1994. All presented with status epilepticus and required endotracheal intubation but subsequently recovered without sequelae. Most children with CSD encephalitis or encephalopathy reported in the literature have had only transient neurologic impairment, although recovery has often taken up to 8 weeks.

V.   Diagnostic Approach

B. henselae **immunoglobulin G antibodies.** Serologic testing is the standard method of diagnosis and should be considered for patients who present with status epilepticus, adenopathy, and a history of feline contact. A single elevated indirect immunofluorescence assay titer or enzyme immunoassay value for IgG antibodies is usually sufficient to confirm CSD, because initiation of a humoral immune response usually precedes or is concurrent with symptom onset. IgG levels rise during the first 2 months after onset of illness, followed by a gradual decline. The sensitivity is reported to be greater than 98%; only 2% to 3% of healthy control subjects have elevated *B. henselae* antibody titers.

B. henselae **DNA polymerase chain reaction.** PCR may be performed on tissue samples (lymph node aspirates, liver or spleen tissue, bone biopsies). It is available on a limited basis at some commercial laboratories and from the Centers for Disease Control and Prevention.

Lumbar puncture. CSF analysis may be normal, but some patients have a mild pleocytosis (fewer than 30 WBCs/mm^3). CSF protein may be slightly elevated, but CSF glucose is normal. PCR assays to exclude other potential causes of encephalitis, such as HSV, enteroviruses, and arboviruses, should be considered.

Abdominal computed tomography. Abdominal CT usually is not warranted but may demonstrate granulomata in the liver and spleen which, as in this case, may help establish the diagnosis.

Central nervous system imaging. Head CT is normal but should be performed to exclude CNS lesions that can cause seizures. MRI of the head may reveal focal or diffuse white matter changes that are not specific for CSD.

Other studies. *B. henselae* can be cultured from blood, lymph nodes, and other tissues, but it grows slowly and requires a 6-week incubation period. A presumptive diagnosis can be made based on microscopic examination of tissues by demonstrating the bacilli with the use of Warthin-Starry silver impregnation staining. The cat-scratch skin test is no longer used. Studies to exclude other causes of encephalopathy should be performed.

VI.   Treatment

In the immunocompetent child with hepatosplenic CSD, the benefit of antimicrobial therapy is unclear, because the illness is self-limited in most cases. Patients who receive rifampin appear to have more rapid resolution of fever, but no controlled trial had been conducted, so the efficacy of any antibiotic regimen in the treatment of hepatosplenic CSD is not known. In a study by Bass et al., a 5-day course of azithromycin hastened resolution of lymphadenopathy, causing an 80% reduction in lymph node volume as assessed by ultrasound during the first month of illness. Trimethoprim-sulfamethoxazole, erythromycin, clarithromycin, doxycycline, ciprofloxacin, and gentamicin may also be effective in treating patients with severe illness. β-Lactam agents appear ineffective despite favorable *in vitro* susceptibility. Immunocompromised patients with CSD should receive one of the following regimens for 6 weeks: (a) erythromycin, clarithromycin, or azithromycin with or without rifampin; (b) doxycycline; or (c) gentamicin.

Experience with antimicrobial therapy in CSD encephalitis is limited to anecdotal reports. Most children appear to recover without CSD-specific therapy. The poor outcome for the patient in this case was probably related to disseminated fungal infection rather than CSD.

VII. References

1. Arisoy ES, Correa AG, Wagner ML, et al. Hepatosplenic cat-scratch disease in children: selected clinical features and treatment. *Clin Infect Dis* 1999;28:778–784.

2. Armengol CE, Hendley JO. Cat-scratch disease encephalopathy: a cause of status epilepticus in school-aged children. *J Pediatr* 1999;134:635–638.

3. Bass JW, Freitas BC, Freitas AD, et al. Prospective randomized double blind placebo-controlled evaluation of azithromycin for treatment of cat-scratch disease. *Pediatr Infect Dis J* 1998;17:447–452.

4. Bass JW, Vincent JM, Person DA. The expanding spectrum of *Bartonella* infections: II. Cat-scratch disease. *Pediatr Infect Dis J* 1997;16:163–179.

5. Carithers HA, Margileth AM. Cat-scratch disease: acute encephalopathy and other neurologic manifestations. *Am J Dis Child* 1991;145:98–101.

6. Margileth AM. Antibiotic therapy for cat-scratch disease: clinical study of therapeutic outcome in 268 patients and review of the literature. *Pediatr Infect Dis J* 1992;11:474–478.

7. Noah DL, Bresee JS, Gorensek MJ, et al. Cluster of five children with acute encephalopathy associated with cat-scratch disease in South Florida. *Pediatr Infect Dis J* 1995;14:866–869.

Case 19-6: 12-Year-Old Boy

I. History of Present Illness

A 12-year-old boy had difficulty rising from a sitting position when asked to do so at a basketball game 2 days before admission. He was able to stand only after several minutes, and he attributed this episode to fatigue. Later that evening, after lying on the couch at home, he again had difficulty standing and required assistance from his mother. He was eventually able to walk upstairs unassisted. His mother found him several minutes later, lying on the floor, staring, open-mouthed, and drooling. He had spontaneous respirations but was unresponsive to verbal stimuli. He was taken to a nearby hospital by ambulance.

On arrival, the patient was somnolent but arousable, with a Glasgow Coma Score of 10. He then experienced an episode of staring, unresponsiveness to verbal stimuli, and right hand shaking that lasted 10 minutes, stopping only after administration of rectal diazepam followed by intravenous lorazepam (0.05 mg/kg) and phenytoin. Unenhanced CT imaging of the head revealed normal-sized ventricles without evidence of midline shift. Opening pressure on the lumbar puncture was 18 mm H_2O. After a CSF sample was sent for laboratory analysis, the patient received ceftriaxone intravenously.

He was transferred to another institution for additional management. Discussion with family members did not reveal a history of fevers, night sweats, vomiting, behavior or personality changes, or ataxia. There was no history of witnessed ingestion or trauma.

II. Past Medical History

The patient was born in Mexico and emigrated to the United States when he was 9 years old. His perinatal history was unremarkable. Specifically, there were no maternal infections during pregnancy. The patient was born at term gestation after an uncomplicated delivery. He had never been hospitalized and did not take any prescription medications. There was no family history of seizures.

III. Physical Examination

T, 36.7°C; RR, 18/min; HR, 60 bpm; BP, 111/67 mm Hg

Height, 50th percentile; weight, 5th percentile

On examination, the patient was somnolent but easily arousable and was able to answer questions appropriately. His appearance was thin but not cachetic. There was no papilledema or scleral icterus. His pupils were symmetrically reactive to light. His neck was supple. There was no hepatomegaly, splenomegaly, or lymphadenopathy. There were no hypopigmented or hyperpigmented skin lesions. The remainder of the physical examination, including the neurologic examination, was normal.

IV. Diagnostic Studies

The complete blood count revealed 11,400 WBCs/mm^3 (86% segmented neutrophils, 9% lymphocytes, and 5% monocytes); hemoglobin, 12.2 g/dL; and platelets 257,000/mm^3. Serum electrolytes, calcium, blood urea nitrogen, and creatinine were normal. The serum glucose was 166 mg/dL, and the phenytoin level was 18.1 mg/L (normal therapeutic range, 10 to 20 mg/L).

Examination of the CSF revealed no WBCs and only 1 red blood cell/mm^3. The protein concentration was 11 mg/dL, and the glucose was 93 mg/dL. There were no organisms on Gram stain of the CSF. An acid-fast stained smear of CSF was negative. An ECG demonstrated sinus bradycardia but was otherwise normal. Echocardiogram and EEG were also normal.

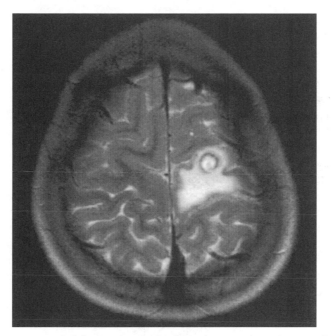

FIG. 19-4. Intravenous gadolinium-enhanced magnetic resonance image of the head (case 19-6).

V. Course of Illness

The patient continued taking phenytoin and did not have any further complex partial seizures. MRI of the head performed with intravenous gadolinium contrast (Fig. 19-4) was considered diagnostic.

DISCUSSION: CASE 19-6

I. Differential Diagnosis

Partial seizures are less common in children than in adults, accounting for about 45% of all childhood seizure disorders. In contrast to adults, most complex partial seizures in children are idiopathic. These typically occur as manifestations of one of the so-called benign focal epilepsy syndromes of childhood. The differential diagnosis in this patient also included early-onset posttraumatic epilepsy, which is associated with partial seizures in the older child. Onset occurs within 24 hours after the injury in 50% of cases. The incidence of traumatic epilepsy is relatively small in closed-head injuries. Infectious causes of partial seizures should always be considered in this age group. Viral encephalitis due to HSV or Epstein-Barr virus is possible. Subacute sclerosing panencephalitis, associated with measles infection, is less likely, but knowledge of the patient's immunization history is important. Parasitic infection of the CNS may result in partial seizures. Neurocysticercosis has a high prevalence in developing areas of Central and South America, and echinococcosis is hyperendemic in areas of South America, central Asia, and the western United States. Tuberculosis with tuberculoma formation in the brain continues to be a problem in some parts of the world. Less common causes of partial seizures in this age group include brain tumors, which are present in fewer than 10% of children with partial seizures. Nevertheless, focal seizures accompanied by a history of headaches may be caused by a CNS tumor. Cerebrovascular disease causing a partial seizure is unlikely unless predisposing factors such as sickle cell disease or an inherited thrombotic disorder (e.g., factor V Leiden mutation, protein C or S deficiency) are present. Bacterial endocarditis with cerebral emboli can cause partial seizures but is usually associated with persistent fever and an abnormal echocardiogram. An important clue to the diagnosis in this case was the patient's history of emigration from Mexico, an area of high prevalence for certain parasitic diseases.

II. Diagnosis

Intravenous gadolinium-enhanced head MRI revealed a 10-mm ring-enhancing lesion in the left parietal white matter with surrounding vasogenic edema and localized mass effect (Fig. 19-4). There was no evidence of elevated intracranial pressure. **These findings were consistent with the diagnosis of neurocysticercosis.** Intravenous dexamethasone, which was started before his arrival at the current institution, was discontinued. Cultures of blood and CSF were negative, and antimicrobial therapy was discontinued. Cysticidal therapy was not recommended. The patient was discharged on phenytoin after a period of observation. On follow-up 1-year later, he had remained seizure-free.

III. Incidence and Epidemiology

Neurocysticercosis is the most common parasitic infection of the CNS. It is caused by the pork tapeworm *Taenia solium.* In the United States, the infection is most common among immigrants from endemic areas and children in contact with these immigrants. The disease is highly endemic in Latin America, Mexico, Eastern Europe, Asia, Africa, and Spain. Cysticercosis can affect humans at any age, including infection by the transplacental route. It is most common during the third and fourth decades of life; only 10% of individuals with neurocysticercosis are children. The estimated serologic prevalence of cysticercosis in Mexican adults is 3.6%, with positive confirmation at autopsy in 1.9%.

T. solium is a gastrointestinal tapeworm (cestode) that causes two types of disease syndromes. Intestinal infection with the adult tapeworm occurs when infective larvae are ingested in undercooked pork. Cysticercosis occurs when humans ingest food contaminated with feces containing *T. solium* eggs. The eggs hatch in the intestine, liberating embryos. The embryos penetrate through the intestinal mucosa and are disseminated by the blood to brain (neurocysticercosis), subcutaneous tissues, muscle, and eye, where they develop into cysticerci. Cysticerci are often 5 mm in diameter, but they may enlarge to 50 mm.

IV. Clinical Presentation

The clinical manifestations in children are different from those in adults. The initial sign of neurocysticercosis in children is usually the new onset of focal or generalized seizures. Rare presentations in children include hemiparesis, increased intracranial pressure with headache and vomiting, encephalitis, meningitis, and simulation of a psychotic illness with delirium or hallucinations. Although some children have several parenchymal cysts, most (75%) have a solitary lesion.

Adolescents and young adults who develop seizures due to neurocysticercosis often have a calcified brain granuloma. The cysticerci remain clinically silent during the natural course of infection, immune reaction, parasite destruction, and granuloma formation. After several years, as evidenced by calcification of the granuloma, the patient develops epilepsy. Adult disease with acute presentation is characterized by multiple brain cysts and an intense immune response. Approximately 30% of adults present with signs of increased intracranial pressure.

V. Diagnostic Approach

Head computed tomography or magnetic resonance imaging. Contrast-enhanced CT and MRI of the head are diagnostic and reveal cysticerci (ring-enhancing) with surrounding edema, granuloma, or calcification. MRI is the best imaging test overall for the diagnosis and should be performed on all patients for whom the clinical history and CT scan suggest the diagnosis of neurocysticercosis. The cysticerci may not be clearly visible on noncontrast CT of the head.

Enzyme-linked immunotransfer blot (EITB). EITB of serum or CSF can assist in confirming a presumptive clinical and radiographic diagnosis. The specificity is approximately 100%. In patients with more than two lesions, the sensitivity is 90%. The test is often negative in patients with a solitary lesion (75% of children).

Stool testing for ova and parasites. All children with neurocysticercosis and their contacts should have their stool examined for *T. solium* ova on three consecutive daily specimens. The source of infection in children is frequently infected stools of family members or other close contacts. Such testing may prevent further exposure and transmission of the disease.

Electroencephalography. An EEG should be performed to assist in localizing seizures in all children with partial seizures.

Lumbar puncture. Examination of the CSF often reveals elevated protein and a mild lymphocytic pleocytosis (mean, 59 WBCs/mm^3).

VI. Treatment

In children, an isolated cystic lesion in the brain parenchyma usually does not require treatment. In these patients, ring enhancement demonstrated on contrast-enhanced CT is associated with inflammation around a dead or dying parasite. Because a solitary lesion usually disappears spontaneously within 2 to 3 months, the use of antihelminthic therapy in this setting is controversial. One study demonstrated faster resolution of solitary lesions and a reduction of late seizure recurrences with albendazole (compared with placebo) in the treatment of neurocysticercosis in 62 children with solitary lesions and focal seizures. Children with the highest risk of chronic seizures are those with a calcified granuloma (indicating a dead parasite) that remains as a permanent sequela of the cysticercus.

Those with multiple lesions or viable cysticerci without radiographic evidence of inflammation need therapy. Albendazole for 28 days is the recommended cysticidal therapy and in most cases results in complete disappearance or significant regression in cyst volume. If albendazole results in only a partial response, praziquantel may be given for 14 days. Individuals whose stool examination reveals adult *T. solium* should be treated with a single dose of praziquantel to prevent transmission.

Initiation of cysticidal therapy may result in cerebral edema. Therefore, dexamethasone should be given 2 days before cysticidal therapy and continued during therapy and shortly after its completion. Of note, dexamethasone lowers plasma levels of praziquantel by as much as 50% but raises the level of albendazole by 50%. Anticonvulsant therapy is also often required.

Neurosurgical resection is used as a last resort for lesions causing significant neurologic impairment. Resolution of lesions with medical management alone is superior and should be attempted first. Brain biopsy should be considered in cases in which the diagnosis remains questionable and the lesion has not resolved.

CNS-imaging studies should be repeated at 2-month intervals (with continued therapy) until the parenchymal brain cysticerci are successfully eliminated. The outcome for neurocysticercosis is generally good. The majority of patients weaned from anticonvulsants remain seizure free. However, there is a 10% mortality rate with neurocysticercosis, and others may have recurrent seizures or deterioration of higher cerebral functions.

VII. References

1. Baranwal AK, Singhi PD, Khandelwal N, et al. Albendazole therapy in children with focal seizures and single small enhancing computerized tomographic lesions: a randomized, placebo-controlled, double blind trial. *Pediatr Infect Dis J* 1998;17:696–700.
2. Hotez PJ. Cestode infections. In: Jenson HB, Baltimore RS, eds. *Pediatric infectious diseases: principles and practice.* Norwalk, CT: Appleton and Lange, 1995;509–516.
3. St. Geme JW III, Maldonado YA, Enzmann D. Consensus: diagnosis and management of neurocysticercosis in children. *Pediatr Infect Dis J* 1993;12:455–461.
4. Sotelo J, del Brutto OH, Penagos P, et al. Comparison of therapeutic regimen of anticysticercal drugs for parenchymal brain cysticercosis. *J Neurol* 1990;237:69–72.
5. Vazquez V, Sotelo J. The course of seizures after treatment for cerebral cysticercosis. *N Engl J Med* 1992;327:696–701.
6. White AC Jr. Neurocysticercosis: a major cause of neurological disease worldwide. *Clin Infect Dis* 1997;24:101–113.

20

Dark Urine

David Munson

APPROACH TO THE PATIENT WITH DARK URINE

I. Definition of the Complaint

Very concentrated urine appears dark in the setting of dehydration, but it is unusual for this to be the primary complaint of the patient. In order for a child or parent to complain of dark urine specifically, there is usually an additional descriptor. The patient may elaborate that the urine is "tea colored," "Coca-Cola colored," bloody, or a particular color. It is these characterizations that help to guide the development of a differential diagnosis. The presence of myoglobin or hemoglobin is frequently responsible for the dark appearance of urine. Porphyria, blackberries, beets, food coloring, and certain medicines such as Pyridium (phenazopyridine) can give urine a reddish appearance. Urate crystals are a common cause of reddish urine in newborns. *Serratia marcescens* can grow on wet diapers and produce "red diaper syndrome." Dark brown or black urine can result from aminoacidopathies such as tyrosinemia.

II. Causes of Dark Urine

The causes of dark urine are most easily grouped by etiology: (a) frank blood; (b) myoglobinuria; (c) infectious; (d) medications; (e) food/dyes; or (g) metabolites (Table 20-1).

III. Clarifying Questions

The generation of an appropriate differential diagnosis for a patient who complains of dark urine is guided by a careful history. Age at onset, associated symptoms, prodromal illness, recurrence of symptoms, available medications in the house, and family history lead to an appropriate workup.

• What is the age of the patient?•

— There are very few causes of dark urine in an infant. Urate crystals associated with dehydration can cause a red tinge to the diaper, and trauma from a catheter or suprapubic tap can cause minor bleeding. Renal vein thrombosis and congenital anomalies should also be considered. Hereditary nephritis typically manifests before 3 years of age. If the patient is an exploring 2-year-old, ingestions should be considered. School age children are classically affected by poststreptococcal glomerulonephritis. Teenagers are more likely than younger patients to experience symptoms of rheumatologic diseases.

• Was there a prodromal illness?

— Acute glomerulonephritis most commonly occurs 10 days after streptococcal pharyngitis. Immunoglobulin A (IgA) nephropathy and benign recurrent hematuria are usually associated with a respiratory tract infection. Influenza and sepsis syndrome have rarely been associated with rhabdomyolysis. Prolonged malaise and weight loss prompt consideration of a chronic disease such as Wilms tumor or Wegener granulomatosis.

TABLE 20-1. *Causes of Dark Urine by Etiology*

Frank hematuria	Acute glomerulonephritis
	Benign recurrent hematuria
	Hereditary nephritis
	Immunoglobulin A nephropathy
	Idiopathic hypercalciuria
	Urolithiasis
	Coagulopathy
	Hemoglobinopathy (sickle cell disease)
	Congenital abnormalities
	Tumor
	Extreme exercise
Myoglobinuria	Rhabdomyolysis (trauma, infection, seizure, exercise, genetically susceptible forms)
Infectious	Hemorrhagic cystitis
	Pseudomonas aeruginosa (green urine)
	Serratia marcescens (nonpathogenic, red diaper syndrome)
Medications	Pyridium
	Rifampin
	Methyldopa
	Phenytoin
	Sulfasalazine
	Phenothiazines
	Ibuprofen
	Deferoxamine
	Metronidazole
	Nitrofurantoin
	Quinine
Foods and dyes	Aniline dyes in candies
	Rhodamine B
	Congo red
	Beets
	Blackberries
Metabolites	Porphyrins
	Bilirubin/biliverdin
	Tyrosinemia

- Is the patient having pain?

  — Flank pain can be an indication of a renal stone and is also sometimes seen with benign recurrent hematuria. Headaches may indicate severe or prolonged hypertension or significant kidney disease. Diffuse muscle pain and tenderness are seen with rhabdomyolysis.

- Has this happened before?

  — Hereditary nephritis usually occurs for the first time before 3 years of age. Benign recurrent hematuria and IgA nephropathy are both recurring illnesses.

- Is the patient complaining of swelling?

  — Edema generally indicates significant kidney disease and may be seen in disorders such as glomerulonephritis and renal vein thrombosis.

- Has there been a change in the pattern of urination?

  — Frequency and urgency are good indications of a urinary tract infection, and hemorrhagic cystitis should move high on the list. New enuresis in a toilet-trained child may be an early indication of urinary tract infection as well. Oliguria is a concerning sign and may indicate progressive glomerulonephritis or severe illness such as sepsis syndrome.

- Is there a family history of similar symptoms?

  — Hypercalciuria usually affects multiple family members. With hereditary nephritis, there should be a positive family history. Some rare metabolic and mitochondrial disorders can manifest as rhabdomyolysis in the setting of exercise or febrile illness in multiple family members.

- Is the patient taking medications? What medications are in the house?

  — Prescribed medications such as ibuprofen, deferoxamine, and Pyridium can discolor the urine. Rifampin, used in the management of tuberculosis and as prophylaxis after exposure to a patient with *Neisseria meningitidis* infection, also colors the urine a red-orange. Because it is important to assess all medications that might be available to a curious child, a thorough inventory of medications used by any household members should be taken.

- Has the child been eating anything that could account for a change in urine color?

  — In an asymptomatic patient, food dyes and some common foods such as beets and blackberries may discolor the urine.

- Has the patient been involved in extreme exercise?

  — In an extreme case, exercise can induce rhabdomyolysis. More commonly, long-distance runners may experience transient frank hematuria. Assessing a teenager's involvement in a sport that involves significant running may clarify the diagnosis. These patients are otherwise asymptomatic.

Case 20-1: 1-Day-Old Boy

I. History of Present Illness

A 36-week gestation newborn boy was admitted to the neonatal intensive care unit due to tachypnea and hypoglycemia. Poor variability of fetal heart tones and nonprogression of labor had complicated the delivery, and a cesarean section was performed. Meconium was noted at delivery, but the baby was vigorous, with Apgar scores of 8 at 1 minute and 9 at 5 minutes. However, he was noted to have significant edema, with the lower extremities being more affected than the upper extremities or face. He also had bilateral hydroceles. The infant was admitted to the intensive care nursery for monitoring of serum glucose and for evaluation of the edema. During the first 24 hours life, he had persistent tachypnea and required supplemental oxygen. He was also noted to have hypertension and intermittent frank hematuria.

II. Past Medical History

The mother was an 18-year-old primigravida woman. Her laboratory values were normal, including a negative rapid plasma reagin test, immunity to rubella, negative hepatitis B status, and a negative screening test for group B *Streptococcus*. The pregnancy had been complicated by gestational diabetes that was controlled with diet. Pregnancy-induced hypertension led to a decision to induce labor at 36 weeks' gestation. The mother had no history of ethanol, drug, or cigarette use during the pregnancy and no history of sexually transmitted diseases. The baby's family history was significant for a paternal uncle with type 1 diabetes and a half brother who died from a brain tumor at the age of 5 years.

III. Physical Examination

T, 37°C; RR, 100 rpm; HR, 148 bpm; BP, 116/69 mm Hg

Weight, 4.5 kg

The general examination was most notable for marked tachypnea, but the infant was alert. He had facial edema, especially of the eyelids. His ears were externally normal, his nares patent, and his palate intact. Cardiac examination revealed normal first and second heart sounds (S1 and S2, respectively) without gallop or murmur. Retractions marked the infant's increased respiratory effort, but there was no nasal flaring or grunting, and the lung fields were clear to auscultation. Abdominal examination revealed a mass on the right side. He had bilateral hydroceles, and there was pitting edema of all extremities, although it was worse in the lower extremities. He had slightly decreased tone but a strong suck and a symmetric Moro reflex.

IV. Diagnostic Studies

The white blood cell (WBC) count was 16,100 cells/mm^3, with 14% band forms, 14% segmented neutrophils, 54% lymphocytes, and 10% monocytes. The hemoglobin was 16.7 g/dL, and the platelet count was 89,000 cells/mm^3. The infant's blood type was A negative, and a Coombs test was negative. Serum electrolytes were normal except for a slightly elevated sodium concentration of 147 mEq/L. Liver function tests showed the following: total bilirubin, 9.9 mg/dL (all unconjugated); alanine aminotransferase (ALT), 79 U/L; aspartate aminotransferase (AST), 101 U/L; alkaline phosphatase, 220 U/L; and γ-glutamyltransferase (GGT), 93 U/L. The albumin concentration was 2.5 mg/dL. An arterial blood gas analysis in room air showed pH, 7.34; carbon dioxide tension (PaCO$_2$), 41 mm Hg; and oxygen tension (PaO$_2$), 63 mm Hg. Urinalysis revealed a specific gravity of 1.015, 3+ protein, and blood. Microscopy showed 21 to 50 red blood cells per high-power field.

V. Course of Illness

An abdominal ultrasound study revealed the cause of hematuria.

DISCUSSION: CASE 20-1

I. Differential Diagnosis

Frank hematuria is an uncommon finding in the neonatal period. As noted earlier, urate crystals can give a pinkish hue to an infant's urine, but this is not usually confused with frank blood. The infant was not exposed to any medications that would give an unusual color to the urine. Microscopic urinalysis provides a quick mechanism to differentiate red blood cells from free hemoglobin or myoglobin. In this case, microscopy indicated that the clinical impression of frank blood was correct. Catheters or suprapubic taps used to obtain urine can result in minor trauma, but they do not usually cause frank hematuria. The remaining constellation of physical findings in this infant directed concern to the kidney. Edema indicates fluid overload, and a palpable abdominal mass could indicate an enlarged kidney or tumor. Although Wilms tumor can manifest as hematuria and an abdominal mass, it would be unlikely to do so this early. Renal vein thrombosis is a rare but known entity in infants; it usually is seen in the setting of a hypercoagulable state, such as infection, maternal diabetes, or hyperviscosity syndrome. Coagulation disorders do not generally present with isolated hematuria. Bleeding from intravenous catheter sites or other procedures would be expected. Congenital kidney anomalies may rarely manifest with hematuria, but they would not commonly make an infant appear ill. Urate crystals and colonization with *S. marcescens* are causes of urine color change that are asymptomatic.

II. Diagnosis

An ultrasound study was obtained to evaluate the possible abdominal mass. A 2-cm clot was seen in the inferior vena cava (IVC) that extended into the right renal vein with enlargement of the right kidney. There was documented flow to and from both kidneys, and collateral circulation provided some flow around the IVC clot. **The diagnosis was renal vein thrombosis, with the predisposing condition being maternal diabetes.**

Captopril was initiated to manage the hypertension, and a hypercoagulation evaluation included antithrombin III levels, protein C and S levels, factor V Leiden mutation screen, and anti-cardiolipin antibodies. These studies were ultimately normal. Urokinase was administered for 3 days via an intravenous catheter in the leg. There was no change in the size of the clot, so a heparin infusion was started and continued for 10 days. The size of the IVC clot decreased, with resolution of the patient's edema. The patient was eventually discharged receiving subcutaneous injections of low-molecular-weight heparin and oral captopril.

III. Incidence and Epidemiology

Thrombotic events are rare in infants, and most are related to the presence of a central venous catheter. In the Canadian and International Registry of Neonatal Thrombosis, 21 cases of renal vein thrombosis, 39 cases of thrombosis of other veins, and 33 arterial thrombotic events were reported from 85 neonatal intensive care units over a 3-year period. Approximately 90% of cases not involving the renal veins were associated with central venous catheters. The cases of renal vein thrombosis were spontaneous, so it appears that this should be considered a separate entity. A nationwide survey in Germany from 1992 to 1994 indicated the incidence of symptomatic renal vein thrombosis to be 2.2 per 100,000 live births. The incidence is higher among premature infants, and most cases appear to occur within the first month of life. Some cases appear to begin *in utero* and can be detected within hours to days after birth.

Renal vein thrombosis is associated with disorders that lead to decreased renal blood flow or increased blood viscosity. Associated conditions include asphyxia, cyanotic heart disease, polycythemia, maternal diabetes, sepsis, and shock. In this instance, the likely etiology was being an infant of a diabetic mother.

There is growing evidence that infants with spontaneous abdominal thrombosis are at significant risk for having a congenital hypercoagulable state. A study in Frankfurt, Germany, found factor V mutations, protein C deficiency, anti-thrombin deficiency, and methylene tetrahydrofolate reductase (MTHFR) mutation in a prospective study of infants younger than 1 year old who presented with symptomatic abdominal clots. Thirteen infants with renal vein thrombosis were identified, and they were found to have an odds ratio of 10.9 for having at least one prothrombotic risk factor.

IV. Clinical Presentation

This infant demonstrated many of the symptoms and physical findings associated with renal vein thrombosis. Obstruction of venous flow can lead to enlargement of the kidney and a palpable abdominal mass. In this case, there was associated obstruction of the IVC, which can lead to cool, mottled, and edematous lower extremities. Renal function is often impaired, leading to diffuse edema and sometimes hypertension. Frank blood, as in this case, should also prompt consideration of thrombosis. Some infants with renal vein thrombosis have bilateral involvement, so evaluation should not be limited to one side. Thrombocytopenia during a thrombotic process results from platelet consumption.

V. Diagnostic Approach

Ultrasonography. Ultrasound is by far the most common procedure, because it is readily available and noninvasive. In addition to assessing renal vein blood flow, enlargement and increased echogenicity of the involved kidney may be seen. There are, however, concerns about the sensitivity of ultrasound for looking at flow in small veins such as those in an infant. A negative ultrasound study in the setting of strong clinical suspicion should not be considered completely reassuring.

Contrast angiography. Angiography has been used infrequently but may be helpful if the diagnosis is uncertain.

Hypercoagulable evaluation. Consideration should also be given to evaluating the infant for a hypercoagulable predisposition. The number of known genetic mutations affecting proteins involved in the coagulation cascade continues to grow. As a result, consultation with a hematologist is recommended to screen for appropriate disorders and to determine the appropriate time for evaluation. Active thrombosis can lead to consumption of many factors and give false results. Evaluation should include determination of factor V mutations, protein C and protein S levels, anti-thrombin activity, anti-cardiolipin antibodies, and homocysteine levels. A hematologist may recommend additional studies.

VI. Treatment

As with diagnostic studies, there is limited information about appropriate treatment for renal vein thrombosis. In the past, renal vein thrombosis was frequently fatal, and recovery of renal function was unusual in those patients who did survive. There are no recent studies evaluating the long-term morbidity associated with renal vein thrombosis. In the Canadian and International Registry of Neonatal Thrombosis, 62% of infants with renal vein thrombosis were treated with supportive care only. The majority of the remaining infants were treated with heparin infusions, as in this case. Many infants with catheter-related clots have been treated with thrombolytic therapy such as tissue plasminogen activator or urokinase, but there is very little information about their utility in renal vein thrombosis. Low-molecular-weight heparin is a relatively new drug available as a subcutaneous injection. It is likely to be useful for outpatient care because of the ease of administration and the low occurrence of bleeding complications. However, its use also is extrapolated from treatment experience with other thrombotic events.

Other management strategies depend on the predisposing condition. Sepsis needs to be considered and evaluated with appropriate cultures and antibiotic coverage. Polycythemia needs to be assessed and an exchange transfusion performed if it is determined to be the cause of the clot. Dehydration should be promptly treated with intravenous fluids, and symptoms of shock need to be managed with appropriate fluid resuscitation and pressor support. If congenital heart disease is suspected, it should be evaluated with a hyperoxia test and echocardiogram.

Lastly, symptoms resulting from the thrombosis itself need to be managed. Renal function should be evaluated periodically, and resolution of the clot should be monitored by ultrasonography. In this case, persistent hypertension was managed with captopril. Survival usually depends on the severity of illness caused by the underlying condition. Long-term consequences of renal vein thrombosis are decreased glomerular flow rate, systemic hypertension, and tubular dysfunction causing impaired urinary concentrating ability and phosphaturia with rickets.

VII.   References

1. Bokenkamp A, von Kries R, Nowak-Gottl U, et al. Neonatal renal venous thrombosis in Germany between 1992 and 1994: epidemiology, treatment and outcome. *Eur J Pediatr* 2000;159:44–48.
2. Brion LP, Berstein J, Spitzer A. Kidney and urinary tract. In: Fanaroff AA, Martin RJ, eds. *Neonatal-perinatal medicine: diseases of the fetus and infant,* 6th ed. St. Louis: Mosby, 1997:1564–1636.
3. Heller C, Schobess R, Kurnik K, et al. Abdominal venous thrombosis in neonates and infants: role of prothrombotic risk factors—a multicentre case-control study. *Br J Haematol* 2000;111:534–539.
4. Monagle P, Michelson AD, Bovill E, et al. Antithrombotic therapy in children. *Chest* 2001;119:s344–s370.
5. Schmidt B, Andrew M. Neonatal thrombosis: report of a prospective Canadian and international registry. *Pediatrics* 1995;96:939–944.
6. Tulassay T, Seri I, Evans J. Renal vascular disease in the newborn. In: Taeusch HW, Ballard RA. *Avery's diseases of the newborn,* 7th ed. Philadelphia: WB Saunders, 1998:1177–1187.
7. Tunnessen WW Jr. *Signs and symptoms in pediatrics,* 3rd ed. Philadelphia: Lippincott Williams & Wilkins, 1999.

Case 20-2: 15-Year-Old Boy

I. History of Present Illness

A 15-year-old boy was well until 12 days before admission. At that time, he complained of a sore throat that resolved spontaneously. Three days later, he noted swelling and tenderness of the right knee that also resolved on its own. There was no associated trauma or redness. One week before admission, he developed "iced tea-colored urine." He did not complain of fever, nausea, vomiting, dysuria, urinary frequency, or urgency. He did have one episode of watery diarrhea. The dark urine continued, and he complained of decreased energy, malaise, and anorexia. He had lost 10 pounds over the course of the last few weeks. Three days before admission, he had developed a nonproductive cough. In his primary physician's office, he had orthostatic hypotension (blood pressure 104/70 mm Hg seated, and 80/40 mm Hg standing). He was hospitalized for further evaluation.

II. Past Medical History

The patient had never been hospitalized or had surgery. He had been treated several times for sinusitis, most recently 3 years earlier. He did not take any medicines and had no allergies. There was no known family history, because the patient is adopted.

III. Physical Examination

T, 36.8°C; RR, 20/min; HR, 82 bpm; BP, 104/54 mm Hg

Weight, 47.5 kg (5th percentile)

On examination, the patient was thin and in no distress. His mucous membranes were moist, his oropharynx clear, and he had no nasal discharge. He had a normal cardiac examination. His breath sounds were slightly coarse and decreased at the bases bilaterally, but he had no wheezes or crackles. He had no hepatomegaly or splenomegaly. His right knee was slightly swollen without erythema or tenderness, and it had full range of motion. He had no significant lymphadenopathy and a normal neurologic examination.

IV. Diagnostic Studies

A complete blood count revealed 8,200 WBCs/mm^3 (3% band forms, 55% segmented neutrophils, 28% lymphocytes, 2% eosinophils, and 15% basophils). His hemoglobin was 7.5 g/dL, and his platelet count was 289,000 cells/mm^3. A reticulocyte count was 3%, and a blood smear demonstrated hypochromia. Serum electrolytes were normal, with the exception of an elevated creatinine concentration of 1.5 mg/dL. Liver enzymes were normal. A chest radiograph was significant for bilateral alveolar infiltrates in a butterfly pattern. Blood, urine, and stool samples were sent for culture. A renal ultrasound study showed increased echogenicity of both kidneys.

V. Hospital Course

On the first day of admission, the patient developed hemoptysis and became anuric. The diagnosis was suggested by the clinical presentation and confirmed by renal biopsy.

DISCUSSION: CASE 20-2

I. Differential Diagnosis

Hemoglobin or myoglobin in the urine causes tea-colored urine. This patient had many additional symptoms to help guide a differential. He complained of a prodrome consisting of a sore throat that lasted 3 days. Classically, poststreptococcal acute glomerulonephritis manifests 10 days after such a prodrome; malaise and anorexia may also be associated with this disease. Symptoms of benign recurrent hematuria and IgA nephropathy may also be brought on by respiratory tract infections. This patient, however, had not had dark urine before. He had no urinary urgency or frequency to indicate hemorrhagic cystitis. Coagulopathies typically cause gum bleeding or spontaneous joint bleeding rather than hematuria and hemoptysis. Teenagers are more likely to have vasculitis than younger children are, and this patient's weight loss speaks to a chronic process. He did not have any other symptoms of lupus, but his past medical history of sinusitis was put together with his new symptoms of tea-colored urine and hemoptysis to derive a diagnosis of Wegener granulomatosis.

II. Diagnosis

The renal biopsy demonstrated severe crescentic glomerulonephritis. Immunofluorescence staining showed pauciimmune glomeruli. **The anti-neutrophil cytoplasmic antibody (ANCA) was positive at a dilution of 1:320 with a cytoplasmic distribution (cANCA), and a diagnosis of Wegener granulomatosis was made.** The patient received plasmapheresis and was treated with intravenous methylprednisone. He was then given a dose of cyclophosphamide and changed to oral prednisone. He was transferred to a hospital closer to his home to continue receiving plasmapheresis every other day.

III. Incidence and Epidemiology

Wegener granulomatosis is a rare vasculitis, and its cause remains unknown. As a result, much of the epidemiology is not well understood, especially in children. The annual incidence of Wegener granulomatosis has been estimated to be approximately 1 in 2 million persons. In the 1990s, corticosteroids and cyclophosphamide became the standard of care, and the 5-year survival rate exceeded 60%. Fifty-six patients with Wegener granulomatosis in Norway were evaluated retrospectively, looking for predictors of survival and organ damage. The youngest patient was 10 years old, but the majority of the patients were adults. Estimates for survival at 1, 5, and 10 years were calculated to be 93%, 79%, and 75%, respectively. In general, the study found that impaired renal function placed patient at higher risk for ultimate end-stage renal disease and death. However, younger patients had a higher rate of recovery of renal function. As a result, it is difficult to predict outcome in children with Wegener granulomatosis. Younger patients were also found to have more nasal and sinus symptomatology and less kidney impairment. Many patients test positive for cANCA, antibodies that are thought to play a role in pathogenesis, perhaps by stimulating neutrophil activity.

IV. Clinical Presentation

Clinical symptoms result from widespread granulomas of arteries and veins. The primary manifestations of Wegener granulomatosis are symptoms of the upper respiratory tract, lungs, and kidneys. Bloody sinusitis, rhinorrhea, and ulceration of the nasal mucosa are common symptoms of respiratory tract involvement and are frequently the first manifestations of the disease. Pulmonary complaints include cough, hemoptysis, and pleuritis. Tea-colored urine or hematuria indicates kidney involvement. Patients also experience generalized symptoms of malaise, anorexia, and weight loss, all of which were reported by this patient. Peripheral symptoms include arthritis, arthralgia, skin ulceration, serous otitis media, conjunctivitis, exophthalmos, corneal ulceration, and hepatitis. None of these symptoms is specific or can be considered pathognomonic. A clustering of these symptoms, especially those affecting the primary organ systems (sinuses, lungs, and kidneys) should prompt evaluation for this disease entity.

V. Diagnostic Approach

Pathology. Biopsies of affected organs provide the strongest basis for making this diagnosis. Affected skin, mucosa, or lung tissue demonstrates granulomas and a necrotizing vasculitis characterized by leukocytic, lymphocytic, and giant cell infiltration. Kidney pathology includes a crescentic glomerulonephritis without immunoglobin deposits (pauciimmune).

Chest radiography or computed tomographic scan of the chest. Nodular lesions or alveolar infiltrates characterize these studies.

Immunology. Most patients have serum that tests positive for cANCA. Combined with progressive glomerulonephritis, a positive cANCA result has a 98% positive predictive value.

Inflammatory markers. Active disease is marked by an elevated erythrocyte sedimentation rate, usually greater than 100 mm/hour.

VI.   Treatment

Immunotherapy has dramatically improved the survival and morbidity associated with this disease. Corticosteroids are the mainstay of therapy. Azathioprine and cyclophosphamide have been used successfully in steroid-resistant disease. Cyclophosphamide can be given as an intravenous pulse every other week, or as daily oral therapy. A study of 56 patients in Norway found that intravenous pulse therapy was ultimately associated with a smaller total dose of cyclophosphamide and fewer days on corticosteroids. Methotrexate has been used with some success as well. Plasmapheresis can be used in acute, life-threatening circumstances.

VII.   References

1. Koldingses W, Nossent H. Predictors of survival and organ damage in Wegener's granulomatosis. *Rheumatology* 2002;41:572–581.
2. Eddy AA. Glomerular disorders. In: Rudolph CD, Rudolph AM, Hostetter MK, et al., eds. *Rudolph's pediatrics,* 21st ed. New York: McGraw-Hill, 2003:1677–1699.
3. Tunnessen WW Jr. *Signs and symptoms in pediatrics,* 3rd ed. Philadelphia: Lippincott Williams & Wilkins, 1999.
4. Yalcindag A, Sundel R. Vasculitis in childhood. *Curr Opin Rheumatol* 2001;13: 422–427.

Case 20-3: 10-Year-Old Boy

I. History of Present Illness

A 10-year-old boy who was previously well developed rhinorrhea with cough and intermittent fever 1 week before admission. For the 4 days before admission, he complained of severe myalgias, followed by weakness and the inability to walk. His urine had become cola-colored, but he had not had any dysuria or increased frequency. He had had no emesis or diarrhea, and he had not complained of headaches. He was initially admitted to a community hospital, where his liver function tests and creatine kinase (CK) concentration became dramatically elevated. His CK more than doubled in 12 hours, and he was then transferred to an academic center.

II. Past Medical History

He had never been hospitalized and had had no surgeries, and he had never before experienced the presenting symptoms. His family history, however, was remarkable. Both his father and a paternal first cousin had similar episodes when they were about 20 years old. The family had recently emigrated from Trinidad.

III. Physical Examination

T, 38.9°C; RR, 20/min; HR, 68 bpm; BP, 120/60 mm Hg; SpO$_2$, 100% in room air

On examination, the patient was in mild distress but was well hydrated. There was no scleral icterus or mucosal pallor. His neck was supple, and his lungs were clear to auscultation bilaterally. His cardiac examination was normal, and the capillary refill time was less than 2 seconds in all of his extremities. His abdomen was benign. His thighs, calves, and arms were all tender. He was able to move his extremities, but only with extreme pain. When pressed, it appeared that his strength was intact. His cranial nerves appeared to be intact as well.

IV. Diagnostic Studies

The patient had a normal electrolyte panel, including a potassium concentration of 4.5 mEq/L and a creatinine level of 0.8 mg/dL. His hepatic function panel was remarkably abnormal: total bilirubin, 0.4 mg/dL; albumin, 3.6 mg/dL; alkaline phosphatase, 274 U/L; ALT, 720 U/L; and AST, 3,480 U/L. His prothrombin and partial thromboplastin times were normal. A urinalysis was significant for 3+ protein and 4+ blood. However, there were minimal red blood cells on microscopy. An electrocardiogram showed normal sinus rhythm. Lactate, pyruvate, plasma amino acids, acylcarnitine, urine organic acids, total and free carnitine, and ketones were all evaluated.

DISCUSSION: CASE 20-3

I. Differential Diagnosis

Hemoglobin or myoglobin most commonly causes cola-colored urine. This patient's prodromal respiratory illness led to consideration of postinfectious glomerulonephritis, although the time course between the prodrome and the urinary changes was short in this case. Respiratory symptoms have also been associated with exacerbation of IgA nephropathy and benign recurrent hematuria, but this patient had never experienced these symptoms before. In addition, the lack of red blood cells on microscopic analysis supported diagnoses consistent with free hemoglobin or myoglobin. He had no other symptoms of sepsis, so diffuse intravascular coagulation syndrome was unlikely. The patient's severe myalgias brings to mind rhabdomyolysis, but an inciting cause would need to be identified. Trauma, strenuous exercise, prolonged seizures, hyperthermia, and toxins such as cocaine or neuroleptics have been associated with rhabdomyolysis, but this patient did not report any of these exposures. True polymyositis is exceptionally rare in children and is usually more chronic. Influenza has been associated with myositis, especially of the gastrocnemius muscle, and it is a rare cause of true rhabdomyolysis. The family history indicated the possibility of a heritable susceptibility to rhabdomyolysis.

II. Diagnosis

The patient's initial CK value was 100,000 U/L, and it ultimately rose to 690,000 U/L. The myocardial bound (MB) fraction was only 26 U/L, making a cardiac cause unlikely. In conjunction with the elevated AST on the hepatic function panel, the diagnosis of rhabdomyolysis was made. The family history made a form of autosomal dominant rhabdomyolysis likely, although no specific defect was found in this case. A heritable defect of the mitochondrial respiratory chain is the most likely metabolic defect leading to myoglobinuria in the setting of a febrile illness.

III. Incidence and Epidemiology

The incidence of rhabdomyolysis is difficult to define because it has a variety of causes (Table 20-2). Autosomal dominant rhabdomyolysis has been reported in the literature only a handful of times. A Swiss family was described in 1997 in which 10 individuals experienced myoglobinuria in the setting of a febrile illness. A variety of pathogens were identified, including *Escherichia coli, Streptococcus pneumoniae,* Epstein-Barr virus, and influenza B virus. Four of the patients had received general anesthesia without incident, and none of the family members had experienced exercise-induced myoglobinuria. A specific mutation was not identified in this family, but muscle biopsy in the index case was consistent with a disorder of cytochrome c oxidase in the respiratory chain. Mutations in the ryanodine receptor have been implicated in some cases of malignant hyperthermia caused by anesthesia. Fatty acid oxidation defects may put some patients at risk for exercise-induced myoglobinuria.

IV. Clinical Presentation

Clinical symptoms specific to rhabdomyolysis consist of a classic triad that includes myalgias, weakness, and dark urine. Myalgias may be severe enough that the patient is unable to walk. On examination, the patient's muscles are tender to palpation. Associated symptoms depend on the cause. Signs and symptoms of shock may accompany trauma, burns, or severe dehydration from strenuous exercise or heat shock. A postictal state is seen after a prolonged seizure. Mental status changes are seen with many of the toxins listed previously. Diabetic ketoacidosis is preceded by a period of polyuria, polydipsia, and polyphagia. Crush injuries are the presenting complaint in patients who have experi-

TABLE 20-2. *Causes of Rhabdomyolysis*

Cause	Examples
Endocrinopathies	Diabetic ketoacidosis, hyperthyroidism
Envenomations	Rattlesnake bite
Infection	Influenza, toxic shock syndrome, Rocky Mountain spotted fever, tetanus
Inherited disorders	Cytochrome *c* oxidase mutation, fatty acid oxidation defects
Hyperthermia	Heat shock
Seizure	Prolonged status epilepticus
Strenuous exercise	Marathon, boot camp
Toxins	Ethanol, cocaine, amphetamines, aspirin, neuroleptics, monoamine oxidase inhibitors, succinylcholine
Trauma	Crush injury, muscle injury

enced this kind of trauma, and the pain from the actual injury obscures the more general symptoms of the developing rhabdomyolysis.

V. Diagnostic Approach

Urinalysis. Urine dipstick tests are positive for blood, but microscopy reveals no red blood cells.

Creatine kinase. CK becomes dramatically elevated, peaking 24 to 36 hours after the onset of rhabdomyolysis. There is no significant elevation of the MB fraction.

Electrolytes and minerals. Potassium and phosphate can become dramatically elevated because of high muscle content spilled into the extracellular compartment. Calcium may drop secondary to the rapid rise in phosphate.

Electrocardiography. If hyperkalemia is present, an electrocardiogram is critical for monitoring the potential for a life-threatening arrhythmia. Peaked T waves are seen, with potassium levels greater than 7 mEq/L. As levels rise above 8 mEq/L, P waves are lost and the QRS widens. At a level of 9 mEq/L, there is further QRS widening and ST-segment depression. Levels greater than 10 mEq/L lead to bradycardia, first-degree atrioventricular node block, and, ultimately, ventricular dysrhythmias and cardiac arrest.

Renal function tests. A rising blood urea nitrogen and creatinine concentrations indicate impaired kidney function, presumably because of precipitation of myoglobin in renal tubules.

VI. Treatment

The inciting event should be identified and, if possible, eliminated. All other elements of therapy are aimed at facilitating the clearance of myoglobin, to prevent renal failure, and preventing severe hyperkalemia. If there is evidence of shock (e.g., crush injury, burns, heat stroke, severe exertion), boluses of isotonic saline in aliquots of 20 mL/kg should be used to restore adequate perfusion. Intravenous fluids are then used to maintain a brisk urine output of at least 4 mL/hr. There should be no potassium in this stock solution. Bicarbonate needs to be added to the intravenous fluids, with the goal of maintaining a urine pH greater than 7. This minimizes precipitation of myoglobin in the kidneys.

If urine output falls, a dose of Lasix (furosemide) can be tried to prevent oliguric renal failure. This may, however, make it more difficult to alkalinize the urine, because the kidney will retain bicarbonate to maintain anionic balance in the face of chloride loss caused by Lasix.

Hypocalcemia may be seen with rhabdomyolysis, so supplemental calcium may be required. Severe hyperkalemia needs to be managed aggressively to prevent an arrhythmia. Kayexalate (sodium polystyrene sulfonate) is a potassium-binding resin that is given by mouth. It is one of the few ways to actually remove potassium from the body. A dose of 1 to 2 g/kg is given with 3mL of sorbitol per gram of resin. Potassium shifts intracellularly in an alkaline environment, so sodium bicarbonate can be used to acutely lower serum potassium levels. Insulin also drives potassium into cells. It should be given as 0.1 U/kg but must be accompanied by 2 mL/kg of 25% dextrose given over 30 minutes to avoid hypoglycemia. Dialysis is the last resort in the face of renal failure and hyperkalemia.

VII. References

1. Brumback RA, Feeback DL, Leech RW. Rhabdomyolysis in childhood. *Pediatr Clin North Am* 1992;39:821–858.
2. Chamberlin MC. Rhabdomyolysis in children: a 3-year retrospective study. *Pediatr Neurol* 1991;7:226–228.

3. Cronan K, Norman ME. Renal and electrolyte emergencies. In: Fleisher GR, Ludwig S, eds. *Textbook of pediatric emergency medicine,* 4th ed. Philadelphia: Lippincott Williams & Wilkins, 2000:811–858.
4. Martin-Du Pan RC, Morris MA, Favre H, et al. Mitochondrial anomalies in a Swiss family with autosomal dominant myoglobinuria. *Am J Med Genet* 1997;69:365–369.

Case 20-4: 7-Year-Old Girl

I. History of Present Illness

A 7-year-old African-American girl with glucose-6-phosphate dehydrogenase (G6PD) deficiency was in good health until 5 days before admission, when she developed cough, rhinorrhea, abdominal pain, and a fever to 40.6°C. Her abdominal pain worsened on the day before admission, and she developed emesis. The family described the emesis as bilious but not bloody. She had had some relief of her pain and fever with ibuprofen. On the day of admission, the patient's symptoms of upper respiratory tract infection had largely resolved, but she was not drinking well and had persistent fevers. She was brought to the emergency department, where she was noted to have bloody urine.

II. Past Medical History

She had had pneumonia at 4 years of age. She did not have any true allergies to medicine, but because of her G6PD deficiency she avoided drugs associated with hemolysis in G6PD deficiency. Her only medication was ibuprofen.

III. Physical Examination

T, 38.5°C; RR, 35/min; HR, 104 bpm; BP, 157/112 mm Hg; SpO$_2$, 93% in room air
Weight, 20.8 kg

On examination, the patient was alert and comfortable. Her sclerae were nonicteric, her nose had no discharge, and her oropharynx was clear with moist mucous membranes. Her tonsils were 2+. Her neck was supple and exhibited shotty cervical and submandibular lymphadenopathy. Her lungs had decreased breath sounds at the bases, with scattered rales and mild end-expiratory wheezing diffusely. Her cardiac examination revealed a hyperdynamic precordium and a II/VI flow murmur at the left lower sternal border. She had no gallop. Her abdomen was soft. Her extremity examination was normal, with no evidence of edema. She had no rash, and her neurologic examination was normal.

IV. Diagnostic Studies

A complete blood count revealed 11,600 WBCs/mm^3, with 1% band forms, 78% segmented neutrophils, 15% lymphocytes, and 4% monocytes. The hemoglobin was 10 g/dL, and the platelet count was 297,000/mm^3. The mean corpuscular volume was 75.8 fL. Her blood urea nitrogen and creatinine concentrations were normal at 8 and 0.6 mg/dL. The remainder of her electrolytes also were normal. A urinalysis revealed moderate ketones, large blood, and 4+ protein. Urine microscopy showed red blood cells too numerous to count, 10 to 20 WBCs per high-power field, and cellular casts. Urine culture was ultimately negative. A complement component C3 level was low at 33 mg/dL (normal range, 88 to 155 mg/dL). A throat swab rapid antigen test was negative for group A *Streptococcus*.

V. Hospital Course

The patient's hypertension was managed with nifedipine. A renal ultrasound study demonstrated mildly enlarged kidneys with increased cortical echogenicity. She had decreased urine output on the second day of hospitalization that required furosemide therapy. A chest radiograph (Fig. 20-1) suggested a diagnostic category that was confirmed by additional testing.

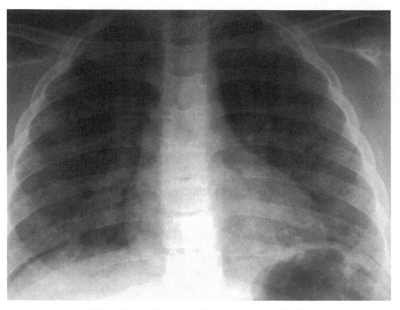

FIG. 20-1. Chest radiograph (case 20-4).

DISCUSSION: CASE 20-4

I. Differential Diagnosis

When this patient presented to the emergency department, the initial concern focused on her fever, cough, and abdominal pain. However, the presence of bloody urine quickly complicated the problem. Attempts to combine all of her symptoms into a single diagnosis led to consideration of her respiratory tract illness as a prodrome. Fever, cough, and abdominal pain could all be the result of a group A *Streptococcus* infection in a school age child. Poststreptococcal glomerulonephritis could then be the cause of bloody urine in this patient. However, glomerulonephritis typically follows the prodrome by 10 days, so the time course does not fit in this case. IgA nephropathy and benign recurrent hematuria can both be triggered by respiratory tract infections. Both are recurrent illnesses, and this patient had never experienced these symptoms before. The patient has G6PD deficiency, and a severe hemolytic event could lead to free hemoglobin in the urine. Such urine, however, is classically cola or tea colored, not frankly bloody. It is possible that the patient has developed hemorrhagic cystitis caused by the same pathogen that led to her other symptoms. However, she had not complained of any change in voiding pattern such as increased frequency or urgency. In addition, the blood and cellular casts on urinalysis strongly supported a diagnosis of glomerulonephritis. High fever, cough, and abdominal pain in a school age child is a classic presentation for pneumonia. The patient's chest radiograph confirmed this suspicion, and so the remaining problem was trying to connect pneumonia with glomerulonephritis. A literature search showed a few case reports of glomerulonephritis associated with *Mycoplasma* infection.

II. Diagnosis

The chest radiograph (Fig. 20-1) showed diffuse bilateral interstitial involvement consistent with an atypical pneumonia. *Mycoplasma pneumoniae* was detected from the nasopharynx by polymerase chain reaction. The low complement level and casts on urinalysis support a diagnosis of glomerulonephritis. Renal biopsy demonstrated a membranoproliferative glomerulonephritis. Specific testing excluded systemic lupus erythematosus, hepatitis B and C, endocarditis, human immunodeficiency virus, and sickle cell disease as possible causes of the glomerulonephritis. The antibiotics were changed to azithromycin. Her respiratory condition improved, and she was discharged on azithromycin and furosemide with plans to follow-up with a blood pressure determination in 1 week. **The diagnosis is membranoproliferative glomerulonephritis and pneumonia caused by *M. pneumoniae*.**

III.   Incidence and Epidemiology

In 1998, Said et al. reported a case series of six children with *M. pneumoniae*-associated nephritis. At that time, 24 total cases had been reported in the literature. The authors suggested that this entity may be more common that the literature would indicate. They reported that between 1991 and 1994, 27% of patients referred to them with acute glomerulonephritis had evidence of *M. pneumoniae* documented by the persistence of anti-*M. pneumoniae* IgM and IgG. Of patients who underwent renal biopsy, the majority had glomerular lesions including membranoproliferative glomerulonephritis, minimal change glomerulonephritis, and endocapillary and extracapillary glomerulonephritis. Other pathologic conditions included tubular interstitial nephritis and acute tubular necrosis. One patient progressed to renal failure, but all other patients quickly regained a normal glomerular filtration rate.

Acute postinfectious glomerulonephritis has been associated with a number of other infections in addition to the classic group A streptococcal disease. *Staphylococcus aureus, S. pneumoniae*, coxsackievirus B4, echovirus 9, influenza A and B, and mumps virus have all been implicated. The mechanism is not clear, but in general it is thought that immune complexes localize to the glomerular wall and activate the complement system, initiating a proliferative and inflammatory response.

IV.   Clinical Presentation

Children with *M. pneumoniae* respiratory tract infection may initially develop malaise, myalgias, headache, and fever—symptoms indistinguishable from those caused by influenza and other viruses that produce respiratory tract disease. Over the next few days, however, the cough worsens, the constitutional symptoms begin to resolve, and the patient begins to feel subjectively better. At this time, auscultation of the chest reveals both wheezing and crackles, leading to the term "walking pneumonia."

Extrapulmonary manifestations of *Mycoplasma* infections include exanthems, hemolysis, central nervous system disease, cardiac disease, hepatitis, pancreatitis, and glomerulonephritis. Renal involvement after *M. pneumoniae* infection is rare. Symptoms of typical *M. pneumoniae* respiratory tract infection, as described previously, generally precede the renal involvement. The glomerulonephritis manifests most commonly with abrupt onset of edema and hematuria. In extreme cases, a patient may experience oliguria, edema, hypertension, azotemia, proteinuria, and hematuria from days to weeks after the initial infection. At least half of children with nephritis remain asymptomatic, with only changes in urinalysis as evidence of kidney involvement. At least half of those who require hospitalization have gross hematuria. This may manifest as grossly bloody, smoky, cola-colored, tea-colored, or rust-colored urine. The hypertension may be severe. Constitutional complaints including malaise, lethargy, anorexia, fever, abdominal pain, and headache are also common.

V.   Diagnostic Approach

Immunology. Serum samples may be sent for determinations of IgG and IgM specific to *M. pneumoniae*, which may be detected by immunofluorescence or enzyme linked immunosorbent assay (ELISA). The IgM is more specific to active current infection, but, in the absence of evidence of other recent infection, IgG may be evidence of the causative agent for glomerulonephritis a few weeks after the initial prodromal illness.

Cold agglutinins. Cold-agglutinating antibodies, or cold agglutinins, are IgM autoantibodies directed against the I-antigen on human red blood cells. They appear within 7 to 10 days after the respiratory tract infection and disappear after approximately 3 weeks. Cold agglutinins are neither sensitive nor specific for *M. pneumoniae* infection. They may be found in other causes of atypical pneumonia. For example, cold agglutinins were detected in 18% of military recruits with adenovirus pneumonia.

***M. pneumoniae* polymerase chain reaction.** This test is available at some institutions to detect *M. pneumoniae* infection. Nasopharyngeal samples are generally positive in affected children. This test has been attempted as a means of detecting *M. pneumoniae* in other tissues (e.g., cerebrospinal fluid, renal biopsy specimens) with varying levels of success.

Complement levels. Approximately 80% to 92% of patients with postinfectious glomerulonephritis have low C3 levels. Many also have low C4 levels.

Urinalysis. Urine dipstick tests are positive for blood and usually are positive for protein. Microscopy reveals red blood cells and cellular casts, as well as hyaline casts.

Renal biopsy. Biopsy is performed infrequently, but in a confusing case the findings of large swollen glomerular tufts, proliferation of mesangial and epithelial cells, and invasion of neutrophils make the diagnosis. IgG and C3 granular deposits may also be seen.

Blood urea nitrogen and creatinine. Both values may be elevated in the acute setting, and they provide vital information in monitoring renal function.

VI. Treatment

The initial approach to treatment focuses on management of severe hypertension. Intravenous hydralazine at 0.15 to 0.3 mg/kg per dose, or oral nifedipine at 0.2 to 0.3 mg/kg per dose, can help to quickly bring blood pressure down. A dose of Lasix as high as 2 mg/kg can be given at the same time. If there is evidence of renal impairment, fluids should be restricted to replace only insensible losses. These fluids should not contain potassium until renal function has improved. The patient should also be placed on a low protein and low sodium diet in the acute phase. The majority of patients recover. Once the patient is discharged to home, blood pressure and hematuria should be evaluated every 4 to 6 weeks for 6 months. If the patient continues to improve, these follow-up studies can be done 3 to 6 months until symptoms resolve. A normal C3 value should be documented approximately 3 months after the acute event.

VII. References

1. Eddy AA. Glomerular disorders. In: Rudolph CD, Rudolph AM, Hostetter MK, et al. *Rudolph's pediatrics,* 21st ed. New York: McGraw-Hill, 2003:1677–1699.
2. George RB, Ziskind MM, Rasch JR, et al. *Mycoplasma* and adenovirus pneumonias: comparison with other atypical pneumonias in a military population. *Ann Intern Med* 1966;65:931–942.
3. McMillan JA, Weiner LB. *Mycoplasma pneumoniae.* In: Long SS, Pickering LK, Prober CG. *Principles and practice of pediatric infectious diseases,* 2nd ed. New York: Churchill Livingstone, 2003:1005–1010.
4. Said MH, Layani MP, Colon S, et al. *Mycoplasma pneumoniae*-associated nephritis in children. *Pediatr Nephrol* 1999;13:39–44.
5. Tunnessen WW Jr. *Signs and symptoms in pediatrics,* 3rd ed. Philadelphia: Lippincott Williams & Wilkins, 1999.
6. Westrhenen R, Weening JJ, Krediet RT. Pneumonia and glomerulonephritis caused by *Mycoplasma pneumoniae. Nephrol Dialysis Transplant* 1998;13:3208–3211.

Subject Index

Page numbers followed by "f" denote figures; those followed by "t" denote tables.